ENDOCRINE

SECRETS

ENDOCRINE

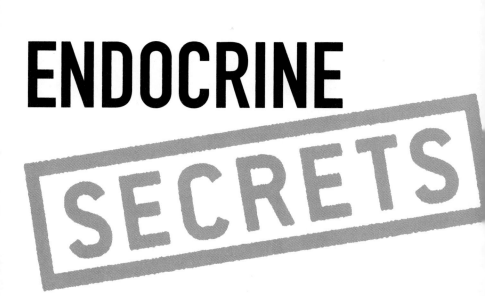

SECRETS

Fourth Edition

Michael T. McDermott, M.D.
Professor of Medicine
Division of Endocrinology, Metabolism, and Diabetes
University of Colorado School of Medicine
Denver, Colorado

ELSEVIER
MOSBY

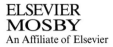

ELSEVIER
MOSBY
An Affiliate of Elsevier

The Curtis Center
170 S Independence Mall W 300E
Philadelphia, Pennsylvania 19106

ENDOCRINE SECRETS   ISBN: 1-56053-611-X
Fourth Edition

NOTICE

Endocrinology is an ever-changing field. Standard safety precautions must be followed, but as new research and clinical experience broaden our knowledge, changes in treatment and drug therapy may become necessary or appropriate. Readers are advised to check the most current product information provided by the manufacturer of each drug to be administered to verify the recommended dose, the method and duration of administration, and contraindications. It is the responsibility of the licensed prescriber, relying on experience and knowledge of the patient, to determine dosages and the best treatment for each individual patient. Neither the publisher nor the author assumes any liability for any injury and/or damage to persons or property arising from this publication.

Previous edition copyrighted 2002, 1998, 1994.

Library of Congress Cataloging-in-Publication Data
Endocrine secrets / [edited by] Michael T. McDermott.—4th ed.
      p.; cm.
   Includes bibliographical references and index.
   ISBN 1-56053-611-X
      1. Endocrinology–Examinations, questions, etc. 2. Endocrine
   glands–Diseases–Examinations, questions, etc. I. McDermott, Michael T., 1952–
   [DNLM: 1. Endocrine Diseases–physiopathology–Examination Questions. WK 18.2 E56
   2005]
   RC649.M36 2005
   616.4'0076–dc22   2004057899

Acquisitions Editor: Linda Belfus
Developmental Editor: Stan Ward
Publishing Services Manager: Joan Sinclair
Project Manager: Cecelia Bayruns

Printed in the United States of America.

Last digit is the print number: 9   8   7   6   5   4   3   2   1

DEDICATION

To those who bring the most light to my life: Libby, Megan, Andi, Mac, Jenny, Scott, Summer, and Maui.

CONTENTS

III. PITUITARY AND HYPOTHALAMIC DISORDERS

IV. ADRENAL DISORDERS

VII. MISCELLANEOUS

CONTRIBUTORS

Arnold A. Asp, M.D., FACP
Gunderson Lutheran Medical Center, LaCrosse, Wisconsin

Jeannie A. Baquero, M.D.
University of Texas Health Sciences Center at San Antonio, San Antonio, Texas

Linda A. Barbour, M.D., M.S.P.H.
Associate Professor of Medicine and Obstetrics and Gynecology, Divisions of Endocrinology, Metabolism, Diabetes, and Maternal-Fetal Medicine, University of Colorado Health Sciences Center, Denver, Colorado

Brenda K. Bell, M.D.
Private practice, Lincoln, Nebraska

Daniel H. Bessesen, M.D.
Associate Professor of Medicine, University of Colorado Health Sciences Center; Chief of Endocrinology, Denver Health Medical Center, Denver, Colorado

Tamis M. Bright, M.D.
Chief, Division of Endocrinology, Texas Tech University Health Sciences Center, El Paso, Texas

Henry B. Burch, M.D.
Department of Medicine, Uniformed Services University of the Health Sciences, Bethesda, Maryland; Endocrine-Metabolic Service, Walter Reed Army Medical Center, Washington, District of Columbia

Reed S. Christensen, M.D.
Assistant Professor of Medicine, Department of Medicine, Uniformed Services University of the Health Sciences, Bethesda, Maryland; Chief, Endocrinology Service, Department of Medicine, Tripler Army Medical Center, Honolulu, Hawaii

Stephen Clement, M.D.
Associate Professor of Medicine, Division of Endocrinology and Medicine; Director, Georgetown Diabetes Center, Georgetown University Medical Center, Washington, District of Columbia

William E. Duncan, M.D., Ph.D.
Chief, Department of Medicine, Walter Reed Army Medical Center, Washington, District of Columbia

James E. Fitzpatrick, M.D.
Associate Professor, Department of Dermatology, University of Colorado Health Sciences Center, Denver, Colorado

Kelly Flesner-Gurley, M.D.
St. John Health System, Tulsa, Oklahoma

William J. Georgitis, M.D.
Clinical Professor, Division of Endocrinology, University of Colorado Health Sciences Center; Regional Director and Chief, Department of Endocrinology and Diabetes, Colorado Permanente Medical Group, Denver, Colorado

Bryan R. Haugen, M.D.
Associate Professor of Medicine, Division of Endocrinology, Metabolism, and Diabetes, University of Colorado Health Sciences Center, Denver, Colorado

James V. Hennessey, M.D.
Associate Professor of Medicine, Brown Medical School; Hallett Center for Diabetes and Metabolism, Providence, Rhode Island

Fred D. Hofeldt, M.D.
Las Cruces, New Mexico

Robert E. Jones, M.D., FACP, FACE
Division of Endocrinology, Metabolism, and Diabetes, Department of Internal Medicine, University of Utah School of Medicine, Salt Lake City, Utah

Wendy M. Kohrt, Ph.D.
Professor of Medicine, Division of Geriatric Medicine, University of Colorado Health Sciences Center, Denver, Colorado

Homer J. LeMar, Jr., M.D.
Chief, Department of Medicine, William Beaumont Army Medical Center, El Paso, Texas

Elliot G. Levy, M.D.
Clinical Professor of Medicine, University of Miami School of Medicine; Endocrinologist in private practice, Miami, Florida

Robert C. McIntyre, M.D.
Department of Surgery, University of Colorado Health Sciences Center, Denver, Colorado

Jonathan R. Parks, M.D.
Private Practice, Fort Bliss, Texas

Christopher D. Raeburn, M.D.
Department of Surgery, University of Colorado Health Sciences Center, Denver, Colorado

Thomas N. Robinson, M.D.
Department of Surgery, University of Colorado Health Sciences Center, Denver, Colorado

Mary H. Samuels, M.D.
Division of Endocrinology, Diabetes and Clinical Nutrition, Oregon Health Sciences Center, Portland, Oregon

Leonard R. Sanders, M.D.
Chairman, Division of Nephrology, Lovelace Health Systems, Albuquerque, New Mexico

Virginia Sarapura, M.D.
Division of Endocrinology, Metabolism, and Diabetes, University of Colorado Health Sciences Center, Denver, Colorado

Robert S. Schwartz, M.D.
Goodstein Professor of Medicine and Head, Division of Geriatric Medicine, University of Colorado Health Sciences Center, Denver, Colorado

Kenneth J. Simcic, M.D., FACP
Assistant Professor of Medicine, University of Texas Health Sciences Center at San Antonio, San Antonio, Texas

Robert H. Slover, M.D.
Barbara Davis Center, University of Colorado Health Sciences Center, Denver, Colorado

Robert C. Smallridge, M.D.
Professor of Medicine, Division of Endocrinology, Mayo Medical School, Jacksonville, Florida

Elizabeth A. Stephens, M.D.
Division of Endocrinology, Metabolism, and Diabetes, Oregon Health Sciences University, Portland, Oregon

Derek J. Stocker, M.D.
Endocrinology Service, Walter Reed Army Medical Center, Washington, District of Columbia

Sharon H. Travers, M.D.
Division of Pediatrics, University of Colorado Health Sciences Center; Children's Hospital of Denver, Denver, Colorado

Terri Ryan-Turek, R.D., C.D.E.
Division of Endocrinology, Metabolism, and Diabetes, University of Colorado Health Sciences Center; Anschutz Center for Advanced Medicine, Denver, Colorado

Robert A. Vigersky, M.D.
Department of Medicine, Uniformed Services University of the Health Sciences, Bethesda, Maryland; Endocrine-Metabolic Service, Walter Reed Army Medical Center, Washington, District of Columbia

Cecilia C.L. Wang, M.D.
Instructor, Division of Endocrinology, Department of Medicine, University of Colorado Health Sciences Center, Denver, Colorado

Katherine Weber, M.D.
Division of Endocrinology, University of Colorado Health Sciences Center, Denver, Colorado

Magaret E. Wierman, M.D.
Division of Endocrinology, Metabolism, and Diabetes, University of Colorado Health Sciences Center; Chief, Division of Endocrinology, Veterans Affairs Medical Center, Denver, Colorado

Susan T. Wingo, M.D.
Amarillo Diagnostic Clinic, Amarillo, Texas

Philip S. Zeitler, M.D.
Associate Professor of Pediatrics, Division of Endocrinology, Department of Pediatrics, University of Colorado Health Sciences Center; Children's Hospital of Denver, Denver, Colorado

PREFACE

A book can provide us with many facts. Better still, for those who are willing, it can make us think, reason, and question. These are the basic tools we need to be good, competent health care providers. But our greatest teachers are our patients. They show us the face, the heart, and the soul of disease and of recovery. It is the truly great providers who understand the enrichment, humility, and wisdom that come from this source. I encourage the readers of this book to study it, and many others as well, to equip them with the basic information to make responsible and, when possible, data-based decisions regarding the evaluation and management of their patients. However, I urge them to learn mostly from their patients, to spend time with them, to show them sincere compassion, and, most of all, to show them respect. We should never fail them in this. They deserve no less than the best of our humanity, and, regardless of the outcome, this is what they will best remember and appreciate.

Michael T. McDermott, M.D.

TOP 100 SECRETS

These secrets are 100 of the top board alerts. They summarize the concepts, principles, and most salient details of endocrinology. They are listed in order of the chapters in which more detailed discussions appear.

1. Type 1 diabetes is caused by the autoimmune destruction of beta cells in approximately 90% of people and results in an absolute deficiency of insulin; type 2 diabetes is the consequence of a combination of insulin resistance and progressive beta-cell failure.

2. Care has been taken to ensure that patients with diabetes are treated to standards that are based on scientific evidence: hemoglobin $A_{1C} < 7\%$, low-density lipoprotein (LDL) cholesterol < 100 mg/dL, blood pressure $< 130/80$ mmHg.

3. Microvascular complications of diabetes mellitus are directly related to hyperglycemia and result from the formation of advanced glycation end products, polyol accumulation, protein kinase C activation, accrual of intracellular glucosamine, and oxidative stress.

4. The propensity for developing vascular disease in type 2 diabetes is likely related to insulin resistance and the pathologic clustering of dyslipidemia and hypertension inherent in this condition.

5. Intensive insulin therapy, or basal/bolus therapy, mimics normal pancreatic insulin secretion; basal insulin is the amount required to regulate hepatic glucose production between meals, while bolus insulin is used to match carbohydrate intake, using a carbohydrate-to-insulin ratio with each meal.

6. Insulin is the best agent for management of hyperglycemia in hospital patients; intravenous insulin infusions are superior to subcutaneous insulin with respect to achieving glycemic control and improving nonglycemic outcomes.

7. Use of "sliding-scale" insulin alone to control blood sugars causes increased rates of hyperglycemia, hypoglycemia, and iatrogenic DKA, which should be avoided.

8. Women who develop gestational diabetes have ~50% risk of developing type 2 diabetes within 5–10 years.

9. Normalizing the hemoglobin A_{1C} prior to pregnancy and during the first 10 weeks of organogenesis can reduce the major malformation rate from 25% to 2–3%.

10. Fasting hypoglycemia often produces neuroglycopenic symptoms and is frequently due to an organic disorder or surreptitious use of insulin or oral hypoglycemic medications.

11. Postprandial (reactive) hypoglycemia usually produces adrenergic symptoms and is most often a functional disorder related to dietary indiscretion or anxiety and stress, but it can occasionally be due to rapid gastric emptying or early type 2 diabetes mellitus.

12. Elevated low-density lipoprotein (LDL) cholesterol and low high-density lipoprotein (HDL) cholesterol are major risk factors for coronary artery disease (CAD), while serum triglyceride levels greater than 1000 mg/dL significantly increase the risk of developing acute pancreatitis.

13. The metabolic syndrome, which is a major CAD risk-factor complex, consists of any three of the following: abdominal obesity, hypertension, hypertriglyceridemia, low HDL cholesterol, insulin resistance, and hyperglycemia.

14. Obesity, defined as a body mass index (BMI) > 30 kg/m^2, is associated with an increased risk of developing related medical illnesses, including diabetes mellitus, hypertension, coronary artery disease, pulmonary emboli, sleep apnea, and osteoarthritis.

15. Diet and exercise to alter energy balance are the mainstays of obesity management, but sibutramine, orlistat, and phentermine are currently Food and Drug Administration (FDA) approved medications that can be used to help overweight and obese patients lose weight.

16. Secondary disorders causing bone loss are present in approximately 30% of women and 64% of men who have osteoporosis.

17. Medications that have been shown to significantly reduce the risk of osteoporotic fractures fall into two main categories: antiresorptive agents and anabolic agents.

18. The pathophysiology of glucocorticoid-induced osteoporosis involves both suppressed bone formation and enhanced bone resorption, accounting for the rapid bone loss often seen in glucocorticoid-treated patients.

19. Treatment is recommended for all postmenopausal women regardless of initial bone mineral density (BMD) and for men or premenopausal women with a BMD T-score < −1.0 when they are being treated or will be treated with >5 mg/day of prednisone (or equivalent) for >3 months.

20. Bone mass measurement of the forearm is the study of choice for patients with hyperparathyroidism.

21. Osteomalacia and rickets result from inadequate or delayed mineralization of bone.

22. The causes of osteomalacia and rickets fall into three categories: (1) abnormal vitamin D supply, metabolism, or action; (2) abnormal phosphate supply or metabolism; (3) a small group of disorders in which there is normal vitamin D and mineral metabolism.

23. Paget's disease is characterized by abnormal bone architecture resulting from an imbalance between osteoblastic bone formation and osteoclastic bone resorption.

24. Bisphosphonates are the most effective treatment for Paget's disease of bone.

25. Although there are over 30 major causes of hypercalcemia, hyperparathyroidism and hypercalcemia of malignancy account for >90%; measuring a serum parathyroid hormone (PTH) level will reliably differentiate these two disorders.

26. Calcimimetics are potentially the most useful drugs for treatment of hypercalcemia caused by hyperparathyroidism, having been shown to frequently normalize serum calcium levels and reduce PTH greater than 40–50%.

27. Primary hyperparathyroidism is associated with hypercalcemia, osteoporosis, nephrolithiasis, and symptoms associated with these conditions.

28. The recommendations for surgery in patients with asymptomatic hyperparathyroidism are as follows: serum calcium > 1 mg/dL above the upper normal limit; hypercalciuria > 400 mg per 24 hours; decreased creatinine clearance < 70% of age matched normal persons; reduced bone density with T-score < –2.5; age < 50 years; calcium nephrolithiasis.

29. Hypercalcemia of malignancy is most often due to tumor production of parathyroid hormone-related peptide (PTHrP), which binds to PTH and PTH/PTHrP receptors to stimulate bone resorption.

30. Hypocalcemia is a frequent problem in intensive care settings and is often a result of intravenous medications.

31. Calcitriol (1,25-dihydroxyvitamin D) is the treatment for hypocalcemia in patients with hypoparathyroidism or renal failure.

32. Stones form because of supersaturation of urinary stone precursors (such as calcium and oxalate), insufficient stone inhibitors (such as citrate), abnormal urine pH, or insufficient urine volume.

33. Therapy of kidney stones includes daily intake of 10–12 eight-ounce glasses of fluid, increased intake of citrate-containing drinks, 1000–1200 mg of calcium, and no more than 2300 mg of sodium and 1gm/kg ideal body weight protein; excessive calcium, oxalate, vitamin D, and grapefruit juice should also be avoided.

34. Replacement with thyroid hormone alone in a hypothyroid patient with coexistent adrenal deficiency may precipitate an acute adrenal crisis.

35. Aldosterone deficiency generally does not occur in hypopituitarism because the principal physiologic regulator of aldosterone secretion is the renin–angiotensin system, not adrenocorticotropic hormone (ACTH) from the hypothalamic–pituitary system.

36. Nonfunctioning pituitary tumors cause symptoms primarily by mass effects, resulting in compression of the pituitary stalk and optic chiasm, invasion of the cavernous sinuses, and erosion into the bony sella turcica.

37. Treatment for nonfunctioning pituitary tumors >1.0 cm is transphenoidal surgery with subsequent radiation therapy or close monitoring for incompletely resected tumors.

38. A prolactin level over 200 ng/mL is almost always indicative of a prolactin-secreting tumor, except when found during late pregnancy.

39. An important consequence of elevated prolactin is decreased bone mineral density, which is not always completely reversible.

40. Acromegaly causes damage to bones, joints, heart, and other organs and is associated with considerable morbidity and excess mortality.

41. The best screening test for acromegaly is an insulin-like growth factor (IGF)-1 level.

58. Congenital adrenal hyperplasia (CAH), the most common inherited disease, is a group of autosomal recessive disorders, the most frequent of which is 21-hydroxylase deficiency.

59. The radioactive iodine uptake (RAIU) is used primarily to determine whether patients with thyrotoxicosis have a high RAIU or a low RAIU disorder.

60. A thyroid scan is used mainly to distinguish among the three main types of high RAIU thyrotoxicosis and to determine whether thyroid nodules are nonfunctioning (cold), eufunctioning (warm), or hyperfunctioning (hot).

61. Older patients with thyrotoxicosis may not have classical hyperadrenergic symptoms and signs but may instead present with weight loss, depression, or heart disease (worsening angina pectoris, atrial fibrillation, congestive heart failure); this picture is often referred to as apathetic thyrotoxicosis.

62. Radioiodine treatment may worsen eye disease in patients with significant proptosis or periorbital inflammation due to Graves' ophthalmopathy; if radioiodine is used, patients should stop smoking and should take a course of oral corticosteroids immediately after the radioiodine treatment.

63. Levothyroxine is the preferred initial treatment for hypothyroidism, and in healthy young patients, it can be started at a dose of 1.6 µg/kg/day.

64. The goal TSH for treatment of primary hypothyroidism is between 0.5 and 2.0 mU/L.

65. Amiodarone-induced thyroid disease (AITD) may be due to iodine-induced hyperthyroidism (type 1 AITD) or destruction-induced thyroiditis (type 2 AITD).

66. Women with type 1 diabetes mellitus have a threefold greater risk of postpartum thyroid disorders than do nondiabetic TPO antibody positive women.

67. Toxic thyroid adenomas are almost never cancerous.

68. Hemorrhagic degeneration of a benign thyroid adenoma causes pain that may radiate to the jaw or ear and be misdiagnosed as a dental abscess or otitis.

69. Thyroglobulin is the most sensitive tumor marker for differentiated thyroid cancer.

70. Suppression of TSH, a thyroid cancer growth factor, with levothyroxine is an important therapeutic intervention in patients with differentiated thyroid cancer.

71. Thyroid storm is treated with antithyroid drugs, cold iodine, beta-blockers, stress glucocorticoid doses, and management of any precipitating factors.

72. Myxedema coma is treated with rapid repletion of the thyroid hormone deficit, stress glucocorticoid doses, and treatment of any precipitating causes.

73. The euthyroid sick syndrome is not a thyroid disorder but is instead a group of changes in serum thyroid hormone and TSH levels that result from cytokines and inflammatory mediators produced in patients with nonthyroidal illnesses.

74. The euthyroid sick syndrome appears to be an adaptive response to reduce tissue metabolism and preserve energy during systemic illnesses, and therefore treatment with thyroid hormone is not currently recommended for this condition.

75. Postpartum thyroiditis occurs in ~5% of normal women and ~25% of women with type 1 diabetes.

76. On average, a woman's thyroid hormone replacement dose for hypothyroidism will increase by 25–50 µg per day during pregnancy, often during the first trimester.

77. The symptoms of hypothyroidism often mimic those of depression, while those of hyperthyroidism may be confused with mania or depression.

78. About 20% of patients admitted to the hospital with acute psychiatric presentations, including schizophrenia and major affective disorders, but rarely dementia or alcoholism, may have mild elevations in their serum T_4 levels, and less often their T_3 levels.

79. Central precocious puberty occurs more frequently in girls than boys; boys with central precocity, however, have a much higher incidence of underlying central nervous system (CNS) pathology.

80. A reduction in testicular volume (below 20 mL) is the most common manifestation of hypogonadism and is seen in nearly all cases of long-standing hypogonadism.

81. The diagnosis of hypogonadism is confirmed with a correctly obtained serum testosterone measurement or semen analysis. Measurement of serum LH and FSH levels then helps to determine whether the hypogonadism is primary (testicular) or secondary (pituitary or hypothalamic).

82. The specific cause of impotence can be diagnosed in 85% of men.

83. The antihypertensive medications that are least likely to cause impotence are angiotensin-converting enzyme (ACE) inhibitors, angiotensin receptor binders (ARBs), and calcium channel blockers.

84. Cysts on ovarian ultrasound do not always signify a diagnosis of polycystic ovary syndrome (PCOS).

85. A serum testosterone > 200 ng/dL or a DHEAS > 1000 ng/mL in a hirsute patient suggests the presence of an androgen-producing ovarian or adrenal tumor.

86. Primary hypothyroidism can cause amenorrhea, galactorrhea, and pituitary enlargement and thus mimics a prolactinoma.

87. Many medications and painful lesions of the chest wall can cause galactorrhea.

88. The common causes of hirsutism are PCOS, CAH, idiopathic/familial hirsutism, and medications.

89. The common causes of virilization are androgen-secreting ovarian or adrenal tumors and CAH.

90. Side effects of anabolic-androgenic steroid abuse include fluid retention, testicular atrophy, oligospermia, azoospermia, gynecomastia, cholestatic hepatitis, peliosis hepatis, benign and malignant hepatic tumors, as well as reduced HDL and higher LDL cholesterol levels.

91. Multiple endocrine neoplasia (MEN) 1 results from a mutation inactivating the menin tumor suppressor on chromosome 11, but routine clinical testing for the mutation is currently impractical.

92. Genetic testing for the RET mutation causing MEN 2 syndromes is now clinically available.

93. Autoimmune polyendocrine syndrome type 1 (APS-1) is a pediatric syndrome marked by hypoparathyroidism, adrenal insufficiency, and mucocutaneous candidiasis.

94. Autoimmune polyendocrine syndrome type 2 (APS-2) consists of adrenal insufficiency, thyroid dysfunction, and diabetes mellitus type 1.

95. Insulinomas most often cause fasting hypoglycemia with neuroglycopenic symptoms.

96. Most patients with carcinoid syndrome have extensive liver metastases that either impair the metabolic clearance of mediators secreted by the primary tumor or secrete the mediators directly into the hepatic vein.

97. A carcinoid crisis can be precipitated when a patient with a carcinoid tumor is given an adrenergic medication or a monoamine oxidase inhibitor.

98. Mucormycosis is more common during diabetic ketoacidosis because the fungi are thermotolerant, grow well in an acid pH, grow rapidly in the presence of high glucose, and are one of the few types of fungi that can utilize ketones as a food substrate.

99. The most common cause of acanthosis nigricans is diabetes associated with insulin resistance and obesity.

100. Aging is associated with losses of muscle mass and bone mass and with increases in fat mass, which may be associated with parallel age-related declines in the production of growth hormone and sex steroid hormones.

DIABETES MELLITUS

Robert E. Jones, M.D., and Stephen Clement, M.D.

1. **What is diabetes mellitus?**

   Diabetes mellitus is a chronic disorder characterized by abnormalities in fuel metabolism, including glucose, lipids, and amino acids. However, abnormalities in glucose tolerance are central in both the diagnosis of diabetes and classic complications of the disease. Because of associated abnormalities in lipid metabolism, people with diabetes are also prone to develop atherosclerosis, especially those with type 2 diabetes. The types of diabetes are summarized in Table 1-1.

TABLE 1-1. TYPES OF DIABETES MELLITUS AND OTHER ABNORMALITIES IN GLUCOSE TOLERANCE	
Clinical Classes	**Distinguishing Characteristics**
Type 1 diabetes mellitus	Due to beta-cell destruction leading to an absolute insulin deficiency. Beta-cell loss may be immune-mediated (90%) or idiopathic (10%). Depending on the rate of beta-cell destruction (rapidly in children and young adults, and more slowly in older adults), all patients eventually require insulin for glucose control and survival. Patients are prone to ketoacidosis.
Type 2 diabetes mellitus	Due to a combination of insulin resistance and relative insulin deficiency. Often associated with obesity or an increase in truncal (visceral) fat. Ketoacidosis is uncommon; may occur during periods of illness or stress. Hypertension and dyslipidemia are frequently associated. Generally does not require exogenous insulin early in course of the illness.
Other types of diabetes	Diabetes associated with specific conditions and syndromes
Gestational diabetes	Any degree of glucose intolerance with onset or first recognition during pregnancy

Adapted from American Diabetes Association: Report of the Expert Committee on the Diagnosis and Classification of Diabetes Mellitus. Diabetes Care 20:1183–1196, 1997.

2. **Describe how diabetes is diagnosed.**

   The currently used diagnostic criteria for abnormalities in glucose tolerance were formulated in 1997 and revised in 2003. The preferred diagnostic test is a fasting plasma glucose (FPG). The FPG must be obtained in the morning before 09:00 hours, since glucose levels may progressively fall during the day and may give a false negative result. The diagnostic criteria are summarized in Table 1-2.

TABLE 1-2. DIAGNOSIS OF DIABETES

		Tests	
Stage	FPG*	Casual Plasma Glucose	OGTT§
Normal	<100 mg/dL (5.5 mmol/L)†		2-hour PG < 140 mg/dL
Prediabetes	Impaired fasting glucose ≥ 100 and <126 mg/dL (7.0 mmol/L)		Impaired glucose tolerance 2-hour PG ≥ 140 mg/dL (7.7 mmol/L) but <200 mg/dL (11.1 mmol/L)
Diabetes	FPG ≥ 126 mg/dL (7.0 mmol/L)	≥200 mg/dL (11.1 mmol/L) plus symptoms‡	2-hour PG ≥ 200 mg/dL (11.1 mmol/L)

FPG = fasting plasma glucose; PG = plasma glucose; OGTT = oral glucose tolerance test.
*The morning FPG is the preferred test for diagnosis, but any one of the three is acceptable. In the absence of unequivocal hyperglycemia with acute metabolic decompensation, one of the three tests should be repeated on a different day to confirm the diagnosis.
†Fasting is defined as no caloric intake for at least 8 hours.
‡Casual refers to any time of the day without regard to the time since the last meal. The classic symptoms of diabetes are polyuria, polydipsia, and unexplained weight loss.
§In nonpregnant individuals, the OGTT should be performed using the equivalent of 75 gm anhydrous glucose dissolved in water. At this point, the OGTT is not recommended for routine clinical use.

3. **Discuss the prevalence of diabetes.**
   The estimated 12 million Americans, or 5.9% of the population, have been diagnosed as having diabetes, and approximately 6 million Americans have diabetes but are unaware of it. The prevalence of type 2 diabetes is increasing dramatically worldwide as the population becomes more sedentary and obese. Labeled as an emerging epidemic by many health organizations, it has been estimated that up to one-third of the population will suffer from diabetes within two decades.

4. **Who should be screened for diabetes?**
   Because many people with type 2 diabetes are either asymptomatic or ignore subtle symptoms of hyperglycemia, screening programs should be established to enhance early detection and thus limit the risk for long-term complications. Table 1-3 summarizes the criteria for testing for diabetes in asymptomatic people.

5. **Describe the effect of genetics on type 1 diabetes.**
   The interplay between genetics and environment in diabetes is complex and still not well understood. Monozygotic twins have a 20–50% concordance for type 1 diabetes. The cumulative risk for siblings of diabetic patients is 6–10% versus 0.6% for the general population. Regarding the effect of parental genes, the offspring of women with type 1 diabetes have a lower risk of disease (2.1%) than the offspring of men with type 1 diabetes (6.1%). The reason for this disparity is unknown. The susceptibility for type 1 diabetes is associated with the genetic expression of

> ### TABLE 1-3. CRITERIA FOR TESTING FOR DIABETES IN ASYMPTOMATIC, UNDIAGNOSED PEOPLE*
>
> Testing should be considered at a younger age or carried out more frequently in asymptomatic people with two or more of the following risk factors (the greater number of risk factors present in an individual, the greater the chance of that individual having or developing diabetes)
>
> - Age > 45 years
> - Overweight (body mass index [BMI] ≥ 25 kg/m^2)
> - Family history of diabetes (i.e., parents or siblings with diabetes)
> - Member of a high-risk ethnic population (African American, Hispanic, Native American, Asian American, and Pacific Islanders)
> - History of gestational diabetes or delivery of infant weighing more than 9 lb
> - Habitual physical inactivity
> - History of hypertension or dyslipidemia (HDL ≤ 35 mg/dL or high triglycerides ≥ 250 mg/dL)
> - Previously identified with either impaired fasting glucose or impaired glucose tolerance (prediabetes)
> - Polycystic ovary syndrome
> - History of vascular disease
>
> *The OGTT or FPG test may be used to diagnose diabetes; however, in clinical settings, the morning FPG test is preferred because of ease of administration, convenience, acceptability, and lower cost.

certain proteins coded by the human leukocyte antigen (HLA) region of the major histocompatibility complex. These proteins are present on the surface of lymphocytes and macrophages and are considered essential for triggering the autoimmune destruction of the beta cells. Although all of the genetic markers (HLA and others) for type 1 diabetes are not known, future progress in this field will allow population screening for genetic susceptibility.

6. **What role does genetics play in the development of type 2 diabetes?**
   The familial clustering of type 2 diabetes suggests a strong genetic component to the disease. Monozygotic twins have a 60–90% concordance for type 2 diabetes. The cumulative risk for type 2 diabetes in siblings of diabetic patients is 10–33% versus 5% for the general population. Offspring of women with type 2 diabetes have a 2- to 3-fold greater risk for developing diabetes than do offspring of men with the disease. The exact mode of inheritance for type 2 diabetes is not known but is thought to be polygenic. Specific mutations that are associated with risk for type 2 diabetes have been identified, but many of these genes are widely found in the population at large. Because type 2 diabetes is so commonly associated with obesity, many investigators suspect that genes that predispose to obesity are associated with type 2 diabetes as well. There appears to be a strong interplay between genetic and environmental influences for causing type 2 diabetes. One illustration of this is the demonstration of higher fasting insulin levels for every weight category in offspring of two parents with type 2 diabetes compared with controls. High insulin levels are a marker for insulin resistance and are predictive of progression to type 2 diabetes.

KEY POINTS: DEFINITIONS RELATED TO DIABETES ✓

1. Diabetes mellitus is characterized by abnormalities in fuel metabolism (glucose, lipids, and amino acids), but the diagnosis centers on documenting abnormal glucose metabolism.

2. In people who are not pregnant, fasting glucose levels > 125 mg/dL (7 mmol/L), or 2-hour glucose level during an oral glucose tolerance test (OGTT) > 199 mg/dL (11.1 mmol/L) or a random glucose ≥ 200 mg/dL (11.1 mmol/L), coupled with the cardinal symptoms of diabetes, are diagnostic of the condition.

3. Type 1 diabetes is caused by the autoimmune destruction of beta cells in approximately 90% of people and results in an absolute deficiency of insulin.

4. Type 2 diabetes is the consequence of a combination of insulin resistance and progressive beta-cell failure.

7. **Discuss the pathogenesis of type 1 diabetes.**

For type 1 diabetes, the primary pathogenic step is the activation of host T lymphocytes against specific antigens present in the patient's own beta cells. These activated T cells orchestrate a slow destruction of the beta cells via the recruitment of T and B lymphocytes, macrophages, and cytokines. Morphologic study of the pancreases of children who died at the onset of diabetes has shown an inflammatory infiltrate of mononuclear cells confined to the islets—called *insulitis*. The final result is the total destruction of the beta cells over a span of years. The finding of high-titer islet-cell antibodies (ICAs) in the serum of a child is highly predictive for progression to type 1 diabetes.

Various antigens that are expressed by the beta cell have been implicated as the target for the autoimmune attack. Candidate antigens include insulin itself and a 64-kDa protein (now recognized as glutamic acid decarboxylase [GAD]). The triggering event for T-cell activation against these autoantigens is unknown but may involve the exposure to some environmental substance that is antigenically similar to the autoantigen. The T cells that are activated against this environmental antigen can then cross-react with the antigen on the beta cells—a process called *molecular mimicry*. Suspected environmental triggers for type 1 diabetes are viruses, toxins, and foods. For example, exposure to cow's milk in the first 6 weeks of life has been implicated in the development of type 1 diabetes in genetically susceptible children. Viruses may trigger type 1 diabetes via molecular mimicry or by direct alteration of the beta cell, causing abnormal expression of autoantigens or by direct destruction of the beta cells.

8. **Describe the pathogenesis of type 2 diabetes.**

Type 1 diabetes is characterized by an absolute insulin deficiency; however, type 2 diabetes is characterized by both a defect in insulin action (insulin resistance) and a relative insulin deficiency. Insulin resistance generally precedes insulin deficiency by several years or decades in most models of type 2 diabetes although recent reports have suggested that a beta-cell defect may be the initiating trigger for both. Elevated levels of fasting or postglucose load insulin levels are the hallmark of insulin resistance. Several quantitative techniques may be used to assess insulin sensitivity or insulin resistance. Examples include: the homeostatic model assessment (HOMA), which describes the relationship between fasting insulin and fasting glucose levels; the frequently sampled intravenous glucose tolerance test; insulin clamps (waist-to-hip ratio), and insulin sensitivity, and the simplest clinical approximation of insulin sensitivity is a measurement of abdominal girth. Figure 1-1 summarizes the natural history of type 2 diabetes.

Not all insulin-resistant patients progress to overt diabetes because normal beta cells can compensate for the increased peripheral demand for insulin. Abnormalities in glucose tolerance begin to appear only after beta-cell failure begins. Loss of first-phase insulin secretion is the initial defect, and as this progresses, the patient displays elevated postprandial glucose levels.

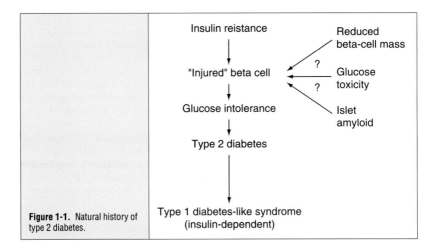

Figure 1-1. Natural history of type 2 diabetes.

Eventually beta-cell death accelerates, and fasting glucose levels rise. It has been estimated that at the time of diagnosis of diabetes, patients have lost nearly 50% of their beta-cell mass.

9. **Describe the metabolic syndrome.**
   The metabolic syndrome has also been called the insulin-resistance syndrome or syndrome X. The components of the metabolic syndrome include obesity, hypertension, hypertriglyc-eridemia, low high-density lipoprotein (HDL) cholesterol levels, and abnormalities in glucose tolerance. A patient may be considered to have the metabolic syndrome if three of the five following criteria are met:
   - Increased waist circumference (>40 in. in men; >35 in. in women).
   - Plasma triglycerides ≥ 150 mg/dL.
   - Plasma HDL cholesterol < 40 mg/dL in men; <50 mg/dL in women.
   - Blood pressure ≥ 130/85 mmHg.
   - Fasting plasma glucose (FPG) ≥ 100 mg/dL.

   Approximately 55 million Americans meet the diagnostic criteria for the metabolic syndrome, and these patients should be screened on a regular basis for diabetes.

10. **What causes beta-cell failure in type 2 diabetes?**
    Type 2 diabetes is associated with a progressive loss of beta-cell mass. In fact, it has been estimated that at the time of diagnosis, patients with type 2 diabetes have lost nearly 50% of their insulin-producing cells. The system of programmed beta-cell death or apoptosis has many possible triggers, but two specific possibilities have been well characterized. Elevated levels of glucose and free fatty acids, collectively called glucolipotoxicity, and chronic increases in certain cytokines, notably tumor necrosis factor alpha (TNF-α) and interleukin 1-beta (IL-1β), have been documented to activate "death" genes (caspases) in beta cells. Both of these conditions have been amply described in subjects with either prediabetes or overt diabetes and clearly contribute to the genesis of type 2 diabetes by reducing the amount of functioning beta cells. On the other hand, there is considerable excitement over the concept of beta-cell preservation and the possibility that the natural history of type 2 diabetes can be altered. There are emerging data that the thiazolidinediones and glucagon-like peptide-1 (GLP-1) may provide either direct or indirect mechanisms to enhance beta-cell survival.

11. **What effect does GLP-1 have on beta-cell function?**
    The L cells in the distal small intestine produce GLP-1, and its secretion is under neurogenic control. Although GLP-1 is a product of the proglucagon gene and was once called "gut

glucagon," its functions in relation to glucose homeostasis are completely unrelated to glucagon. The beta-cell-independent actions of GLP-1 include suppressing glucagon secretion, delaying gastric emptying, and enhancing satiety through a direct effect on the central nervous system (CNS). The direct actions of GLP-1 or its analogs on beta cells portend its possible therapeutic value. GLP-1 augments glucose-dependent insulin secretion and, in effect, acts to resensitize the islets to a glucose challenge without causing hypoglycemia. In addition, GLP-1 is the only compound shown to stimulate insulin gene expression. Perhaps the most exciting aspects of GLP-1 physiology center on its abilities to induce beta-cell differentiation from pancreatic ductal cells and protection of beta cells from apoptosis.

Unfortunately, the extremely short half-life of GLP-1 (1–3 minutes) limits its therapeutic usefulness. On the other hand, GLP-1 analogs that are more resistant to enzymatic degradation by dipeptidyl peptidase IV (DPP IV) are being developed as are inhibitors of DPP IV. A new class of compounds, GLP-1 receptor agonists, shows particular promise. Exendin-4, derived from Gila monster saliva, is the best-described member of this class and shows great promise in clinical trials.

12. **Can diabetes be prevented?**

Several recent trials that have enrolled subjects at high risk for developing type 2 diabetes (e.g., subjects with either prediabetes, a history of gestational diabetes, or obesity) have documented the potential beneficial effects of thiazolidinediones (TRIPOD Study), metformin (DPP), alpha-glucosidase inhibitors (STOP-NIDDM), and intestinal lipase inhibitors (XENDOS) in reducing the rate of progression to overt diabetes. However, subjects participating in the lifestyle modification arm (diet and exercise) of the Diabetes Prevention Program (DPP) fared the best with a 60% reduction in the risk of developing diabetes. Provocative post-hoc analyses of the HOPE and WOSCOPS trials documented an approximate 30% reduction in diabetes risk with ramipril and pravastatin, respectively. However, the American Diabetes Association does not recommend pharmacotherapy for type 2 diabetes prevention due to a lack of long-term data on effectiveness and costs.

Prevention of type 1 diabetes has proven to be more challenging because it is less common than type 2 diabetes, and the recognition of people at risk is very difficult. Identifying people in the "prediabetic" phase of type 1 diabetes requires serial measurements of beta-cell function and close monitoring of immunologic markers. All of these factors have confounded the selection of an appropriate cohort, but the DPT-1 study overcame many of these obstacles. Unfortunately, the results of the study were disappointing. In contrast, short-term studies targeting early intervention with either monoclonal antibodies or peptide immunomodulators in patients who have already presented with type 1 diabetes, have shown some modest benefit in preserving residual beta-cell function.

13. **Describe the Diabetes Control and Complications Trial (DCCT) model for management of type 1 diabetes.**

The DCCT showed a 34–76% reduction in clinically meaningful diabetic microvascular complications (retinopathy, neuropathy, and nephropathy) in subjects randomized to intensive diabetes therapy compared to subjects assigned to standard diabetes management. The only major adverse effect of intensified control was a threefold higher risk of severe hypoglycemia. The implementation of intensive therapy requires that the patients should monitor their blood glucose 4–8 times a day and use an insulin regimen that involves multiple insulin injections per day or an insulin pump.

Intensive therapy is best managed by a specialized team consisting of a certified diabetes educator (CDE), nurse, dietitian, behavorial medicine specialist, and a physician who has specialized training in intensive therapy. Patients must be involved in their own management and should be in frequent contact with the diabetes team in order that appropriate adjustments (food, insulin, and exercise) can be incorporated into their regimen.

Based on the results of the DCCT, the American Diabetes Association recommends, "Patients should aim for the best level of glucose control they can achieve without placing themselves at undo risk for hypoglycemia or other hazards associated with tight control."

14. **What are insulin analogs?**

Insulin analogs are recombinant proteins that are based on the structure of insulin but have undergone selected amino acid substitutions or additions. These amino acid alterations are designed to either enhance or protract the subcutaneous absorption of the molecule without altering its biologic properties. Native human insulin (regular) exists as a molecular hexamer that must be progressively broken down into dimers and then monomers prior to absorption. Amino acid substitutions in the carboxy terminal region of the beta-chain of insulin tend to destabilize hexamer formation and enhance the rate of absorption. Examples of these analogs are insulins lispro (Humalog), aspart (NovoLog), and glulisine (Apidra). These insulins are excellent for premeal (prandial) use, and because they also have a shorter duration of action in comparison to native human insulin (regular), they provide better mealtime coverage with a lower risk of postmeal hypoglycemia. On the other hand, basal insulin should have both a peak-less action profile and a prolonged duration of action. The only available bioengineered basal insulin is insulin glargine (Lantus). The mechanisms for protraction of glargine absorption center around the addition of two arginines to the carboxy terminus of the beta-chain that in turn lowers the isoelectric point of the molecule from 7 to 4 and promotes hexamer formation. Once injected, insulin glargine is buffered to a physiologic pH and forms a microprecipitate at the site of injection that is slowly absorbed.

15. **Describe the approach to the patient with a labile glucose profile.**

A careful history that searches for causes of glucose variability is essential for optimizing a diabetes regimen. The presence and cause of hypoglycemic reactions are crucial information because hypoglycemia often leads to overtreatment with carbohydrate, causing hyperglycemia. Hypoglycemia also may blunt the patient's ability to respond to subsequent hypoglycemic episodes in the ensuing 24 hours. A common strategy for optimizing a diabetes regimen is as follows:

- Address and abolish causes of hypoglycemia.
- Optimize the fasting glucose.
- Fine-tune the regimen to optimize the preprandial and postprandial glucose readings.

KEY POINTS: TREATMENT OF DIABETES ✓

1. While several different classes of medications may reduce the risk of progression from prediabetes to overt diabetes, the current recommendations focus on lifestyle interventions, including weight loss and increased physical activity.

2. The cornerstones of diabetes therapy are patient empowerment, disease state education, medical nutrition therapy, appropriate levels of physical activity, pharmacotherapy, and attention to cardiac risk factors (control of hypertension, treatment of dyslipidemias, and smoking cessation).

3. Patients with type 1 diabetes are always treated with insulin.

4. Patients with type 2 diabetes are managed by medications that address insulin resistance and insulin deficiency.

5. Care has been taken to ensure that patients with diabetes are treated to standards that are based on scientific evidence: hemoglobin A_{1C} < 7%, LDL cholesterol < 100 mg/dL, blood pressure < 130/80 mmHg.

16. **Is intensive diabetes therapy cost-effective?**

Analyses of the cost-effectiveness of intensive therapy suggest that the potential reduction in cost for treating diabetic complications (laser photocoagulation, dialysis, hospitalization for amputations, and rehabilitation) justifies the cost of personnel and supplies to support intensive diabetes therapy. The risk–benefit ratio for intensive therapy may be less favorable for prepubertal children, patients with far advanced complications, and patients with coronary or cerebral vascular disease.

17. **What is amylin?**

Amylin is a beta-cell hormone that is co-secreted with insulin but is structurally distinct from insulin. Under normal circumstances, amylin acts to reduce postprandial glucose excursions by delaying gastric emptying through a neurogenic mechanism and suppressing glucagon secretion. In addition to an absolute insulin deficiency, patients with type 1 diabetes also have a complete deficiency of amylin, and patients with type 2 diabetes taking insulin have clearly reduced amylin responses to meals. Pramlintide (Symlin) is a synthetic analog of amylin, and mealtime replacement of amylin using pramlintide in subjects who required insulin was shown to modestly reduce hemoglobin A_{1C} levels while promoting weight loss. Symlin is presently pending FDA approval.

18. **What is the United Kingdom Prospective Diabetes Study (UKPDS)?**

The UKPDS is the largest and longest prospective study on type 2 diabetes ever conducted. Investigators recruited 5102 patients with newly diagnosed type 2 diabetes in 23 centers within the UK between 1977 and 1991. Patients were followed for an average of 10 years to determine the impact of intensive therapy using pharmacologic agents versus dietary therapy alone. The study also tested the efficacy of intensive blood pressure control versus "less tight blood pressure control." The results of the study showed a significant reduction in microvascular complications in patients randomized to the intensive therapy arm. Tight blood pressure was associated with a reduction in both microvascular and macrovascular events. When the entire cohort of patients was studied together, the mean hemoglobin A_{1C} level for the duration of the study was a strong positive predictor of all diabetes-related endpoints, including death, amputation, myocardial infarction, and stroke.

19. **Based on the UKPDS and other studies, describe the optimal treatment for type 2 diabetes.**

Because type 2 diabetes is a heterogeneous disorder and patients may have other comorbid illnesses, treatment must be individualized. The most common mistake in management is to label type 2 diabetes as "borderline" or to neglect treatment completely. Patients with fasting glucose levels $\geq$ 126 mg/dL or postprandial glucose levels > 200 mg/dL, even though asymptomatic, are at risk for diabetic complications.

The optimal treatment strategy for type 2 diabetes is one that normalizes blood glucose levels by increasing insulin sensitivity, normalizes blood pressure, and normalizes the lipid profile. The lifestyle interventions of diet and exercise can dramatically enhance insulin sensitivity in sufficiently motivated patients. The initial intervention should include providing a specific prescription for an aerobic exercise program. Insulin sensitivity can be enhanced with a program as simple as brisk walking for 20 minutes daily. The exercise program should fit the patient's lifestyle and schedule. An optimal program is one in which the patient can be part of a supervised exercise group. Dietary intervention should include an initial evaluation by a dietitian and personalized follow-up visits or classes. The goal should be modest but for steady weight loss (if appropriate). Target levels for key tests are as follows: hemoglobin A_{1C} < 7%, blood pressure $\leq$ 130/80 mmHg, and low-density lipoprotein (LDL) cholesterol $\leq$ 100 mg/dL.

20. **Describe the current paradigms for diabetes management.**

The cornerstones of diabetes management are patient education and patient empowerment. Diabetes is a self-management illness and requires that the patient be educated in self-glucose monitoring, nutrition therapy, exercise, and the proper use of medications. Similarly, the patient must be taught how to recognize and treat hypoglycemia. Diabetes educators are crucial in these endeavors, and it is clear that a well-educated patient can make immense contributions to their own management.

The medical regimen for type 1 diabetes is straightforward. Because these patients are completely insulin deficient, they must be managed with insulin. The most physiologic replacement regimen has been described as the "basal-bolus" technique and can be accomplished either by using a continuous subcutaneous insulin infusion (insulin pump) or by using an injection of basal insulin and the prandial injection of a rapid-acting insulin analog.

Because of the dual defects (insulin resistance and insulin deficiency) and the progressive nature of beta-cell failure in type 2 diabetes, management of these patients is very different. Several factors may influence initial treatment. Patients who present with profound hyperglycemia (glucose levels > 300 mg/dL; 16.7 mmol/L) will respond quickly to insulin therapy, and once the effects of acute glucotoxicity have been resolved, they may be managed with oral agents alone. Metformin is the initial drug of choice for obese patients whereas sulfonylureas are preferred for lean patients with type 2 diabetes. Nonetheless, these patients will eventually fail initial therapy, and a second oral agent will be required. If the patient has been on an insulin sensitizer, such as metformin or a thiazolidinedione, an insulin secretogogue should be added. Conversely, if the patient has failed a secretogogue, adding an insulin sensitizer is appropriate. This simple approach has proven to be very successful and has prompted the introduction of fixed dose combination medications—Glucovance (glyburide + metformin) and Metaglip (glipizide + metformin); however, employing these medications as initial therapy may hinder the titration of individual components. Another fixed dose combination medication, Avandamet (metformin + rosiglitazone), only addresses the insulin-resistance side of the equation but has been very effective without a risk of hypoglycemia. Most patients ultimately fail dual therapy and either need to have a third oral agent added to their regimen (thiazolidinedione, sulfonylurea, and metformin) or need to be placed on insulin. Eventually, however, many patients with type 2 diabetes require exogenous insulin.

21. **What are the classes of oral diabetes medications? How do they work?**
Several classes of diabetes medications are available for optimizing glycemic control in people with type 2 diabetes. Sulfonylureas (glyburide, glipizide, and glimepiride) and meglitinides (repaglinide and nateglinide) enhance the secretion of endogenous insulin through membrane-associated receptors. Metformin, the only available member of the biguanide class, reduces hepatic gluconeogenesis, thereby indirectly increasing peripheral insulin sensitivity. The alpha-glucosidase inhibitors, miglitol and acarbose, slow the absorption of dietary carbohydrates by inhibiting the intestinal brush border enzymes that breakdown polysaccharides into absorbable monosaccharides. The thiazolidinediones, pioglitazone and rosiglitazone, are true insulin sensitizers and directly enhance insulin action in muscle and fat cells. While not all of the actions of thiazolidinediones are completely understood, they appear to initiate their action by binding to nuclear peroxisome proliferator-activated receptor-gamma (PPARγ) receptors. Oral agents may be used as monotherapy or may be used in various combinations to achieve desired glucose levels. Table 1-4 summarizes the sites of action of various drugs used to treat type 2 diabetes.

TABLE 1-4. SITE OF ACTION OF VARIOUS DRUGS FOR TYPE 2 DIABETES				
Drug	Pancreas	Liver	Muscle/Fat	Gastrointestinal Tract
Sulfonylureas	X			
Meglitinides	X			
Metformin		X		
Thiazolidinediones		X	X	
α-Glucosidase inhibitors				X

22. **What is basal insulin therapy?**

When fasting glucose levels exceed 160 mg/dL or hemoglobin A_{1C} is greater than 8.4%, fasting or basal hyperglycemia contributes more to hyperglycemic exposure than does postprandial hyperglycemia. Fasting hyperglycemia is due to poorly regulated hepatic glucose production and is a significant contributor to subacute glucotoxicity that can further impair insulin secretion and action. The basic concept underpinning basal insulin therapy is to reduce fasting hyperglycemia to appropriate target levels using either a bedtime injection of NPH insulin or a single daily injection of insulin glargine. In order to enhance endogenous prandial insulin production, sulfonylureas are often continued, although this remains somewhat controversial despite the observations that this combination results in somewhat better overall glycemic control with lower insulin requirements. Because of its effects on endogenous glucose production, metformin has also been frequently used in combination with insulin. One recent study has achieved hemoglobin A_{1C} levels less than 7% in over half of subjects who were placed on either bedtime NPH or insulin glargine as basal insulin, which was added to their preexisting oral agent regimen. While both NPH and insulin glargine were equally effective in lowering glucose levels to preselected targets (fasting glucose ≤ 100 mg/dL), the rate of hypoglycemia was substantially lower in subjects receiving insulin glargine. The key to success with basal insulin therapy is to aggressively titrate the dose of insulin in order to achieve target fasting glucose levels. Because of the inexorable loss of beta-cell function in type 2 diabetes, initiating insulin as basal insulin therapy eases the transition to physiologic (basal-bolus) insulin replacement.

23. **Have standards of care been established for the medical care of patients with diabetes mellitus?**

Yes. Both the American Diabetes Association (ADA) and the American Association of Clinical Endocrinologists (AACE) publish minimal standards of diabetes care. While both groups have minor differences in absolute target values, they agree that it is crucial to address glycemic control and the risk factors for diabetes complications. These comprehensive standards are evidence-based and are regularly updated. For example, the standards state that patients should have a complete history and physical examination at the initial visit. Laboratory testing should include a fasting lipid profile and hemoglobin A_{1C} level. Annual surveillance for complications should include an annual physical examination, ophthalmologic examination, and a screen for microalbuminuria. Overall glycemic control (hemoglobin A_{1C}) should be assessed at least semiannually in all patients and quarterly in insulin-treated patients and patients with poorly controlled type 2 diabetes. Published targets include a hemoglobin A_{1C} of <7.0% (ADA) or ≤ 6.5% (AACE), LDL cholesterol < 100 mg/dL, and blood pressure < 130/80 mmHg. Unfortunately, a recent report indicates that only 7% of people with diabetes are treated to all of these goals.

WEBSITE

Centers for Disease Control and Prevention. Available at http://www.cdc.gov/health/diabetes.html

BIBLIOGRAPHY

1. American Diabetes Association: Standards of medical care in diabetes. Diabetes Care 27(Suppl 1):S15–S35, 2004.
2. Bell DSH: β-cell rejuvenation with thiazolidinediones. Am J Med 115(8A):20S–23S, 2003.
3. Chandra J, Zhivotovsky B, Zaitsev S, et al: Role of apoptosis in pancreatic β-cell death in diabetes. Diabetes 50(Suppl 1):S44–S47, 2000.
4. DeFronzo RA: Pharmacologic therapy for type 2 diabetes mellitus. Ann Intern Med 131:281–303, 1999.

5. Diabetes Control and Complications Trial Research Group: The effect of intensive treatment of diabetes on the development and progression of long-term complications in insulin-dependent diabetes mellitus. N Engl J Med 329:977–986, 1993.

6. Edelman SV, Weyer C: Unresolved challenges with insulin therapy in type 1 diabetes: Potential benefit of replacing amylin, a second β-cell hormone. Diabetes Technol Therapeut 4:175–189, 2002.

7. Egan JM, Bulotta A, Hui H, Perfetti R: GLP-1 receptor agonists are growth and differentiation factors for pancreatic islet beta cells. Diabetes Metab Res Rev 19:114–123, 2003.

8. Expert Committee on the Diagnosis and Classification of Diabetes Mellitus: Report of the expert committee on the diagnosis and classification of diabetes mellitus. Diabetes Care 20:1183–1196, 1997.

9. Expert Committee on the Diagnosis and Classification of Diabetes Mellitus: Follow-up report on the diagnosis of diabetes mellitus. Diabetes Care 26:3160–3167, 2003.

10. Garber AJ: Benefits of combination therapy of insulin and oral hypoglycemic agents. Arch Intern Med 163:1781–1782, 2003.

11. Knowler WC, Barrett-Conner E, Fowler SE, et al: Reduction in the incidence of type 2 diabetes with lifestyle intervention or metformin. N Engl J Med 346:393–403, 2002.

12. Pimenta W, Korytkowski M, Mitrakou A, et al: Pancreatic beta-cell dysfunction as the primary as the primary genetic lesion in NIDDM: Evidence from studies in normal glucose-tolerant individuals with a first-degree NIDDM relative. JAMA 273:1855–1861, 1995.

13. Reaven G: Role of insulin resistance in human disease. Diabetes 37:1595–1607, 1988.

14. Riddle MC: Timely initiation of basal insulin. Am J Med 116(3A):3S–9S, 2004.

15. Saydah SH, Fradkin J, Cowie CC: Poor control of risk factors for vascular disease among adults with previously diagnosed diabetes. JAMA 291:335–342, 2004.

16. Tuomilehto J, Lindstrom J, Eriksson JG, et al: Prevention of type 2 diabetes by changes in lifestyle among subjects with impaired glucose tolerance. N Engl J Med 344:1343–1350, 2001.

17. UK Prospective Diabetes Study (UKPDS) Group: Intensive blood-glucose control with sulphonylureas or insulin compared with conventional treatment and risk of complications in patients with type 2 diabetes (UKPDS 33). Lancet 352:857–858, 1998.

18. Vajo Z, Fawcett J, Duckworth WC: Recombinant DNA technology in the treatment of diabetes: Insulin analogs. Endocr Rev 22:706–717, 2001.

CHAPTER 2

ACUTE AND CHRONIC COMPLICATIONS OF DIABETES

Robert E. Jones, M.D., and Stephen Clement, M.D.

1. **What causes the most common acute complications of diabetes?**
   Acute complications of diabetes are a direct result of abnormalities in the plasma glucose level; hyperglycemia or hypoglycemia. Hypoglycemia results from an imbalance between the medication for diabetes treatment (insulin or oral agent) and the patient's food intake or exercise.

2. **Describe the symptoms of hyperglycemia.**
   Initial symptoms of hyperglycemia are increased thirst (polydipsia), increased urination (polyuria), fatigue, and blurry vision. If uncorrected, hyperglycemia eventually may lead to diabetic ketoacidosis (DKA) or hyperglycemic hyperosmolar nonketotic syndrome (HHNS). DKA and HHNS have traditionally been considered to be distinct entities. In actuality, they represent parts of a spectrum of a disease process characterized by varying degrees of insulin deficiency, overproduction of counter-regulatory hormones and dehydration. In some situations, features of DKA and HHNS may occur concurrently.

3. **Describe the symptoms of hypoglycemia.**
   Because the brain depends almost entirely on glucose for normal function, a dramatic fall in circulating glucose can lead to confusion, stupor, or coma.

4. **What is DKA?**
   DKA is a state of uncontrolled catabolism triggered by a relative or absolute deficiency in circulating insulin. The triad of DKA is metabolic acidosis (pH < 7.35), hyperglycemia (blood glucose level usually >250 mg/dL), and positive ketones in the urine or blood. The relative or absolute deficiency of insulin is accompanied by a reciprocal elevation in counter-regulatory hormones (glucagon, epinephrine, growth hormone, and cortisol), causing increased glucose production by the liver (gluconeogenesis) and catabolism of fat (lipolysis). Lipolysis provides the substrate (free fatty acids) for the uncontrolled production of ketones by the liver. The production of ketones leads to acidosis and elevation of the anion gap, which almost always occur in DKA.

5. **What causes DKA?**
   Any disorder that alters the balance between insulin and counter-regulatory hormones can precipitate DKA. A minority of cases occurs in people (generally older) not previously diagnosed with diabetes. Most cases (up to 80%) of DKA, however, occur in people with previously diagnosed diabetes owing to inadequate insulin or intercurrent illness. DKA is most often associated with type 1 (insulin-dependent) diabetes. However, it also may occur in the older patients with type 2 (non–insulin-dependent) diabetes, particularly when associated with a major intercurrent illness.

6. **What illnesses may trigger DKA?**
   The most common illnesses that may trigger DKA are infection and myocardial infarction. Even local infections, such as urinary tract infections or prostatitis, have precipitated DKA. Other triggering events include severe emotional stress, trauma, and exogenous medications (i.e., corticosteroids, pentamidine) or hormonal changes (i.e., preovulation) in women.

7. **How can deficiencies in education trigger DKA?**

Many patients with recurrent episodes of DKA have deficient knowledge about their insulin regimen or have not been taught how to test their urine for ketones or how to handle diabetes during times of illness.

8. **Discuss the signs and symptoms of DKA.**

Signs and symptoms suggestive of DKA are rapid or Kussmaul respirations, an acetone odor on the breath, nausea and vomiting, and diffuse abdominal pain (30% of patients). Other important features of the history are symptoms of infection, ischemic heart disease, other possible precipitating factors, and pattern of insulin use.

9. **How is DKA diagnosed?**

Prompt diagnosis is essential, because delays may lead to increased morbidity and mortality. Levels of serum electrolytes and glucose should be determined before initiating intravenous (IV) fluids in any patient who appears to be dehydrated. Dehydrated patients should routinely be asked if they have any symptoms suggestive of diabetes.

The diagnosis should be suspected if the patient presents with marked hyperglycemia (glucose > 300 mg/dL) and metabolic acidosis. An elevated anion gap (>13 mEq/L) is usually, but not always, present. The finding of elevated ketones in the blood or urine in the above setting confirms the diagnosis.

10. **When should treatment for DKA be initiated?**

If blood or urine ketones are negative and DKA is strongly suspected, treatment with fluids and insulin should still be initiated. During the course of treatment, the blood and urine ketone tests will become positive. This "delay" in positivity for measured ketones is due to a limitation of the laboratory test for ketones, which detects only acetoacetate. The predominant ketone in untreated DKA is beta-hydroxybutyrate. As DKA is treated, acetoacetate becomes the predominant ketone, causing the test for ketones to turn positive.

11. **What lab tests are recommended in the first hour of treatment?**

1. Obtain baseline electrolytes, blood urea nitrogen (BUN), creatinine, glucose, urinalysis, urine/blood ketone measurements, and electrocardiogram (ECG).
2. Obtain an arterial blood gas if the patient appears ill or tachypneic or if the serum bicarbonate is low (<10 mEq/L).
3. Start a flow sheet for recording fluid intake, output, and laboratory data (Fig. 2-1).
4. Look for a precipitating event for DKA (e.g., infection, myocardial infarction).

12. **Summarize the strategy for fluid and potassium administration in the first hour.**

Fluids: Give normal saline, 15 cc/kg/h (~1 L/h for 70 kg).

Potassium (K): Look at the T waves on the ECG. If the T waves are peaked or normal, no potassium is necessary initially. If T waves are low or if U waves are present (denoting hypokalemia), add 40 mEq/L of potassium chloride (KCl) to each liter of IV fluids.

13. **How is insulin administered during the first hour of treatment?**

Give a bolus with 10–20 units IV, followed by a continuous infusion of 5–10 units per hour (0.1 unit/kg/h). The insulin drip is mixed by adding 500 units of regular insulin to 1 L of normal saline (concentration: 0.5 units/mL). Run the first 50 mL through the IV tubing into the sink before hooking up to the patient. Use only regular insulin for IV administration.

14. **With what assessments should the second hour of treatment begin?**

1. Assess the patient's breathing, vital signs, alertness, level of hydration, and urine output.
2. Obtain repeat values for electrolytes, glucose, and urine/blood ketones.

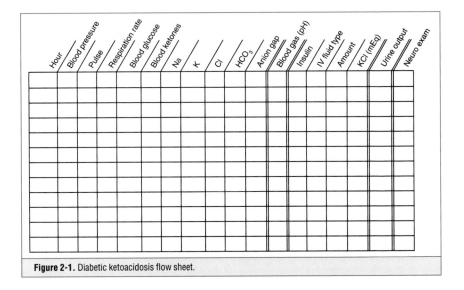

Figure 2-1. Diabetic ketoacidosis flow sheet.

15. **Summarize the strategy for fluid and potassium administration in the second hour of treatment.**
    Fluids: Continue normal saline at approximately 1 L/h.
    Potassium: Adjust KCl supplement in fluids to maintain the serum potassium at 4–5 mEq/L. Anticipate a need for 40 mEq/L replacement per hour as therapy continues.

16. **How is insulin administered during the first hour of treatment?**
    Continue the infusion of regular insulin. If the serum glucose drops to <250 mg/dL, change fluids to 5–10% dextrose with saline. The insulin infusion rate may be doubled if the serum glucose does not decline. The optimal rate of glucose decline is 100 mg/dL/h. The serum glucose level should not be allowed to fall to <250 mg/dL during the first 4–5 hours of treatment.

17. **Outline the basic steps in treatment during the third and subsequent hours.**
    1. Assess the patient and repeat lab tests as mentioned earlier (question 14).
    2. *Fluids:* Adjust infusion rate based on the patient's state of hydration. Consider changing to 0.45% saline if the patient is euvolemic and hypernatremic.
    3. *Potassium:* Adjust supplement in fluids as noted earlier.
    4. *Insulin:* Continue infusion as long as acidosis is present; supplement with dextrose as needed.

18. **When can the insulin infusion be discontinued?**
    Follow the anion gap. Once the anion gap corrects to normal, the pH is ≥7.3, or the serum bicarbonate is ≥18 mEq/L, the patient can be given a subcutaneous dose of regular or lispro insulin to cover a meal. The insulin infusion can be discontinued 30 minutes after the insulin dose. If the patient is unable to eat, give 5 units of regular or lispro insulin, continue the dextrose solution, and give supplemental regular or lispro insulin every 4 hours based on the blood glucose level (e.g., 5–15 units every 4 hours).

19. **What other interventions may be needed in the treatment of DKA?**
    1. Consider replacing *phosphate* as potassium phosphate, 10–20 mEq/h in the IV fluids if the initial serum phosphorus is <1.0 mg/dL.

2. *Sodium bicarbonate* replacement is not recommended unless other causes of severe acidosis are present (e.g., sepsis, lactic acidosis) or the arterial pH is very low (<6.9). If used, dilute in IV fluids and give over 1 hour.

20. **Which patients are at risk for cerebral edema during an episode of DKA? How are they treated?**
Patients with new-onset diabetes and young age are at risk for cerebral edema. If the patient suddenly develops a headache or becomes confused during therapy, give mannitol, 1 mg/kg, immediately.

21. **What is HHNS?**
In 1957, Sument and Schwarts described a syndrome of marked diabetic stupor with hyperglycemia and hyperosmolarity in the absence of ketosis. Since their description, the syndrome has been given a number of names, including nonketotic hyperosmolar coma, diabetic hyperosmolar state, hyperosmolar nonacidotic diabetes, and hyperglycemic hyperosmolar nonketotic syndrome (HHNS).

22. **What are the signs of HHNS?**
- Marked hyperglycemia (serum glucose > 600 mg/dL).
- Hyperosmolarity (serum > 320 mOsm/L).
- Arterial pH > 7.3.

23. **Who is at risk for HHNS? Why?**
The syndrome occurs primarily in elderly patients with or without a history of type 2 diabetes and is always associated with severe dehydration. Polyuria and polydipsia often occur days to weeks before presentation of the syndrome. Elderly people are predisposed to the syndrome because they have a higher prevalence of impaired thirst perception. Impaired renal function, also common in the elderly, prevents clearance of excess glucose in the urine. Both factors contribute to dehydration and marked hyperglycemia.

24. **Why is metabolic acidosis often not seen in HHNS?**
The absence of metabolic acidosis is due to the presence of circulating insulin and/or lower levels of counter-regulatory hormones. These two factors prevent lipolysis and ketone production. Hyperglycemia, once triggered, leads to glycosuria, osmotic diuresis, hyperosmolarity, cellular dehydration, hypovolemia, shock, coma and, if untreated, death.

25. **What is the most common presenting symptom of HHNS?**
Altered mental status is the most common reason patients are brought to the hospital. An effective osmolarity of >340 mOsm/L is required for coma to be attributed to the syndrome. To calculate the effective osmolarity, the following equation is used:

$$\text{effective osmolarity} \geq 2\,[\text{measured Na (mEq/L)}] + \text{glucose (mg/dL)}/18.$$

The serum sodium (Na) and potassium levels are measured in mEq/L; the serum glucose in mg/dL. "Effective osmolarity" refers to the true osmolarity seen by the cell. Because urea is freely permeable through membranes, it does not contribute to this condition and is not used in the equation.

26. **List other possible causes of impaired mental state.**
If the impairment in mental status is out of proportion to the effective osmolarity, another cause should be sought. For other causes of altered mental state, keep in mind the mnemonic AEIOU TIPSS:

A = **A**lcohol   **O** = **O**verdose
E = **E**ncephalopathy   **U** = **U**remia
I = **I**nfection

T = **T**rauma   S = **S**yncope
I = **I**nsulin   S = **S**eizures
P = **P**sychosis

27. **What other neurologic signs may suggest HHNS?**
    Other neurologic signs include bilateral or unilateral hypo- or hyperreflexia, seizures, hemipare-sis, aphasia, positive Babinski sign, hemianopsia, nystagmus, visual hallucinations, acute quad-riplegia, and dysphagia. Fever is *not* part of the syndrome and, if present, should suggest an infectious component to the illness. Other physical features are those of profound dehydration. The physical exam and other tests should be performed to search for possible precipitating fac-tors, such as infection, myocardial infarction, cerebrovascular events, pancreatitis, gastroin-testinal hemorrhage, or exogenous medications.

28. **What is the hallmark laboratory finding in patients with HHNS?**
    The hallmark laboratory finding is marked hyperglycemia (often >1000 mg/dL). The serum sodium is often factitiously low due to hyperglycemia. To correct for this factor, the following formula is used:

    $$\text{corrected Na} = \text{serum Na} + \frac{1.6\,(\text{serum glucose} - 100)}{100}$$

    Other laboratory abnormalities include elevated BUN and creatinine, hypertriglyceridemia, and leukocytosis.

29. **What is the first step in the treatment of HHNS?**
    After the diagnosis is made, attention should be directed to replacing the patient's fluid deficit. The fluid deficit is usually severe, ranging from 9 to 12 L. The most critical issue in fluid replacement is having an accurate means of monitoring the level of hydration and response to therapy. In the pres-ence of renal insufficiency or cardiac disease, monitoring may require central venous line access. In the patient with an altered mental state, an indwelling urinary catheter is also usually required.

30. **Should isotonic or hypotonic fluids be used?**
    Despite some controversy, the authors recommend isotonic (0.9%) saline at a rate of approxi-mately 1–2 L over the first hour until the blood pressure normalizes. After the first hour, the flu-ids may be changed based on the measured serum sodium level. If the serum sodium is between 145 and 165 mEq/L, a change to half normal saline should be considered to replace the free water deficit. If the serum sodium is lower than 145 mEq/L, isotonic saline should be con-tinued. Replacement of one-half of the calculated fluid deficit over the initial 5–12 hours is rec-ommended, with the balance of the deficit replaced over the subsequent 12 hour.

KEY POINTS: ACUTE COMPLICATIONS OF DIABETES ✓

1. DKA, HHNS, and hypoglycemia are the major acute complications.

2. DKA and HHNS are treated with vigorous fluid/electrolyte replacement and insulin.

3. Hypoglycemia is acutely treated with supplemental glucose and correction of possible predisposing factors.

31. **Is continuous IV infusion of insulin helpful in the treatment of HHNS?**
    The use of a continuous IV insulin infusion, as described for DKA, has been found to be useful for reducing the glucose levels at a predictable rate. Care must be taken not to induce hypo-glycemia.

32. **Summarize the management of electrolytes in patients with HHNS.**
The replacement of other electrolytes, including potassium, is identical to the protocol for DKA.

33. **Discuss therapy-related causes of hypoglycemia in diabetes mellitus.**
For diabetic patients on sulfonylureas or insulin, hypoglycemia is an occupational hazard of the therapy. Particularly in type 1 diabetes, it is impossible to mimic the peaks and troughs of a normal insulin secretory pattern with intermittent subcutaneous insulin injections. Even a perfectly designed insulin regimen can lead to hypoglycemia when the patient even slightly decreases food intake, delays a meal, or exercises slightly more than usual. Menstruating women can experience hypoglycemia at the time of menses due to a rapid fall in estrogen and progesterone. Elderly patients given a sulfonylurea for the first time may respond with severe hypoglycemia.

34. **What other factors may contribute to the development of hypoglycemia?**
In addition to "misadventures" in therapy, patients with diabetes may develop hypoglycemia as a result of a number of other contributing disorders (Table 2-1).

TABLE 2-1.   CAUSES OF POSTABSORPTIVE (FASTING) HYPOGLYCEMIA

1 Drugs: especially insulin, sulfonylureas, or alcohol
2 Critical organ failure: renal, hepatic or cardiac failure; sepsis; inanition
3 Hormonal deficiencies: cortisol, growth hormone or both; glucagon + epinephrine
4 Non-beta-cell tumor
5 Endogenous hyperinsulinism: beta-cell tumor (insulinoma); functional beta-cell hypersecretion; autoimmune hypoglycemia; ? ectopic insulin secretion
6 Hypoglycemias of infancy and childhood

From Cryer PE, Gerich JE: Hypoglycemia in insulin-dependent diabetes mellitus: Insulin excess and defective glucose counterregulation. In Rifkin H, Porte E (eds): Ellenberg and Rifkin's Diabetes Mellitus: Theory and Practice, 4th ed. New York, Elsevier, 1990, pp 526–546.

---

35. **Are some diabetic patients more susceptible to hypoglycemia than others?**
Yes. Some type 1 diabetic patients have a defect in glucose counter-regulation. When the blood glucose is lowered experimentally, counter-regulatory hormones (glucagon and epinephrine, among others) normally are released. These hormones stimulate glycogenolysis and gluconeogenesis by the liver, resulting in a reversal of hypoglycemia. In some patients with type 1 diabetes, this hormone release is blunted, leading to severe hypoglycemia or delayed recovery from hypoglycemia.

36. **Explain "hypoglycemia unawareness."**
Defective counter-regulation is often associated with hypoglycemia unawareness, in which the patient reports having none of the typical neurogenic warning symptoms of hypoglycemia. In contrast, the predominant signs and symptoms are due to decreased delivery of glucose to the brain—so-called neuroglycopenic symptoms (Table 2-2). The cognitive impairment associated with neuroglycopenia may prevent the patient from responding appropriately to self-treat the hypoglycemia. The result may be a traumatic automobile accident, seizure, coma, or death.

37. **Can hypoglycemia unawareness be prevented?**
It was previously thought that the development of hypoglycemic unawareness or defective counter-regulation was an unpreventable manifestation of autonomic neuropathy due to diabetes. However, recent studies suggest that this disorder may be the body's maladaptation to

TABLE 2-2. CLINICAL MANIFESTATIONS OF HYPOGLYCEMIA	
Neurogenic	Neuroglycopenic
Diaphoresis	Cognitive impairment
Palpitations	Fatigue
Tremor	Dizziness/faintness
Arousal/anxiety	Visual changes
Pallor	Paresthesias
Hypertension	Hunger
	Inappropriate behavior
	Focal neurologic deficits
	Seizures
	Loss of consciousness
	Death

From Cryer PE, Gerich JE: Hypoglycemia in insulin-dependent diabetes mellitus: Insulin excess and defective glucose counterregulation. In Rifkin H, Porte D (eds): Ellenberg and Rifkin's Diabetes Mellitus: Theory and Practice, 4th ed. New York, Elsevier, 1990, pp 526–546.

previous episodes of hypoglycemia. A single episode of hypoglycemia has been shown to reduce autonomic and symptomatic responses to hypoglycemia on the following day in normal subjects and in patients with type 1 diabetes. In contrast, meticulous prevention of hypoglycemia has been shown to reverse the defective counter-regulation and reestablish the neurogenic symptoms after 3 months. Thus, meticulous attention to prevent hypoglycemia in patients without established autonomic neuropathy may be beneficial in reversing hypoglycemic unawareness.

38. **How is hypoglycemia treated?**
   Once detected, hypoglycemia is easily self-treated by the patient. For mild hypoglycemia (blood glucose: 50–60 mg/dL), 15 gm of simple carbohydrate, such as 4 oz of unsweetened fruit juice or nondietetic soft drink, are sufficient. For more profound symptoms of hypoglycemia, 15–20 gm of simple carbohydrate should be ingested quickly and followed by 15–20 gm of a complex carbohydrate, such as crackers or bread.

39. **What should be done if the patient is unconscious?**
   Patients who are unconscious should not be given liquids. More viscous sources of sugar (e.g., honey, glucose gels, cake icing in a tube) can be carefully placed inside the cheek or under the tongue. Alternatively, 1 mg of glucagon may be injected intramuscularly. Glucagon indirectly causes the blood glucose level to increase via its effect on the liver. In the hospital setting, IV dextrose (D-50) is probably more accessible than glucagon and results in a prompt return of consciousness.

40. **Discuss the role of education in treating hypoglycemia.**
   Instruction in the use of glucose gels and glucagon should be an essential part of training for people living with insulin-treated diabetic patients. Patients and family members should be instructed not to overtreat hypoglycemia, particularly if it is mild. Overtreatment leads to subsequent hyperglycemia. Patients should also be instructed to test blood glucose level when symptoms occur to confirm hypoglycemia whenever feasible. If testing is not possible, it is best to

treat first. Patients on medication should be instructed to test blood glucose level before driving a vehicle. If the glucose level is lower than a preset level (e.g., <125 mg/dL), the patient should be instructed to ingest a small source of carbohydrate before driving.

41. **Summarize the common long-term complications of diabetes mellitus.**
Although patients with diabetes are susceptible to an extensive array of medical complications, most of these problems can be attributed to particular susceptibility to damage to the eye (retinopathy), kidney (nephropathy), peripheral nerves (neuropathy), and blood vessels (atherosclerosis). The first three categories of complications are relatively specific for diabetes and are associated with pathologic endothelial changes, such as basement membrane thickening and increased vascular permeability. For this reason, retinopathy, nephropathy, and neuropathy have been categorized as *microvascular complications* of diabetes. The increased susceptibility to atherosclerosis and its ensuing complications are categorized as *macrovascular complications*.

42. **What basic mechanism underlies the development of long-term diabetic complications?**
Hyperglycemia is the major force underlying the microvascular complications of diabetes and has been implicated in the excessive risk of atherosclerosis seen in patients with insulin resistance. However, it is difficult to ascribe all of these observations to glucotoxicity alone.

43. **What other mechanisms may be involved?**
   - *Mass-action driven nonenzymatic glycation of proteins:* These proteins ultimately form advanced glycosylation end products (AGEs), which are associated with altered protein function. AGEs have been found in the connective tissue of blood vessels and in the renal glomerular matrix and have been shown to modify low-density lipoprotein (LDL) composition.
   - *Enzymatic conversion of glucose to sorbitol by the enzyme aldose reductase in the eyes and peripheral nerves:* Because the cellular clearance of sorbitol is extremely slow, it accumulates as an osmotically active molecule. This accumulation is associated with neuronal myoinositol depletion.
   - Excess of intracellular glucosamine, another product of glucose, which been linked to endothelial dysfunction and to impaired insulin action.
   - Activation of protein kinase C (PKC) by glucose.
   - Hyperglycemia-driven oxidative stress and subsequent activation of poly(ADP-ribose) polymerase (PARP) has been tied to glycemic injury and may serve, in part, to increase substrate flux into glucosamine, polyol, and AGE formation, as well as promoting PKC activation.

44. **Name the most common type of diabetic neuropathy.**
Distal symmetric polyneuropathy.

45. **Summarize the symptoms of distal symmetric polyneuropathy.**
The disorder is usually discovered on routine physical exam by the finding of loss of vibration sense in the toes and loss of ankle reflexes. Light touch and pinprick sensation are subsequently lost. Common associated symptoms are numbness and paresthesias of the feet, especially at night. The paresthesias may evolve to severe knife-like or burning pain, which can be quite disabling.

46. **Explain the basic pathophysiology of distal symmetric polyneuropathy.**
Pathologically, the nerves show axonal degeneration. Sensory loss or pain in the hands may also occur but more commonly is a manifestation of entrapment neuropathy, such as carpal tunnel syndrome. Entrapment neuropathies are common in patients with diabetes and may result from increased susceptibility of these nerves to external pressure.

KEY POINTS: ACUTE COMPLICATIONS OF DIABETES ✓

1. The chronic complications of diabetes are classified into microvascular and macrovascular categories.

2. Microvascular complications (retinopathy, neuropathy, and nephropathy) are directly related to hyperglycemia and result from the formation of advanced glycation end products, polyol accumulation, PKC activation, accrual of intracellular glucosamine, and oxidative stress.

3. Macrovascular complications (coronary artery, cerebrovascular, and peripheral vascular disease) are probably related to insulin resistance and the pathologic clustering of dyslipidemia and hypertension inherent in diabetes.

4. Ample data suggest that intensive glycemic control delays the development and progression of the microvascular complications.

5. Stringent control of lipids, blood pressure, and other modifiable risk factors is a cost-effective way of diminishing the probability of developing macrovascular disease, as well as its attendant morbidities.

47. **What causes the foot problems in patients with diabetics?**
Loss of nerve fibers for proprioception can result in an abnormal gait, leading to "pressure spots" on the foot that are signaled by the presence of a thick callus. If untreated, the callus may ulcerate and become infected. Neuropathy, vascular disease, and predisposition to infection are the primary pathogenic components for the increased incidence of foot injury and amputation in patients with diabetes.

48. **How are foot problems treated surgically?**
Revascularization of the foot using distally placed in situ saphenous bypass grafts often results in healing of limb-threatening foot infections or gangrene.

49. **How common is diabetic autonomic neuropathy (DAN)? How does it affect survival rates?**
Depending on the degree of sophistication of testing, up to 90% of people with diabetes can be found to have some degree of autonomic dysfunction. However, less than 50% of affected people are symptomatic. Patients with clinically significant autonomic neuropathy have a less than 50% 10-year survival rate. Both the sympathetic and parasympathetic nervous systems may be affected by DAN, and because the neuropathies in diabetes initially damage nerves with the longest axons, patients with DAN also have readily apparent peripheral neuropathy.

50. **Describe the classic signs of DAN.**
Classic signs of DAN are unexplained resting tachycardia and postural hypotension. Usual causes, such as fever, hypoglycemia, and hyperthyroidism, are absent. Gastrointestinal symptoms from DAN are secondary to a lack of peristalsis in the stomach (gastroparesis) or intestine. Symptoms include early satiety, bloating, nausea, belching, abdominal distension, constipation, or diarrhea. Urinary retention or overflow incontinence may indicate autonomic neuropathy involving the urinary bladder. Erectile dysfunction is a frequent symptom of autonomic neuropathy in diabetic men.

51. **How is DAN diagnosed?**
A lack of R-R variation on the electrocardiogram during deep breathing or during the Valsalva maneuver is often used to confirm the diagnosis. Postural hypotension can be diagnosed by

documenting a fall in upright blood pressure without a concurrent increase in pulse rate. The diagnosis of gastroparesis is usually made by demonstrating prolonged gastric emptying using standardized radiolabeled meals, but even mild hyperglycemia (glucose > 150 mg/dL) at the time of the test may functionally slow gastric emptying. Urinary and erectile problems are elicited by the history.

52. **Describe the characteristics of nonproliferative diabetic retinopathy.**
Significant diabetic retinopathy may progress without symptoms. The initial visible lesions are microaneurysms that form on the terminal capillaries of the retina. Increased permeability of the capillaries is manifested by the leaking of proteinaceous fluid, causing hard exudates. Dot-and-blot hemorrhages result from the leaking of red blood cells. These findings by themselves do not lead to visual loss and are categorized as nonproliferative retinopathy (Table 2-3).

TABLE 2-3.   CLINICAL MANIFESTATIONS OF EYE DISEASE

Nonproliferative diabetic retinopathy
Nonproliferative diabetic retinopathy
- Retinal microaneurysms
- Occasional blot hemorrhages
- Hard exudates
- One or two soft exudates

Preproliferative diabetic retinopathy
- Presence of venous beading
- Significant areas of large retinal blot hemorrhages
- Multiple cotton-wool spots (nerve fiber infarcts)
- Multiple intraretinal microvascular abnormalities

Proliferative diabetic retinopathy
- New vessels on the disc (NVD)
- New vessels elsewhere on the retina (NVE)
- Preretinal or vitreous hemorrhage
- Fibrous tissue proliferation

High-risk proliferative diabetic retinopathy
- NVD with or without preretinal or vitreous hemorrhage
- NVE with preretinal or vitreous hemorrhage

Diabetic macular edema
- Any thickening of retina <2 disc diameters from center of macula
- Any hard exudate <2 disc diameters from center of macula with associated thickening of the retina
- Any nonperfused retina inside the temporal vessel arcades
- Any combination of the above

From Centers for Disease Control: The Prevention and Treatment of Complications of Diabetes Mellitus. Division of Diabetes Translation, Department of Health and Human Services, Atlanta, 1991.

53. **Describe the characteristics of proliferative retinopathy.**
Proliferative retinopathy (Table 2-3) develops when the retinal vessels are further damaged, causing retinal ischemia. The ischemia triggers new, fragile vessels to develop, a process termed neovascularization. These vessels may grow into the vitreous cavity and may bleed into preretinal areas or vitreous, causing significant vision loss. Loss of vision also may result from retinal detachment secondary to the contraction of fibrous tissue, which often accompanies neovascularization. Diabetic macular edema occurs when fluid from abnormal vessels leaks into the macula. It is detected with indirect funduscopy by the finding of a thickened retina near the macula and is commonly associated with the presence of hard exudates.

54. **How common is diabetic retinopathy?**
Over a lifetime, up to 70% of patients with type 1 diabetes may develop proliferative retinopathy. In type 2 diabetes, 2% of patients may have significant nonproliferative and even proliferative retinopathy or macular edema at the time of diagnosis of diabetes. This may be due to the long asymptomatic (and undiagnosed) period of hyperglycemia that often occurs in people with type 2 diabetes.

55. **What are the risk factors for development of diabetic retinopathy?**
- Duration of diabetes.
- Level of glycemic control.
- Hypertension.
Diabetic nephropathy is strongly associated with proliferative retinopathy in type 1 diabetes and insulin-treated type 2 diabetes.

56. **List the other ophthalmologic complications of diabetes.**
Cataracts and open-angle glaucoma.

57. **How serious a problem is diabetic nephropathy?**
Diabetic nephropathy is currently the leading cause of end-stage renal disease in the United States. The onset and progression of disease follow a relatively predictable pattern, described as stages I–V.

58. **Describe stage I of diabetic nephropathy.**
Stage I is characterized by renal hypertrophy and an increase in glomerular filtration rate (GFR). Patients with a sustained GFR > 125 cc/minute are at particularly high risk for progression of disease.

59. **What findings define stage II diabetic nephropathy?**
Stage II nephropathy is defined by demonstration of histologic changes in the glomerulus, which are distinctive for diabetes.

60. **Describe stage III of diabetic nephropathy.**
Stage III is marked by mildly elevated urinary albumin excretion (microalbuminuria) on a 24-hour or timed urine collection. Normal urinary albumin is less than 30 mg/day. Microalbuminuria is defined as the excretion of 30–300 mg/day. Patients with microalbuminuria are at markedly increased risk for progression to clinical nephropathy. Hypertension is commonly present at this stage, particularly in patients with type 2 diabetes.

61. **Describe stage IV of diabetic nephropathy.**
Stage IV is defined by Dipstix-positive proteinuria, as measured by routine urinalysis. The urinary albumin excretion in this stage is >300 mg/day or total protein >500 mg/day. Hypertension is invariably present. During this stage, proteinuria increases, and GFR declines slowly but steadily.

62. **Define stage V of diabetic nephropathy.**
Stage V nephropathy is end-stage renal disease.

63. **What is the risk that a diabetic person will develop nephropathy?**
Patients with type 1 diabetes are at highest risk for nephropathy, which affects approximately 30%. The risk of nephropathy is about 10 times less for type 2 patients, but because of the overwhelming prevalence of type 2 diabetes, this group currently outnumbers type 1 patients with end-stage renal disease.

64. **What factors affect the development of diabetic nephropathy?**
In addition to glycemic control, genetic factors play a key role in determining the risk for diabetic nephropathy. Genes that code for essential hypertension appear to increase the risk. Known risk factors for diabetic nephropathy are listed in the following along with their risk ratio (RR):
   1. A family history of hypertension (RR ≥ 3.7).
   2. Sibling with diabetic nephropathy (RR > 4.0).
   3. Black race (RR ≥ 2.6 versus white race).
   4. History of smoking (RR ≥ 2.0).
   5. History of poor glycemic control (RR ≥ 1.3–2.0).

65. **What are the characteristics of macrovascular disease in diabetes?**
Patients with diabetes are at two- to fourfold increased risk for both cardiovascular disease (CVD) and peripheral vascular disease compared with the nondiabetic population. Women with diabetes have as high a risk for CVD as men. The commonly identified risk factors for CVD—smoking, hypercholesterolemia, and hypertension—adversely affect CVD risk in diabetic persons.

66. **Which factors specific to diabetes increase the risk for CVD?**
The blood in diabetic patients has been found to have increased platelet aggregation, decreased red cell deformability, and reduced fibrinolytic activity. The glycation of lipoproteins may lead to decreased clearance by the liver and increased atherosclerosis. The blood vessels themselves have distinct abnormalities. Long-standing diabetes predisposes the arteries to calcification.

67. **How important is glycemic control in preventing the chronic complications of diabetes mellitus?**
As discussed in Chapter 1, the DCCT, Kumamoto study, and UKPDS have established that improving glycemic control effectively reduces the risk of developing microvascular complications (retinopathy, neuropathy, and nephropathy) in patients with type 1 and type 2 diabetes mellitus. The UKPDS also demonstrated that glycemic control with metformin reduced the risk of macrovascular disease (coronary artery and cerebrovascular disease), and that control with either sulfonylureas or insulin produced a similar, although not statistically significant, trend for coronary artery disease. Based on these data, the American Diabetes Association recommends that glycemic control be sufficient to maintain the fasting blood glucose level below 120 mg/dL and the hemoglobin A_{1C} below 7%.

68. **What treatments are effective for sensory loss due to diabetic neuropathy?**
There is no known treatment for sensory loss from diabetic neuropathy. Educational programs addressing proper foot care and prevention of foot injury have been shown to reduce the incidence of serious foot lesions. Routine foot examination and early referral to a podiatrist or vascular surgeon for patients with foot lesions are considered essential to prevent limb loss.

69. **How is painful diabetic neuropathy treated?**
Medications tried with mixed success for treatment of painful neuropathy include nonsteroidal anti-inflammatory drugs, tricyclic antidepressants, anticonvulsant medications, mexiletine, and topical capsaicin. The most effective drug currently available is gabapentin (Neurontin); the

starting dose is 300 mg two or three times a day with titration up to a dose of 600 mg three times a day, as needed.

70. Discuss the management of postural hypotension.
Postural hypotension from autonomic neuropathy is improved by the use of supportive stockings to prevent venous pooling in the legs. Fludrocortisone is effective but must be used cautiously to prevent worsening of hypertension or edema. Other drugs that have demonstrated benefit include clonidine, octreotide, and midodrine.

71. How are the symptoms of gastroparesis treated?
The symptoms of diabetic gastroparesis can be improved by reducing fiber and fat in the diet, decreasing meal size, and increasing exercise. Metoclopramide has been shown to increase gastrointestinal motility and reduce symptoms in patients with diabetic gastroparesis.

72. Describe the treatment for diabetic retinopathy.
Early detection is essential for successful treatment of diabetic complications. For retinopathy, this approach requires annual examination (including dilation of the fundus) by a trained specialist, usually an ophthalmologist. If preproliferative or proliferative retinopathy or significant macular edema is detected, laser therapy may be indicated, which can prevent significant vision loss. Vitrectomy or retinal surgery may be required for restoration of vision loss due to vitreous hemorrhage or retinal detachment.

73. How is diabetic nephropathy managed?
The progression of diabetic nephropathy can be slowed by aggressive treatment of hypertension. Angiotensin-converting enzyme (ACE) inhibitors are the agents of choice because they have been shown to have beneficial effects independent of blood pressure control. Other antihypertensive agents are also beneficial, but their effects appear to be more closely related to the degree of blood pressure control. The recommended blood pressure goal is 130/80 mmHg. ACE inhibitors have also been shown to attenuate the decline in renal function in normotensive, normoalbuminemic patients with type 2 diabetes. Based on this type of information, one study concluded that treating all type 2 diabetic patients would be a cost-effective strategy; further study of this important question is warranted. Some, but not all, studies have shown that a low-protein diet (<0.6 gm/kg/day) can also reduce progression of renal disease in diabetic patients.

74. How can macrovascular disease be prevented in the diabetic population?
Cardiovascular risk factor reduction should be initiated at the first visit and should be pursued as aggressively in diabetic patients as in patients with known coronary artery disease. Aggressive blood pressure control is strongly supported by recent randomized controlled trials; the currently recommended blood pressure goal is 130/80 mmHg. ACE inhibitors have been reported to be more effective than other antihypertensive agents in preventing CVD events and thus are currently the antihypertensive agents of choice. Control of hyperlipidemia should be pursued just as aggressively; the recommended goal for LDL cholesterol is 100 mg/dL. Improving glycemia often causes a dramatic reduction in the triglyceride level and a modest reduction in LDL cholesterol. If goals for lipids are not achieved through glycemic control, diet, and exercise, then antihyperlipidemic drug therapy should be considered. Smoking should be strongly discouraged, while exercise and weight loss (if overweight) should be encouraged. Low-dose aspirin therapy is also recommended; additionally, specific antiplatelet therapy may be considered.

75. Does aggressive lipid-lowering therapy improve cardiac outcomes in diabetic patients?
Yes. The Scandinavian Simvastatin Survival Study compared the outcome of 4242 patients with a previous myocardial infarction or angina pectoris and elevated total cholesterol. Patients were randomized to aggressive lipid-lowering therapy with simvastatin or placebo. A post-hoc

subgroup analysis of the 202 diabetic participants showed a 55% reduction in major coronary events, including myocardial infarction, in the simvastatin-treated group. At 5.4 years, total mortality was also reduced by 43%. Statistically significant beneficial results were also reported with pravastatin in the CARE and LIPID studies. Based on these reports, aggressive lipid-lowering therapy should be advocated in all diabetic patients, particularly those with known coronary artery disease.

76. **Does improved glycemic control in hospitalized patients affect outcome?**
Adults with diabetes are six times more likely to be hospitalized than those without diabetes and have a 30% longer length of stay. Under any circumstances, poorly controlled diabetes is a catabolic condition, and in hospitalized people with diabetes who are under physiologic stress, catabolism is certainly detrimental. In addition, leukocytes and immune function are impaired by hyperglycemia. A recent randomized prospective study designed to assess whether lowering blood glucose levels to 80–110 mg/dL in patients admitted to an intensive care unit using insulin influenced outcomes. In-hospital mortality was reduced 34%; sepsis was reduced 46%; hemodialysis rate was reduced 41%; transfusions were reduced 50%; and critical-illness related polyneuropathy was reduced 44%. Another study demonstrated a reduction in deep sternal infections with improved glycemic control in people with diabetes undergoing open-heart surgery. The Diabetes and Insulin–Glucose Infusion in Acute Myocardial Infarction (DIGAMI) study demonstrated significant reductions in mortality in diabetic patients treated with insulin during and after hospitalization for acute myocardial infarction.

BIBLIOGRAPHY

1. American Diabetes Association: Hypertension management in adults with diabetes. Diabetes Care 27(Suppl 1):S65–S67, 2004.
2. American Diabetes Association: Dyslipidemia management in adults with diabetes. Diabetes Care 27(Suppl 1):S68–S71, 2004.
3. American Diabetes Association: Nephropathy in diabetes. Diabetes Care 27(Suppl 1):S79–S83, 2004.
4. American Diabetes Association: Retinopathy in diabetes. Diabetes Care 27(Suppl 1):S84–S87, 2004
5. American Diabetes Association: Hyperglycemic crises in diabetes. Diabetes Care 27(Suppl 1):S94–S102, 2004.
6. CDC Cost-effectiveness Group: Cost-effectiveness of intensive glycemic control, intensified hypertension control, and serum cholesterol level reduction for type 2 diabetes. JAMA 287:2542–2551, 2002.
7. Chrysant SG: The ALLHAT study: Results and clinical implications. Q J Med 96:771–773, 2003.
8. Clement S, Braithwaite SS, Magee MF, et al: Management of diabetes and hyperglycemia in hospitals. Diabetes Care 27:553–591, 2004.
9. Collins R, Armitage J, Parish S, et al: MRC/BHF heart protection study of cholesterol-lowering with simvastatin in 5963 people with diabetes: A randomized placebo-controlled trial. Lancet 361:2005–2016, 2003.
10. Folwaczny C, Wawarta R, Otto B, et al: Gastric emptying of solid and liquid meals in healthy controls compared with long-term type-1 diabetes mellitus under optimal glucose control. Exp Clin Endocrinol Diabetes 111:223–229, 2003.
11. Fritsche A, Stefan N, Häring H, et al: Avoidance of hypoglycemia restored hypoglycemia awareness by increasing β-adrenergic sensitivity in type 1 diabetes. Ann Intern Med 134:729–736, 2001.
12. Haffner SM, Lehto S, Ronnemaa T, et al: Mortality from coronary heart disease in subjects with type 2 diabetes and in nondiabetic subjects with and without prior myocardial infarction. N Engl J Med 339:229–234, 1998.
13. Hollenberg NK: Treatment of the patient with diabetes mellitus and risk of nephropathy. Arch Intern Med 164:125–130, 2004.
14. Kitabchi A, Wall BM: Management of diabetic ketoacidosis. Am Fam Physician 60:455–464, 1999.
15. Magee MF, Bhatt BA: Management of decompensated diabetes. Diabetic ketoacidosis and hyperglycemic hyperosmolar syndrome. Crit Care Clin 17:75–106, 2001.
16. Pyörälä K, Pederson TR, Kjekshus J, et al: Cholesterol lowering with simvastatin improves prognosis of diabetic patients with coronary heart disease: A subgroup analysis of the Scandinavian Simvastatin Survival Study (4S). Diabetes Care 20:614–620, 1997.

17. Reusch JEB: Diabetes, microvascular complications, and cardiovascular complications: What is it about glucose? J Clin Invest 112:986–988, 2003.

18. Ritz E, Orth SR: Nephropathy in patients with type 2 diabetes mellitus. N Engl J Med 341:1127–1133, 1999.

19. Van den Berghe G, Wouters P, Weekers F, et al: Intensive insulin therapy in the surgical intensive care unit. N Engl J Med 342:1301–1308, 2000.

20. Vinik AI, Mehrabyan A: Diagnosis and management of diabetic autonomic neuropathy. Compr Ther 29:130–145, 2003.

CHAPTER 3

INTENSIVE INSULIN THERAPY

Elizabeth A. Stephens, M.D., and Terri Ryan-Turek, R.D., C.D.E.

1. **What is intensive insulin therapy (IIT)?**
   IIT, or basal-bolus therapy, is the utilization of multiple daily injections (MDIs) of insulin (both long- and rapid-acting formulations) or an insulin pump in an effort to mimic normal pancreatic function. IIT is complex, as it often requires 3–6 injections per day but is only one aspect of intensive therapy.

2. **List the other critical components of intensive therapy.**
   - Frequent self-monitored blood glucose (SMBG).
   - Establishment of targeted blood glucose (BG) levels.
   - Understanding of diet composition, specifically carbohydrate content.
   - Use of carbohydrate/insulin ratios.
   - Use of correction factors (CFs) for the adjustment of insulin according to food intake and glucose levels.

3. **Summarize studies that support optimal diabetes management to decrease chronic complications from diabetes mellitus.**
   The Diabetes Control and Complications Trial (DCCT), evaluating patients with type 1 diabetes, and the United Kingdom Prospective Diabetes Study (UKPDS), evaluating patients with type 2 diabetes, documented that intensive glycemic control leads to significantly reduced rates of complications, including progression of retinopathy, nephropathy, and neuropathy. The UKPDS trial also evaluated blood pressure control using angiotensin-converting enzyme (ACE)-inhibitors and beta-blockers in patients with type 2 diabetes and found that both agents effectively improve cardiovascular outcomes.

4. **Which patients are candidates for IIT?**
   All people with diabetes should be considered as potential candidates for IIT. However, the degree of intensification must be based on each patient's personal situation and abilities. Patients' characteristics that predict greater success with IIT include motivation, willingness to perform frequent SMBG (up to 6–10 times/day) and record results, time to spend with the dietitian and educator, and the ability to recognize and treat hypoglycemia/sick days appropriately and a supportive network of family and/or friends. In addition, implementation of IIT requires a cohesive diabetes team that is available for frequent interaction and discussion about results from monitoring, insulin adjustments, and other issues.

5. **What is an insulin pump?**
   An insulin pump is a battery-operated device composed of a pump reservoir (which holds the insulin) connected to an "infusion set," which ends in a cannula that is inserted into the skin and changed every 2–3 days to prevent infection. Insulin is delivered through this system in microliter amounts continuously over 24 hours. The user is responsible for setting basal rates and determining bolus doses, depending on the meal ingested and the results of SMBG. Currently, five companies offer insulin pumps in the United States. Each pump has special features and functions that are unique and help with the flexibility of pump use. To learn more about each of these pumps, contact the companies listed in Table 3-1.

TABLE 3-1. COMPANIES OFFERING INSULIN PUMPS		
Company Name	**Phone**	**Website**
Animas	1-877-937-7867	www.animascorp.com
Dana-Diabecare	1-866-342-2322	www.theinsulinpump.com
Deltec	1-800-826-9703	www.delteccozmo.com
Disetronic	1-800-280-7801	www.disetronic-usa.com
Medtronic/MiniMed	1-800-MiniMed	www.minimed.com

6. **What are the patients' responsibilities before insulin pump therapy can be initiated?**
   - Commitment to devote at least 2–3 months to pump initiation, including multiple meetings with the diabetes team before, during, and after the pump is initiated.
   - Monitoring of SMBG values at least 4–10 times per day, keeping logs of readings, insulin doses and food consumed, and faxing/mailing of information to the team.
   - Watching the pump training video and practicing pump functions at least 2–3 times before wearing the pump.
   - Willingness to perform verifications to ensure that basal rates are set appropriately.

7. **Describe the benefits of insulin pump therapy.**
   Benefits include a reduction in frequency of hypoglycemia due to a more predictable absorption of insulin, ability to compensate for the dawn phenomenon by adjustment in the basal rate, improved flexibility of lifestyle, and the ability to administer very small amounts of insulin (as little as 0.05 units).

8. **What risks are associated with pump use?**
   Risks associated with pump use, including weight gain and hypoglycemia, are similar to any therapy that results in an overall lowering of BG values. A unique risk to pump therapy is for diabetic ketoacidosis (DKA). This can occur with any interruption of insulin delivery, since pumps only provide rapid-acting insulin.

9. **Explain the difference between basal and bolus insulin coverages.**
   Basal insulin coverage is the insulin required to manage BG fluctuations due to hepatic glucose production. Basal coverage is usually accomplished with injections of long-acting insulin preparations or with the basal infusion function on the insulin pump. *Bolus insulin coverage* is the insulin required to manage glucose excursions following meals, accomplished by injections of rapid-acting, or short-acting, insulin preparations or using the bolus function on the insulin pump. Bolus insulin doses are estimated for each meal based on the amount of insulin required to cover the carbohydrate in the meal, as well as a high BG CF.

10. **What are the currently available long-acting insulins?**
    - Long-acting analog: insulin glargine (Lantus).
    - Long-acting human insulin: ultralente human insulin (Humulin U).
    - Intermediate-acting insulins: neutral protamine Hagedorn (NPH) and insulin lente (Humulin L).
    - Premixed insulin analogs: biphasic insulin lispro (Humalog Mix 75/25) and biphasic insulin aspart (NovoLog Mix 70/30)
    - Premixed biphasic human insulins: Humulin 70/30, Novolin 70/30, and Humulin 50/50.

11. **How are long-acting insulins used with an MDI regimen?**
Ideally, basal insulin should cover background insulin needs only, independent of food intake and exercise. Basal insulin is approximately 50% of a patient's total daily dose (TDD) of insulin. Premixed "biphasic" insulin preparations combine either a rapid-acting insulin analog or regular human insulin with a crystalline protaminated form of the analog or regular human insulin in an attempt to imitate basal and bolus therapy with fewer injections.

12. **What are the currently available bolus insulins?**
   - Rapid-acting analogs: insulin lispro (Humalog) and insulin aspart (NovoLog).
   - Short-acting human insulins: regular human insulin (Humulin or Novolin R) and regular buffered insulin (Velosulin).

13. **Describe the pharmacodynamics of the bolus and basal insulins.**
   See Table 3-2.

TABLE 3-2. PHARMACODYNAMICS OF ADMINISTERED INSULIN PREPARATIONS			
	Insulin Onset	Peak*	Duration* (Hours)
Humalog	5–15 minutes	1–2 hours	3.5–5
NovoLog	10–20 minutes	1–3 hours	3–5
Regular	30–60 minutes	2–4 hours	6–8
Lantus	1–4 hours	None	22–24
NPH or Lente	1–4 hours	6–12 hours	12–20
Ultralente	3–5 hours	10–16 hours	18–24

*The peak and duration of insulin action are variable, depending on the injection site (regular and long-acting), duration of diabetes, renal function, smoking status, and other factors.

14. **When should bolus insulin be taken?**
   - 5–10 minutes before meals and snacks when glucose is in the normal range (80–120 mg/dL).
   - 15–30 minutes before meals if the premeal BG is >120 mg/dL. (Supplemental bolus insulin [CF] is added to meal insulin when the BG is elevated.)
   - Immediately after eating, if gastroparesis or an intercurrent illness is present.
   - Upon arrival of food, if unfamiliar with meal size, content, or timing (i.e., in restaurant or hospital).
   - 30–45 minutes before meals if using regular or Velosulin human insulin.

15. **When should basal insulin be taken?**
   - Insulin glargine is taken at bedtime if a dawn phenomenon is present.
   - Insulin glargine may be taken at any consistent time, approximately every 24 hours. (Insulin glargine cannot be mixed with other insulins.)
   - An ultralente dose may be split into half and injected with breakfast and dinner insulin.
   - NPH or lente insulin is given in the morning and at bedtime to avoid nocturnal hypoglycemia.

16. **Define carbohydrate counting. How is it used with IIT?**
   Carbohydrate counting is a tool used to match bolus insulin doses to food intake because carbohydrates have the greatest effect on BG levels. The peak of bolus insulin analogs should match

the peak of BG following carbohydrate digestion and absorption (~1–3 hours, depending on the fat and fiber content of the meal).

17. **List common foods that contain dietary carbohydrates.**
Starch: cereals, grains, beans, bread, rice, pasta, and starchy vegetables.
Sugar: lactose (milk and yogurt), fructose (fruit and fruit juice), and sucrose (table sugar and desserts).
Fiber: cellulose and hemicellulose, lignins, gums, or pectins.

18. **How are carbohydrates counted?**
Calculating the number of carbohydrates may initially require measuring and weighing commonly eaten foods. Nutrition labels on the package (Table 3-3) state the number of grams of carbohydrates based on the serving size. Carbohydrate reference books are available at bookstores or through the American Dietetic Association www.eatright.org or the American Diabetes Association (ADA) www.diabetes.org. Software programs are available for PDAs or on-line. Many restaurant chains provide nutrition brochures.

TABLE 3-3. NUTRITION FACTS ON LABELS	
Serving size: 10 crackers (30 gm)	Dietary fiber: 1 gm
Servings per container: 8	Sugars: 3 gm
Calories: 140	Protein: 2 gm
Total fat: 6 gm	Vitamin A: 0%
Saturated fat: 1 gm	Vitamin C: 0%
Cholesterol: 0 mg	Calcium: 2%
Sodium: 260 mg	Iron: 6%
Total carbohydrate: 20 gm	

19. **Explain the carbohydrate-to-insulin (C:I) ratio.**
The C:I ratio is used to estimate how many grams of carbohydrate each unit of rapid-acting insulin will cover (e.g., 20:1 = 20 gm of carbohydrate consumed requires 1 unit of meal insulin).

20. **How do you determine an initial C:I ratio?**
Ratios are based on a patient's weight and TDD of insulin, which usually indicates the patient's sensitivity to insulin. An MDI regimen of basal insulin and premeal injections of rapid-acting insulin must be previously (or concurrently) implemented before establishing a C:I ratio. A person must be taught to count carbohydrates before using a C:I ratio safely.
1. Add the patient's TDD of insulin on *current* therapy.
2. Consider the hemoglobin AIC value A_{1C} (ADA target is < 7%).
3. Frequency of hypoglycemia and comorbidities.
4. Divide the TDD of insulin into 1650 and multiply the result by 0.33: C:I = (1650/TDD) × 0.33.

21. **Give an example of an initial C:I ratio in changing to basal and bolus insulins.**
- 35 units of Humulin 70/30 premixed insulin in the morning.
- 15 units of Humulin 70/30 premixed insulin before the evening meal.
- TDD = 50 units (A_{1C} of 8.5% with 2–3 nocturnal hypoglycemic episodes per week).
- 1650/50 = 33 × 0.33 = 11.
- C:I = 11:1.
  In this example, 1 unit of rapid-acting insulin will be given for every 11 gm of carbohydrate eaten.

22. **How do you adjust the C:I ratio once the initial ratio has been established?**
Fine-tuning of a C:I ratio is based on BG records before meals and 2 hours after meals. The desired premeal BG is 80–120 mg/dL for most patients using IIT. A C:I ratio is correct if the BG increases by approximately 30–50 mg/dL over the premeal value at the 2-hour postprandial reading and returns to the range of 80–120 mg/dL by about 5 hours after the bolus insulin is given (Fig. 3-1).

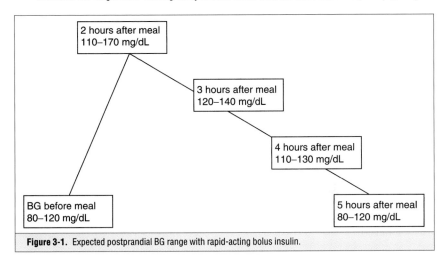

Figure 3-1. Expected postprandial BG range with rapid-acting bolus insulin.

23. **What are common causes of high BG?**
- Missing an injection of insulin
- Decreased activity
- Underestimating carbohydrates
- Menstrual cycle
- Stress, illness, or infection
- Steroids or other medications

24. **What are the mysterious or random causes of high BG readings?**
- *Dawn phenomenon:* Rise in BG in predawn hours due to increased growth hormone and cortisol production.
- *Shower or nap phenomenon:* Unexplained increase in BG when tested before and after a shower or nap.
- *Bad insulin phenomenon:* High BG occurs when insulin denatures if exposed to moderate-to-extreme temperatures (i.e., using a mail-order pharmacy, traveling with insulin).
- *Bubble-in-the-infusion-set-tubing phenomenon:* Air bubbles in the tubing of an insulin pump infusion set should be removed by disconnecting and priming the air out. In addition, when the infusion set is disconnected for showering or other purposes, gravity may cause the insulin to back up into the tubing, leaving a bubble. Holding the pump higher than the infusion site when reconnecting or repriming the tubing will avoid these bubbles.

25. **What causes high prandial BG readings that are difficult to explain?**
- *Coffee phenomenon (caffeine):* Rise in BG after drinking coffee (including black) is seen in many patients' records (mechanism unknown but may involve increases in epinephrine and/or free fatty acid mobilization).
- *Cereal phenomenon:* Rise in BG seen by patients consuming cereal, which requires a lower C:I (more insulin).
- *Food-on-the-fingers phenomenon:* High BG from residual food or dextrose on fingers when testing (patient must wash hands).
- *Chinese food or pizza phenomenon:* High BG from a meal high in fat, which requires more insulin and a split dose.

42. Glycoprotein-secreting pituitary tumors include gonadotropinomas (luteinizing hormone [LH]- or follicle-stimulating hormone [FSH]-secreting) and thyroid-stimulating hormone (TSH)-secreting pituitary adenomas (TSHomas).

43. Hyperthyroid patients with detectable serum TSH should always be evaluated for inappropriate TSH secretion (either a TSH-tumor or thyroid hormone resistance).

44. Screening biochemical tests for Cushing's syndrome can be misleading, and repeated testing or more extensive confirmatory testing is often needed.

45. Most patients with endogenous Cushing's syndrome have a small pituitary tumor producing ACTH.

46. Rapid changes in body water or distribution can cause severe neurologic dysfunction and are reflected clinically by hyponatremia or hypernatremia. Treatment requires a clear understanding of changes in plasma sodium, plasma osmolality, and effective circulating volume.

47. Identification of growth abnormalities requires accurate height measurements and plotting against appropriate standards.

48. Growth abnormalities are most commonly due to normal growth variants or chronic medical problems; hormonal abnormalities are less common causes.

49. Chronic abuse of supraphysiologic growth hormone doses may lead to features of acromegaly; osteoarthritis; irreversible bone and joint deformities; increased vascular, respiratory, and cardiac abnormalities; hypogonadism; diabetes mellitus; and abnormal lipid metabolism.

50. Spontaneous hypokalemia in a hypertensive patient should suggest the possibility of primary or secondary hyperaldosteronism.

51. The best screen for primary hyperaldosteronism is a plasma aldosterone/plasma renin activity (PA/PRA) ratio > 20.

52. Episodic headache, diaphoresis, and palpitations in a hypertensive patient suggest pheochromocytoma.

53. Pheochromocytomas are 10% bilateral, 10% extra-adrenal, 10% familial, and 10% malignant.

54. Features suggesting that an adrenal tumor is malignant are size > 6 cm; evidence of local invasion or metastases to the liver or lung; and high levels of urinary 17 ketosteroids, homovanillic acid, or plasma dopamine.

55. Incidentally discovered adrenal masses should be evaluated for evidence of malignancy (size > 6 cm or progressive growth) and excess hormone secretion (cortisol, aldosterone, androgens, catecholamines).

56. Adrenal insufficiency should be suspected in outpatients who have received supraphysiologic doses of glucocorticoids for >1 month, ICU patients who are hemodynamically unstable despite aggressive fluid resuscitation or have septic shock, or any patient with signs or symptoms suggesting adrenal insufficiency.

57. Adrenal crisis should be treated aggressively using normal saline with 5% dextrose, intravenous glucocorticoids (dexamethasone if treating before drawing random cortisol and ACTH, hydrocortisone afterwards), other supportive care, and a search for the precipitating illness.

26. **How is supplemental insulin added for high BG before meals?**
Supplemental insulin (high BG correction factor) is used to reduce a high BG detected before meals. A high blood glucose CF is a formula based on the person's insulin sensitivity. A CF estimates the "expected" decrease in BG per unit of administered insulin under normal circumstances. Davidson et al. described a "1500 rule" for regular insulin and an "1800 rule" for bolus insulin analogs. Instead, we average the two formulas and begin with a "1650 rule," which decreases the time needed for fine-tuning the CF. The initial CF is estimated by dividing 1650 by the TDD. The CF must then be adjusted based on each patient's records and is, therefore, only a starting point.

27. **Give an example of determining an initial CF.**
   - 14 units of insulin glargine at 12 noon + 5 units Humalog before each meal.
   - TDD = 29 units (A_{1C} of 7.2% with 1–2 hypoglycemic episodes per week).
   - 1650/29 = 56.9.
   - Begin with a CF of 60:1.
   In this example, 1 unit of rapid-acting insulin will lower the BG about 60 mg/dL; therefore, 1 extra unit will be taken (in addition to the meal insulin dose) for each 60 mg/dL that the premeal BG is over the premeal goal of 100 mg/dL.

28. **Give an example of CF usage.**
   To determine the amount of extra insulin needed if the BG is out of the target range before a meal, subtract the goal BG (100 mg/dL) from the actual BG and divide by the CF.
   - CF is 60:1.
   - Preprandial BG is 220 mg/dL.
   - Calculation: 220 – 100 mg/dL = 120 mg/dL above target.
   - Calculation: 120 (mg/dL)/60 = 2 units of insulin.
   In this example, 2 units of rapid-acting insulin will be added to the meal bolus to return the BG to the target range.

29. **When is a CF used?**
   - It is recommended that high BG corrections be taken before meals or at least 5 hours after the last bolus due to the duration of action of the bolus insulin analogs.
   - Hypoglycemia may occur from the accumulation of active insulin with frequent BG corrections.
   - A CF is more effective if it is taken 15–30 minutes prior to eating. This time frame allows the insulin to begin working before the BG rises further due to the meal.

30. **What can be done for a high postprandial BG reading?**
   - If a postprandial BG is dangerously high (i.e., > 300 mg/dL) or a patient insists on making high BG corrections less than 5 hours, since the last bolus or during the night, they should be instructed how to take a partial correction for safety.
   - Using one-half of the usual premeal CF to lower the BG to the target level is safest between meals.
   - A target level of 150 mg/dL (expected BG level 2 hours postprandial) rather than a target BG of 100 mg/dL is used in the correction calculation between meals.

31. **Provide an example of using a ½ CF.**
   1. BG before dinner = 100 mg/dL.
   2. BG 2 hours after dinner = 300 mg/dL.
   3. "Expected" BG 2 hours after dinner = ~130–150 mg/dL.
   4. Calculation: 300 – 150 mg/dL = 150 mg/dL above target.
   5. CF is 60:1.
   6. Calculation: 150/60 = 2.5 units (full CF).
   7. The premeal insulin is still active for about 3 more hours; therefore, use ½ CF.

8. Calculation of ½ CF: 2.5 (units)/2 = 1.3 units.

In this example, 1.3 units with an insulin pump or 1 unit with a syringe or insulin pen should be given 2 hours after the meal to bring the postprandial BG into the target range. BG should be rechecked within 2 hours to avoid a severe low glucose.

KEY POINTS: IIT ✓

1. Studies have clearly demonstrated that optimal diabetes management decreases chronic complications.

2. IIT, or basal/bolus therapy, is required to mimic normal pancreatic function.

3. Basal insulin is physiologic insulin required to manage BG fluctuations due to hepatic glucose production.

4. Bolus insulin is matched to carbohydrates using a carbohydrate-to-insulin ratio.

5. Supplemental bolus insulin reduces the BG to within normal limits when a high glucose CF is used.

32. **Calculate an initial basal rate for insulin pump therapy.**
    - An established C:I ratio and CF on MDI is critical for a smooth transition to pump therapy.
    - To calculate an initial basal rate, take the current TDD of insulin on MDI and reduce it by 25% (or other appropriate reduction, depending on current A_{1c} and number of hypoglycemic episodes).
    - Use 50% of the reduced dose as the total basal dose to be given over 24 hours.
    - Start with one basal rate for 24 hours (divide the total basal dose by 24). [Initial basal rate per hour = $(TDD \times .75)/(2 \times 24)$.]
    - The remaining 50% will be used as bolus doses for meals based on carbohydrate counting.

33. **Calculate an example of an initial basal rate for insulin pump therapy.**
    1. Current TDD of insulin is: <u>50</u> units
       - 25% reduction of TDD = <u>37.5</u> or
       - 10% reduction of TDD = _____ or
       - ____ reduction of TDD = _____
    2. Reduced dose = <u>37.5</u>/2 = <u>18.75</u> units as total basal
    3. Total basal insulin = <u>18.75</u>/24 = <u>0.78</u> U/h

    In this example, the initial basal rate will be 0.8 U/h. Basal rate adjustments will then be made based on testing and recording BG profiles throughout the day.

34. **When are nighttime basal rate adjustments made?**
    Nighttime basal rates should be adjusted before the daytime basal rates are verified. Testing is typically done during the first week of insulin pump therapy. Testing is then repeated if a significant weight change occurs, if an exercise routine is begun or altered, following hormonal changes (i.e., puberty, menopause), or prn.

35. **List recommendations to follow during the nighttime basal rate verification process.**
    - Assess basal rate accuracy on three different nights.
    - Eat evening meal early, preferably before 7 PM (or begin the test period ~5 hours after eating).
    - If a patient typically eats high-fat meals or is unsure of their carbohydrate counting skills, choose a meal that they frequently eat or one for which they are confident of the carbohydrate amount.

- Avoid meals with more than 15–20 gm of fat, 10 gm of fiber, and alcohol on testing nights.
- Avoid any food or insulin bolus after the evening meal.
- Avoid exercise other than typical activity.
- Monitor BG before and 2 hours after the evening meal, at 12 midnight, at 3 AM, and at 6 AM.
- Stop the test if BG < 70 mg/dL or >250 mg/dL during the basal test and treat the abnormal BG.

36. **How are nighttime basal rate adjustments made?**
    - If BG levels change by more than 20–30 mg/dL during overnight monitoring, adjust the basal rate for the next night by 0.1 U/h, starting 1 hour before the glucose change was seen.
    - Changes are made until the fasting BG in the morning is within the target range (80–120 mg/dL).
    - Daytime basal rates are verified next, usually 1–2 weeks after pump initiation or as needed.

37. **Describe the procedure for making daytime basal rate adjustments.**
    - Having the patient skip breakfast and check their BG levels every hour from 7 AM to 12 noon will verify the morning basal rate.
    - If BG levels change by more than 20–30 mg/dL during this time, adjust the basal rate for the next day by 0.1 U/h, starting 1 hour before the glucose change was seen.
    - Once the morning basal rate is set, have the patients skip their other meals (on separate days) and follow the same monitoring and adjustment procedures to confirm the afternoon and evening basal rate(s).

38. **What is the recommended carbohydrate for the treatment of hypoglycemia?**
    Dextrose should be taken for a BG of <70 mg/dL. Dextrose is the first ingredient in the following products: glucose tablets and gel, candies (SweetTarts, Smarties, Sprees, Pixie Stix, and Runts).

39. **How does the use of rapid-acting insulin impact the treatment of hypoglycemia with MDI and pump therapy?**
    With a shorter duration of effect, rapid-acting insulin analogs require less dextrose to raise the BG than was previously needed with regular insulin.
    - If the last rapid-acting insulin dose was 1–3 hours earlier, 15 gm dextrose should be taken.
    - If the last rapid-acting insulin dose was > 4 hours earlier, only 5–10 gm dextrose may be required.
    - After 15–20 minutes, the patients should wash their hands and test their BG again.
    - If the repeat BG is < 70 mg/dL, additional dextrose should be taken.

40. **Why does rebound hyperglycemia occur after hypoglycemia?**
    - Overtreatment with an inappropriate amount of carbohydrate.
    - No treatment (i.e., sleeping through a low glucose episode) resulting in counter-regulatory hormone release and increased hepatic glycogenolysis.
    - Treatment with a food that contains fat will delay digestion and absorption, thereby prolonging hypoglycemia and causing counter-regulatory hormone release with subsequent hepatic glycogenolysis.

41. **Discuss the use of glucagon to treat severe hypoglycemia.**
    All patients undergoing MDI or pump therapy should be given a glucagon emergency kit prescription and a demonstration. Glucagon is used to raise BG when a person is unable to swallow. This may occur either as a result of a seizure or unconsciousness. Family members should receive instruction and the patient should be able to demonstrate the procedure to a third party (coworker or neighbor).

BIBLIOGRAPHY

1. American Diabetes Association: Implications of the United Kingdom Prospective Diabetes Study. Diabetes Care 23(Suppl 1):26:S28–S32, 2003.

2. Diabetes Control and Complications Trial Research Group: The effect of intensive treatment of diabetes on the development and progression of long-term complications in insulin-dependent diabetes mellitus. N Engl J Med 329:977–986, 1993.

3. Hirsch IB: Intensive treatment of type 1 diabetes. Med Clin North Am 82:689, 1998.

4. Shichiri M, Kishikawa H: Long-term results of the Kumamoto study of optimal diabetes control in type 2 diabetic patients. Diabetes Care 23(Suppl 2):B21, 2000.

RECOMMENDED PATIENT READING

1. Walsh J, Roberts R: Pumping insulin. San Diego, Torrey Pines Press, 2000.

2. Walsh J, Roberts R: Using Insulin. San Diego, Torrey Pines Press, 2003.

CHAPTER 4

INPATIENT MANAGEMENT OF DIABETES AND HYPERGLYCEMIA

Kelly Flesner-Gurley, M.D.

1. **What evidence supports more intensive management of blood sugars in the hospital setting?**
   Numerous studies have now demonstrated the correlation between glycemic control and outcomes. Suboptimal glycemic control in hospitalized patients with diabetes has multiple adverse consequences, including volume and electrolyte abnormalities, immune suppression, and poor wound healing. There is a clear association between poorly controlled diabetes and increased susceptibility to complications, prolonged hospital stay, and increased mortality.

2. **Besides diabetic ketoacidosis (DKA) and hyperosmolar state, in what specific patient populations have studies shown improved mortality outcomes with aggressive intravenous insulin therapy?**
   Acute myocardial infarction: IV insulin infusions followed by subcutaneous insulin for 3 months improved long-term survival rates by 28% at 3.4 years.
   Coronary artery bypass surgery: IV insulin infusions used for the first 3 postoperative days decreased absolute mortality in hyperglycemic patients by 57%.
   Critically ill patients in ICU settings: Controlling blood sugar in the range of 80–110 mg/dL decreased hospital mortality by 34%.

3. **What specific outcomes were improved by treating patients with IV insulin infusions in the three categories mentioned in question 2?**
   Intravenous insulin infusions were shown to reduce the incidence of deep sternal wound infections by 66%, sepsis by 46%, acute renal failure by 41%, transfusions by 50%, and critical illness polyneuropathy by 44%. Length of hospital stay and cost were also reduced.

4. **Apart from glycemic regulation, how may insulin improve metabolic regulation and outcomes?**
   Some explanation may lie with the intrinsic anti-inflammatory properties of insulin. By regulation of nuclear factor-$\kappa\beta$, insulin suppresses tumor necrosis factor alpha (TNFα) and antagonizes macrophage migration inhibitory factor (MIF), two proinflammatory cytokines. Insulin also inhibits inflammatory growth factors (activator protein-1 and early growth response gene-1). In addition, insulin stimulates endothelial nitric oxide synthase, which provides beneficial effects on oxidation and inflammation. Last, insulin inhibits lipolysis, thus lowering free fatty acids. These effects cause favorable alterations in myocardial and skeletal muscle metabolism.

5. **Despite all the evidence to support better glycemic control, why is poor glycemic control so common in hospitalized patients?**
   Many patient factors, such as infection, fever, steroids, stress, and inactivity, exacerbate hyperglycemia in the hospital setting. However, three major physician issues are even more responsible:
   - Fear of hypoglycemia.
   - Lack of understanding of how to appropriately use insulin.
   - Underappreciation of the importance of glycemic control, causing the care of diabetes to become a secondary issue.

6. **What can we do to help prevent hypoglycemia?**
   - Use physiologic insulin orders.
   - Hold prandial insulin or hypoglycemic agents when patients have an interruption of their nutritional source.
   - For patients who have an unexpected interruption of their nutritional source and the hypo-glycemic agent has already been given, one can increase blood glucose (BG) monitoring and provide a supplemental D5 infusion if needed.

7. **What should the glycemic targets be for hospitalized patients?**
   Intensive care unit: 80–110 mg/dL.
   Noncritical care units: preprandial, 90–130 mg/dL; peak postprandial, <180 mg/dL.
   Prelabor: preprandial, 100 mg/dL; 1-hour postprandial, <120 mg/dL.
   Labor and delivery: 100 mg/dL.

8. **What is the best agent available for inpatient management of diabetes?**
   Insulin, given physiologically as an intravenous infusion or subcutaneously with basal and nutri-tional coverage.

9. **Explain the role of oral agents in hospital patients.**
   In the inpatient setting, oral agents are limited to patients who took them prior to admission, with minimal elevations of BG; who are able to eat; and who do not have other contraindications. If the fasting BG is >180 mg/dL, oral agents are unlikely to control hyperglycemia.

10. **What are the contraindications of the various oral agents?**
    Metformin is contraindicated for patients with renal dysfunction (serum creatinine > 1.5 mg/dL in males and >1.4 mg/dL in females), hypotension, sepsis, myocardial infarction, congestive heart failure (CHF), and hypoxia. In patients with symptomatic CHF undergoing a procedure requiring IV contrast, it must be discontinued at the time of the procedure and held for 48 hours after and until renal function is considered normal. Thiazolidinediones are contraindicated in patients with CHF or abnormal liver function; they can also cause fluid retention and take many weeks to produce maximal glucose-lowering effects. Sulfonylureas must be held for any patient in whom oral ingestion is prohibited (NPO status). Of note, glipizide is associated with less hypoglycemia than glyburide in renal insufficiency.

11. **List the indications for intravenous insulin therapy.**

DKA	After organ transplantation
Hyperosmolar state	Labor and delivery
Critical illness	Total parenteral nutrition
Prolonged NPO status	Uncontrolled hyperglycemia exacerbated by illness or
Perioperative period	steroids
Acute myocardial infarction	Any illness requiring prompt glucose control
Coronary artery bypass surgery	Dose-finding strategy
Stroke	

12. **Why is the intravenous route superior to the subcutaneous route?**
    The intravenous route surpasses the subcutaneous route with respect to rapidity, flexibility, and overall ability to achieve glycemic control. Although there seems to be a fear of intra-venous insulin, it is actually safer than subcutaneous insulin since patients are monitored more closely, the delivery is more physiologic, and the hypoglycemia that may occur is short-lived compared with the prolonged hypoglycemia that may result from "stacking" subcuta-neous insulin.

KEY POINTS: TARGET GLUCOSE LEVELS FOR HOSPITALIZED PATIENTS ✓

1. Intensive care unit: 80–110 mg/dL.

2. Non–critical care units: preprandial, 90–130 mg/dL; peak postprandial, <180 mg/dL.

3. Prelabor: preprandial, 100 mg/dL; 1-hour postprandial, <120 mg/dL.

4. Labor and delivery: 100 mg/dL.

13. **At what rate should an insulin infusion be started?**
For an unstressed normoglycemic adult of average body mass index (BMI), an insulin infusion is commonly initiated at 1 U/h and adjusted as needed. Another method that can be used to estimate the initial hourly requirement is to divide ~50% of the previous total daily dose by 24. Alternatively, a weight-based insulin dose may be calculated, using 0.02 U/k/h as a starting rate. Lower and higher initiation rates may be required in certain clinical conditions. The prime determinants of the initial hourly intravenous requirements are the initial BG and BMI.

14. **How should you adjust the intravenous insulin infusion rate?**
The serum half-life of insulin is about 4–5 minutes, but insulin action lasts about 1 hour. Adjustments are made based on the BG level and the rate of hourly change in response to the current insulin rate. An appropriate rate of change is ~80 mg/dL per hour. If the BG does not change by at least 60 mg/dL after 1 hour, the rate should be increased. Conversely, if the BG is dropping >100 mg/dL per hour, the rate should be decreased. Factors, such as interruption of dextrose or other feedings, steroids, and pressors, acutely affect the rate of infusion. The best way to manage intravenous insulin infusions is through implementation of physiologic infusion algorithms (Table 4-1). When an algorithm is

TABLE 4-1. ALGORITHMS FOR CONTROL OF BLOOD GLUCOSE IN HOSPITAL PATIENTS

Algorithm 1		Algorithm 2		Algorithm 3		Algorithm 4	
BG	U/h	BG	U/h	BG	U/h	BG	U/h
<60 mg/dL = hypoglycemia (see the following for treatment)							
<70	Off	<70	Off	<70	Off	<70	Off
70–109	0.2	70–109	0.5	70–109	1	70–109	1.5
110–119	0.5	110–119	1	110–119	2	110–119	3
120–149	1	120–149	1.5	120–149	3	120–149	5
150–179	1.5	150–179	2	150–179	4	150–179	7
180–209	2	180–209	3	180–209	5	180–209	9
210–239	2	210–239	4	210–239	6	210–239	12
240–269	3	240–269	5	240–269	8	240–269	16
270–299	3	270–299	6	270–299	10	270–299	20
300–329	4	300–329	7	300–329	12	300–329	24
330–359	4	330–359	8	330–359	14	>330	28
>360	6	>360	12	>360	16		

selected, it is imperative to provide in-service teaching of pharmacy, nursing, and physician staff and to obtain feedback to improve any deficiencies.

15. Give general guidelines for an insulin infusion protocol.
Standardized guidelines for intravenous insulin infusion (not appropriate for DKA or hyperosmolar state) may look much as follows:

Goal BG = _____(usually 80–180 mg/dL):

- *Standard drip*: 100 units/100 mL in 0.9% NaCl via an infusion device.
- Surgical patients who have received an oral diabetes medication within 24 hours should start when BG > 120 mg/dL. All other patients can start when BG is ≥70 mg/dL.
- Insulin infusions should be discontinued when a patient is eating *and* has received the first dose of subcutaneous insulin. (Continue drip until 2 hours after rapid insulin is given or 4 hours after long-acting insulin is given.)
- Most patients need 5–10 gm of glucose per hour, given in D_5W or D_5W ½NS at 100–200 mL\h or equivalent (e.g., TPN, enteral feeds).46

16. How is the infusion initiated?
- *Algorithm 1:* Start here for most patients.
- *Algorithm 2:* For patients not controlled with algorithm 1; start here for patients who have undergone coronary artery bypass grafting or solid organ or islet cell transplant, patients receiving glucocorticoids, and patients with diabetes who received >80 U/day of insulin as outpatients.
- *Algorithm 3:* For patients not controlled with algorithm 2. *No patients start here without authorization from the endocrine service.*
- *Algorithm 4:* For patients not controlled with algorithm 3. *No patients start here.*
Patients not controlled with the above algorithms need an endocrine consult.

17. Describe the criteria for moving from one algorithm to another.
Moving up: Algorithm failure is defined as BG outside the goal range (see the above-mentioned goal), and the BG does not change by at least 60 mg/dL within 1 hour.
Moving down: When BG is < 70 mg/dL × 2.

18. How often should patients be monitored?
Goal BG = 80–180 mg/dL:
- Check capillary BG every hour until it is within goal range for 4 hours; then decrease to every 2 hours for 4 hours. If the patient remains stable, decrease to every 4 hours.
- Hourly monitoring may be indicated for critically ill patients even if they have stable BG.

19. Describe the treatment of hypoglycemia (BG < 60 mg/dL).
1. Discontinue insulin drip.
2. Give $D_{50}W$ IV:
   - if the patient is awake, 25 mL (½ ampule);
   - if the patient is not awake, 50 mL (1 ampule).
3. Recheck BG every 20 minutes and repeat 25 mL of $D_{50}W$ IV if it is <60 mg/dL. Restart drip once BG is >70 mg/dL for 2 checks. Restart drip with lower algorithm (see *Moving down* in question 17).

20. When should the physician be notified?
- For any BG change greater than 100 mg/dL in 1 hour.
- For BG > 360 mg/dL.
- For hypoglycemia that has not resolved within 20 minutes of administering 50 mL of $D_{50}W$ IV and discontinuing the insulin drip.

21. **How do I transition the patient off the insulin drip?**
     To maintain adequate blood insulin levels, it is imperative to continue the insulin infusion for 1–2 hours after the rapid- or short-acting insulin has been given or 2–4 hours after intermediate- or long-acting insulin has been given. Once the patient can tolerate oral intake, discontinue other excess dextrose to avoid additive hyperglycemia. A starting subcutaneous basal insulin dose can be calculated by giving ~40–50% of the previous 24-hour IV insulin requirement. The subcutaneous prandial insulin dose can be calculated by giving ~20–40% of the previous 24-hour insulin requirement divided between meals.

22. **What is a "sliding-scale"? How is it different from correction-dose insulin?**
     Sliding-scale insulin refers to a set amount of insulin administered for hyperglycemia without regard to the timing of food, other pre-existing treatment, or individual response to insulin. Problems cited with sliding-scale regimens include lack of any modification throughout the hospital stay and treating hyperglycemia instead of preventing it. Correction-dose insulin, on the other hand, is an important adjunct to scheduled insulin and correcting hyperglycemia as you adjust the scheduled doses.

23. **Why do endocrinologists get so upset when patients are managed on sliding-scale regimens alone for blood sugar control?**
     Although sliding-scale insulin regimens continue to be prescribed for the majority of inpatients with diabetes, evidence shows that they provide no benefit. In fact, when used without a standing dose of scheduled insulin, they are associated with an increased rate of hyperglycemic episodes, hypoglycemic episodes, and iatrogenic DKA.

KEY POINTS: INPATIENT MANAGEMENT OF DIABETES AND HYPERGLYCEMIA ✓

1. Evidence shows that controlling BG in hospitalized patients improves outcomes.

2. Insulin is the best agent for management of hyperglycemia in hospital patients.

3. Intravenous insulin infusions have been shown to be superior to subcutaneous insulin with respect to achieving glycemic control and improving nonglycemic outcomes.

4. Use of sliding-scale insulin alone to control blood sugars should be avoided.

24. **How do I write the admit orders if I do not know whether the patient will require insulin?**
     All patients should have either a plasma or a capillary BG determination as part of their initial assessment. If BG is high, scheduled BG checks should be ordered. If the patient is critically ill, an insulin infusion should be started if two BG checks are >100 mg/dL. If the patient is on the ward and has two BG checks >170 mg/dL or any BG check >300 mg/dL, scheduled subcutaneous insulin should be started.

25. **What are the goals of effective insulin therapy in the hospital?**
     Effective insulin therapy must provide both basal and nutritional coverage to achieve glycemic goals. In addition, patients also require correction-dose insulin to correct hyperglycemia as the scheduled dose is adjusted. Patients who are conscious, eating, and experienced should continue self-management in the hospital. Limiting factors in the outpatient setting, such as cost of medications, ability to check BG, or ability to comprehend multiple daily injections (MDI), do not

apply to the inpatient. Therefore, doctors can take advantage of newer, more physiologic insulins, and patients can be managed with more flexibility in timing of meals and less hypoglycemia.

26. **How should you write orders for scheduled subcutaneous insulin for hospital patients?**

The best way to order insulin subcutaneously is with an MDI regimen or subcutaneous insulin pump. Writing the actual order is a three-step process: (1) choose the scheduled basal insulin dose, (2) choose the scheduled prandial insulin dose, and (3) order correction-dose insulin.

27. **How do you choose the scheduled basal insulin dose?**

Basal insulin can be provided by intermediate insulin (NPH, lente, or ultralente), given two times a day or occasionally at bedtime, or by long-acting insulin (glargine) given once daily. Since NPH, lente, and ultralente result in increased variability and peaks of insulin action that may exceed basal needs and cause hypoglycemia, many prefer to transition patients to once-daily insulin glargine while they are in the hospital. (Pregnancy is an exception.) Basal insulin generally accounts for 40–50% of the daily insulin requirement. Therefore, the basal dose is ~40–50% of the prior daily dose requirement or ~0.2–0.3 U/k/day.

28. **How do you choose the prandial dose for patients already taking insulin?**

Prandial insulin can be provided by giving either regular insulin 30–40 minutes before meals or rapid-acting insulin 0–15 minutes before meals. Rapid-acting insulins (lispro and aspart) allow more dosing flexibility with less hypoglycemia and are preferable for the inpatient setting. In the outpatient setting, the total daily prandial dose is calculated as ~50% of the total daily insulin dose. Because patients often do not eat consistently in the hospital, a safe starting estimate of prandial dose is ~20–40% of the total daily dose divided among the meals.

29. **How do you choose the prandial dose for patients who previously have not taken insulin?**

Most patients who have not previously taken insulin require about 1 unit of short- or rapid-acting insulin for every 10–15 gm of carbohydrate eaten. A safe starting point is to schedule 4–5 units per meal for patients with type 1 diabetes and 6–8 units per meal for patients with type 2 diabetes.

30. **How do you choose the correction dose of insulin?**

Rapid-acting insulin should be given with meals in addition to the prandial dose to correct for preprandial hyperglycemia, with a goal of using less supplemental insulin each day as you titrate the scheduled dose upward. For more insulin-sensitive patients with type 1 diabetes, a safe starting point is to correct by giving 1 unit of insulin to lower glucose by 50 mg/dL if BG is above 150 mg/dL. For more insulin-resistant patients, a starting point is to correct by giving 1 unit to lower glucose by 25–30 mg/dL if BG is above 150 mg/dL. Figure 4-1 shows a sample order sheet.

31. **What is the general rule for insulin delivery to diabetic patients scheduled for hospital procedures?**

Diabetic patients should be scheduled for procedures early in the morning. The usual insulin/oral agents should be given to all patients on the night before a procedure to ensure normal morning glycemia.

32. **What two questions should be asked before writing orders for patients who may not be eating because of nausea or NPO status during the perioperative period?**

1. Does the patient have insulin deficiency? (Insulin deficiency is defined as type 1 diabetes, history of pancreatic dysfunction, insulin use > 5 years, or diabetes > 10 years.)
2. How long will the patient be on NPO status?

BG Monitoring: ☐ Before meals and at bedtime. ☐ ___ hours after meals. ☐ 2-3 AM

Goal Premeal BG = 80-150 mg/dl

	Breakfast	Lunch	Dinner	Bedtime
Prandial Insulin Orders	Give____units of: ☐ Lispro (Humalog) ☐ Aspart (Novolog) ☐ Regular	Give ____units of: ☐ Lispro (Humalog) ☐ Aspart (Novolog) ☐ Regular	Give____units of: ☐ Lispro (Humalog) ☐ Aspart (Novolog) ☐ Regular	
Basal Insulin Orders	Give ____units of: ☐ NPH ☐ Lente ☐ Ultralente ☐ Glargine		Give ____units of: ☐ NPH ☐ Lente ☐ Ultralente ☐ Glargine	Give ____units of: ☐ NPH ☐ Lente ☐ Ultralente ☐ Glargine

Suggested Lag Times for Prandial Insulin:

Aspart/Lispro: 0-15 minutes before eating

Regular: 30 minutes before eating

For BG < 60 mg/dL

    A. If patient can take PO, give 15 grams of fast-acting carbohydrate

        (4 oz fruit juice/non diet soda, 8 oz nonfat milk, or 3-4 glucose tablets).

    B. If patient cannot take PO, give 25 mL of D50 as IV push.

    C. Check finger capillary glucose every 15 minutes and repeat above if BG < 80.

Premeal "correction dose" algorithm for hyperglycemia: To be administered in addition to scheduled insulin dose to correct premeal hyperglycemia.

    ☐ Lispro   ☐ Aspart

☐ **Low Dose Algorithm**
(For pts on ≤ 40 U insulin/day)

☐ **Medium Dose Algorithm**
(For pts on 40-80 U of insulin/day)

Premeal BG	Additional Insulin	Premeal BG	Additional Insulin
150-199	1 unit	150-199	1 unit
200-249	2 units	200-249	3 units
250-299	3 units	250-299	5 units
300-349	4 units	300-349	7 units
> 349	5 units	> 349	8 units

☐ **High Dose Algorithm**
(For pts requiring > 80 U insulin/day)

☐ **Individualized Algorithm**

Premeal BG	Additional Insulin	Premeal BG	Additional Insulin
150-199	2 unit	150-199	
200-249	4 units	200-249	
250-299	7 units	250-299	
300-349	10 units	300-349	
> 349	12 units	> 349	

Figure 4-1. Sample order sheet for insulin administration to hospitalized patients.

33. **What orders are appropriate for patients with insulin deficiency during the preoperative period?**

Basal insulin is required at all times, even when patients are not eating. When long-acting insulin glargine is used, the current dose can usually be continued and only the prandial insulin doses withheld. If intermediate insulin is used, because of the peaking effect, the dose should be lowered from two-thirds to one-half. Correction-dose insulin can be used every 4–6 hours as needed. For patients with diabetes/hyperglycemia who still have endogenous insulin production, the basal insulin dose should be lowered and is sometimes not required; oral hypoglycemic agents should be withheld that day. Correction-dose insulin can be used every 4–6 hours as needed.

34. **What approach is appropriate when a prolonged NPO status is anticipated?**
    When a prolonged NPO status is anticipated (>12–24 hours), an insulin infusion is recommended.

35. **Discuss the postoperative orders for diabetic patients.**
    After surgery, if the patient is not eating well, low-dose insulin glargine can be started at 0.2 U/kg body weight per day with correction-dose insulin as needed. For patients "grazing" all day and not eating consistent meals, regular short-acting correction-dose insulin is preferred over rapid-acting insulin.

36. **Characterize hyperglycemia induced by steroids.**
    Classically, glucocorticoid use causes minimal elevations of fasting BG levels but exaggerates postprandial BG excursions and increases insulin resistance.

37. **How is steroid-induced hyperglycemia best treated?**
    Because of the effects described earlier, patients can often be treated with supplemental prandial insulin alone. If basal insulin is needed, a 12-hour insulin, such as NPH, during the day works well as does a scheduled regimen using 70% prandial and 30% basal. Of course, uncontrolled patients can be managed well on variable-rate insulin infusions.

38. **How should hyperglycemic patients on TPN or enteral feeding be treated?**
    A variable-rate insulin infusion is the quickest way to achieve BG stabilization. When the TPN infusion is constant, 70–100% of the total number of units used in the insulin infusion over the previous 24 hours can be added to the subsequent TPN bag. Other options for TPN or enteral feeds include basal insulin to match the timing of the feeding. Caution must be used in this setting; if feeding is discontinued, glucose must be infused until the subcutaneous insulin has dissipated.

39. **How should daily insulin doses be adjusted?**
    Assessing daily BG trends and adjusting scheduled insulin doses are the keys to better glucose control. The fasting BG is affected mainly by the basal insulin, while premeal BGs are affected by both prandial and basal insulins. To assess prandial insulin doses, check BG 2 hours after eating; postprandial BG values should be 30–50 mg/dL above the preprandial BG values and less than 180 mg/dL.

40. **Are daily doses adjusted as often as they should be?**
    Amazingly, many studies show that, although adverse finger-stick BG measurements are repeatedly recorded, most often providers take no action to adjust scheduled insulin doses. This finding is likely attributable to physicians' erroneous assumption that the sliding-scale is taking care of the problem!

41. **How do I decide what orders to give the patient when he or she is sent home?**
    As previously stated, it is more effective to manage the inpatient with basal-bolus therapy using more physiologic insulin. Once the patient is stable for discharge, the physician, with the help of the diabetes educator, can reassess the regimen. Factors, such as cost of medications, the patient's ability to monitor and self-manage, previous control of diabetes, and contraindications to medications, need to be evaluated. One can also use the calculated inpatient TDD to change insulin back to a split mix if needed. In general, once- and twice-daily insulin regimens are no longer suitable for type 1 patients. Patients whose TDD requirements are <0.3 U/kg body weight per day can be considered for transition to an oral regimen.

42. **How can the hospital system work to improve glycemic outcomes?**
    A team approach, including physicians, nurses, pharmacists, and diabetes educators, has been shown to decrease length of stay and cost of care. In the hospital system, patients with new-onset diabetes or insulin resistance can be identified for appropriate follow-up and education. In

one study, 60% of patients with a random BG > 126 mg/dL during hospitalization were found to have diabetes at follow-up testing. During the hospital stay, home regimens can be reassessed and improved. Most importantly, the patients are watching how physicians manage their blood sugars. It is extremely significant for patients to see that the physician *can* control the blood sugar, and that the physician considers control important.

BIBLIOGRAPHY

1. Aljada A, Dandona P: Effect of insulin on human aortic endothelial nitric oxide synthase. Metabolism 49:147–150, 2000.

2. Aljada A, Ghanim H, Mohanty P, et al: Insulin inhibits the proinflammatory transcription factor early growth response gene-1 (*Erg*-1) expression in mononuclear cells (MNC) and reduces plasma tissue factor (TF) and plasminogen activator inhibitor-1 (PAI-1) concentrations. J Clin Endocrinol Metab 87:1419–1422, 2002.

3. American Association of Clinical Endocrinologists, Consensus Development Conference on Inpatient Diabetes and Metabolic Control: Position Statement, December 2003.

4. Bhattacharyya A: Inpatient management of diabetes mellitus and patient satisfaction. Diabetic Med 19:412–416, 2002.

5. Braithwaite SS: Hospital management of hyperglycemia. Grand Rounds Lecture, July 2003.

6. Brown G, Dodek P: Intravenous insulin nomogram improves blood glucose control in the critically ill. Crit Care Med 29(9):1714–1719, 2001.

7. Clement S, Braithwaite S, Magee M, et al: Management of diabetes and hyperglycemia in hospitals. Diabetes Care 27:553–597, 2004.

8. Dandona P, Aljada A, Bandyopadhyay A: The potential therapeutic role of insulin in acute myocardial infarction in patients admitted to intensive care and in those with unspecified hyperglycemia. Diabetes Care 26:516–519, 2003.

9. Furnary AP, Gao G, Grunkmeier GL, et al: Continuous insulin infusion reduces mortality in patients with diabetes undergoing coronary artery bypass grafting. J Thorac Cardiovasc Surg 125:1007–1021, 2003.

10. Gearhart J, Duncan JL, Replogle WH, et al: Efficacy of sliding-scale insulin therapy: a comparison with prospective regimens. Fam Pract Res J 14:313–322, 1994 (Medline).

11. Ghanim H, Mohanty P, Aljada A, et al: Insulin reduces the pro-inflammatory transcription factor, activation protein-1 (AP-1), in mononuclear cells (MNC) and plasma matrix metalloproteinase-9 (MMP-9) concentration. Diabetes 50 (Suppl 1):A408, 2001 (abstract).

12. Golden SH, Pert-Vigilance C, Kao WHL, Brancati FL: Perioperative glycemic control and the risk of infectious complications in a cohort of adults with diabetes. Diabetes Care 22:1408–1414, 1999.

13. Greci LS, Kailasam M, Malkani S, et al: Utility of Hb A1c levels for diabetes case finding in hospitalized patients with hyperglycemia. Diabetes Care 26:1064–1068, 2003.

14. Hirsch IB: Insulin in the Hospital Setting. New York, Adelphia Inc., 2002.

15. Lebovitz HE (ed): Therapy for Diabetes Mellitus and Related Disorders, 3rd ed. Alexandria, VA, American Diabetes Association, 1998.

16. Lilley SH, Levine GL: Management of hospitalized patients with type 2 diabetes mellitus. Am Fam Physician 57:1079–1088, 1998.

17. Levetan CS, Macgee MF: Hospital management of diabetes and hyperglycemia. Acute Compl Diabetes 29(4):745–770, 2000.

18. Levetan CS, Passaro M, Jablonski K, et al: Unrecognized diabetes among hospitalized patients. Diabetes Care 21:246–249, 1998.

19. Metchick LN: Inpatient management of diabetes mellitus. Am J Med 113:317–323, 2002.

20. Queale WS, Seidler AJ, Brancati FL: Glycemic control and sliding scale insulin use in medical inpatients with diabetes mellitus. Arch Intern Med 157: 545–552, 1997.

21. Umpierrez GE, Isaacs SD, Bazargan N, et al: Hyperglycemia: An independent marker of in-hospital mortality in patients with undiagnosed diabetes. J Clin Endocrinol Metab 87:978–982, 2002.

22. Van den Berghe G: Insulin therapy for the critically ill patient. Clin Cornerstones 5(2):56–63, 2003.

23. Van den Berghe G, Wouters P, Weekers F, et al: Intensive insulin therapy in critically ill patients. N Engl J Med 345:1359–1367, 2001.

CHAPTER 5

DIABETES IN PREGNANCY

Linda A. Barbour, M.D., M.S.P.H.

1. **How does normal pregnancy affect fuel metabolism?**
   Pregnancy is a complex metabolic state that involves dramatic alterations in the hormonal milieu (increases in estrogen, progesterone, prolactin, cortisol, human chorionic gonadotropin, placental growth hormone, and human placental lactogen) in order for the mother to provide the necessary nutrients for the growing fetal–placental unit.

2. **Summarize the changes in the first trimester of pregnancy.**
   Metabolically, the first trimester is characterized by increased insulin sensitivity and accelerated starvation with an increased turnover of maternal metabolic fuels and an earlier transition from carbohydrate to fat utilization in the fasting state. Pregnant women deplete their glycogen stores quickly and switch from carbohydrate to fat metabolism within 12 hours, often becoming ketonemic.

3. **Summarize the changes in the second and third trimesters.**
   The second and third trimesters, in contrast, are characterized by insulin resistance, with a nearly 50% decrease in insulin-mediated glucose disposal (assessed by the hyperinsulinemic-euglycemic clamp technique) and a 200–300% increase in insulin secretion in late pregnancy. These changes shunt necessary fuels to meet the metabolic demands of the fetus, which requires 80% of its energy as glucose, while maintaining euglycemia in the mother. Women usually have lower fasting levels of plasma glucose and fasting hypoinsulinemia because continued shunting of carbohydrate to the fetus in the unfed state results in an increase in maternal free fatty acids and ketones. However, due to the placental hormone-mediated insulin resistance in the fed state, they demonstrate modestly elevated postprandial glucose excursions associated with maternal hyperinsulinemia.

4. **Is glucose the only fuel altered in normal pregnancy?**
   No. Amino acids, triglycerides, cholesterol, and free fatty acids are also increased; the increase in free fatty acids may further accentuate the insulin resistance of pregnancy.

5. **Explain the effect of the metabolic changes in pregnancy on diabetes management in the first trimester.**
   Diabetes should optimally be under tight control before conception. During the first trimester, nausea, accelerated starvation, and increased insulin sensitivity may place the mother at risk for hypoglycemia. This risk is especially high at night because of prolonged fasting and continuous fetal glucose utilization. Women with type 1 diabetes mellitus must have a bedtime snack and usually need to have their evening dose of NPH insulin lowered and moved from suppertime to bedtime to avoid early morning hypoglycemia. Severe hypoglycemia occurs in 30–40% of pregnant women with type 1 diabetes in the first 20 weeks of pregnancy, most often between midnight and 8:00 AM. Diabetic women who have gastroparesis or hyperemesis gravidarum are at the greatest risk for daytime hypoglycemia. During the first trimester, glycemic control just above the normal range (hemoglobin A_{1C} [HbA1C] < 7.0%) may thus be safer than "normal" and may decrease the risk of fetal hypoglycemia.

6. **How do metabolic changes in pregnancy affect the management of diabetes in the second and third trimesters?**
   After 20 weeks, peripheral insulin resistance increases insulin requirements. It is not unusual for a pregnant woman to require twice as much insulin as she did before pregnancy. Postprandial hyperglycemia is the strongest risk factor for macrosomia. Therefore, tight glucose control in women with preexisting diabetes usually requires short-acting insulin with each meal with frequent monitoring to allow appropriate insulin dosage adjustments.

7. **What is the most important recommendation in counseling a diabetic woman who wants to become pregnant?**
   The most important recommendation in preconception counseling is the need for optimal glucose control before conception. Unplanned pregnancies occur in about two-thirds of women with diabetes, making it critical that the primary care physician, endocrinologist, or obstetrician-gynecologist address preconception care in women of child-bearing age. In a retrospective study, <40% of women attempted to achieve optimal glycemic control before becoming pregnant. Four times as many fetal and neonatal deaths and congenital abnormalities occurred in a group of women who did not receive prenatal counseling in comparison with those who did.

8. **Why is maintenance of glucose control essential for the well-being of the fetus?**
   The maintenance of normal glucose control is the key to prevention of complications, such as fetal malformations in the first trimester, macrosomia in the second and third trimesters, and neonatal metabolic abnormalities. Hyperglycemia modulates the expression of an apoptosis regulatory gene as early as the preimplantation blastocyst stage in the mouse, resulting in fetal wastage that can be prevented by treating with insulin. This finding may account for the high risk of first-trimester loss in pregnant women with poor glycemic control.

9. **Describe the relationship between HbAlC and the teratogenic effects of hyperglycemia.**
   Epidemiologic and prospective studies have shown that the level of HbA1C in the 6 months before conception and during the first trimester correlates with the incidence of major malformations, such as neural tube and cardiac defects. The neural tube is completely formed by 4 weeks and the heart by 6 weeks after conception; many women do not even know that they are pregnant at these times. It has been demonstrated that women with a normal HbA1C at conception and during the first trimester have no increased risk, while women with a HbA1C of > 12% have up to a 25% risk of major malformations.

10. **How has the incidence of congenital abnormalities in the offspring of diabetic mothers changed over the past decade?**
    The incidence of congenital abnormalities in the offspring of diabetic mothers in the early era of insulin use was 33%. Over the past decade, with the advent of home glucose monitoring and more rigid objectives, this percentage has fallen to <10% of offspring. The randomized prospective Diabetes Control and Complications Trial (DCCT) has shown that timely institution of intensive therapy for blood glucose is associated with rates of spontaneous abortion and congenital malformations that are similar to those in the nondiabetic population.

11. **What are the risks if a woman conceives while taking an oral hypoglycemic agent?**
    Oral hypoglycemic agents, such as sulfonylureas and metformin, do not appear to be teratogenic. A retrospective series of 332 women with type 2 diabetes treated with diet, insulin, or oral sulfonylureas during the first 8 weeks of gestation found no significant adverse effects. However, no trials of adequate sample size have addressed the risks of oral hypoglycemics during embryogenesis. Women who are actively trying to become pregnant should be switched to

insulin during the preconception period because it may take some time to determine the ideal insulin dose prior to the critical time of embryogenesis.

12. **How is glyburide different from the other sulfonylureas?**
Glyburide is the only sulfonylurea shown not to cross the placenta or to significantly affect fetal insulin levels. In the only large randomized prospective trial, however, it was not given until after 24 weeks to women with gestational diabetes.

13. **Can oral hypoglycemic agents be continued in pregnancy?**
It is recommended that oral hypoglycemic agents be avoided during pregnancy with the possible exception of glyburide, which should be limited to use in the second and third trimesters based on one large randomized controlled trial in women with gestational diabetes.

14. **Summarize the evidence related to the role of metformin during pregnancy.**
Metformin has been continued during the first trimester in nonrandomized studies of women with polycystic ovary syndrome (PCOS) and spontaneous fetal loss. It may decrease first-trimester loss in patients with PCOS. It has been continued throughout pregnancy in ~100 patients, and in one trial of 28 patients was shown to decrease the incidence of gestational diabetes. However, in a retrospective series, in which 50 pregnant women were treated with metformin, 68 women with a sulfonylurea, and 42 with insulin, there was a higher incidence of preeclampsia in the metformin group, as well as an increase in perinatal mortality. Metformin does cross the placenta, and until the results of a multicenter trial investigating the risks of metformin in pregnancy is completed, women should be counseled that it is not yet approved in pregnancy. If used at all, it should be restricted to the first trimester in patients with PCOS who are taking it to improve first-trimester loss rates.

15. **How should hypertensive women who take angiotensin-converting enzyme (ACE) inhibitors or have risk factors for coronary artery disease be counseled in the preconception period?**
Women should be counseled that ACE inhibitors are contraindicated in the second and third trimesters of pregnancy because of the risk of fetal anuria. Although first-trimester exposure alone has not been shown to cause problems, women who are actively trying to conceive and who have no history of infertility should probably be switched to a safer agent before pregnancy (calcium channel blocker, methyldopa, hydralazine). A woman who receives treatment with an ACE inhibitor for significant diabetic nephropathy and is not actively trying to conceive should be told to stop her ACE inhibitor as soon as she misses a period and to obtain a pregnancy test. At that time she can be switched safely to an alternative agent.

16. **How does pregnancy affect the morbidity and mortality of coronary artery disease in diabetic women?**
The morbidity and mortality rates of coronary artery disease are high in pregnant women with diabetes. Cardiac status should be assessed with functional testing before conception in women possessing any additional cardiac risk factors, such as hyperlipidemia, hypertension, smoking, advanced maternal age (> 35 years), or a strong family history. Pregnancy causes a 25% increase in cardiac output, a significant decrease in systemic vascular resistance (which can shunt blood away from the coronary arteries), and an increase in oxygen consumption, all of which decrease the ability of maternal coronary blood flow to meet the demands of the myocardium. Myocardial demands are even higher at labor and delivery, and activation of catecholamines can cause myocardial ischemia.

17. **Should statins be discontinued before conception?**
Yes. Data about their safety during human pregnancy are inadequate, and animal data are concerning. However, if a woman has severe hypertriglyceridemia, which places her at high risk for

pancreatitis, it may be necessary to continue fibrate therapy if a low-fat diet and fish oils are not effective or tolerated.

18. **Should diabetic women take folic acid supplements before conception?**
All women should take folic acid supplements (1 mg/day) before conception.

19. **Summarize the effect of smoking during pregnancy.**
Smoking continues to be the leading cause of low-birth-weight infants in patients with and without diabetes and places the infant at increased risk for respiratory infections, reactive airway disease, and sudden infant death syndrome. Smoking cessation efforts need to be intensified before conception, since agents, such as the nicotine patch and Wellbutrin, are not approved for use during pregnancy.

20. **How does pregnancy affect diabetic nephropathy?**
Proteinuria increases in pregnancy, and women with proteinuria often become nephrotic due to the increased glomerular filtration rate (GFR) of protein during pregnancy. In some patients, the proteinuria can become massive and results in significant edema, hypoalbuminemia, and a hypercoagulable state. While women with mild renal insufficiency are not at an appreciable risk for irreversible progression of their nephropathy, those with more severe renal insufficiency (creatinine > 2.5 mg/dL) have a 30–50% risk of a permanent pregnancy-related decline in GFR.

21. **Does nephropathy increase the risk of preeclampsia?**
Preeclampsia complicates ~20% of pregnancies in women with preexisting diabetes, and the risk is much higher in women with hypertension or renal disease. The risk of developing preeclampsia in women with nephropathy is > 50%. The preeclampsia may be severe. Women with nephropathy are also at higher risk of having preterm and low-birth-weight infants. Therefore, women with diabetic nephropathy should be counseled to have children when their diabetes is optimally controlled and preferably early in the course of their nephropathy.

22. **How does renal transplantation affect the outcome in pregnant women?**
Women who have had a successful renal transplant at least 1–2 years ago and who have good renal function, adequate blood pressure control, and a low requirement for antirejection medications have a much more favorable outcome than women with severe renal disease who have not received a transplant.

23. **Summarize the effects of pregnancy on diabetic retinopathy.**
Proliferative retinopathy may progress during pregnancy either from the institutution of tight control or due to increases in growth factors, blood volume, cardiac output, the hypercogulable state of pregnancy, and anemia. It is imperative, therefore, that retinopathy be optimally treated with laser therapy before pregnancy. It is unusual for women with only background retinopathy to progress significantly during pregnancy.

24. **What is the White Classification of diabetes in pregnancy?**
Priscilla White observed that the patient's age at onset of diabetes, duration of diabetes, and severity of complications, including vascular disease, nephropathy, and retinopathy, significantly influenced maternal and perinatal outcomes. In 1949, she developed a classification scheme based on these parameters. The initial scheme was developed for women with type 1 diabetes; there is no separate classification for type 2 diabetes.

25. **Why is the White Classification used by obstetricians?**
Its predictive value allows identification of patients at greatest risk for obstetric complications during pregnancy so that physicians can intensify management and fetal surveillance. In the updated classification (Table 5-1), pregestational diabetic women are designated by the letters B, C, D, F, R, T, and H according to duration of diabetes and complications.

TABLE 5-1.	MODIFIED WHITE CLASSIFICATION OF PREGNANT DIABETIC WOMEN			
Class	Age at Onset (Years)	Duration (Years)	Type of Vascular Disease	Insulin Need
Gestational diabetes				
A1	Any	Pregnancy	None	None
A2	Any	Pregnancy	None	Yes
Pregestational diabetes				
B	≥20	<10	None	Yes
C	10–19 *or*	10–19	None	Yes
D	<10 *or*	≥20	Benign retinopathy	Yes
F	Any	Any	Nephropathy	Yes
R	Any	Any	Proliferative retinopathy	Yes
T	Any	Any	Renal transplant	Yes
H	Any	Any	Coronary artery disease	Yes

26. **What are the goals of glucose control for pregnant women with diabetes?**
    The goals of blood glucose control during pregnancy are rigorous. Optimally, the premeal whole blood glucose should be < 95 mg/dL, the 1-hour postprandial glucose < 140 mg/dL, and the 2-hour postprandial glucose < 120 mg/dL. Since macrosomia is more strongly related to the postprandial glucose excursions, pregnant diabetic women need to monitor premeal and postprandial glucose values regularly. Type 1 diabetic patients usually require 3–4 injections per day or an insulin pump to achieve adequate control during pregnancy. Short-acting insulins, such as lispro or aspart, may be especially helpful in women with hyperemesis or gastroparesis because they can be dosed after a successful meal and still be effective.

27. **Discuss the role of the insulin pump during pregnancy.**
    Experience using the insulin pump in the treatment of type 1 diabetes in pregnancy is increasing. A nonrandomized trial in which 24 women began insulin pump therapy during pregnancy and were compared with 12 women using the pump before pregnancy and 24 women treated with multiple insulin injections found no deterioration of glycemic control. Maternal and perinatal outcomes were similar. However, 2 of 24 women who began using the pump in pregnancy developed ketoacidosis from pump failure; therefore, it may be optimal to begin pump therapy before pregnancy, given the steep learning curve involved in its use and the continuous changes that must be made in dosing basal and bolus insulins.

28. **Discuss the role of glargine during pregnancy.**
    Insulin glargine (Lantus) is not yet approved in pregnancy due to concerns about its potential mitogenic effects and higher affinity for the IGF-1 receptor. However, it does not cross the placenta, and no evidence indicates reproductive toxicity or embryotoxicity. If a patient without proliferative retinopathy is doing well on insulin glargine, it is probably not necessary to switch her to another insulin during pregnancy.

29. **How common is hypoglycemia in pregnant women with type 1 diabetes?**
    Maternal hypoglycemia is common and often severe in pregnant women with type 1 diabetes. In one series, hypoglycemia requiring assistance occurred in 71% of patients, with a peak incidence at 10–15 weeks. One-third of the women had at least one episode resulting in seizures,

loss of consciousness, or injury, any of which may have long-term effects on the offspring, including neuropsychological defects. Current data suggest that the counter-regulatory hormonal response to hypoglycemia is diminished in pregnancy. The physician must have a low threshold for bringing the expectant mother into the hospital to optimize education and glycemic control. Occasional monitoring in the middle of the night is recommended in women with type 1 diabetes because of the increased risk of nocturnal hypoglycemia, especially if they have hypoglycemia unawareness.

30. **Discuss special concerns in pregnant women with type 2 diabetes.**
Women with type 2 diabetes may be able to achieve optimal glycemic control with twice-daily injections; however, postprandial hyperglycemia has been recently shown to be better treated with three daily injections of a rapid-acting insulin, even in gestational diabetes. Failure to achieve optimal control in early pregnancy in women with any type of preexisting diabetes may have teratogenic effects or lead to early fetal loss. Poor control later in pregnancy increases the risk of intrauterine fetal demise, macrosomia, and metabolic complications in the newborn. An early dating ultrasound is necessary to accurately determine the gestational age of the fetus and a formal anatomy scan at 18–20 weeks should be performed to evaluate for fetal anomalies. A fetal echocardiogram should be offered at 20–22 weeks if the HbA1C was elevated during the first trimester.

31. **What is the risk of diabetic ketoacidosis (DKA) in pregnancy?**
Pregnancy predisposes to accelerated starvation, which can result in ketonuria after an overnight fast. DKA may thus occur at lower glucose levels (often referred to as "euglycemic DKA") due to the increased glomerular glucose filtration, continuous glucose utilization by the fetal–placental unit, and increased volume of distribution of glucose due to a 30–40% expansion of plasma volume. Women also have a lower buffering capacity due to the progesterone-induced respiratory alkalosis, which results in a compensatory metabolic acidosis. A rapid switch from carbohydrate metabolism to lipolysis occurs in pregnant women who have depleted their glycogen stores after a 12-hour fast, resulting in a starvation ketoacidosis.

32. **How should the risk of DKA be managed?**
Any pregnant women with type 1 diabetes who is unable to keep down food or fluids should check urine ketones at home; and, if the results are positive, a chemistry panel should be ordered to rule out an anion gap, even if the maternal glucose is <200 mg/dL. Often the only precipitant for DKA in pregnancy is nausea and vomiting, but the possibility of an infection, particularly pyelonephritis, should be aggressively investigated. Women with type 2 diabetes and even women with gestational diabetes can also develop DKA, especially in the context of prolonged fasting, infections, use of beta agonists for preterm labor, or steroids to promote fetal lung maturity.

33. **How does maternal DKA affect the fetus?**
In a study of 20 consecutive cases of DKA, only 65% of the fetuses were alive on admission to the hospital. Risk factors for fetal loss included DKA presenting later in pregnancy (32 weeks versus 24 weeks), high insulin requirements, and longer duration of DKA. Electrolyte disturbances and fetal hypoxemia are additional risk factors for fetal death. The fetal heart rate, therefore, must be monitored continuously until the acidosis has resolved.

34. **What must the physician remember about DKA in pregnant women?**
Pregnant women unable to take oral nutrients require an additional 100–150 gm/day of intravenous glucose to meet the metabolic demands of the fetal–placental unit. Without adequate carbohydrate (often a D10 glucose solution is needed), fat will be burned for fuel and the patient in DKA will remain ketotic.

KEY POINTS: DIABETES IN PREGNANCY ✓

1. Although hyperglycemia is a major teratogen, the fetal malformation rate can be decreased from 25% to the normal baseline risk with optimal glycemic control prior to pregnancy and during the first 10 weeks of gestation.

2. DKA may occur at glucose levels < 200 mg/dL in pregnancy and may also occur in women with gestational diabetes.

3. Inadequately controlled gestational diabetes in the mother may place the fetus at risk for developing childhood obesity and glucose intolerance.

4. Women who develop gestational diabetes have ~50% risk of developing type 2 diabetes within 5–10 years.

5. Pregnancy does not usually accelerate the progression of diabetic nephropathy unless severe; however, proteinuria, diabetic retinopathy, and autonomic neuropathy may worsen.

6. Insulin requirements often decrease in the first trimester placing the mother at high risk of severe hypoglycemia, but requirements may double in the late second and third trimesters due to the insulin resistance of pregnancy.

35. **What is gestational diabetes?**
    Gestational diabetes mellitus (GDM) is a glucose-intolerant state with onset or first recognition during pregnancy. The incidence of GDM ranges from 2% to 14% of pregnancies throughout the world and is highest in ethnic groups that have a higher incidence of type 2 diabetes (Hispanic Americans, African Americans, Native Americans, and Pacific Islanders).

36. **How is GDM diagnosed?**
    The criteria for diagnosis in the United States have recently changed. The Carpenter and Coustan criteria have been adopted by the American Diabetes Association (ADA) and the Fourth International Workshop—Conference on Gestational Diabetes. Screening recommendations have been stratified according to low-risk status, average-risk status, and high-risk status of GDM. Most obstetricians employ universal screening of all women at 24–28 weeks, which is a reasonable approach, especially in a population that contains ethnic groups with a higher prevalence of GDM.

37. **Summarize the recommendations for low-risk status.**
    Low-risk status requires no glucose testing, but this category is limited to women meeting *all* of the following criteria: age < 25 years; weight normal before pregnancy; member of an ethnic group with a low prevalence of GDM; no known diabetes in first-degree relatives; no history of abnormal glucose tolerance; and no history of poor obstetric outcome or macrosomic infant.

38. **What are the recommendations for high-risk status?**
    High-risk status requires glucose testing as soon as pregnancy is diagnosed and again at 24–28 weeks if the early testing is normal. Women meeting *any* of the following criteria should be tested early: obesity; personal history of GDM or previous macrosomic infant; glycosuria; or strong family history of diabetes. Women with a fasting blood glucose > 125 mg/dL or a random or postprandial glucose > 200 mg/dL meet the criteria for diabetes, and this diagnosis precludes the need for any glucose challenge. All other high-risk women should be given a 50-gm glucose challenge (Glucola test) or proceed directly to a 100-gm oral glucose tolerance test (OGTT) as soon as they establish prenatal care. If initial testing is normal, repeat testing should be done at 24–28 weeks gestation.

39. **How should women of average risk be approached?**
    Women who do not fall in the low-risk or high-risk category should receive a 50-gm glucose challenge at 24–28 weeks. If the results are positive, they should undergo diagnostic testing with a 100-gm, 3-hour OGTT.

40. **Describe the 50-gm glucose challenge.**
    The 50-gm glucose challenge is the accepted screen for the presence of GDM in the United States, but a positive result must be followed by a diagnostic 100-gm, 3-hour OGTT. A positive screen is in the range of 130–140 mg/dL. The sensitivity and specificity of the test depend on what threshold value is chosen, and the cutoff may be selected according to the prevalence of GDM in the population being screened. The test does not have to be performed during a fasting state, but a serum sample must be drawn exactly 1 hour after administering the oral glucose.

41. **Describe the 100-gm, 3-hour OGTT.**
    The 100-gm, 3-hour test must be performed after 3 days of an unrestricted carbohydrate diet and while the patient is fasting. A positive test requires that two values be met or exceeded. One abnormal value should be followed with a repeated 3-hour test 1 month later because a single elevated value increases the risk of macrosomia and one-third of patients ultimately meet the diagnostic criteria for GDM (Table 5-2).

TABLE 5-2.	CRITERIA FOR A POSITIVE 100-GM OGTT
Fasting glucose	95 mg/dL
1-hour glucose	180 mg/dL
2-hour glucose	155 mg/dL
3-hour glucose	140 mg/dL

42. **Summarize the risks to the mother with GDM.**
    The immediate risks to the mother with GDM are an increased incidence of cesarean section (~30%), preeclampsia (~20–30%), and polyhydramnios (~20%), which can result in preterm labor. The long-term risks to the mother are related to recurrent GDM pregnancies and the substantial risk of developing type 2 diabetes mellitus.

43. **What factors increase the risk of subsequently developing type 2 diabetes?**
    Women with GDM have an extremely high risk (~50%) of developing type 2 diabetes in the subsequent 5–10 years. Risk factors include fasting hyperglycemia, GDM diagnosed prior to 24 weeks of gestation (preexisting glucose intolerance), obesity, membership in an ethnic group with a high prevalence of type 2 diabetes, and impaired glucose tolerance at 6 weeks postpartum. Women with GDM in multiple pregnancies also have a higher risk of developing type 2 diabetes.

44. **What factors may reduce the risk of developing type 2 diabetes?**
    Counseling with regard to diet, weight loss, and exercise is essential and is likely to improve insulin sensitivity, given the findings of the Diabetes Prevention Study. Such dietary modifications should be adopted by the family, since the infant is also at risk for developing obesity and the metabolic syndrome. Whether or not medications that may improve insulin sensitivity (metformin and thiazolidinediones) can be used in this group of high-risk patients to prevent the development of type 2 diabetes is under current investigation. One trial demonstrated that the use of a thiazolidinedione versus placebo postpartum decreased the rate of developing type 2 diabetes in 30 months from 12.1% to 5.4% in the 133 women randomized.

45. What is the incidence of complications in the infant of a mother with GDM?
Even with the advent of screening and aggressive management of GDM, the incidence of neonatal complications ranges from 12% to 28%.

46. Summarize the basic mechanism behind complications related to GDM.
Excessive transfer of glucose, amino acids, and free fatty acids from mother to fetus induces fetal hyperglycemia, which results in fetal pancreatic islet hypertrophy and beta-cell hyperplasia with consequent fetal hyperinsulinemia.

47. What is the most common complication of GDM?
The most common complication is macrosomia (Fig. 5-1). Increased fat synthesis by the fetus leads to adiposity and visceromegaly, which place the mother at increased risk of requiring a cesarean section and the infant at risk for shoulder dystocia. The excessive supply of nutrients causes an increase in fetal abdominal girth disproportionate to other body measurements, resulting in a difficult delivery.

48. What other complications may result from GDM?
- *Shoulder dystocia* can result in Erb's palsy, clavicular fractures, fetal distress, low APGAR scores, and even birth asphyxia when unrecognized.
- If mothers have poor glycemic control, *respiratory distress syndrome* may occur in up to 30% of infants due to decreased lung surfactant synthesis.
- *Cardiac septal hypertrophy* may be seen in 35–40%.
- With extremely poor glucose control, there is also an increased risk of *fetal mortality* as a result of fetal acidemia and hypoxia.
- Common *metabolic abnormalities* in the infant of a mother with GDM include neonatal hypoglycemia from sustained hyperinsulinemia, deficient lipolysis, and increased peripheral glucose uptake, as well as hypocalcemia, polycythemia, and hyperbilirubinemia.

49. Explain the fetoplacental glucose steal phenomenon.
Fetal hyperinsulinemia may cause exaggerated fetal siphoning of glucose from the mother, which blunts the maternal postload glucose peaks. This fetoplacental glucose steal phenomenon can actually decrease maternal glucose concentrations on an OGTT, leading to an illusion of improved glucose control. Maternal glucose monitoring alone may not accurately reflect the fetal metabolic situation when fetal hyperinsulinemia is present.

50. How is the glucose steal phenomenon managed?
It has become increasingly common to evaluate excessive fetal growth by measuring fetal abdominal circumference at 28–32 weeks and to intensify maternal medical therapy for fetuses whose abdominal

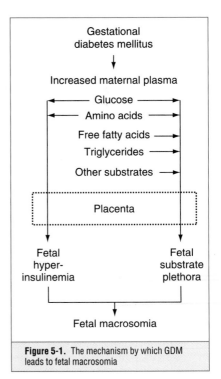

Figure 5-1. The mechanism by which GDM leads to fetal macrosomia

circumference is above the 70th percentile. Women with GDM who require medical therapy or with suboptimal glycemic control should undergo fetal surveillance at ~32 weeks' gestation, and an earlier delivery should be considered after fetal lung maturity is confirmed by amniocentesis. An estimated fetal weight of > 4500 gm carries such a high risk of shoulder dystocia that an elective cesarean section is usually recommended.

51. **Discuss the long-term sequelae of GDM in offspring of affected mothers.**
The long-term sequelae of GDM for offspring are much more controversial. Proliferation of fetal adipocytes and pancreatic beta cells may be responsible for "programming" the later development of obesity and the metabolic syndrome. Reports of an increased risk of adolescent obesity and type 2 diabetes are compelling. The incidence of childhood type 2 diabetes was ~10-fold higher in Pima Indian offspring born to mothers with diabetes compared with offspring whose mothers did not develop diabetes until after pregnancy. Furthermore, despite a similar incidence of obesity at 20 years of age between the two groups of offspring, the incidence of type 2 diabetes was ~70% at age 25–29 years in the offspring of diabetic mothers compared with ~10% in the offspring of prediabetic mothers.

52. **How does in utero hyperglycemia affect the long-term sequelae of GDM?**
In utero hyperglycemia appears to be an independent risk factor for the development of childhood glucose intolerance. Elevated insulin levels in amniotic fluid (owing to fetal hyperinsulinemia as a result of maternal hyperglycemia) predicted teenage obesity in one study, independently of fetal weight, and one-third of these offspring had impaired glucose tolerance by 17 years of age. Fetal imprinting appears to occur in this intrauterine environment of nutrient excess and may contribute to the growing incidence of type 2 diabetes as children with impaired glucose tolerance become mothers themselves, perpetuating the cycle.

53. **What causes women to get GDM?**
GDM is caused by abnormalities in at least three aspects of fuel metabolism: insulin resistance, increased hepatic glucose production, and impaired insulin secretion.

54. **Explain the cause of insulin resistance.**
Insulin resistance is thought to be due primarily to the effects of increased production of human placental lactogen and placental growth hormone. Women developing GDM have a lower pregravid insulin sensitivity compared with matched control groups, and some abnormalities may persist after delivery.

55. **What causes increased hepatic glucose production?**
Increased hepatic glucose production results from inadequate insulin suppression of excessive hepatic gluconeogenesis. Beta-cell sensing of glucose is also abnormal and is manifested as an inadequate insulin response for a given degree of hyperglycemia.

56. **Summarize the role of impaired insulin secretion.**
Impaired insulin secretion renders the woman unable to meet the requirement for greater insulin production necessitated by the insulin resistance and increased hepatic glucose production. These same pathophysiologic disorders, which are in large part genetically determined, make the patient with GDM more likely to develop type 2 diabetes mellitus later in life when weight gain and aging often contribute further to insulin resistance and impaired insulin secretion. Pregnancy can be thought of as a "stress test" for the development of type 2 diabetes, since the marked insulin resistance of pregnancy necessitates a 2- to 3-fold increase in insulin secretion that the beta cell may not be able to achieve, resulting in a clinically evident abnormality in glucose metabolism.

57. **What is the best therapy for women with GDM?**

Women with GDM should be taught home glucose monitoring to ensure that glycemic goals are met throughout the duration of pregnancy. The best therapy for GDM depends entirely on the extent of the glucose intolerance and on the mother's response. In at least half of the cases, diet alone maintains the postprandial blood glucose values within the target range but is more likely to fail if fasting hyperglycemia exists. Since postprandial glucose levels have been most strongly associated with the risk of macrosomia (De Viciana 1995), modest carbohydrate restriction to 35–40% of total calories may be helpful to blunt the postprandial glucose excursions. Women with a body mass index (BMI) > 30 kg/m^2 may benefit from a 30–34% caloric restriction to ~25 kcal/kg, which has been shown to reduce hyperglycemia and plasma triglycerides with no increase in ketonuria.

58. **Discuss the role of oral diabetes medication in the management of GDM.**

None of the oral diabetes medications (sulfonylureas, metformin, acarbose, or thiazolidinediones) are currently approved for use in pregnancy. However, in a multicenter trial, 400 women with GDM were randomized to receive either insulin or glyburide after 24 weeks' gestation. Maternal glycemic control, macrosomia, neonatal hypoglycemia, and neonatal outcomes were not different between the groups. Most importantly, the cord serum insulin concentrations were similar between the two groups, and glyburide was not detected in the cord serum of any infant tested (Langer 2000).

59. **When should insulin be used to treat GDM?**

Women who have fasting blood glucose levels > 95 mg/dL, 1-hour postprandial glucose levels > 140 mg/dL, or 2-hour postprandial glucose levels > 120 mg/dL should be started on insulin therapy. Those who are unwilling to start insulin may be candidates for glyburide therapy. Women with a fetus that is large for gestational age, as demonstrated by ultrasound, are also candidates for medical management. GDM can usually be treated with twice-daily injections of NPH and regular insulin, but occasionally postprandial glycemic excursions are so excessive that mealtime injections of a short-acting insulin are necessary. Hypoglycemia tends to be an infrequent occurrence in such patients because of their underlying insulin resistance.

60. **What is the role of exercise in patients with GDM?**

Moderate exercise is well tolerated in pregnancy. Fetal safety has been established if the maternal heart rate is maintained < 140 beats/minute at durations of 30 minutes and if the mother is well hydrated and does not get overheated. Two of three trials in pregnancy have shown that exercise three times a week can achieve glycemic control and infant birth weights that are similar to those seen in women who are treated with insulin. Establishing a regular routine of modest exercise during pregnancy may also have long-lasting benefits for the mother with GDM, who clearly has an appreciable risk of developing type 2 diabetes in the future. Home glucose monitoring must be continued throughout pregnancy to determine whether or not insulin therapy is necessary.

61. **When is a controlled exercise program contraindicated?**

Women at risk for preterm labor or conditions predisposing to growth restriction are not candidates for a controlled exercise program.

62. **What important postpartum management issues should be addressed in women with pregestational or gestational diabetes?**

Critical issues in the postpartum period include maintenance of glycemic control, diet, exercise, weight loss, blood pressure management, breast-feeding, contraception, and postpartum thyroiditis. The majority of women, even those who have been extremely compliant and have had optimal glycemic control during pregnancy, experience a dramatic worsening of glucose control after delivery. Furthermore, many quit seeking medical care for their diabetes. The postpartum period is relatively neglected as both the new mother and her physician relax their vigilance. However, this period offers a unique opportunity to institute health habits that can have highly beneficial effects on the quality of life of both the mother and her infant.

63. **Explain the value of diet and exercise in the postpartum period.**
A weight loss program consisting of diet and exercise should be instituted for women with GDM to improve insulin sensitivity and prevent the development of type 2 diabetes.

64. **Discuss the importance of monitoring during the postpartum period.**
Home glucose monitoring should be continued in the postpartum period because insulin requirements drop almost immediately and often dramatically at this time, increasing the risk of hypoglycemia. In women with a history of GDM, glycemic status should be reassessed at 6 weeks after delivery. Hyperglycemia generally resolves in the majority of patients during this interval but may persist in up to 10%. At the minimum, a fasting blood glucose should be performed to determine whether the woman has persistent diabetes (glucose > 125 mg/dL) or impaired fasting glucose (glucose of at least 100 mg/dL). A 75-gm, 2-hour glucose tolerance test is recommended by the ADA and ACOG, since a 2-hour value of at least 200 mg/dL establishes a diagnosis of diabetes and a 2-hour value of at least 140 mg/dL but less than 200 mg/dL makes the diagnosis of impaired glucose tolerance. The majority of women with persistent impaired glucose tolerance will be missed if only a fasting blood glucose level is checked.

65. **Why is diagnosis of impaired glucose tolerance of critical importance?**
The importance of diagnosing impaired glucose intolerance lies in its value in predicting the future development of type 2 diabetes. In one series, a diagnosis of impaired glucose tolerance was the most potent predictor of the development of type 2 diabetes in women with a history of GDM; 80% of such women developed diabetes in the subsequent 5–7 years. Intensified efforts promoting diet, exercise, and weight loss should be instituted in such patients given that the Diabetes Prevention Trial demonstrated a > 50% reduction in the development of type 2 diabetes with diet and exercise in a different population of patients with impaired glucose tolerance.

66. **Summarize the role of ACE inhibitors in the postpartum period.**
Women who are candidates for an ACE inhibitor can be started on enalapril, which has not been shown to appear in breast milk at appreciable concentrations.

67. **Should women with GDM breast-feed their infants?**
Women should be encouraged to breast-feed unless difficulties in glycemic control arise. None of the oral agents are approved for use during breast-feeding. It appears that the sulfonylureas and metformin cross into breast milk. It is recommended that insulin be continued in diabetic mothers who choose to breast-feed. Women with a history of GDM who breast-feed appear to have a lower incidence of developing type 2 diabetes. Breast-feeding also appears to decrease the risk of infant obesity and impaired glucose tolerance. In a woman with type 1 diabetes, an additional 300–400 kcal/day is needed to maintain weight with breast-feeding. The mother also needs to make sure that her calcium intake is at least 1500 mg/day.

68. **How common is postpartum thyroiditis? When does it appear?**
Women with type 1 diabetes have been reported to have a 25% incidence of postpartum thyroiditis. Hyperthyroidism can occur in the 2- to 4-month postpartum period, and hypothyroidism may present in the 4- to 8-month period. Given the significance of this disorder, measurement of thyroid-stimulating hormone (TSH) should be offered in all type 1 patients at 6 months after delivery and before this time if a patient has symptoms.

69. **Summarize the long-term follow-up of nondiabetic women with a history of GDM.**

    In nondiabetic women with a history of GDM, fasting glucose levels should be measured once or twice a year, depending on individual risk factors for developing type 2 diabetes. Risk factors include fasting hyperglycemia in pregnancy, insulin requirement in pregnancy, obesity, strong family history, and degree of abnormality on their postpartum glucose tolerance test.

70. **Which contraceptive agents can be used by women with diabetes or a history of GDM?**

    It should be documented at every visit that women are using or have been offered an effective birth control method. The vast majority of contraceptive methods are relatively safe in women with diabetes who do not have poorly controlled hypertension or hypertriglyceridemia and who are not at increased risk for thromboembolic disease. Triglycerides should be measured after the initiation of oral contraceptives in all women with diabetes or a history of GDM because of the significant incidence of hypertriglyceridemia and the associated risk of pancreatitis with oral estrogen use.

71. **Summarize the role of low-dose combined oral contraceptives.**

    Low-dose combined oral contraceptives have been shown to be effective and have minimal metabolic effects in women with diabetes. The Ortho Evra patch and Nuva Ring have not been studied to determine whether they offer even fewer metabolic side effects. In a retrospective cohort of 904 women with GDM, combined oral contraceptives did not influence the development of type 2 diabetes.

72. **What other contraceptive options are appropriate?**

    Progestational agents, such as Depo-Provera or norethindrone, are also alternatives, although they may slightly affect carbohydrate tolerance. There is no increase in pelvic inflammatory disease with the use of intrauterine devices in women with well-controlled type 1 or type 2 diabetes after the postinsertion period. Therefore, this may be an attractive choice in older women who do not desire future pregnancies.

BIBLIOGRAPHY

1. American Diabetes Association: Preconception care of women with diabetes. Diabetes Care 26:S91–S93, 2003.
2. American Diabetes Association: Gestational diabetes mellitus. Diabetes Care 26:S103–S105, 2003.
3. Artal R: Exercise: The alternative therapeutic intervention for gestational diabetes. Clin Obstet Gynecol 46:479–487, 2003.
4. Barbour LA: New concepts in insulin resistance of pregnancy and gestational diabetes: Long-term implications for mother and offspring. J Obstet Gynaecol 24:545–549, 2003.
5. Barbour LA, Shao J, Qiao L, et al: Human placental growth hormone causes severe insulin resistance in transgenic mice. Am J Obstet Gynecol 186:512–517, 2002.
6. Buchanan TA, Xiang AH, Peters RK, et al: Preservation of pancreatic beta-cell function and prevention of type 2 diabetes by pharmacological treatment of insulin resistance in high-risk Hispanic women. Diabetes 51:2796–2803, 2002.
7. Carrapato MRG: The offspring of gestational diabetes. J Perinat Med 31:5–11, 2003.
8. Catalano PM, Kirwan JP, Haugel-de Mouzon S, King J: Gestational diabetes and insulin resistance: Role in short- and long-term implications for mother and fetus. J Nutr 133:1674S–1683S, 2003.
9. Conway DL, Langer O: Effects of new criteria for type 2 diabetes on the rate of postpartum glucose intolerance in women with gestational diabetes. Am J Obstet Gynecol 191:610–614, 1999.
10. Dabelea D, Knowler WC, Pettett DJ: Effect of diabetes in pregnancy on offspring: Follow-up research in the Pima Indians. J Mat Fet Med 9:83–88, 2000.
11. Diabetes Control and Complications Research Group: Pregnancy outcomes in the diabetes control and complications trial. Am J Obstet Gynecol 177:1165–1171, 1996.

12. Diabetes Prevention Program Research Group: Reduction in the incidence of type 2 diabetes with lifestyle intervention or metformin. N Engl J Med 346:393–403, 2002.

13. Gabbe SG, Holing E, Temple P, Brown ZA: Benefits, risks, costs, and patient satisfaction associated with insulin pump therapy for the pregnancy complicated by type 1 diabetes mellitus. Am J Obstet Gynecol 182:1283–1291, 2000.

14. Gestational diabetes. ACOG Practice Bull 30:525–538, 2001.

15. Glueck CJ, Wang P, Goldenberg N, Sieve-Smith L: Pregnancy outcomes among women with polycystic ovary syndrome treated with metformin. Human Reprod 17:2858–2864, 2002.

16. Glueck CJ, Wang P, Kobayashi S, et al: Metformin therapy throughout pregnancy reduces the development of gestational diabetes in women with polycystic ovary syndrome. Fert Steril 77:520–525, 2002.

17. Hellmuth E, Damm P, Molsted-Pederson L: Oral hypoglycemic agents in 118 diabetic pregnancies. Diabetic Med 17:507–511, 2000.

18. Hofmann T, Horstmann G, Stammberger I: Evaluation of the reproductive toxicity and embryotoxicity of insulin glargine (LANTUS) in rats and rabbits. Int J Toxicol 21:181–189, 2002.

19. Jakubowicz DJ, Iuorno MJ, Jakubowicz S, et al: Effects of metformin on early pregnancy loss in the polycystic ovary syndrome. J Clin Endocrinol Metab 87:524–529, 2002.

20. Kenshole A, Ray J, Keely E: Type 1 and type 2 diabetes. In Lee RV, Rosene-Montella K, Barbour LA, et al (eds): Medical Care of the Pregnant Patient. Philadelphia, American College of Physicians, 2000, pp 253–272.

21. Kim C, Newton KM, Knopp RH: Gestational diabetes and the incidence of type 2 diabetes. Diabetes Care 25:1862–1868, 2002.

22. Kjos SL: Postpartum care of the woman with diabetes. Clin Obstet Gynecol 43:75–90, 2000.

23. Kjos SL, Peters RJ, Xiang A, et al: Predicting future diabetes in Latino women with gestational diabetes. Diabetes 44:586–591, 1995.

24. DeViciana M, Major CA, Morgan MA, et al: Postprandial versus preprandial blood glucose monitoring in women gestational diabetes requiring insulin therapy. N Engl J Med 333:1237–1241, 1995.

25. Buchanan TA, Kjos SI, Montoro MN, et al: use of fetal ultrasound to select metabolic therapy for pregnancies complicated by mild gestational diabetes. Diabetes care 17:275–283, 1994.

26. Langer O, Conway DL, Berkus MD, et al: A comparison of glyburide and insulin in women with gestational diabetes. N Engl J Med 343:1134–1138, 2000.

27. Martorell R, Stein AD, Schroeder DG: Early nutrition and later adiposity. J Nutr 131:874S–880S, 2001.

28. Petitt DJ, Ospina P, Kolaczynski JW, Jovanovic L: Comparison of an insulin analog, insulin aspart, and regular human insulin with no insulin in gestational diabetes mellitus. Diabetes Care 26:183–186, 2003.

29. Reece EA, Homko CJ: Why do diabetic women deliver malformed infants? Clin Obstet Gynecol 43:32–45, 2000.

30. Rossing K, Jacobsen P, Hommel E, et al: Pregnancy and progression of diabetic nephropathy. Diabetologia 45:36–41, 2002.

31. Sabai BM, Caritis S, Hauth J, et al: Risks of preeclampsia and adverse neonatal outcomes among women with pregestational diabetes mellitus. Am J Obstet Gynecol 182:364–369, 2000.

32. Stamm CA, Barbour LA, McGrefor JA: Effective birth control for women with medical disorders. In Lee RV, Rosene-Montella K, Barbour LA, et al (eds): Medical Care of the Pregnant Patient. Philadelphia, American College of Physicians, 2000, pp 19–33.

33. Temple RC, Aldridge VA, Sampson MJ et al: Impact of pregnancy on the progression of diabetic retinopathy in type 1 diabetes. Diabetic Med 18:573–577, 2001.

34. Weiss PAM, Scholz HS, Haas J, Tamussino KF: Effect of fetal hyperinsulinism on oral glucose tolerance test results in patients with gestational diabetes mellitus. Am J Obstet Gynecol 184:470–475, 2001.

35. Yamashita H, Shao J, Friedman JE: Physiologic and molecular alterations in carbohydrate metabolism during pregnancy and gestational diabetes. Clini Obstet Gynecol 43:87–98, 2000.

CHAPTER 6

HYPOGLYCEMIA

Michael T. McDermott, M.D., and Fred D. Hofeldt, M.D.

1. **Define hypoglycemia.**
   Hypoglycemia is currently defined as a blood glucose value of less than 50 mg/dL (2.8 mmol/L). Clinically, hypoglycemia is defined by Whipple's triad: low plasma glucose level, symptoms consistent with hypoglycemia, and resolution of symptoms with correction of the low glucose level.

2. **What are the important clinical symptoms of hypoglycemia?**
   The symptoms of hypoglycemia can be divided into two categories as follows. *Adrenergic symptoms* are catecholamine-mediated and include diaphoresis, palpitations, apprehension, anxiety, headaches, and weakness. *Neuroglycopenic symptoms* include reduced intellectual capacity, confusion, irritability, abnormal behavior, convulsions, and coma.

3. **What is the importance of the timing of symptoms in relation to food intake?**
   The timing of symptoms is helpful in determining the etiology of the hypoglycemia. *Fasting hypoglycemia* refers to low blood glucose that occurs more than 5 hours after a meal, especially after missed meals or an overnight fast. This type frequently produces symptoms of neuroglycopenia and often results from an organic etiology. *Postprandial hypoglycemia* (reactive hypoglycemia) occurs within 5 hours of the previous meal. It is usually associated with adrenergic symptoms and is thought to arise from a functional disorder. Although this separation is important for clinical classification, it is artificial and patients may have mixed-component symptoms.

4. **What causes fasting hypoglycemia?**
   See Table 6-1.

5. **What causes postprandial or reactive hypoglycemia?**
   See Table 6-2.

6. **What are the artifactual causes of hypoglycemia?**
   Pseudohypoglycemia occurs in certain chronic leukemias when the leukocyte counts are markedly elevated. This artifactual hypoglycemia reflects utilization of glucose by leukocytes after the blood sample has been drawn. Pseudohypoglycemia may also occur with hemolytic anemia or polycythemia through similar mechanisms. Other artifactual hypoglycemias may be seen with improper sample collection or storage, errors in analytic methodology, or confusion between whole-blood and plasma glucose values. Plasma glucose is about 15% higher than corresponding whole-blood glucose values.

7. **When hypoglycemia occurs, what counter-regulatory events spare glucose for brain metabolism?**
   Glucagon and epinephrine are the dominant counter-regulatory hormones. Other hormones that respond to hypoglycemic stress are norepinephrine, cortisol, and growth hormone, but their effects are delayed. The metabolic effects of glucagon and epinephrine are immediate; stimulation of hepatic glycogenolysis and later gluconeogenesis results in increased hepatic glucose production. Glucagon appears to be the most important counter-regulatory hormone during

TABLE 6-1. CAUSES OF FASTING HYPOGLYCEMIA

Pancreatic disorders
- Islet beta-cell hyperfunction (adenoma, carcinoma, hyperplasia, nesidioblastosis)
- Islet alpha-cell hypofunction or deficiency

Hepatic disorders
- Severe liver disease (cirrhosis, hepatitis, carcinomatosis, circulatory failure, ascending cholangitis)
- Enzyme defects (glycogen-storage disease, galactosemia, hereditary fructose intolerance, familial galactose and fructose intolerance, fructose-1,6-diphosphatase deficiency)

Pituitary-adrenal disorders
- Hypopituitarism
- Addison's disease
- Congenital adrenal hyperplasia

Nonpancreatic neoplasms
- Mesodermal tumors (spindle-cell fibrosarcoma, leiomyosarcoma, mesothelioma, rhabdomyosarcoma, liposarcoma, neurofibroma, reticulum-cell sarcoma)
- Adenocarcinoma (hepatoma, cholangiocarcinoma, gastric carcinoma, adrenocortical carcinoma, cecal carcinoma)

Unclassified causes
- Excessive loss or utilization of glucose and/or deficient substrate (prolonged or strenuous exercise, fever, lactation, pregnancy, renal glycosuria, diarrheal states, chronic starvation)
- Ketotic hypoglycemia of childhood (idiopathic hypoglycemia of childhood)

Exogenous causes
- Iatrogenic (related to treatment with insulin or oral hypoglycemic agents)
- Factitious insulin, sulfonylurea or meglitinide use (seen especially in paramedical personnel)
- Pharmacologic (Akee nut, salicylates, antihistamines, monoamine oxidase inhibitors, propranolol)
- Phenylbutazone, pentamidine, phentolamine, alcohol, ACE-inhibitors

acute hypoglycemia. If glucagon secretion is decreased or absent, epinephrine serves as the principal counter-regulatory hormone.

8. **Which conditions cause islet beta-cell hyperfunction?**
The insulinoma syndrome is caused by a pancreatic islet cell adenoma in 75–85% of cases. Multiple adenomas (adenomatosis) are present in about 10% of cases. Carcinomas cause 5–6% of cases, and an additional 5–10% have islet-cell hyperplasia.

9. **If other family members have pancreatic tumors, what condition is suggested?**
Multiple endocrine neoplasia type 1 (MEN-1) occurs as an autosomal dominant condition characterized by functioning and nonfunctioning pituitary tumors, parathyroid hyperplasia, and islet-cell tumors, most commonly insulinomas and gastrinomas (Zollinger-Ellison syndrome). When

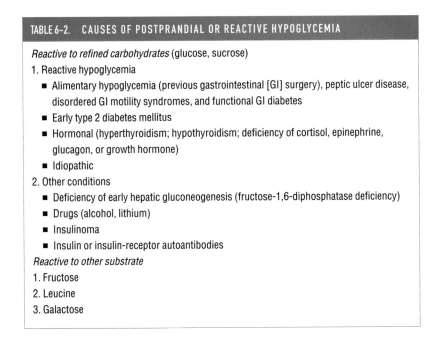

TABLE 6-2. CAUSES OF POSTPRANDIAL OR REACTIVE HYPOGLYCEMIA

Reactive to refined carbohydrates (glucose, sucrose)
1. Reactive hypoglycemia
   - Alimentary hypoglycemia (previous gastrointestinal [GI] surgery), peptic ulcer disease, disordered GI motility syndromes, and functional GI diabetes
   - Early type 2 diabetes mellitus
   - Hormonal (hyperthyroidism; hypothyroidism; deficiency of cortisol, epinephrine, glucagon, or growth hormone)
   - Idiopathic
2. Other conditions
   - Deficiency of early hepatic gluconeogenesis (fructose-1,6-diphosphatase deficiency)
   - Drugs (alcohol, lithium)
   - Insulinoma
   - Insulin or insulin-receptor autoantibodies

Reactive to other substrate
1. Fructose
2. Leucine
3. Galactose

MEN-1 is suspected, family members should be screened for its components. However, only about 5–10% of insulinomas are associated with MEN-1.

10. **Which laboratory tests are useful in evaluation of fasting hypoglycemia?**
    Simultaneous measurement of fasting blood glucose and insulin levels during the occurrence of symptoms is the most important laboratory test. Other potentially important tests include C-peptide, proinsulin, sulfonylurea levels, renal and liver function, insulin antibody levels, and plasma cortisol.

11. **What is hyperinsulinemic hypoglycemia?**
    Hyperinsulinemic hypoglycemia refers to an episode of hypoglycemia associated with an elevated serum insulin level and insulin-to-glucose ratio (I/G ratio > 0.33). Hyperinsulinemic hypoglycemia suggests islet beta-cell hyperfunction (insulinoma, hyperplasia) or the factitious use of insulin or hypoglycemic agents. Hypoinsulinemic hypoglycemia points to a cause not mediated by insulin.

12. **How do you distinguish an insulinoma from factitious hypoglycemia?**
    Insulinomas are characterized by elevated insulin and C-peptide values, and proinsulin levels that may be as much as 80% of total insulin (normal: 10–20%). Factitious insulin administration is identified by finding elevated serum insulin but decreased levels of C-peptide and proinsulin, since endogenous insulin secretion is suppressed. Circulating insulin antibodies are also evidence of insulin administration. Factitious sulfonylurea or meglitinide ingestion is suggested by finding elevated insulin and C-peptide but normal proinsulin levels. Drug screens are usually necessary for verification.

13. **When an insulinoma work-up is inconclusive, what additional studies may be performed?**
    A supervised 48-hour fast with measurements of glucose and insulin every 6 hours, and any time the patient becomes symptomatic, will unmask the hypoglycemia in most patients with

insulinomas. Hypoglycemia is usually evident within 24 hours of fasting. Exercise often evokes hypoglycemia in the patient with insulinoma who remains asymptomatic after 48 hours of fasting.

14. **What procedures are helpful to localize the cause of pancreatic islet-cell hyperinsulinemia?**
Ultrasound, celiac angiography, aortography, and abdominal CT scan are frequently insensitive and localize only about 60% of insulinomas. Some insulinomas are extremely small (less than a few millimeters) and easily escape detection. Endoscopic ultrasonography may be useful in these cases. Transhepatic portal venous sampling may localize occult tumors and help to distinguish between an isolated insulinoma and diffuse disease (adenomatosis or hyperplasia). Intraoperative ultrasound is also useful for localizing pancreatic tumors.

15. **If surgical resection is not possible or the patient has metastatic or inoperable carcinoma, adenomatosis or hyperplasia, what medications may control the hypoglycemia?**
Diet (frequent feeding and snacks) is the cornerstone of medical management. The most commonly used medication is diazoxide, which inhibits insulin release. Phenytoin, propranolol, verapamil, and octreotide have also been used. Various chemotherapeutic agents can be used for islet-cell carcinoma.

16. **What is the leading cause of childhood hypoglycemia?**
Although hyperinsulinemic hypoglycemia in children can result from the same diseases that cause this condition in adults, nesidioblastosis is the leading cause in newborns and infants. Nesidioblastosis is a type of islet-cell hyperplasia in which primordial pancreatic ductal cells remain undifferentiated islet cells capable of polyhormonal secretion (insulin, gastrin, pancreatic polypeptide, and glucagon).

KEY POINTS: HYPOGLYCEMIA ✔

1. Fasting hypoglycemia often produces neuroglycopenic symptoms and is frequently due to an organic disorder or surreptitious use of insulin or oral hypoglycemic medications.

2. Patients with fasting hypoglycemia should be tested during a symptomatic episode or a 48-hour supervised fast with measurements of serum glucose, insulin, and C-peptide and a drug screen for sulfonylureas and meglitinides.

3. Treatment of fasting hypoglycemia involves correction of the underlying disorder or multiple frequent feedings and/or medications, such as diazoxide.

4. Postprandial (reactive) hypoglycemia usually produces adrenergic symptoms and is most often a functional disorder related to dietary indiscretion or anxiety and stress but occasionally is due to rapid gastric emptying or early type 2 diabetes mellitus.

5. Treatment of reactive hypoglycemia involves primarily dietary changes and management of any existing sources of excess anxiety and stress.

17. **Which inherited disorders may be associated with hypoinsulinemic hypoglycemia in infants and young children?**
Hypoinsulinemic hypoglycemia in infants and young children suggests an inherited disorder of intermediary metabolism, such as the glycogen storage diseases, gluconeogenic disorders (deficiencies of fructose-1,6-diphosphatase, pyruvate carboxylase, and phosphoenolpyruvate

carboxykinase), galactosemia, hereditary fructose intolerance, maple syrup urine disease, carnitine deficiency, and ketotic hypoglycemia.

18. **List the other possible causes of hypoglycemia in children.**
    - Hormonal deficiencies (glucagon, growth hormone, thyroid, and adrenal hormones).
    - Accidental drug overdose, especially with salicylates and alcohol.

19. **Which drugs most commonly cause hypoglycemia in adults?**
    Drugs are the most common cause of hypoglycemia in adults. Responsible drugs include insulin, the diabetic oral agents, angiotensin-converting enzyme (ACE)-inhibitors, ethanol, propranolol, and pentamidine. An extensive list of drugs associated with hypoglycemia in 1418 cases is included in the reference by Seltzer.

20. **How does alcohol cause hypoglycemia?**
    Ethanol can cause hypoglycemia 6–36 hours after ingestion of even modest amounts (100 gm). Alcohol acutely inhibits hepatic gluconeogenesis through alterations of the cytosol $NADH_2/NAD$ ratio. Hypoglycemia from alcohol ingestion generally occurs only in patients who also have impaired glycogenolysis due to depletion of hepatic glycogen stores from fasting or chronic malnutrition. It is, therefore, the combination of acutely impaired gluconeogenesis and ineffective glycogenolysis that results in alcohol-induced hypoglycemia.

21. **What non–islet-cell tumors cause hypoglycemia?**
    Hypoglycemia can occur with mesenchymal tumors (mesothelioma, fibrosarcoma, liposarcoma, rhabdomyosarcoma, leiomyosarcoma, hemangiopericytoma), adenocarcinomas (liver, adrenal, breast, genitourinary), pheochromocytomas, carcinoid tumors, and hematologic malignancies (leukemia, lymphomas, myeloma).

22. **By what mechanisms do non-islet-cell tumors cause hypoglycemia?**
    The mechanisms vary according to the tumor type but include glucose utilization by some large tumors; malnutrition with fat and muscle wasting; production of catabolic cytokines, such as tumor necrosis factor; and production of insulin-like growth factors (IGF-1 and IGF-2) that bind to insulin receptors to promote hypoglycemia. Rarely does a tumor secrete insulin.

23. **What autoimmune syndromes are associated with hypoglycemia?**
    Autoantibodies directed against insulin receptors or insulin itself may provoke hypoglycemia. Antireceptor antibodies bind directly to the insulin receptor and thereby mimic insulin action in tissues. Anti-insulin antibodies bind circulating insulin and sometimes dissociate from insulin at inappropriate times, often during the early postprandial fasting period. This process acutely raises serum-free insulin levels, causing hypoglycemia. This disorder has been observed most often in Japanese patients, usually in association with other autoimmune diseases, such as Graves' disease, rheumatoid arthritis, systemic lupus erythematosus, and type 1 diabetes mellitus.

24. **What other endocrine disorders are associated with hypoglycemia?**
    Hypoglycemia may be seen in patients with anterior pituitary insufficiency due to deficient secretion of growth hormone, adrenocorticotropic hormone, and thyroid-stimulating hormone. In addition, primary adrenal insufficiency and primary hypothyroidism may be associated with either fasting or reactive hypoglycemia.

25. **When is hypoglycemia attributed to underlying medical illness?**
    Frequently, medically ill patients have multiple reasons for developing hypoglycemia, including renal failure, hepatic dysfunction, medications, and poor dietary intake. Hepatic failure leads to hypoglycemia because of the liver's role in gluconeogenesis and glycogenolysis. The hypoglycemia of congestive heart failure, sepsis, and lactic acidosis is also likely due to hepatic

dysfunction. Starvation states, such as anorexia nervosa and protein calorie malnutrition, also cause hypoglycemia.

26. **How is reactive hypoglycemia diagnosed?**

Reactive hypoglycemia occurs within 5 hours of food intake (usually between 2–4 hours). The diagnosis is made by eliminating other causes of the symptoms and documenting hypoglycemia during the occurrence of symptoms. The supervised 48-hour fast can exclude an insulinoma. The oral glucose tolerance test probably no longer plays a role in the diagnosis.

27. **What conditions cause reactive hypoglycemia?**

Reactive hypoglycemia can be caused by gastrointestinal disorders (alimentary hypoglycemia), hormone deficiencies, and early type 2 diabetes mellitus. However, the vast majority of patients have idiopathic reactive hypoglycemia with no underlying cause apparent. Most patients with idiopathic reactive hypoglycemia have a delayed discharge of insulin (dysinsulinism) that occurs inappropriately after postprandial glucose levels have peaked and are already beginning to fall. Hypoglycemia following meals can also occur in patients with insulinomas, pheochromocytomas, the insulin autoantibody syndrome described earlier, and with the use of lithium. Reactive hypoglycemia also has been noted in some patients who consume gin-and-tonic cocktails. In this type of hypoglycemia, the alcohol impairs epinephrine and growth hormone counter-hormonal responsiveness to the hypoglycemic stress.

28. **What conditions should be considered in the patient self-diagnosed with hypoglycemia?**

This type of hypoglycemia may be more correctly termed idiopathic postprandial syndrome. Whipple's triad is usually not fulfilled, in that chemical hypoglycemia cannot be demonstrated during symptoms. Frequently, underlying neuropsychiatric disease, anxiety, or situational stress reactions are the real culprits of the episodic symptoms, which the patient characterizes or self-diagnoses as reactive hypoglycemia. Although hypoglycemic disorders are uncommon, symptoms suggestive of hypoglycemia are quite common.

BIBLIOGRAPHY

1. Arem R: Hypoglycemia associated with renal failure. Endocrinol Metab Clin North Am 18:103–121, 1989.
2. Arky RA: Hypoglycemia associated with liver disease and ethanol. Endocrinol Metab Clin North Am 18:75–90, 1989.
3. Field JB: Hypoglycemia: Definitions, clinical presentation, classification, and laboratory tests. Endocrinol Metab Clin North Am 18:27–44, 1989.
4. Flanagan D, Wood P, Sherwin R, et al: Gin and tonic and reactive hypoglycemia. J Clin Endocrinol Metab 83:796–800, 1998.
5. Haymond MW: Hypoglycemia in infants and children. Endocrinol Metab Clin North Am 18:211–252, 1989.
6. Hirshberg B, Livi A, Bartlett DL, et al: Forty-eight hour fast: The diagnostic test for insulinoma. J Clin Endocrinol Metab 85:3222–3226, 2000.
7. Hofeldt FD: Reactive hypoglycemia. Endocrinol Metab Clin North Am 18:185–201, 1989.
8. Palardy J, Haurarkova J, Lepage R, et al: Blood glucose measurements during symptomatic episodes in patients with suspected postprandial hypoglycemia. N Engl J Med 321:1421–1425, 1989.
9. Rosch T, Lightdale CJ, Botet JF, et al: Localization of pancreatic endocrine tumor by endoscopic ultrasonography. N Engl J Med 326:1726–1736, 1992.
10. Seltzer HS: Drug-induced hypoglycemia. Endocrinol Metab Clin North Am 18:163–183, 1989.
11. Service FJ: Hypoglycemic disorders. N Engl J Med 332:1144–1152, 1995.
12. Shapiro ET, Bell GI, Polonsky KS, et al: Tumor hypoglycemia: Relationship to high molecular weight insulin-like growth factor II. J Clin Invest 85:1672–1679, 1990.
13. Whipple AO: The surgical therapy of hyperinsulinism. J Int Chir 3:237–276, 1938.

LIPID DISORDERS

Michael T. McDermott, M.D.

CHAPTER 7

1. **What are the major lipids in the bloodstream?**
   Cholesterol and triglycerides (TGs) are the major circulating lipids. Cholesterol is utilized by all cells for the synthesis and repair of membranes and intracellular organelles and by the adrenal glands and gonads as a substrate to synthesize adrenal and gonadal steroid hormones. TGs are an energy source that can be stored as fat in adipose tissue or burned as fuel by muscle and other tissues.

2. **What are lipoproteins?**
   Cholesterol and TGs are not water-soluble and thus cannot be transported through the circulation as individual molecules. Lipoproteins are large spherical particles that package these lipids into a core surrounded by a shell of water-soluble proteins and phospholipids. Lipoproteins serve as vehicles that transport cholesterol and TGs from one part of the body to another.

3. **What are the major lipoproteins in the bloodstream?**
   Chylomicrons, very-low-density lipoproteins (VLDL), low-density lipoproteins (LDL), and high-density lipoproteins (HDL) are the major circulating lipoproteins. Their functions are shown in the following:

Lipoprotein	Function
Chylomicron	Transport exogenous TG from the gut to adipose tissue and muscle
VLDL	Transport endogenous TG from the liver to adipose tissue and muscle
LDL	Transport cholesterol from the liver to peripheral tissues
HDL	Transport cholesterol from peripheral tissues to the liver

4. **What are the apoproteins?**
   Apoproteins are located on the surface of the lipoproteins. They function as ligands for binding to lipoprotein receptors and as cofactors for metabolic enzymes. Their functions are listed in the following:

Apoprotein	Function
Apoprotein A	Ligand for peripheral HDL receptors
Apoprotein B	Ligand for peripheral LDL receptors
Apoprotein E	Ligand for hepatic receptors for remnant particles
Apoprotein C-II	Cofactor for lipoprotein lipase (LPL)

5. **Name other enzymes and transport proteins that are important in lipoprotein metabolism.**
   See Table 7-1.

TABLE 7-1. ENZYMES AND TRANSPORT PROTEINS IMPORTANT IN LIPOPROTEIN METABOLISM

Enzyme/Protein	Function
HMG CoA reductase	The rate-limiting enzyme in hepatic cholesterol synthesis
LPL	Removes TG from chylomicrons and VLDL in adipose tissue, leaving remnant particles
Hepatic lipase (HL)	Removes additional TG from remnant particles in the liver, converting them into LDL
LCAT	Esterifies cholesterol molecules on the surface of HDL, drawing them into the HDL core
CETP	Shuttles esterified cholesterol back and forth between HDL and LDL

6. **How are TGs metabolized?**
   TGs come from the diet (exogenous) or hepatic synthesis (endogenous). They are transported by chylomicrons (exogenous TG) and VLDL (endogenous TG) to adipose tissue and muscle, where LPL and cofactor apoprotein C-II break down TGs into fatty acids and monoglycerides. Fatty acids then enter adipose cells to be stored as fat or muscle cells to be burned as fuel. The remnant particles return to the liver, where HL converts VLDL remnants into LDL.

7. **How is LDL metabolized?**
   LDL transports cholesterol from the liver to peripheral tissues, where LDL receptors bind the apoprotein B-100 molecule. LDL is next internalized and degraded to make free cholesterol available for intracellular needs. Excess LDL is cleared from the circulation by the scavenger system.

8. **Explain briefly the metabolism of HDL.**
   HDL docks on peripheral tissues that have apoprotein A receptors. Cholesterol attaches to the HDL surface, where it is esterified and drawn into the HDL core by lecithin-cholesterol acetyl-transferase (LCAT). Cholesterol ester transfer protein (CETP) then shuttles cholesterol back and forth between HDL bound for the liver and outgoing LDL to ensure the proper distribution of cholesterol destined for peripheral utilization or hepatic disposal (see Fig. 7-1).

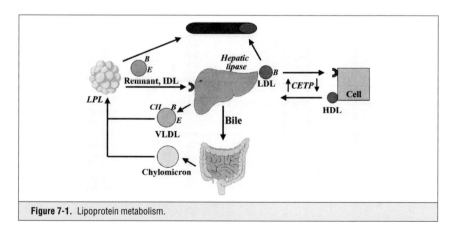

Figure 7-1. Lipoprotein metabolism.

9. **Describe the pathogenesis of the atherosclerotic plaque and arterial thrombosis.**

LDL can be modified by oxidation. Scavenger macrophages located beneath the intimal surface of arteries engulf oxidized LDL, becoming lipid-laden foam cells, which secrete growth factors that stimulate smooth muscle cell proliferation. These developing plaques also secrete cytokines that attract inflammatory cells, which secrete proteolytic enzymes that erode the fibromuscular plaque cap, making it prone to rupture. When rupture occurs, platelets aggregate and release chemicals that promote vasoconstriction and initiate thrombus formation, which may ultimately occlude the artery.

10. **Are elevated serum TG levels harmful?**

Serum TG levels that exceed 200 mg/dL appear to be associated with atherosclerosis. High TG levels are often accompanied by low HDL cholesterol levels and by small, dense LDL particles that are more easily oxidized and therefore more atherogenic. Elevated TG levels are also frequently associated with the metabolic syndrome. It is unclear whether atherosclerosis results directly from elevated TG or from the associated metabolic changes that accompany hypertriglyceridemia. TG values greater than 1000 mg/dL significantly increase the risk of developing acute pancreatitis.

11. **What is the metabolic syndrome?**

The metabolic syndrome (also called the dysmetabolic syndrome) is a constellation of associated disorders that is diagnosed when a patient has any three of the following: elevated fasting glucose, insulin resistance, high TG, low HDL, hypertension, and abdominal obesity (waist > 40 inches in men, >35 inches in women). This condition carries a very high risk for atherosclerotic vascular disease.

12. **What is lipoprotein(a)?**

Apoprotein(a) has approximately 85% amino-acid sequence homology with plasminogen. When an apoprotein(a) molecule attaches to apoprotein B on the surface of an LDL particle, the new particle is referred to as lipoprotein(a). Excessive lipoprotein(a) promotes atherosclerosis, possibly because it is easily oxidized and engulfed by macrophages and/or because it inhibits thrombolysis.

13. **What are the primary dyslipidemias?**

Primary dyslipidemias are inherited disorders of lipoprotein metabolism. The major primary dyslipidemias and their lipid phenotypes are:

Primary Dyslipidemia	Phenotype
Familial hypercholesterolemia (FH)	↑↑Cholesterol
Polygenic hypercholesterolemia	↑Cholesterol
Familial combined hyperlipidemia (FCH)	↑Cholesterol and ↑TG
Familial dysbetalipoproteinemia (FDL)	↑Cholesterol and ↑TG
Familial hypertriglyceridemia (FHT)	↑↑TG

14. **What is FH?**

Familial hypercholesterolemia (FH) is an inherited disease characterized by extreme elevations of serum cholesterol but normal serum TG levels. The disorder is caused by genetic mutations resulting in absent or deficient LDL receptors or defective apoprotein B that cannot bind to LDL receptors. Homozygous patients often have serum cholesterol levels of 800–1200 mg/dL and die of coronary artery disease (CAD) before age 20 years. Heterozygotes have cholesterol levels of 300–600 mg/dL and often manifest CAD before age 50 years. Tendon xanthomas are characteristic of this disorder.

15. **What is FCH?**

Familial combined hyperlipidemia (FCH) is an inherited disorder characterized by variable elevations of both serum cholesterol and TG levels. The condition results from excessive hepatic apoprotein B synthesis, with increased numbers of apoprotein B containing VLDL and LDL particles. Affected patients typically have elevations of both cholesterol and TG, although the levels of each may vary greatly over time. These patients are prone to develop premature CAD.

16. **What is FDL?**

Familial dysbetalipoproteinemia (FDL) is an inherited condition characterized by significant and relatively balanced elevations of both serum cholesterol and TG. It is also referred to as type III hyperlipidemia. This disorder results from an abnormal apoprotein E phenotype (E2/E2), which binds poorly to hepatic receptors resulting in impaired clearance of circulating VLDL remnants by the liver. Affected patients often develop premature CAD. Planar xanthomas in the creases of the palms and soles of the feet are a characteristic finding in patients with this disorder.

17. **What is polygenic hypercholesterolemia?**

Polygenic hypercholesterolemia, which is characterized by mild-to-moderate elevations of serum cholesterol alone, is the most common type of inherited hypercholesterolemia. This condition generally occurs when one or more mild defects of cholesterol metabolism combine to elevate the serum cholesterol level. Affected patients have an increased risk of developing CAD.

18. **What is FHT?**

Familial hypertriglyceridemia (FHT) is an inherited condition characterized by moderate-to-severe elevations of serum TG with normal serum cholesterol levels. The disorder results from excessive hepatic TG synthesis, producing TG-enriched VLDL particles. It is not known to be associated with a high risk of CAD. However, if serum TG levels are sufficiently elevated, affected individuals are at an increased risk for the development of acute pancreatitis.

19. **How do you distinguish among FCH, FDL, and FHT?**

Because FCH and FDL are characterized by combined elevations of both cholesterol and TGs, additional tests may be necessary to make the distinction. Patients with FCH have increased serum apoprotein B levels, whereas patients with FDL have an E2/E2 apoprotein E phenotype and a broad beta-band on lipoprotein electrophoresis. Since FCH and FHT may both present with isolated hypertriglyceridemia, an apoprotein B measurement, which will only be elevated in FCH, can help to distinguish these two disorders. Family studies are also quite helpful.

20. **Name the secondary dyslipidemias.**

The secondary dyslipidemias are serum lipid elevations that result from systemic diseases, such as diabetes mellitus, hypothyroidism, nephrotic syndrome, renal disease, obstructive liver disease, and dysproteinemias. Lipids also may be increased by medications, such as beta blockers, diuretics, estrogens, progestins, androgens, retinoids, corticosteroids, cyclosporin A, phenothiazines, anticonvulsants, and certain antiviral agents used in the treatment of HIV infection. These disorders usually improve when the primary condition is treated or the offending drugs are discontinued.

KEY POINTS: CAUSES OF LIPID DISORDERS ✓

1. Elevated LDL cholesterol is a major risk factor for CAD.

2. Low HDL cholesterol is also a significant risk factor for CAD.

3. High serum TGs may not directly cause atherosclerosis but are often associated with an atherosclerotic profile, consisting of low HDL, small dense LDL particles, insulin resistance, hypertension, and abdominal obesity.

4. Serum TG levels greater than 1000 mg/dL significantly increase the risk of developing acute pancreatitis.

5. Inflammation within the atherosclerotic plaque plays a major role in plaque rupture and the occurrence of acute coronary events.

21. **What is the cause of severe elevations of serum TGs?**
TG levels above 1000 mg/dL pose a very high risk for the development of acute pancreatitis, a condition with a mortality rate of up to 10%. Most patients with such severe TG elevations have a primary TG disorder, such as FHT, FCH, or FDL combined with a secondary disorder, most commonly poorly controlled diabetes mellitus, alcohol abuse, estrogen use, or the use of HIV medications.

22. **Summarize the revised (2004) CAD risk stratification from the Adult Treatment Panel III (ATP III) of the National Cholesterol Education Program (NCEP).**
High Risk
1. Known CAD
2. CAD Risk Equivalents
   a. Peripheral arterial disease
   b. Cerebral arterial disease
   c. Abdominal aortic aneurysm
   d. Diabetes mellitus
   e. 2+ risk factors with CAD 10-year risk > 20%
Moderately High Risk
2+ risk factors with CAD 10-year risk = 10–20%
Moderate Risk
2+ risk factors with CAD 10-year risk < 10%
Low Risk
0–1 risk factors with CAD 10-year risk < 10%

Risk factors: Smoking; hypertension ($\geq$ 140/90); HDL < 40 mg/dL; Age $\geq$ 45 years (men), $\geq$ 55 years (women); CAD in first-degree relative (< 55 years [men], < 65 years [women])
CAD 10-year risk calculation: www.nhlbi.nih.gov/guidelines/cholesterol

23. **What are the revised (2004) lipoprotein treatment goals from the ATP III?**

Patient Risk	LDL Cholesterol (mg/dL)	Non-HDL Cholesterol (mg/dL)
High risk	< 70 mg/dL	< 100 mg/dL
Moderately high risk	< 100 mg/dL	< 130 mg/dL
Moderate risk	< 130 mg/dL	< 160 mg/dL
Low risk	< 160 mg/dL	< 190 mg/dL

24. **What treatment approaches are recommended for lipoproteins above these goals?**
    - LDL cholesterol < 30 mg/dL above risk stratified goal: therapeutic lifestyle change (TLC).
    - LDL cholesterol > 30 mg/dL above risk stratified goal: medications to lower lipids.

25. **Summarize TLC as recommended by the ATP III.**

Component	Goals
Total fat	25–35% of total calories
Saturated fat	<7% of total calories
Polyunsaturated fat	<10% of total calories
Monounsaturated fat	<20% of total calories
Carbohydrate	50–60% of total calories
Protein	15% of total calories
Total calories	Adjust to achieve and maintain ideal body weight
Dietary fiber	20–30 gm/day
Physical activity	Expend at least 200 kcal/day

26. **What medications most effectively lower serum LDL cholesterol?**

Medication	LDL Reduction (%)
Statins	20–60
Ezetimibe	20–25
Bile acid resins	15–25
Niacin	15–25

27. **How do the currently available statin medications differ?**
    The statins inhibit HMG CoA reductase, the rate-limiting enzyme in cholesterol synthesis. Some statins are "natural" (simvastatin, pravastatin; fungal derived) and the others are synthetic. Some are more hydrophilic (pravastatin, rosuvastatin), while the others are more lipophilic. The main differences of clinical interest, however, are their LDL-lowering potencies. A randomized controlled trial involving 2240 patients (STELLAR) reported the following results for the four most commonly used agents:

Medication	Doses (mg)	LDL Reduction (%)	HDL Increase (%)
Pravastatin	10–40	20–30	3–6
Simvastatin	10–80	28–46	5–7
Atorvastatin	10–80	37–51	2–6
Rosuvastatin	10–40	46–55	8–10

28. **What medications significantly lower TGs?**

Medication	TG Reduction (%)
Fibrates	30–50
Niacin	20–30
Statins	10–20
Fish oils	Variable

29. **What medications most effectively raise serum HDL cholesterol levels?**

Medication	HDL Increase (%)
Niacin	10–25
Fibrates	10–20
Statins	5–10

Medications that inhibit CETP have been shown to raise HDL cholesterol levels by as much as 50–60%; these agents are currently in preclinical trials.

30. **Once a statin is being used, how effective are subsequent dose increments?**
The initial statin dose will produce the greatest LDL cholesterol reduction. Each subsequent doubling of the statin dose will, on average, result only in an additional 6% decrease in serum LDL cholesterol. This "6% rule" is derived from numerous prospective studies.

31. **How effective and safe are combinations of lipid-lowering medications?**
For severe cholesterol elevations, the addition of ezetimibe, niacin or a bile acid resin to a statin will often reduce serum LDL cholesterol by an additional 20%, compared to only 6% when the statin dose is doubled. These combinations are generally safe to use but side effects can be additive. For elevations of both cholesterol and TG, adding a fibrate to a statin can lower the serum TG level up to 50%. However, the risk of myositis and frank rhabdomyolysis increases. Fenofibrate appears to be significantly safer than gemfibrozil when combination with a statin is considered necessary.

32. **Is aggressive reduction of serum LDL cholesterol with medication an effective strategy for primary prevention of CAD?**
Three large randomized controlled trials (WOSCOPS [pravastatin], AFCAPS [lovastatin], and HPS [simvastatin]) all clearly demonstrated that lowering serum LDL cholesterol with statin therapy in patients with elevated serum cholesterol levels but no prior history of CAD significantly reduces the risk of developing a first myocardial infarction and the need for coronary revascularization procedures.

33. **Is aggressive reduction of serum LDL cholesterol with medication an effective strategy for secondary prevention in patients with established CAD?**
Four large randomized controlled trials (4S [simvastatin], CARE [pravastatin], LIPID [pravastatin], and HPS [simvastatin]) demonstrated that treating patients with hypercholesterolemia and existing CAD significantly reduces the risk of recurrent myocardial infarctions, cardiovascular death, strokes, and the need for revascularization procedures. The AVERT trial [atorvastatin]

reported that aggressive LDL cholesterol reduction was more effective in reducing ischemic events than was coronary angioplasty.

34. **Can established CAD lesions be reduced by lipid-lowering therapy?**
Angiographic studies have demonstrated that aggressive lipid-lowering programs can halt progression or induce regression of coronary lesions in patients with known CAD (FATS) or previous bypass surgery (Post CABG Study).

35. **Do interventions that raise serum HDL cholesterol or lower serum TG have a significant effect on coronary events?**
Two large randomized controlled trials examined the effects of gemfibrozil in dyslipidemic patients without (HHS) and with (VA-HIT) known CAD. In both studies, a 6–8% increase in HDL cholesterol associated with a 30–40% reduction in serum TG significantly lowered the incidence of subsequent major CAD events.

KEY POINTS: TREATMENT OF LIPID DISORDERS ✔

1. Statins are the most effective LDL cholesterol-lowering agents, but additional LDL reduction can be achieved by adding ezetimibe, niacin, and bile acid resins.

2. Fibrates are the most effective TG-lowering agents, but additional reductions can be achieved by adding niacin, fish oils, and high-dose statins.

3. Combined statin and fibrate therapy may be needed when both cholesterol and TGs are significantly elevated; in such patients, it is advisable to use fenofibrate and low statin doses. Creatine kinase (CK) levels should be closely monitored.

4. The ATP III recommends LDL goals of <100 mg/dL for patients with CAD or CAD equivalents, <130 mg/dL for patients with 2 or more CAD risk factors, and <160 mg/dL for patients with 0–1 CAD risk factors.

5. The ATP III recommends non-HDL cholesterol goals of 30 mg/dL above the LDL cholesterol goals in patients whose serum TG levels are >200 mg/dL after the LDL goal has been achieved.

36. **Should all high-risk patients be treated with lipid-lowering therapy regardless of LDL cholesterol level?**
Two large randomized controlled trials, the HPS [simvastatin] and ASCOT [atorvastatin] showed that patients at high risk of CAD events by virtue of a past history of CAD, non-CAD vascular disease, diabetes mellitus, or hypertension had a significant reduction in CAD events in response to statin therapy even when their initial LDL cholesterol levels were not elevated. In the HPS, patients whose initial serum LDL cholesterol level was <100 mg/dL had a significant 24% reduction in events. Whether lipid-lowering therapy should be routinely recommended in all such patients is currently a subject of debate.

37. **Is measurement of inflammatory markers a useful tool in CAD risk assessment?**
Inflammation within an atherosclerotic plaque makes the plaque more likely to rupture, precipitating an acute ischemic event. Highly sensitive C-reactive protein (hsCRP), a nonspecific marker of inflammation, appears to predict CAD risk, as well as do LDL cholesterol levels. Measurement of LDL cholesterol and hsCRP together has even greater predictive value. This information can be useful to providers when making decisions about which patients to treat more aggressively but should not be performed routinely in all patients. Effective LDL reduc-

tion has been shown to reduce hsCRP levels. Other markers, such as myeloperoxidase (MPO) and glutathione peroxidase 1 (GTX-1), are currently under investigation.

38. Should we be utilizing measurements of lipoprotein size and number?
Lipoprotein size and number can now be assessed by a variety of commercially available techniques, such as a nuclear magnetic resonance (NMR). The analyses provide additional information about the atherogenicity of a lipoprotein profile, but the cost-effectiveness and utility of such information has not yet been demonstrated. Decisions regarding the need for treatment and the choice of agents can be made based on the clinical risk factor profile and standard lipid profile in the majority of patients. Therefore, these additional tests should be limited to situations in which they are likely to have a clear impact on the choice and aggressiveness of therapy.

39. How should the patient with severe hypertriglyceridemia be managed?
Serum TG levels above 1000 mg/dL must be lowered quickly because of the high risk of precipitating acute pancreatitis. Medications alone are not effective when TG levels are this high. Patients must immediately be placed on a very low fat (less than 5% fat) diet until the TG level is less than 1000 mg/dL. Such a diet lowers serum TG approximately 20% each day. Contributing factors, most commonly poorly controlled diabetes mellitus, alcohol abuse, estrogen use, and HIV medications, must simultaneously be addressed. Once serum TG levels are less than 1000 mg/dL, the most effective medications to further reduce serum TG are the fibrates. If these medications do not lower serum TG sufficiently, niacin, fish oils, or a statin may be added to the regimen.

BIBLIOGRAPHY

1. Balk EM, Lau J, Goudas LC, et al: Effects of statins on non-lipid serum markers associated with cardiovascular disease. Ann Intern Med 139:670–682, 2003.
2. Brown G, Albers JJ, Fisher LD, et al: Regression of coronary artery disease as a result of lipid-lowering therapy in men with high levels of apolipoprotein B. N Engl J Med 323:1289–1296, 1990 (FATS).
3. Cannon CP et al: Intensive versus moderate lipid lowering with statins after acute coronary syndromes. (Prove It Trial) N Engl J Med 350:1495–1504, 2004.
4. Criqui MG, Heiss G, Cohn R, et al: Plasma triglyceride level and mortality from coronary artery disease. N Engl J Med 328:1220–1225, 1993.
5. Downs JR, Clearfield M, Weis S, et al: Primary prevention of acute coronary events with lovastatin in men and women with average cholesterol levels: Results of AFCAPS/TexCAPS. Air Force/Texas Coronary Atherosclerosis Prevention Study. JAMA 279:1615–1622, 1995 (AFCAPS).
6. Executive Summary of the Third Report of The National Education Program (NCEP) Expert Panel on Detection, Evaluation, and Treatment of High Blood Cholesterol in Adults (Adult Treatment Panel III). JAMA 285: 2486–2497, 2001.
7. Grundy SM et al: Implications of recent clinical trials for the National Cholesterol Education Program Adult Treatment Panel III Guidelines. Circulation 110:227–239, 2004.
8. Heart Protection Collaborative Group: MRC/BHF Heart Protection Study of cholesterol lowering with simvastatin in 20,536 high-risk individuals: A randomized placebo-controlled trial. Lancet 360: 7–22, 2002 (HPS).
9. Henkin Y, Como JA, Oberman A: Secondary dyslipidemia: Inadvertent effects of drugs in clinical practice. JAMA 267:961–968, 1992.
10. Jones PH, Davidson MH, Stein EA, et al: Comparison of the efficacy and safety of rosuvastatin versus atorvastatin, simvastatin, and pravastatin across doses. Am J Cardiol 93:152–160, 2003 (STELLAR).
11. Knopp RH: Drug treatment of lipid disorders. N Engl J Med 341:498–511, 1999.
12. Kreisberg RA, Oberman A: Medical management of hyperlipidemia/dyslipidemia. J Clin Endocrinol Metab 88:2445–2461, 2003.
13. Lipid Study Group: Prevention of cardiovascular events and death with pravastatin in patients with coronary heart disease and a broad range of initial cholesterol levels. N Engl J Med 339:1349–1357, 1998 (LIPID).

14. Nissen SE et al: Effect of intensive compared with moderate lipid-lowering therapy on progression of coronary atherosclerosis (reversal trial). JAMA 291:1071–1080, 2004.

15. Manninen V, Elo MO, Frick MH, et al. Lipid alteration and decline in the incidence of coronary heart disease in the Helsinki Heart Study. JAMA 260:641–651, 1988 (HHS).

16. Pitt B, Waters D, Brown WV, et al: Aggressive lipid-lowering therapy compared with angioplasty in stable coronary artery disease. N Engl J Med 341:70–76, 1999 (AVERT).

17. Post Coronary Artery Bypass Graft Trial Investigators: The effect of aggressive lowering of low-density lipoprotein cholesterol levels and low-dose anticoagulation on obstructive changes in saphenous-vein coronary-artery bypass grafts. N Engl J Med 336:153–162, 1997.

18. Ridker PM, Hennekens CH, Buring JE, Rifai N: C-reactive protein and other markers of inflammation in the prediction of cardiovascular disease in women. N Engl J Med 342:836–843, 2000.

19. Rubins HB, Robins SJ, Collins D, et al: Gemfibrozil for the secondary prevention of coronary heart disease in men with low levels of high-density lipoprotein cholesterol. N Engl J Med 341:410–418, 1999 (V-HIT).

20. Sacks FM, Pfeffer MA, Moye LA, et al: The effect of pravastatin on coronary events after myocardial infarction in patients with average cholesterol levels. N Engl J Med 335:1001–1009, 1996 (CARE).

21. Scandinavian Simvastatin Survival Study Group: Randomized trial of cholesterol lowering in 4444 patients with coronary heart disease: The Scandinavian Simvastatin Survival Study (4S). Lancet 344:1383–1389, 1994.

22. Scanu AM: Lipoprotein(a) and atherosclerosis. Ann Intern Med 115:209–218, 1991.

23. Schectman G, Hiatt J. Dose–response characteristics of cholesterol-lowering drug therapies: Implications for treatment. Ann Intern Med 125:990–1000, 1996.

24. Sever PS, Dahlof B, Poulter NR, et al: Prevention of coronary and stroke events with atorvastatin in hypertensive patients who have average or lower than average cholesterol concentrations, in the Anglo-22. Scandinavian Cardiac Outcomes Trial-Lipid Lowering Arm (ASCOT-LLA): A multicenter randomized controlled trial. Lancet 361:1149–1158, 2003.

25. Shepherd J, Cobbe SM, Ford I, et al: Prevention of coronary heart disease with pravastatin in men with hypercholesterolemia. N Engl J Med 333:1301–1307, 1995 (WOSCOPS).

26. Third Report of The National Education Program (NCEP) Expert Panel on Detection, Evaluation, and Treatment of High Blood Cholesterol in Adults (Adult Treatment Panel III) final report. Circulation 106:3143–3421, 2002.

CHAPTER 8

OBESITY

Daniel H. Bessesen, M.D.

1. **Define the terms overweight and obesity.**
   Obesity is a degree of overweight that is associated with increases in morbidity and mortality. In 1998, the National Heart Lung and Blood Institute (NHLBI) of the National Institutes of Health published guidelines on the diagnosis and treatment of overweight and obesity. The expert panel advocated using specific body mass index (BMI) cut-off points to diagnose both conditions. The BMI is calculated by dividing a person's weight in kilograms by height in meters squared. A BMI (kg/m^2) of 25 or less is normal; 25–29.9, overweight; 30–34.9, mild obesity; 35–39.9, moderately obese; and > 40, severe or morbid obesity.

2. **Does fat distribution affect the assessment of risk in an overweight or obese patient?**
   Yes. The BMI not only determines the health risks of obesity but also the distribution of fat. Accumulation of excessive adipose tissue in a central- or upper-body distribution (android or male pattern) is associated with a greater risk of adverse health consequences than lower-body obesity (gynoid or female pattern). It appears that it is the absolute amount of central fat that confers adverse health risks.

3. **Explain the role of waist circumference in risk stratification.**
   For this reason, the waist circumference is now the favored measure for risk stratification based on fat distribution. High risk is conferred in men by a waist circumference greater than 40 in. (> 102 cm) and in women by a waist circumference greater than 35 in. (> 88 cm). Waist circumference is most useful for risk stratification of people whose BMI is between 25 and 30 kg/m^2. In this intermediate-risk area, those with an increased waist circumference should undertake greater efforts directed at preventing further weight gain, while those with a smaller waist circumference can be reassured that their weight does not pose major health hazards.

4. **How is waist circumference measured?**
   Waist circumference should be measured with a tape measure at the level of the iliac crest parallel to the floor at the end of a relaxed expiration.

5. **What adverse health consequences are associated with obesity?**
   Obesity has clearly been associated with diabetes, hypertension, hyperlipidemia, coronary artery disease, degenerative arthritis, gallbladder disease, and cancer of the endometrium, breast, prostate, and colon. The incidence of these conditions rises steadily as body weight increases (Figs. 8-1 and 8-2). It is surprising how risks increase with even modest gains in weight. Health risks are magnified with advancing age and a positive family history of obesity-related diseases.

6. **Summarize the economic consequences of obesity.**
   An NIH publication from 2003 estimated the direct and indirect health care costs due to obesity as $122.9 billion for the year 2001. In addition, NIH estimated that Americans pay $33 billion for weight loss products and services, many of which provide little or no benefit. These costs suggest that obesity accounts for 5.5–7% of national health expenditures in the United States.

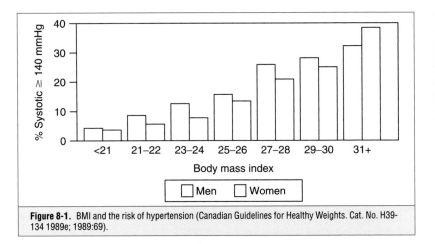

Figure 8-1. BMI and the risk of hypertension (Canadian Guidelines for Healthy Weights. Cat. No. H39-134 1989e; 1989:69).

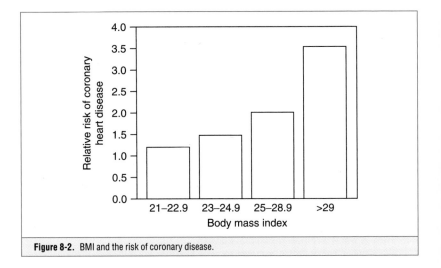

Figure 8-2. BMI and the risk of coronary disease.

7. **What are the psychological complications of obesity?**
Situational depression and anxiety related to obesity are common. The obese person may suffer from discrimination that contributes further to difficulty with poor self-image and social isolation. Severely obese people may avoid leaving their home for fear of ridicule. It may be difficult in some patients to determine whether depression is accelerating weight gain or whether weight gain is exacerbating an underlying depression, but treating both conditions may improve quality of life. It may be difficult or impossible for a care provider who has never experienced discrimination based on obesity to understand the scope of these effects.

8. **How common is obesity?**
Obesity has reached epidemic proportions in the United States. The National Health and Nutrition Examination Survey (NHANES) conducted by the federal government uses direct measures of height and weight in a representative sample of Americans to estimate the

prevalence of obesity. The most recent NHANES data published in 2002 showed that in 1999–2000, 30.5% of adults, over 61 million people were obese as defined as a BMI > 30 kg/m^2. The prevalence of overweight was found to be 64.5%. The prevalence of extreme obesity (BMI > 40 kg/m^2) was found to be 4.7%. Levels of childhood overweight have nearly tripled since 1970 with roughly 15% of children and teens age 6–19 years now being overweight.

9. **What has caused this dramatic rise in the prevalence of obesity?**
The prevalence of obesity has risen over such a short period; it seems that the primary culprit is a changing environment that promotes increased food intake and reduced physical activity. This statement should not be taken to mean, however, that body weight is not subject to physiologic regulation. The control of body weight is complex with multiple interrelated systems controlling caloric intake, macronutrient content of the diet, energy expenditure, and fuel metabolism.

10. **Describe the current model for obesity as a chronic disease.**
Professionals are increasingly viewing obesity as a chronic metabolic disease much like diabetes or hypertension. This model requires a conceptual shift from the previous widely held belief that obesity is simply a cosmetic or behavioral problem. Development of obesity requires a period of positive energy balance; that is, energy intake must exceed energy expenditure. Maintaining energy balance is one of the most important jobs of any organism. Between ages 20 and 60 years, the average human eats over 32 tons of food. A sustained negative imbalance between energy intake and expenditure is potentially life threatening within a relatively short time. To maintain energy balance, the organism must assess energy stores within the body; assess the nutrient content of the diet; determine whether the body is in negative energy or nutrient balance; and adjust hormone levels, energy expenditure, nutrient movement, and consumptive behavior in response to these assessments.

11. **Do abnormal genes cause obesity?**
Obesity is clearly more common in people who have family members who are also obese. The problem of human obesity involves an interaction between genetic susceptibility and environmental triggers. The genes that we possess to regulate body weight evolved somewhere between 200,000 and 1 million years ago. The environmental factors controlling nutrient acquisition and habitual physical activity were dramatically different then. While a few cases of human obesity caused by single gene mutations have been found, most human obesity appears to be polygenic involving probably 10–30 genes in any individual. Genetics appears to be responsible for 20–40% of the variance in weight in most populations.

12. **What is leptin?**
Leptin is a hormone secreted by adipose tissue. It was discovered in 1994. Its name comes from the Greek word *leptos* meaning thin. Leptin was cloned from the *ob/ob* mouse model of obesity that was first described in 1950. The obese phenotype of this mouse model is due to a genetic mutation that produces leptin deficiency. In *ob/ob* mice, the administration of recombinant leptin produces sustained weight loss through both decreases in food intake and increases in energy expenditure. The weight loss occurs largely from fat mass with little loss in lean body mass.

13. **Discuss the role of leptin in human obesity.**
Although leptin is also produced in humans, there have been only three cases in which leptin deficiency was identified as a cause of human obesity out of thousands of people studied. Many studies have shown that leptin levels are actually increased in obese compared with lean humans, suggesting that either leptin does not have a major role in reducing food intake in humans or that obese humans have leptin resistance. Leptin is secreted by adipose tissue in proportion to its mass. It appears to be a reliable marker of total body adiposity and is highly correlated with other markers of body fat. Recent studies in which recombinant human leptin was administered to obese humans found that this hormone did not substantially reduce weight.

14. **Explain how the melanocortin system is involved in weight regulation.**
    An unexpected but potentially important role of the melanocortin system in body weight regulation was uncovered from studies of obesity in the agouti mouse, so named because of its yellow coat. The gene defect in this mouse model involves a peptide (agouti) that competes with alpha melanocortin (MSH) for binding to MSH receptors. The identification of this pathway has highlighted the role of MSH receptors, particularly the MC4-R subtype, in the regulation of body weight. Various lines of research now have clearly shown that alpha-MSH made in the hypothalamus inhibits food intake, while the natural antagonist agouti-related peptide (AGRP), also made in the hypothalamus, stimulates food intake. Several companies now have drugs that interact with the MC4-R as antagonists. These drugs decrease food intake in rats and reduce body weight. There is hope that they may be useful in treating human obesity in the future.

15. **What is ghrelin?**
    Ghrelin is a hormone produced by the stomach and proximal small intestine that appears to regulate both growth hormone secretion and appetite. Ghrelin levels rise before meals and promptly fall after the ingestion of nutrients. Self-reports of hunger seem to mirror serum ghrelin levels. Twenty-four hour ghrelin levels rise when people go on a calorically restricted diet and are dramatically reduced after gastric bypass surgery.

16. **Does a decrease in energy expenditure play a role in the development of obesity?**
    The development of obesity requires an imbalance between caloric intake and caloric expenditure. For fat mass to increase, there must be an imbalance between the amount of fat deposited compared with the amount of fat oxidized. One possibility is that people become obese because of a reduction in their energy expenditure.

17. **Explain the three components of energy expenditure.**
    1. *Basal metabolic rate* (BMR): The amount of energy that is needed to keep sodium and potassium where they belong, to keep the body warm, to pump blood, to breathe, and to perform other basic functions.
    2. *Energy expended in activity* (EA): The most variable component. It can account for as little as 10–20% of total energy expenditure in people who are bedridden or as much as 60–80% of total energy expenditure in training athletes. EA increases with planned physical activity or with activities of daily living, such as stair climbing or even fidgeting. The unconscious component of physical activity has been termed nonexercise activity thermogenesis (NEAT) and may be a regulated parameter.
    3. *Thermic effect of food* (TEF): A relatively small component of energy expenditure that represents the increase in energy expenditure after consumption of a meal.

18. **Explain the concept of energy balance.**
    Total energy expenditure equals total daily caloric intake when an individual is in energy balance. Total energy expenditure is, in general, linearly related to lean body mass. Studies using indirect calorimetry have shown that obese people clearly consume more calories than lean people. The obese peson who says that he or she eats only a small salad may be telling the truth in the short term, but over longer periods high caloric intakes are required to maintain the obese state. However, the role of alterations in energy expenditure in the development of obesity and the response to dieting is less clear. Increasing evidence suggests that obesity is associated with a relative reduction in energy expended with physical activity. Evidence in favor of this hypothesis comes from the Pima Indians, as well as Caucasian obese, and reduced obese people. The role that reductions in BMR play in weight gain is more controversial. Suffice it to say that regardless of the absolute level of expenditure, obesity results from failure to couple energy intake to energy expenditure accurately.

19. **What options are available for treating the obese patient?**

The treatment options for an overweight or obese patient include diet, exercise, pharmacotherapy, surgery, and combinations of these modalities. The specific modality should be based on the individual's BMI and associated health problems. A more aggressive treatment approach is warranted in those whose BMI is higher and those with adverse health consequences.

Behavioral approaches can be advocated for all overweight and obese patients. Pharmacologic treatment should be considered in those whose BMI is greater than 27 kg/m^2 in the presence of medical complications or greater than 30 kg/m^2 in the absence of medical complications. Surgical treatment should be reserved for those with a BMI greater than 40 kg/m^2.

20. **What is the goal of a weight loss program?**

Before discussing the treatment options with a patient, it is important to decide the goal of the treatment program. Increasing evidence suggests that many obese people have unrealistic expectations about the amount of weight that they might lose through a weight loss program. Most obese people would like to achieve ideal body weight and are disappointed if they lose only 5–10% of their initial weight. These desires stand in stark contrast to the magnitude of weight loss that has been seen with all treatment modalities short of gastric bypass surgery. The most effective diet, exercise, or drug treatment programs available give roughly a 10% weight loss in most people.

21. **Is a 10% reduction helpful in terms of health improvement?**

This degree of weight reduction has been associated with improvements in health-related measures, such as lower blood pressure, reductions in low-density lipoprotein (LDL) cholesterol levels, improved functional capacity, and a markedly reduced risk of developing diabetes. However, a 10% weight reduction will be disappointing to most patients unless the goal of the weight reduction program is clearly discussed in advance. It is important to help the patient adopt more realistic goals for a diet and exercise program. Most experts now believe that a sustained 5–10% weight loss (e.g., a weight loss of 11–12 lb for someone who initially weighed 220 lb) is a realistic goal with probable medical benefits. Alternatively, prevention of further weight gain may be a reasonable and attainable goal, or the health care provider may encourage the patient to focus on eating and activity habits and not on a weight goal at all.

22. **How can a patient's readiness to change his or her diet or physical activity be assessed?**

Stages of change theory can help the clinician focus counseling activities within the context of a brief office visit. Prochazka has hypothesized six, predictable stages through which a person passes before he or she is able to change long-standing behaviors, such as diet, physical activity patterns, or smoking: precontemplative, contemplative, planning, action, maintenance, and relapse. Identifying the stage that the patient is in and targeting counseling efforts to that stage may improve the effectiveness of the counseling activities.

23. **Define the precontemplative stage.**

In this stage people are not even thinking about changing their behavior. The issue is generally lack of perceived benefits to behavior change. For such people, perhaps a simple statement about the association between obesity and adverse health consequences may be appropriate, similar to what would be said about smoking cessation.

24. **What is the contemplative stage?**

People in this stage acknowledge the potential benefits of behavior change but have not yet decided what they are going to do. They are "thinking about it." The important issues to discuss during this stage are perceived barriers to behavior change. Lack of time, lack of money, or a lack of a sense of control may be preventing progress.

25. **Explain the planning stage.**
People in this stage have decided that they are going to change their behavior and are developing strategies to do so. They are "reading the book." People in the planning stage need support and encouragement. They may request and benefit from specific suggestions to guide behavior change.

26. **What happens in the action stage?**
People in this stage have finished reading the book and have embarked on a behavior change program. They are usually excited, maybe even zealous. Sometimes they are seen at an initial visit and may be looking for your support of their current diet or exercise program. People in the action stage also benefit from encouragement, support, and the provision of objective evidence of the effects, either positive or negative, of their current approach.

27. **Define the maintenance stage.**
People in this stage are on an established program that has become second nature. They may need to work on relapse prevention. The counseling time should be spent in looking for situations in which the patient may slip back into older habits and planning strategies to avoid these pitfalls.

28. **What happens in the relapse stage?**
People in this stage have reverted to a previous pattern of behavior. They may feel like they will always fail. They may say, "I've tried diets. They never work for me." People in the relapse stage feel frustrated and may make the care provider feel frustrated as well. Counseling time should acknowledge and reward previous successes. The discussion should also explore what happened in the previous efforts. Can the patient learn from past efforts? Why did the patient fail? Were expectations too high? Were the changes too great? Where did the patient succeed? What would be reasonable new goals?

29. **Discuss the role of diet in the treatment of the obese patient.**
The mainstays of dietary modification in weight loss therapy have been diets low in fat and reduced in calories. Evidence in favor of this approach has recently come from the Diabetes Prevention Project and the Finnish Diabetes Prevention Trial. Whatever intervention the clinician makes must be lifelong to be beneficial; therefore, it must be tolerable to the patient. The clinician should assess the current diet with a good nutritional history, which may involve a verbal 24- or 72-hour diet recall. Alternatively, the patient may keep a written 7-day food diary. Assessing meal pattern is important, as many people skip breakfast and eat lunch erratically. Attention should be paid to how often the person eats out, especially fast food. Then the clinician needs to make suggestions for slow, gradual change. Simple dietary suggestions include eating three meals per day, eating only at meal times, and eating only one serving. These suggestions help patients to focus on what they are eating, emphasizing making good food choices and controlling portion size.

30. **Should patients be encouraged to attend a commercial weight loss program?**
Yes. Most people know what they should eat. The problem is that they either do not pay attention to what they eat or do not find a "good diet" palatable. Many of the settings in which care is provided do not allow the teaching of sophisticated behavioral modification techniques. The use of commercial programs, such as Weight Watchers, can provide reasonable nutritional counseling along with social support. Many patients are surprised at the cost of these programs, which may be a deterrent to their continued use. However, this kind of program involves no risk and may be cheaper in the long term than pharmacologic treatment. The scientific literature supports the notion that for many people commercial weight loss programs are a reasonable option.

KEY POINTS: OBESITY ✓

1. Obesity is defined as a BMI > 30 kg/m^2.

2. A 5–10% weight loss is a good goal with known health benefits.

3. Three recent randomized controlled clinical trials show that over 6–12 months there are no adverse effects on lipids from the Atkins diet plan.

4. Sibutramine, orlistat, and phentermine are currently FDA-approved medications to help overweight and obese patients lose weight.

5. The average weight loss following gastric bypass surgery is 30%.

31. **How are meal replacements useful in a weight loss program?**
For some people it is difficult to control calories through self-design of healthy meals. Often time is not available for food preparation, and convenience overrides health concerns. For such people, meal replacements, which are reduced-calorie, nutritionally complete meals, are a reasonable option with scientifically proven effectiveness if used as a long-term strategy. In fact, this approach is currently used in the NIH Look Ahead Trial, which is examining the health effects of long-term weight loss.

32. **What is the Atkins diet? Does it work?**
The Atkins diet is a severely carbohydrate-restricted (< 20 gm/day during the induction phase) plan that is quite popular. The idea behind the diet is that hyperinsulinemia is harmful because it promotes fat storage and hunger. Dr. Atkins reasoned that because insulin goes up as dietary carbohydrate increases, carbohydrate should be restricted. The severe carbohydrate restriction produces what Atkins called "benign dietary ketosis," which he argued suppresses appetite. The diet has very few other restrictions. Several recent studies support the idea that most people lose a moderate amount of weight on this diet, actually more than a control group lost on a more traditional low-fat diet. These studies also showed no adverse effects on blood lipid levels.

33. **Describe the Zone diet.**
The Zone diet contains 30% protein, 30% fat, and 40% carbohydrate. The goal is not weight loss per se but rather "optimizing" health. Dr. Sears' thesis is that foods are like drugs in that they have dose-response curves. Therefore, one can optimize metabolism (in particular, eicosanoid levels) by eating a diet that has optimal ratios of fat, carbohydrate, and protein. Too much carbohydrate is bad because of hyperinsulinemia. Diets containing too little carbohydrate (ketogenic diets) are bad because they promote muscle breakdown, increase counter-regulatory hormones, and as a result increase the production of "bad eicosanoids." Like Atkins, Sears believes that the excessive emphasis on low-fat, high-carbohydrate diets is partly responsible for the increased prevalence of obesity.

34. **Discuss the Ornish diet.**
Dr. Dean Ornish was looking for an alternative to bypass surgery for patients with coronary artery disease that was based on nutrition and lifestyle change. His target audience is not obese people but rather those with known coronary artery disease. The Ornish diet is not a weight loss diet. It is a "lifestyle change program" incorporating diet (specifically, a very low-fat [10% fat, 10% protein] vegetarian diet) with group interactions designed to increase physical activity and decrease "type A" behaviors. Group psychological support, smoking cessation, yoga-based physical activities, and meditation are part of this program. As currently practiced, it is a labor-intensive program for the care provider and participants. Ornish and his collaborators have reported the 5-year follow-up on a cohort of 20 patients who were on the program compared

with 15 controls. The subjects experienced a dramatic reduction in anginal events and angiographic evidence of regression of coronary artery disease.

35. **What is the South Beach diet?**

This dietary program was developed by a cardiologist in Florida, who advocates a diet somewhat restricted in carbohydrate, especially refined carbohydrates, but believes that low glycemic index carbohydrate sources are beneficial. He advocates increased consumption of monounsaturated fats, omega-3 fatty acids, and nuts. He gave these principles to several chefs from fashionable restaurants in South Beach. The dietary principals are reasonable; the recipes look quite appetizing; and the program is very clearly defined. It seems like a reasonable, more tolerable version of several other popular diet books, including the Atkins diet, the glucose revolution, and the Zone diet.

36. **Do any of the popular diet books emphasize good behavioral approaches to weight loss?**

The most reputable text for patients on this subject is *The LEARN Manual for Weight Control* by Dr. Kelly Brownell. This book represents the best of his behavioral weight loss program. However, many patients find it a little dull. Two recent books address behavioral issues in dieting: *The Personality Type Diet* by Dr. Robert Kushner and *The Ultimate Weight Solution* by Dr. Phil McGraw address these issues in a more reader-friendly manner. Both books give reasonable and readable advice about a variety of important behavioral topics related to diet and exercise and can reasonably be recommended to patients.

37. **What should a clinician do when a patient wants to go on a "fad diet"?**

1. The clinician may pick and promote one of the popular diet programs. However, because no one is really sure what the right program is, this approach may not be the best. Probably no single program is right for all patients.
2. The clinician may try to dissuade people from participating in any of these programs. This approach is certainly the easiest and most common option. In fact, fad diets are not currently promoted or even accepted by reputable groups, such as the American Heart Association, the American Diabetes Association, or the National Institutes of Health. However, it is also hard to ignore the often-heard testimonials to the effectiveness of these diets and the growing body of randomized controlled clinical trials that support their use.
3. The third, and perhaps the most acceptable, approach is to try to understand the principles underlying these diets and provide information and encouragement to patients in their efforts to take control of their health. A clinician may even want to select one or two of these books to share with patients who ask. The discussion should also focus on realistic goals. Patients can be provided with objective data on which to evaluate their program (e.g., fasting lipid and glucose levels, blood pressure, weight, waist circumference, percent body fat). The mood should be kept positive yet realistic.

38. **What drugs are available to treat obesity?**

- Phentermine (Adipex-P, Fastin, Ionamin)
- Orlistat (Xenical)
- Sibutramine (Meridia)
- Bupropion (Wellbutrin)

39. **Discuss the relationship between phentermine and amphetamine.**

Phentermine is chemically related to amphetamine and works predominantly on the neurotransmitter norepinephrine to reduce appetite. The addictive effects of amphetamine are thought to be due to its actions on the neurotransmitter dopamine. Phentermine has substantially fewer dopaminergic effects than amphetamine and thus minimal potential for addiction. It is, however, a central stimulant and can cause hypertension, tachycardia, nervousness, headache, difficulty sleeping, and tremor in some people.

40. **Is phentermine effective? How much does it cost?**
It achieves some weight loss compared with placebo in 50–60% of those who take it, with the average weight loss being in the 5–8% range. The average cost is about $30/month.

41. **Discuss the side effects of phentermine.**
No evidence indicates that phentermine used alone is associated with cardiac valvular and pulmonary vascular toxicity. Phentermine is still on the market but is approved by the Food and Drug Administration (FDA) only for 3-month use. There are no long-term studies of its safety and efficacy. However, it has been in widespread clinical use longer than any other weight loss agent, and there has been no evidence of serious side effects.

42. **How does orlistat work? What is the usual dose? How much does it cost?**
Orlistat is a pancreatic lipase inhibitor. It reduces the absorption of fat by roughly 30% by inhibiting the enzyme responsible for fat digestion. It is given as 120 mg three times a day with meals. The average wholesale price for this drug is $120/month.

43. **What are the side effects of orlistat?**
Since it is not absorbed into the bloodstream, orlistat is not associated with primary pulmonary hypertension, cardiac valvular disease, or other systemic side effects. Some patients like the fact that it is not an appetite suppressant. The main side effects are due to the malabsorption of fat. Patients who eat a high-fat meal experience greasy stools and may even have problems with incontinence of stool. If the patient chooses to skip the medication, he or she can eat a high-fat meal without side effects and without the benefit that the medication would otherwise provide. The FDA has approved orlistat for long-term use, and there is no specific mention in the package insert of when it should be stopped.

44. **How effective is orlistat?**
The average weight loss seen is about 7–8%. This medication may be preferred in people currently using a serotonin-specific reuptake inhibitor (SSRI).

45. **How does sibutramine work?**
Sibutramine is a combination norepinephrine and serotonin reuptake blocker. Unlike fenfluramine and dexfenfluramine, it has no serotonin-releasing action and therefore is pharmacologically more like the SSRIs that are widely prescribed for the treatment of depression.

46. **How effective is sibutramine? How much does it cost?**
Taken at doses ranging from 10 to 15 mg/day, sibutramine produces weight losses in the range of 5–8%. Sibutramine is currently available for roughly $100/month.

47. **Discuss the side effects of sibutramine.**
Sibutramine has been associated with an increase in blood pressure in some people, particularly at the higher doses. It should not be used in people with poorly controlled hypertension. Blood pressure should be monitored closely after initiation of this medicine. The most common side effects are dry mouth, headache, nervousness, and difficulty falling asleep. However, these side effects are generally well tolerated. Sibutramine has been widely used, and no evidence indicates that its use is associated with serious side effects, such as valvular heart disease or pulmonary hypertension. The FDA has approved it for 1-year treatment, with longer use to be decided by physician and patient. Two-year safety and efficacy data have been published.

48. **Discuss the role of bupropion in the treatment of obesity.**
Preliminary information suggests that bupropion may produce gradual weight loss over as long as 1 year in some people. Currently, there is no weight loss indication for bupropion, but the manufacturer is pursuing one. While this drug should not currently be prescribed for weight

reduction, if patients already are taking a different antidepressant and do not want to use orlistat, it may be reasonable to discuss switching to bupropion with their psychiatrist. More data are needed before bupropion can be generally recommended as a weight loss medication.

49. **How long will a medication need to be taken?**
    In the past, the FDA allowed only short-term use of weight-loss medicines. However, experts now feel that obesity is a chronic illness just like diabetes or high blood pressure, and that a medicine used to promote weight loss will work only as long as it is taken. In other words, if a patient loses weight with a specific medication and then stops its use, he or she is likely to regain the lost weight. The same principle applies when someone goes on a diet for a period of time then stops the diet. In general, if a primary care provider and a patient decide to try a weight loss medication, it should be taken for a minimum of 3 months to determine whether the patient will lose at least 5–8% of his or her weight. Then some form of chronic use should be considered, given the available information about the risks and potential benefits of the medications.

50. **Discuss the role of exercise in a weight loss program.**
    Increased physical activity appears to be a central part of a successful weight loss program. While exercise does not produce much added weight loss over diet alone in the short run, it appears to be extremely important in maintaining the reduced state. The National Weight Control Registry is a group of 1000 people who have been identified because they have successfully lost 30 lb and kept it off for at least 1 year. They self-report 2000 calories/week of planned physical activity. A discussion of physical activity should begin with a physical activity history. Ask about the frequency of engaging in planned physical activity. Then ask about hours per day of television viewing, computer time, and other sedentary activities. Finally, discuss activities of daily living, including work-related activities. Assess the individual's readiness to change physical activity.

51. **Explain the exercise recommendation of the American College of Sports Medicine.**
    The American College of Sports Medicine recommends, "all Americans should accumulate at least 30 minutes of moderate physical activity on most days of the week." There are three important points here:
    1. *Accumulate:* Three 10-minute bouts of exercise in a day are as good as one 30-minute bout.
    2. *Moderate physical activity:* Monitoring and achieving a target heart rate are not necessary. Most people are able to make a subjective assessment of what constitutes moderate physical activity.
    3. *On most days of the week:* Frequent activity appears to be important. The goal is to make physical activity part of everyday life.

52. **Does exercise have health benefits other than weight loss?**
    A growing body of evidence indicates that fitness conveys health benefits independent of weight loss. In addition, increasing physical activity is the number-one priority of the Healthy People 2010 national goals.

53. **What are pedometers? How are they used?**
    Pedometers are small devices that clip to the waistband of clothing. They can be used both to assess usual physical activity and to make and monitor physical activity goals. The usual number of steps taken by an average person is 6000/day. The recommended level of steps to prevent weight gain is 10,000 steps/day. The average for people in the National Weight Control Registry is 12,000.

54. **Discuss the role of surgical treatment in the management of the obese patient.**
    Gastric bypass surgery, gastric banding, and other related procedures have the highest level of success in the treatment of serious obesity, as well as the highest rate of complications.

Procedures can be performed in an open technique or, now commonly, by laparoscopic means. The success rate for gastric bypass is roughly 85%, with most patients losing 30% of their pre-operative weight. The weight loss appears to last for more than 15 years, the longest follow-up currently available. Weight loss is consistently greater with gastric bypass than with banding. The complication rate, however, is not trivial, with roughly 20% of patients experiencing some form of postoperative morbidity, including persistent vomiting, wound infections, dehiscence, depression, and pulmonary complications, to name a few.

55. Does surgical treatment confer benefits other than weight loss?
Diabetes resolves in 83% of patients with preoperative diabetes. Sleep apnea, gastroesophageal reflux, infertility, and other health problems also are substantially improved postoperatively.

56. What is a very low-calorie diet (VLCD)? When should its use be considered?
A VLCD is a nutritionally complete diet of 800 kcal/day that produces rapid weight loss. Experienced teams in supervised settings should administer VLCDs. When VLCDs are used in this manner, complications are rare. The long-term results with VLCDs are no better than with other dietary programs. For this reason, their usefulness is limited. They may be helpful for the patient who needs a short-term weight loss to reduce the risk of a diagnostic or surgical procedure.

WEBSITES

1. http://www.nhlbi.nih.gov/guidelines/obesity/ob_home.htm

2. http://www.niddk.nih.gov/health/nutrit/pubs/statobes.htm

BIBLIOGRAPHY

1. Agatston A: The South Beach Diet. New York, Random House, 2003.
2. Bessesen DH, Kushner R: Evaluation and Management of Obesity. Philadelphia, Hanley & Belfus, 2002.
3. Bray GA, Greenway FL: Current and potential drugs for treatment of obesity. Endocrine Rev 20:805–875, 1999.
4. Brolin RE: Bariatric surgery and long-term control of morbid obesity. JAMA 288:2793–2796, 2002.
5. Brownell KD: The LEARN Program for Weight Control, 7th ed. Dallas, American Health, 1997.
6. Changon YC, Rankinen T, Snyder EE, et al: The human obesity map: The 2002 update. Obesity Res 11:313–367, 2003.
7. Flegal KM, Carroll MD, Ogden CL, Johnson CL: Prevalence and trends in obesity among US adults, 1999–2000. JAMA 288:1723–1727, 2002.
8. Foster GD, Wyatt HR, Hill JO, et al: A randomized trial of a low-carbohydrate diet for obesity. N Engl J Med 348:2082–2090, 2003.
9. Hensrud DD: Pharmacotherapy for obesity. Med Clin North Am 84:463–476, 2000.
10. Heshka S, Anderson JW, Atkinson RL, et al: Weight loss with self-help compared with a structured commercial program: A randomized trial. JAMA 289:1792–1798, 2003.
11. Heymsfield SB, Van Mierlo CA, Van Der Knaap HC, et al: Weight management using a meal replacement strategy: Meta and pooling analysis from size studies. Int J Obesity Relat Metab Disord 27:537–549, 2003.
12. Knowler WC, Barrett-Conner E, Fowler SE, et al: Reduction in the incidence of type 2 diabetes with lifestyle intervention or metformin. N Engl J Med 346:393–403, 2002.
13. Kushner RF, Kushner N: Dr. Kushner's Personality Type Diet. New York, St. Martin's Press, 2003.
14. Mantzoros CS: The role of leptin in human obesity and disease: A review of current evidence. Ann Intern Med 130:671–680, 1999.
15. McGraw P: The Ultimate Weight Solution. New York, Simon & Schuster, 2003.

16. National Institutes of Health: The practical guide to the identification, evaluation and treatment of overweight and obesity in adults. Obesity Res 6(Suppl 12), 1998.

17. Obesity Issue. JAMA 282:1493–1596, 1999.

18. Quinn RD: Five-year self-management of weight using meal replacements: Comparison with matched controls in rural Wisconsin. Nutrition 16:344–348, 2000.

19. Reaven GM: Importance of identifying the overweight patient who will benefit the most by losing weight. Ann Intern Med 138:420–423, 2003.

20. Rosenbaum M, Leibel RL, Hirsch J: Obesity. N Engl J Med 337:396–407,1997.

21. Samaha FF, Iqbal N, Seshadri P, et al: A low-carbohydrate as compared with a low-fat diet in severe obesity. N Engl J Med 348:2074–2081, 2003.

22. Schwartz MW, Woods SC, Porte D, et al: Central nervous system control of food intake. Nature 404:661–671, 2000.

23. Thompson D, Wolf AM: The medical care cost burden of obesity. Obesity Rev 2:189–197, 2001.

24. Tuomilehto J, Lindstrom J, Eriksson JG, et al: Prevention of type 2 diabetes mellitus by changes in lifestyle among subjects with impaired glucose tolerance. N Engl J Med 344:1343–1350, 2001.

25. Wadden TA, Foster GD: Behavioral treatment of obesity. Med Clin North Am 84:441–461, 2000.

OSTEOPOROSIS

Michael T. McDermott, M.D.

CHAPTER 9

1. **What is osteoporosis?**
   Osteoporosis is a skeletal disorder characterized by compromised bone strength, predispos-ing to an increased risk for the development of fragility fractures. This definition emphasizes the critical role of bone strength, which is determined by both bone mass and bone quality, and the importance of fractures, which cause the major morbidity and mortality from this condition.

2. **What is a fragility fracture?**
   A fragility fracture is one that occurs spontaneously or following minimal trauma, defined as falling from a standing height or less. Fractures of the vertebrae, hips, and distal radius (Colles' fracture) are characteristic, but any fracture may occur. Osteoporosis accounts for approxi-mately 1.5 million fractures in the United States each year.

3. **What are the complications of osteoporotic fractures?**
   Vertebral fractures cause loss of height, anterior kyphosis (dowager's hump), reduced pul-monary function, and an increased mortality rate. Approximately one-third of all vertebral frac-tures are painful but two-thirds are asymptomatic. Hip fractures are associated with permanent disability in nearly 50% of patients and with a 20% excess mortality rate compared to the age-matched nonfracture population.

4. **What factors contribute most to the risk of developing an osteoporotic fracture?**
   1. Low bone mass (2-fold risk increase for every standard deviation decrease of bone mass).
   2. Age (2-fold risk increase for every decade in age above age 60 years at same bone mass level).
   3. Previous fragility fracture (5-fold risk increase if there has been a previous fracture).
   4. Propensity to fall.

5. **What are the currently accepted indications for bone mass measurement?**
   - Age > 65 years.
   - Estrogen deficiency plus one risk factor for osteoporosis.
   - Vertebral deformity, fracture, or osteopenia by x-ray.
   - Primary hyperparathyroidism.
   - Glucocorticoid therapy, ≥ 5 mg/day of prednisone for ≥ 3 months.
   - Monitoring the response to an FDA-approved osteoporosis medication.

6. **How is bone mass currently measured?**
   The most accurate and widely used methods in current practice are dual energy x-ray absorp-tiometry (DEXA), computed tomography (CT), and ultrasound (US). In my opinion, DEXA offers the best accuracy and precision with the least radiation exposure in most patients.

Central densitometry measurements (spine and hip) are the best predictors of fracture risk and have the best precision for longitudinal monitoring. Peripheral densitometry measurements (heel, radius, hands), however, are more widely available and less expensive.

7. **How do you read a bone densitometry report?**

   T-score: The number of standard deviations (SDs) the patient is below or above the mean value for young normal subjects (peak bone mass). The T-score is a good predictor of the fracture risk.

   Z-score: The number of SDs the patient is below or above the mean value for age-matched normal subjects. The Z-score indicates whether or not the patient's bone mass is appropriate for age or whether other factors are likely to account for excessively low bone mass.

   Absolute bone mineral density (BMD): The actual bone density value expressed in gm/cm^2. This is the value one should use to calculate percent changes in bone density during longitudinal follow-up.

8. **How is the diagnosis of osteoporosis made?**

   The diagnosis of osteoporosis is made when a patient has a characteristic osteoporotic fracture or when the following World Health Organization (WHO) criteria for BMD are met at any skeletal site:

T-score ≥ -1	Normal
T-score between -1 and -2.5	Osteopenia
T-score ≤ -2.5	Osteoporosis

9. **What are the major risk factors for developing low bone mass?**

Nonmodifiable	Modifiable
Age	Low calcium intake
Race (Caucasian, Asian)	Low vitamin D intake
Female gender	Estrogen deficiency
Early menopause	Sedentary lifestyle
Slender build	Cigarette smoking
Positive family history	Alcohol excess (> 2 drinks/day)
	Caffeine excess (> 2 servings/day)
	Medications (glucocorticoids, excess thyroxine)

10. **What other conditions must be considered as causes of low bone mass?**

Osteomalacia	Celiac disease
Osteogenesis imperfecta	Idiopathic hypercalciuria
Hyperparathyroidism	Multiple myeloma
Hyperthyroidism	Rheumatoid arthritis
Hypogonadism	Renal failure
Cushing's syndrome	Mastocytosis

11. **Outline a cost-effective evaluation to rule out these possibilities.**

    A complete history and physical examination should always be performed. Afterward the following tests should be adequate in most patients:

    - Complete blood count with erythrocyte sedimentation rate.
    - Serum calcium, phosphate, alkaline phosphatase, and creatinine.
    - Serum TSH.
    - Serum testosterone (men).
    - 24-hour urine calcium and creatinine.

KEY POINTS: PREVALENCE AND RISK FACTORS FOR OSTEOPOROSIS ✓

1. Approximately 10 million Americans have osteoporosis and are therefore at high risk of developing fragility fractures; this condition affects both women and men.

2. The major risk factors for fragility fractures are low bone mass, a previous fragility fracture, advancing age, and the propensity to fall.

3. Secondary disorders causing bone loss are present in approximately 30% of women and 64% of men who have osteoporosis.

4. Patients who have a fragility fracture or low bone mass should have a complete history and physical examination and a limited number of key, cost-effective laboratory tests to identify any underlying responsible disorders.

12. **What is the best way to determine if a patient has had a previous vertebral fracture?**
Since two-thirds of vertebral fractures are asymptomatic, current or previous back pain may not be reported. A history of 2 in. or more of height loss or the presence of dorsal kyphosis on physical examination are highly suggestive. However, lateral thoracic and lumbar spine films or morphometric x-ray absorptiometry are the most accurate ways to detect existing vertebral fractures.

13. **What are the most significant risk factors for sustaining a fall from the upright position?**
   - Use of sedatives.
   - Visual impairment.
   - Cognitive impairment.
   - Lower extremity disability.
   - Obstacles to ambulation in the home.

14. **What nonpharmacologic measures are useful for preventing and treating osteoporosis?**
   1. Adequate calcium intake:
      - 1000 mg/day, premenopausal women and men.
      - 1500 mg/day, postmenopausal women and men ≥ age 65 years.
   2. Adequate vitamin D intake: 400–800 U/day.
   3. Adequate exercise: aerobic and resistance.
   4. Smoking cessation.
   5. Limitation of alcohol consumption to 2 drinks/day or less.
   6. Limitation of caffeine consumption to 2 servings/day or less.
   7. Fall prevention.

15. **How do you clinically assess a patient's dietary calcium intake?**
The major bioavailable sources are dairy products and calcium-fortified fruit drinks. Ask their daily intake of these products and assign the following approximate calcium contents for their responses:

Milk	300 mg/cup
Cheese	300 mg/oz
Yogurt	300 mg/cup
Fruit juice with calcium	300 mg/cup

Add 300 mg for the general nondairy diet for a reasonable estimate of daily intake.

16. **How do you ensure an adequate intake of calcium and vitamin D?**
    Encourage the consumption of low-fat dairy products using the estimated calcium contents shown above. Any shortfalls in dietary calcium intake should be supplemented with calcium tablets or elixirs. Calcium carbonate and calcium citrate have different solubilities in water but both dissolve readily in acid and are well absorbed when taken with meals. Multivitamins contain 400 units of vitamin D per tablet; one or two tablets per day is sufficient for most patients.

17. **When should medical therapy be initiated for the prevention and treatment of osteoporosis?**
    Nonpharmacologic measures are appropriate for all individuals who want to reduce their risk of developing osteoporosis. The National Osteoporosis Foundation further recommends that pharmacologic therapy be considered in patients with a T-score of −2.0 or less and in patients with a T-score of −1.5 or less in the presence of other osteoporotic risk factors. Patients who have had vertebral, hip, or distal radius fractures should be considered for pharmacologic therapy regardless of their bone density.

18. **Describe bone remodeling.**
    Bone remodeling is the process by which old bone is removed and new bone is formed (see Fig. 9-1). Osteoclasts are multinucleated giant cells that attach to bone surfaces where they secrete acid and proteolytic enzymes that dissolve underlying bone, leaving a resorption pit. Osteoblasts then move in and secrete osteoid, which is subsequently mineralized with calcium and phosphate crystals (hydroxyapatite), refilling the resorption pit with new bone. Bone remodeling occurs throughout the skeleton as an adaptation to changing mechanical stresses on bone (Fig. 9-1).

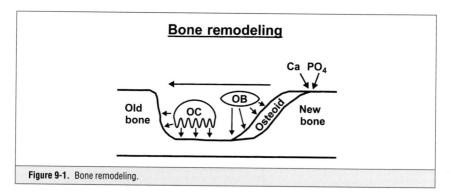

Figure 9-1. Bone remodeling.

19. **How do the pharmacologic agents for the prevention and treatment of osteoporosis work?**
    Medications for osteoporosis fall into two main categories: those that inhibit bone resorption (antiresorptive agents) and those that stimulate bone formation (anabolic agents).

Antiresorptive Agents	Anabolic Agents
Bisphosphonates	Parathyroid hormone (PTH)
Raloxifene	Growth hormone/growth factors
Calcitonin	Sodium fluoride
Estrogens	Strontium

20. **Which bisphosphonates are used in the treatment of osteoporosis?**
    - Alendronate (Fosamax): 10 mg/day or 70 mg/week orally.
    - Risedronate (Actonel): 5 mg/day or 35 mg/week orally.
    - Etidronate (Didronel): 200 mg 2 times a day for 14 days every 3 months orally.
    - Pamidronate (Aredia): 30 mg every 3 months intravenously.

    Only two (alendronate, risedronate) are FDA-approved for the treatment of osteoporosis; both have proven antifracture efficacy at the spine and the hip. Patients should take them in the morning on an empty stomach with a full glass of water and then remain upright and take nothing by mouth for 30 minutes afterwards. Etidronate or pamidronate may be considered in patients who are unable to tolerate one of these FDA-approved oral agents.

21. **How effective are the bisphosphonates in reducing the risk of fragility fractures?**
    Alendronate and risedronate have been demonstrated to significantly reduce both vertebral and hip fractures in randomized controlled trials (RCTs) involving women with postmenopausal osteoporosis (PMO) and previous vertebral fractures. Alendronate reduced vertebral fractures by 47% and hip fractures by 51% after 3 years of treatment (FIT-1 trial). Risedronate reduced vertebral fractures by 65% after 1 year and by 41% after 3 years (VERT-NA trial) and reduced hip fractures by 40% (HIP trial) after 3 years of treatment. Compelling fracture reduction data are not available for etidronate or pamidronate.

22. **Discuss the use of raloxifene in the management of osteoporosis.**
    Raloxifene (Evista), a selective estrogen receptor modulator (SERM), is an estrogen agonist in bone and an antagonist in the breast and uterus. It was shown in a large RCT to reduce vertebral fractures by 50% in women with PMO but no previous vertebral fractures and by 30% in those with prior vertebral fractures (MORE trial). The dose is 60 mg every day. Side effects can include hot flashes, leg cramps, and a modestly increased risk of venous thrombosis. Raloxifene may also reduce the risk of breast cancer and coronary artery disease (CAD). RCTs (RUTH, STAR) are in progress to evaluate these potential effects.

23. **Does calcitonin also reduce osteoporotic fractures?**
    Calcitonin nasal spray (Miacalcin) was reported to reduce vertebral fractures by 33% in women with PMO in a large RCT (PROOF trial). The effective dose is 200 units intranasally every day. Side effects are uncommon, consisting mainly of nasal congestion and skin rashes. Calcitonin may also have modest analgesic effects in some patients with recent vertebral fractures.

24. **Briefly discuss the issues regarding hormone replacement therapy (HRT).**
    The Women's Health Initiative (WHI) is an ongoing RCT investigating the effects of HRT (Premarin + Provera) and estrogen replacement therapy (ERT; Premarin alone) in women who have an intact uterus (HRT) or a previous hysterectomy (ERT). The HRT arm was stopped after 5 years because of mild increases in the occurrence of CAD events (29%), invasive breast cancer (26%), strokes (41%), and venous thromboembolic events (110%). However, vertebral fractures and hip fractures were both reduced by 34%. The ERT arm was also recently stopped, and the data are now being analyzed. As a result of this and other studies, HRT and ERT are no longer recommended for the prevention or treatment of osteoporosis or CAD. HRT and ERT may still be useful for the treatment of hot flashes in the first few years after menopause.

25. **How could PTH be an anabolic agent for treating osteoporosis?**
    Persistently elevated serum PTH levels, as occur in primary hyperparathyroidism, promote osteoclastic bone resorption and bone loss. However, intermittent daily pulses of exogenous PTH actually stimulate new osteoblastic bone formation with a resultant increase in both cortical

and trabecular bone mass. Intact PTH is an 84-amino-acid peptide. Since only the first 13 amino acids are necessary for binding to PTH receptors, smaller fragments, such as teriparatide (1–34 PTH), can be injected daily to produce this effect.

26. **Does teriparatide effectively and safely reduce fractures in osteoporotic patients?**

    Teriparatide (Forteo), given as 20 μg subcutaneously every day for 18 months to women with PMO, increased vertebral bone mass by 10% and reduced vertebral fractures by 65% and nonvertebral fractures by 53% in a large multicenter RCT. Significant hypercalcemia did not occur and side effects were uncommon. Transient orthostatic hypotension sometimes develops in the first few weeks of therapy but can be minimized by administering the dose at bedtime in affected individuals.

27. **Are other anabolic agents available for treating osteoporosis?**

    Strontium ranelate was shown in an RCT involving 1649 postmenopausal osteoporotic women to increase bone mass by 14% in the spine and 8% in the hip and to reduce the risk of new vertebral fractures by 49% in the first year and by 41% after 3 years of use. Sodium fluoride, given as a low-dose slow-release formulation, also increases bone mass and has been demonstrated to reduce fractures, whereas the higher doses used in earlier studies lack proven fracture efficacy and have excessive side effects. Neither strontium nor fluoride is currently FDA-approved for use in osteoporosis. Growth hormone, IGF-1 and HMG CoA reductase inhibitors (statins) are other agents with apparent anabolic effects on bone, but none have yet been adequately tested for antifracture efficacy or safety in humans.

28. **Are combinations of osteoporosis medications more effective than single agents?**

    Combinations of antiresorptive agents increase bone mass more than do single agents used alone. However, fracture data are not yet available for such regimens. While it may seem intuitive that greater bone mass gains would result in fewer fractures, experts have raised the concern that over-suppression of bone resorption could impair the removal of older bone to such an extent that bone strength might ultimately be reduced. Combinations of anabolic and antiresorptive agents used concurrently have disappointingly shown no greater effects on BMD compared to single agents alone. Additional studies investigating sequential use of various agents are currently in progress.

29. **Should BMD be monitored in patients on osteoporosis therapy?**

    BMD is commonly monitored by practitioners, but it is critical that one understands the expected BMD changes and the least significant change (LSC) for the measurements. The antiresorptive agents increase BMD during the first 18–24 months of therapy, after which BMD tends to stabilize; however, this does not represent a loss of medication effectiveness, since fracture protection persists. The long-term response pattern to anabolic agents has not yet been fully defined but will likely be similar. The LSC is the amount of BMD change that must occur to exceed the precision error of the instrument of measurement. This typically is 2.7–3.0% in the spine and 5.7–6.0% in the hip. These figures should be calculated for each instrument used in patient care; standard equations are available for this calculation.

30. **What markers are available to assess bone remodeling and how are they used?**

Bone Formation	Bone Resorption
Serum alkaline phosphatase	Urine or serum *N*-telopeptides
Serum osteocalcin	Urine or serum pyridinoline crosslinks

Elevation of one or more biomarkers at baseline predicts an increased risk of future bone loss and fragility fracture development. A 50% reduction of biomarkers 3–6 months after therapy is initiated verifies compliance and predicts an increase in bone mass and reduction in fracture risk. However, marked variability in biomarker measurement limits the utility of this tool.

KEY POINTS: PREVENTION AND TREATMENT OF OSTEOPOROSIS ✓

1. Nonpharmacologic measures that are important for both the prevention and treatment of osteoporosis include adequate calcium and vitamin D nutrition, regular exercise, fall prevention, discontinuation of smoking, and limitation of alcohol and caffeine intake.

2. Pharmacologic interventions for osteoporosis fall into two main categories: antiresorptive agents and anabolic agents.

3. The antiresorptive agents currently approved by the FDA increase BMD and decrease the risk of vertebral fractures; alendronate and risedronate have also been reported to decrease the risk of hip fractures.

4. Teriparatide, the only anabolic agent currently approved by the FDA, increases BMD and reduces the risk of both vertebral and nonvertebral fractures.

5. Combination therapy with two antiresorptive agents increases BMD to a slightly greater extent than does monotherapy. But no fracture data exist to verify the overall effectiveness of such regimens.

6. Combination therapy with antiresorptive and anabolic agents does not appear to increase BMD more than either type of agent used alone, but sequential regimens are under investigation and appear promising.

31. **What is the role of vertebroplasty and kyphoplasty following vertebral fractures?**
Vertebroplasty is a procedure in which a trochar is inserted into a collapsed vertebra and cement (methylmethacrylate) is infused under pressure to re-expand the vertebral body. Kyphoplasty differs in that the vertebra is first expanded with a balloon, and cement is then infused under low pressure to avoid extra-vertebral extrusion of the cement. These procedures are useful in relieving chronic pain from vertebral fractures and may help to reduce the development of progressive kyphosis.

32. **How common is osteoporosis in men?**
Approximately 1–2 million men in the United States have osteoporosis by bone densitometry criteria. Worldwide, approximately 30% of hip fractures occur in men. Men have a substantially higher risk of having a hip fracture than they do of developing prostate cancer and have a higher mortality rate after hip fractures than do women. Elderly men have a 25% lifetime risk of sustaining any type of fragility fracture. BMD screening is recommended for all men who have significant risk factors for osteoporosis and in otherwise healthy men at age 70 years and older.

33. **How is the diagnosis of osteoporosis made in men?**
The presence of a fragility fracture establishes the diagnosis, provided no other metabolic bone disease can be identified as the culprit. However, bone densitometry criteria for the diagnosis of osteoporosis in men without fragility fractures have not been firmly established. Most experts propose that we should use the same criteria as those employed in women (T-score < –2.5), and

that a normal male reference database should be used to calculate the T-scores. Better data comparing the fracture risk for the various BMD levels and the cost-benefit ratios of treatment at each level are clearly needed.

34. **What are the causes of osteoporosis in men?**
Osteoporosis in men very often occurs as a consequence of another condition or disorder. The more common underlying conditions include hypogonadism, alcohol abuse, glucocorticoid use, and idiopathic hypercalciuria. The use of GnRH analogs to lower serum testosterone levels for the treatment of prostate cancer also frequently causes substantial bone loss and increases the risk of fractures in men.

35. **How effective is pharmacologic therapy in men with osteoporosis?**
Oral bisphosphonates and teriparatide improve BMD in men, as well as they do in women. Testosterone replacement increases BMD in men with low serum testosterone levels (but not in those with normal values) and is therefore recommended only in hypogonadal men. Thiazide diuretics improve BMD in men with idiopathic hypercalciuria. Bisphosphonate therapy has been shown to prevent bone loss in men taking GnRH analogs for prostate cancer.

36. **How can falls be prevented?**
1. Sedatives should be minimized or discontinued.
2. Visual impairment should be corrected.
3. Ambulatory aids should be used when appropriate.
4. Make the home "fall-proof": adequate lighting, carpeting, handrails, nonslip surfaces in bathrooms, removal of clutter and other obstacles to walking.

BIBLIOGRAPHY

1. Adams JS, Song CF, Kantorovich V: Rapid recovery of bone mass in hypercalciuric, osteoporotic men treated with hydrochlorothiazide. Ann Intern Med 130(8):658–660, 1999.
2. Barrett-Connor E, Grady D, Sashegyi A, et al: Raloxifene and cardiovascular events in osteoporotic postmenopausal women. Four-year results from the MORE (multiple outcomes of raloxifene evaluation) randomized trial. JAMA 287:847–857, 2002.
3. Black DM, Cummings SR, Karpf DB, et al: Randomized trial of effect of alendronate on risk of fracture in women with existing vertebral fractures. Lancet 348:1535–1541, 1996 (FIT 1).
4. Black DM, Greenspan SL, Ensrud KE, et al: The effects of parathyroid hormone and alendronate alone or in combination in postmenopausal osteoporosis. N Engl J Med 349:1207–1215, 2003.
5. Bonnick S, Johnston CC, Kleerekoper M, et al: Importance of precision in bone density measurements. J Clin Densitom 4:1–6, 2001.
6. Cauley JA, Thompson DE, Ensrud KC, et al: Risk of mortality following clinical fractures. Osteoporos Int 11:556–561, 2000.
7. Chesnut CH, Silverman S, Andriano K, et al: A randomized trial of nasal spray salmon calcitonin in postmenopausal women with established osteoporosis: the Prevent Recurrence of Osteoporotic Fractures Study. Am J Med 109:267–276, 2000 (PROOF).
8. Cummings SR, Eckert S, Krueger KA, et al: The effect of raloxifene on risk of breast cancer in postmenopausal women. Results from the MORE randomized trial. JAMA 281:2189–2197, 1999.
9. Cummings SR, Palermo L, Browner W, et al: Monitoring osteoporosis therapy with bone densitometry. JAMA 283:1318–1321, 2000.
10. Ettinger B, Black DM, Mitlak BH, et al: Reduction of vertebral fracture risk in postmenopausal women with osteo porosis treated with raloxifene. JAMA 282:637–645, 1999 (MORE).
11. Faulkner KG, Orwoll E: Implications in the use of T-scores for the diagnosis of osteoporosis in men. J Clin Densitom 5:87–93, 2002.
12. Finkelstein JS, Hayes A, Hunzelman JL, et al: The effects of parathyroid hormone, alendronate or both in men with osteoporosis. N Engl J Med 349:1216–1226, 2003.

13. Garnero P, Hausherr E, Chapuy M-C, et al: Markers of bone resorption predict hip fracture in elderly women: The EPIDOS prospective study. J Bone Miner Res 11:1531–1538, 1996.

14. Harris ST, Watts NB, Genant HK, et al: Effects of risedronate treatment on vertebral and nonvertebral fractures in women with postmenopausal osteoporosis. A randomized controlled trial. JAMA 282:1344–1352, 1999 (VERT-NA).

15. Hatano T, Oishi Y, Furuta A, et al: Incidence of bone fracture in patients receiving luteinizing hormone-releasing hormone agonists for prostate cancer. BJU Int 86:449–452, 2000.

16. Hui SL, Slemenda CW, Johnston Jr CC: Age and bone mass as predictors of fracture in a prospective study, J Clin Invest 81:1804–1809, 1988.

17. Klotzbuecher CM, Ross PD, Landsman PB, et al: Patients with prior fractures have an increased risk of future fractures: A summary of the literature and statistical synthesis. J Bone Miner Res 15:721–739, 2000.

18. Lindsay R, Cosman F, Lobo RA, et al: Addition of alendronate to ongoing hormone replacement therapy in the treatment of osteoporosis: A randomized, controlled clinical trial. J Clin Endocrinol Metab 84:3076–3081, 1999.

19. Lindsay R, Silverman SL, Cooper C, et al: Risk of new vertebral fracture in the year following a fracture. JAMA 285:320–23, 2001.

20. Looker AC, Orwoll ES, Johnston Jr CC, et al. Prevalence of low femoral bone density in older U.S. adults from NHANES III. J Bone Miner Res 12:1761–1768, 1997.

21. McClung MR, Geusens P, Miller PD, et al: Effect of risedronate on the risk of hip fracture in elderly women. N Engl J Med 344:333–340, 2001 (HIP).

22. Melton III LJ, Orwoll ES, Wasnich RD: Does bone density predict fractures comparably in men and women? Osteoporos Int 12(9):707–709, 2001.

23. Meunier PJ, Roux C, et al: The effects of strontium ranelate on the risk of vertebral fracture in women with postmenopausal osteoporosis. N Engl J Med 350:459–468, 2004.

24. Miller PD, Bonnick SL, Johnston Jr CC, et al: The challenges of peripheral bone density testing. Which patients need additional central density skeletal measurements? J Clin Densitom 1:211–217, 1998.

25. Mittan D, Lee S, Miller E, et al: Bone loss following hypogonadism in men with prostate cancer treated with GnRH analogs. J Clin Endocrinol Metab 87:3656–3661, 2002.

26. Miller PD, Zapalowski C, Kulak CAM, Bilezikian JP: Bone densitometry: The best way to detect osteoporosis and to monitor therapy. J Clin Endocrinol Metab 84:1867–1871, 1999.

27. Neer RM, Arnaud CD, Zanchetta JR, et al: Effect of parathyroid hormone (1–34) on fractures and bone mineral density in postmenopausal women with osteoporosis. N Engl J Med 344:1434–1441, 2001.

28. Orwoll ES: Osteoporosis in men. Osteoporosis 27:349–367, 1998.

29. Orwoll E, Ettinger M, Weiss S, et al: Alendronate for the treatment of osteoporosis in men. N Engl J Med 343:604–610, 2000.

30. Orwoll E, Scheele WH, Paul S, et al: The effect of teriparatide [human parathyroid hormone (1–34)] therapy on bone density in men with osteoporosis. J Bone Miner Res 18:9–17, 2003.

31. Rea JA, Li J, Blake GM, et al: Visual assessment of vertebral deformity by X-ray absorptiometry: A highly predictive method to exclude vertebral deformity. Osteoporos Int 11:660–668, 2000.

32. Rittmaster RS, Bolognese M, Ettinger MP, et al: Enhancement of bone mass in osteoporotic women with parathyroid hormone followed by alendronate. J Clin Endocrinol Metab 85:2129–2134, 2000.

33. Rosen CJ, Rackoff RJ: Emerging anabolic treatments for osteoporosis. Rheum Dis Clin North Am 27:215–233, 2001.

34. Siris ES, Miller PD, Barrett-Conner E, et al: Identification and fracture outcomes of undiagnosed low bone mineral density in post-menopausal women: Results from the National Osteoporosis Risk Assessment (NORA). JAMA 286:2815–2822, 2001.

35. Smith MR, McGovern FJ, Zietman AL, et al: Pamidronate to prevent bone loss during androgen-deprivation therapy for prostate cancer. N Engl J Med 345:948–955, 2001.

36. Snyder PJ, Peachey H, Hannoush P, et al: Effect of testosterone treatment on bone mineral density in men over 65 years of age. J Clin Endocrinol Metab 84:1966–1972, 1999.

37. Tinetti ME, Speechley M, Ginter SF: Risk factors for falls among elderly persons living in the community. N Engl J Med 19 (26):1701–1707, 1998.

38. Writing Group for the Women's Health Initiative Investigators: Risk and benefits of estrogen plus progestin in healthy postmenopausal women. Principle results from the women's health initiative randomized controlled trial. JAMA 288:321–333, 2002 (WHI).

CHAPTER 10

GLUCOCORTICOID-INDUCED OSTEOPOROSIS

Michael T. McDermott, M.D.

1. **How common is glucocorticoid-induced osteoporosis (GIOP)?**
   GIOP is presently the most common cause of drug-induced osteoporosis. Significant bone loss and skeletal fractures may occur within 6 months of starting glucocorticoid therapy, and up to 50% of people on chronic glucocorticoid treatment develop an osteoporotic fracture.

2. **What are the important determinants of bone loss with glucocorticoid therapy?**
   Bone loss is related mainly to the dose and the duration of glucocorticoid therapy. Glucocorticoid doses ≥ 7.5 mg of prednisone (or equivalent) are associated with the greatest risk. However, a large cohort study showed a significantly increased fracture risk even in those whose median prednisolone doses had been as low as 2.5 mg per day. Decreased bone mass and an increased fracture risk have even been demonstrated in patients using only inhaled glucocorticoids.

3. **Explain the pathogenesis of GIOP.**
   Glucocorticoids adversely affect both phases of bone remodeling (Fig. 10-1). They impair bone formation by promoting cell death (apoptosis) of existing osteoblasts and by reducing the development of new osteoblasts, partly through inhibitory effects on local growth factors, such as IGF-1. They simultaneously increase bone resorption through various mechanisms, such as decreasing the production of sex steroids and osteoprotegerin, an endogenous inhibitor of bone resorption.

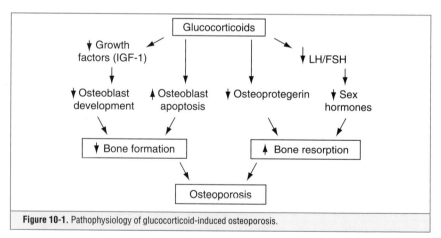

Figure 10-1. Pathophysiology of glucocorticoid-induced osteoporosis.

4. **What are the BMD criteria for a diagnosis of GIOP?**
   The ideal BMD criteria for the diagnosis of GIOP are still being debated but the best existing evidence suggests that the fracture risk per BMD decrement does not differ between GIOP and primary osteoporosis. Accordingly, the same BMD criteria are currently used to diagnose osteoporosis in these patients as in those who are not taking glucocorticoids. However, because of the rapidity of bone loss in this condition, active treatment should be considered at an earlier stage (T-score ≤ −1.0).

KEY POINTS: PREVALENCE AND PATHOPHYSIOLOGY OF GIOP ✓

1. Glucocorticoid-induced osteoporosis is the most common type of drug-induced osteoporosis.

2. High doses and prolonged use of glucocorticoids produce greater risk, but all doses of oral glucocorticoids and even inhaled steroids appear to increase the risk of osteoporotic fractures.

3. The pathophysiology of glucocorticoid-induced osteoporosis involves both suppressed bone formation and enhanced bone resorption, which account for the rapid bone loss often seen in glucocorticoid-treated patients.

5. **In which patients on glucocorticoids should BMD be tested?**
   Patients starting glucocorticoid therapy (prednisone dose ≥ 5 mg/day or equivalent) with planned duration of treatment ≥3 months or on existing treatment for ≥3 months.

6. **When should BMD be tested?**
   1. BMD of the spine and/or hip should be measured at initiation of glucocorticoid therapy or as soon as possible thereafter.
   2. Repeat BMD every 6–12 months as long as glucocorticoid therapy is continued.

7. **What measures should be instituted in all patients on glucocorticoids?**
   All glucocorticoid-treated patients should be advised to consume adequate calcium (1500 mg/day; combination of dietary intake plus supplements) and vitamin D (800 U/day), exercise regularly (aerobic and resistance), stop smoking, and limit alcohol and caffeine consumption.

8. **Which medications are effective in preventing and treating GIOP?**
   Bisphosphonates increase spine BMD by an average of 4.6% in patients with GIOP, according to a large meta-analysis. The mean increments for calcitonin and fluoride were 2.3% and 2.9%, respectively. Teriparatide has been shown to improve spine BMD by 9.8% in glucocorticoid-treated women who were also on hormone replacement therapy. Fracture data are only available for the bisphosphonates, which have been reported to decrease the incidence of vertebral fractures by 40–70% (Fig. 10-2).

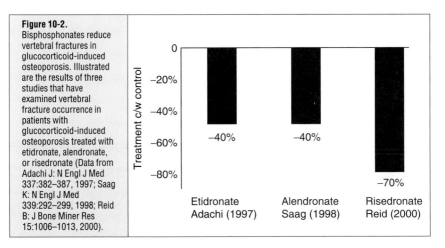

Figure 10-2. Bisphosphonates reduce vertebral fractures in glucocorticoid-induced osteoporosis. Illustrated are the results of three studies that have examined vertebral fracture occurrence in patients with glucocorticoid-induced osteoporosis treated with etidronate, alendronate, or risedronate (Data from Adachi J: N Engl J Med 337:382–387, 1997; Saag K: N Engl J Med 339:292–299, 1998; Reid B: J Bone Miner Res 15:1006–1013, 2000).

9. **Which glucocorticoid-treated patients should receive active intervention?**
   - Postmenopausal women (all).
   - Men and premenopausal women with T-score ≤ –1.0.

10. **What are the current first-line agents for active intervention?**
    Bisphosphonates: oral (alendronate, risedronate, etidronate) or intravenous (pamidronate).

11. **When should teriparatide be considered?**
    Teriparatide should be considered in patients with very low BMD, existing fragility fractures, and inadequate response to bisphosphonates.

KEY POINTS: PREVENTION AND TREATMENT OF GIOP ✔

1. Bone mineral density (BMD) testing is recommended before initiation of glucocorticoid therapy in patients who will receive ≥ 5 mg/day of prednisone (or equivalent) for ≥ 3 months duration and every 6–12 months thereafter as long as glucocorticoid therapy is continued.

2. Treatment is recommended for all postmenopausal women regardless of initial BMD and for men or premenopausal women with a BMD T-score ≤ –1.0 who are treated or will be treated with ≥5 mg/day of prednisone (or equivalent) for ≥ 3 months.

3. Both antiresorptive and anabolic agents improve BMD in patients with glucocorticoid-induced osteoporosis, while alendronate, risedronate, and etidronate have all been shown to reduce the occurrence of fragility fractures.

12. **When should calcitonin be considered?**
    Calcitonin should be considered in patients with intolerance or contraindication to bisphosphonates.

13. **When should gonadal steroids be considered?**
    Gonadal steroids may be considered in combination with other agents or alone in post-menopausal women and hypogonadal men (low serum testosterone).

14. **List the indications for thiazide diuretics.**
    - If urine calcium > 300 mg/day in men.
    - If urine calcium > 250 mg/day in women.

BIBLIOGRAPHY

1. Adachi JD, Bensen WG, Brown J, et al: Intermittent etidronate therapy to prevent corticosteroid-induced osteoporosis. N Engl J Med 337:382–387, 1997.

2. Adachi JD, Olszynski WP, Hanley DA, et al: Management of corticosteroid-induced osteoporosis. Semin Arthritis Rheum 29: 228–251, 2000.

3. Adinoff AD, Hollister JR: Steroid-induced fractures and bone loss in patients with asthma. N Engl J Med 309:265–268, 1983.

4. American College of Rheumatology Ad Hoc Committee on Glucocorticoid-induced Osteoporosis: Recommendations for the prevention and treatment of glucocorticoid-induced osteoporosis. 2001 update. Arthritis Rheum 44:1496–1503, 2001.

5. Amin S, LaValley MP, Simms RW, Felson DT: The comparative efficacy of drug therapies used for the management of corticosteroid-induced osteoporosis: A meta-regression. J Bone Miner Res 17:1512–1526, 2002.

6. Canalis E: Glucocorticoid-induced osteoporosis. Curr Opin Endocrinol Diabetes 7:320–324, 2000.

7. Isreal E, Banerjee TR, Fitzmaurice GM, et al: Effects of inhaled glucocorticoids on bone density in premenopausal women. N Engl J Med 345:941–947, 2001.

8. Lane NE, Sanchez S, Modin GW, et al: Parathyroid hormone treatment can reverse corticosteroid-induced osteoporosis. Results of a randomized controlled clinical trial. J Clin Invest 102:1627–1633, 1998.

9. Manolagas SC, Weinstein RS: New developments in the pathogenesis and treatment of steroid-induced osteoporosis. J Bone Miner Res 14:1061–1066, 1999.

10. Reid DM, Hughes RA, Laan RF, et al: Efficacy and safety of daily risedronate in the treatment of cortico-steroid-induced osteoporosis in men and women: A randomized trial. European corticosteroid-induced osteoporosis treatment study. J Bone Miner Res 15:1006–1103, 2000.

11. Rubin MR, Bilezikian JP: The role of parathyroid hormone in the pathogenesis of glucocorticoid-induced osteoporosis: A re-examination of the evidence. J Clin Endocrinol Metab 87: 4033–4041, 2002.

12. Saag KG, Emkey R, Schnitzer TJ, et al: Alendronate for the prevention and treatment of glucocorticoid-induced osteoporosis. N Engl J Med 339:292–299, 1998.

13. Selby PL, Halsey JP, Adams KRH, et al: Corticosteroids do not alter the threshold for vertebral fracture. J Bone Miner Res 15:952–956, 2000.

14. Van Staa TP, Leufkens HGM, Abenhaim L, et al: Use of oral corticosteroids and risk of fractures. J Bone Miner Res 15:993–1000, 2000.

15. Van Staa TP, Leufkens HGM, Cooper C: Use of inhaled corticosteroids and risk of fractures. J Bone Miner Res 16:581–588, 2001.

CHAPTER 11

MEASUREMENT OF BONE MASS

William E. Duncan, M.D., Ph.D.

1. **Why measure bone mass?**

   Bone mass is measured by bone mineral densitometry to establish the diagnosis of osteo-porosis, to predict the risk of subsequent fractures, and to monitor changes in bone mass during therapy for osteoporosis. No clinical finding, laboratory test, or other radiographic exam-ination can reliably identify individuals with osteoporosis. Standard roentgenograms are not sensitive indicators of bone loss, as they do not reliably indicate osteoporosis until 30–40% of the bone mineral is lost. However, while bone densitometry can determine if there is low bone mass, it cannot determine its cause. Thus, bone densitometry must be used along with a complete clinical evaluation, laboratory testing, and other diagnostic studies to determine the cause of and the most appropriate treatment for osteoporosis.

2. **Is bone mass the only factor that determines if a bone will fracture?**

   While a decreased bone mass is the primary determinant of whether a bone will fracture, bone architecture (connectivity and remodeling) and bone geometry are also important factors contributing to bone strength. The relationship between bone mass and fracture risk is more pow-erful than the relationship between serum cholesterol concentration and coronary artery disease. A decrease in bone mass of 1 SD doubles the risk of fracture. In comparison, a decrease in the cho-lesterol concentration of 1 SD increases the risk of coronary artery disease by only 20–30%.

3. **How does bone densitometry measure bone mass?**

   All bone densitometry techniques measure the amount of calcium present in bone utilizing an ionizing radiation source, either from a radionuclide or from x-rays, and a radiation detector. Bone densitometry is based on the principle that bone will absorb a beam of radiation in propor-tion to its bone mineral content. The bone mineral content of the bone (or a region of interest within a bone) is then divided by the measured area. The result is the bone mineral density in grams per unit area (gm/cm^2). This bone mineral density is not a true volumetric density (gm/cm^3) but rather an areal density. In this chapter, bone mass and bone density are used interchangeably and synonymously.

4. **What techniques are available to measure bone mass?**

   The techniques available to measure bone mass include single-photon absorptiometry (SPA), single-energy x-ray absorptiometry (SEXA), dual-photon absorptiometry (DPA), dual-energy x-ray absorptiometry (DXA), quantitative computed tomography (QCT), and radiographic absorptiometry (RA). Another technique, quantitative ultrasound (QUS), transmits ultrasound waves through the bone. The more complex and dense the bone structure, the greater the attenuation of the ultrasound wave. Thus, QUS may determine both density and structure of the bone. Table 11-1 compares several of these bone mass measurement techniques.

5. **What is the preferred method for measuring bone mass?**

   DXA is the preferred method for measuring bone mass in the United States. In 1997, 89% of bone density tests were performed using DXA. DXA can measure the bone mass of the spine, hip, or wrist—the most common sites for osteoporotic fractures.

TABLE 11-1.   COMPARISON OF BONE MASS MEASUREMENT TECHNIQUES

Method	Sites Measured	Precision Error* (%)	Accuracy Error[†] (%)	Radiation Dose (μSV)
SPA	Forearm, calcaneus	1–2	2–5	<1
DXA	PA spine	1	5–8	1
	Lateral spine	2–3	5–10	5
	Proximal femur	1–2	5–8	1
	Total body	1	1–2	3
QCT	Single-energy (spine)	2–4	5–10	60
	Dual-energy (spine)	4–6	3–6	90
	Peripheral (radius)	0.5–1.0	0.5	<2
QUS	Calcaneus	0.3–3.8	—	0
	Patella	<2	—	0

*The error around repeated measurements (reproducibility or coefficient of variation).
[†]A measure of the agreement between the test result and true value (accuracy)

6. **Discuss the advantages and disadvantages of DXA.**
   DXA has the best correlation with fracture risk, requires relatively short scanning times (< 5 minutes) and has the ability to measure bone mass in all areas of the skeleton with high accuracy and reproducibility (precision) and with low radiation exposure. This method does not require replacement of the radioactive source. One drawback of DXA is the initial cost of the equipment.

7. **What are the indications for the measurement of bone mass?**
   Because of the cost, widespread bone density screening for osteoporosis is not recommended at this time. However, individuals at high risk for osteoporosis should be considered for bone mineral density testing. The National Osteoporosis Foundation recommendations for bone mineral density testing are listed as:
   ■ Women ≥ 65 years of age (regardless of risk factors).
   ■ Postmenopausal women < 65 years of age who have at least one risk factor for osteoporosis other than being Caucasian, postmenopausal, and female.
   ■ Postmenopausal women who present with fractures.
      Other indications for measurement of bone mass include x-ray findings suggestive of osteoporosis or vertebral deformity, glucocorticoid therapy for more than 3 months, primary hyperparathyroidism, and monitoring the response to or effectiveness of drug therapy for osteoporosis.

8. **What do bone densitometry results mean?**
   The bone densitometry report gives the absolute bone mass measurements (in gm/cm^2), which do not provide clinically useful information unless these values are compared with those of reference populations. To do so, the bone mineral density report usually provides two scores: a T-score and a Z-score (Fig. 11-1).

9. **What are T-scores?**
   The T-score is the number of standard deviations above or below the mean bone mass of a normal young adult gender-matched population. This population represents the optimal or peak bone mass for the patient. A patient whose bone mass is 1 SD below that of the young reference population has a T-score of −1.0. At the spine, 1 SD is about 10%. Thus, someone with a T-score of −1.0 has lost about 10% of his or her bone mass. Because the T-score is a measure of bone loss, this value is used to diagnose osteoporosis.

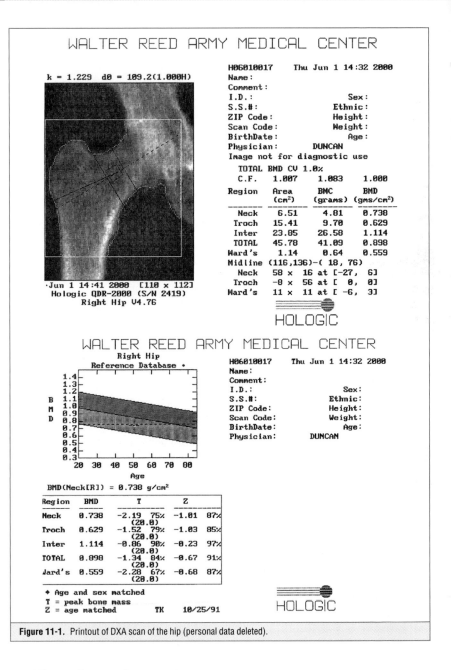

Figure 11-1. Printout of DXA scan of the hip (personal data deleted).

10. **Why are Z-scores important?**

The Z-score is the number of standard deviations above or below the mean bone mass of an age- and gender-matched reference population. The Z-score is used to determine if the measured bone mass is appropriate for the patient's age. A Z-score less than expected for a given individual (e.g., less than −2.0) should prompt a search for associated medical or lifestyle conditions (either current or in the past) that may have accelerated bone loss or prevented the patient from reaching peak bone mass in early adulthood.

11. **How is bone mass classified?**
In 1994, the World Health Organization (WHO) developed criteria for the diagnosis of osteoporosis and osteopenia in postmenopausal white women using T-scores from any skeletal site. A T-score greater than −1.0 is defined as normal bone mass, a T-score between −1.0 and −2.5 is defined as low bone mass (or osteopenia), and a T-score less than −2.5 is defined as osteoporosis. Established (or severe) osteoporosis was defined as a T-score less than −2.5 with one or more osteoporotic fractures.

12. **What are the problems with the WHO classification?**
There are several caveats about using the WHO classification criteria. These criteria were derived from data pertaining to white postmenopausal women. Thus, applying these definitions to other ethnic groups or to men should be done with caution. The WHO criteria were also not intended to apply to premenopausal women. The WHO criteria were developed from studies using DXA. Therefore, applying the WHO criteria to bone mass measurements obtained with other technologies (such as QUS) may be misleading. Finally, these definitions were developed as general guidelines for diagnosis and were not intended to require or restrict therapy for individual patients.

13. **How are bone density measurements interpreted in men and non-Caucasians?**
The criteria by which a densitometric diagnosis of osteoporosis can be made in males and in non-Caucasians is extremely controversial since it is unclear if fractures occur at the same bone mineral density in Caucasian women as they do in men and non-Caucasians. Pending additional studies, the International Society for Clinical Densitometry has recommended that osteoporosis in these groups be diagnosed at or below a T-score of −2.5 using a gender but not a race-adjusted normative database.

14. **Discuss how bone mass measurements are used to determine the need for treatment of osteoporosis.**
The healthcare provider should use information from bone mass testing in conjunction with knowledge of the patient's specific medical and personal history to determine the best treatment. The bone mineral density results should not be used as the sole determinant for treatment decisions. The National Osteoporosis Foundation has proposed that women with T-scores less than −2.0 by central DXA in the absence of risk factors for osteoporosis, women with T-scores less than −1.5 by central DXA with one or more risk factors, or women with a prior vertebral or hip fracture should be treated for osteoporosis.

15. **Which bone(s) should be selected for measurement of bone mass?**
It is possible to measure the bone mass of several bones (Fig. 11-2). Measurement of bone mass at any skeletal site has value in predicting fracture risk. However, the bone density of the hip is the best predictor of hip fractures (the most serious osteoporotic fracture). Hip-bone mass also predicts fractures at other sites, as well as do bone mass measurements at those sites. For these reasons, the hip is the preferred site for measurement of bone mass. While there is significant concordance between skeletal sites in predicting bone mass, there is still enough discordance in bone mass at various sites to not rely on single bone mass measurements to diagnose osteoporosis. Thus, bone mass should be measured at both the hip and the posteroanterior (PA) spine, and the diagnosis of osteoporosis should be based on the lowest T-score.

16. **What is the role for measurement of forearm bone mass?**
Measurement of peripheral bone mass (e.g., the forearm) generally adds little to the evaluation of an individual with postmenopausal osteoporosis, although the forearm appears to be the best site to assess the effects on bone of excess parathyroid hormone activity seen with primary

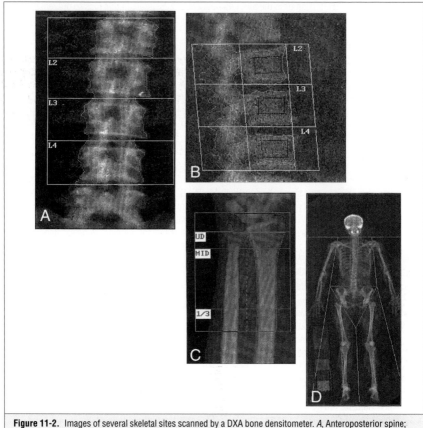

Figure 11-2. Images of several skeletal sites scanned by a DXA bone densitometer. *A*, Anteroposterior spine; *B*, lateral spine; *C*, forearm; *D*, whole body.

hyperparathyroidism. In addition, measurement of forearm bone mass should be done when the hip and spine cannot be accurately measured or when a patient is over the weight limit for the DXA table. Peripheral bone mass measurements have not yet been shown to be useful for monitoring the effects of therapy for osteoporosis.

KEY POINTS: MEASUREMENT OF BONE MASS ✓

1. Direct measurement of bone mass is the only way to diagnose osteoporosis. No clinical finding, laboratory test, or other radiographic examination can reliably identify people with a low bone mass.

2. The preferred technique for diagnosis of osteoporosis is DXA of the spine and hip.

3. The diagnosis of osteoporosis is made using the WHO criteria of a T-score less than or equal to −2.5.

4. Bone mass measurement of the forearm is the study of choice for patients with hyperparathyroidism.

17. **How often should bone mass measurements be repeated?**
The frequency of bone density measurements is determined, in part, by the precision error (or reproducibility) of the technique. The precision of bone mass measurements by DXA is 1.0% for spine and 1–2% for the femoral neck. This means that the smallest difference between two bone mass measurements that is significant is a change of 2.83% at the spine and 5.66% at the femoral neck. In contrast, the average amount of early postmenopausal bone loss from the spine is 1–2% per year. Therefore, to obtain statistically meaningful results, postmenopausal women should not undergo measurements of spine bone mass by DXA more often than once every 1.4 years. Measurement of bone mass every 6 months is recommended for patients in whom glucocorticoid therapy is being initiated because a more rapid rate of bone loss may occur than observed in postmenopausal women.

18. **What conditions limit the accuracy of bone mass measurements?**
Several factors may limit the accuracy of PA spine mass measurements: degenerative changes, oral contrast taken for other radiographic studies, and osteophytes artificially elevate the measured bone density. Anatomic distortions that affect the accuracy of these measurements may also result from lumbar disc disease, compression fractures, scoliosis, prior surgical intervention, or vascular calcifications in the overlying aorta, which are common in the elderly. Likewise, previous surgery on the hip may alter bone mass.

19. **Interpret the bone mineral density results from the following four patients.**
Each patient is a white postmenopausal woman. The bone mass was measured at any skeletal site.

Patient 1	T-score = –0.9	Z-score = +0.2
Patient 2	T-score = –2.0	Z-score = –0.9
Patient 3	T-score = –3.0	Z-score = –1.4
Patient 4	T-score = –3.0	Z-score = –2.5

Interpretation:
Patient 1   This woman has a normal bone mass.
Patient 2   This woman has a low bone mass (osteopenia) that is appropriate
for her age (the Z-score is greater than –2.0).
Patient 3   This woman has osteoporosis that is appropriate for her age.
Patient 4   This woman has osteoporosis with bone loss that is greater than expected for her age.
This bone density finding should prompt a thorough evaluation to rule out secondary causes of osteoporosis (such as hyperthyroidism, malabsorption, Cushing's syndrome, hypogonadism, vitamin D deficiency, excessive alcohol consumption, celiac disease, and use of certain drugs).

WEBSITES

1. National Osteoporosis Foundation: http://www.nof.org

2. International Society for Clinical Densitometry: http://www.iscd.org

BIBLIOGRAPHY

1. Binkley N, Schmeer P, Wasnich R, Lenchik L: What are the criteria by which a densitometric diagnosis of osteoporosis can be made in males and noncaucasians? J Clin Densitom 5(Suppl):S19–S27, 2002.

2. Blake G, Fogelman I: Dual energy x-ray absorptiometry and its clinical applications. Semin Musculoskelet Radiol 6:207–218, 2002.

3. Genant HK, Engelke K, Fuerst T, et al: Noninvasive assessment of bone mineral and structure: State of the art. J Bone Miner Res 11:707, 1996.

4. Gluer CC, Genant HK, Hans D, et al: Quantitative ultrasound techniques for the assessment of osteoporosis: Expert agreement on current status. J Bone Miner Res 12:1280, 1997.

5. Hamdy R, Petak S, Lenchik L: Which central dual x-ray absorptiometry skeletal sites and regions of interest should be used to determine the diagnosis of osteoporosis? J Clin Densitrom 5(Suppl): S11–S18, 2002.

6. Lenchik L, Kiebzak G, Blunt B: What is the role of serial bone mineral density measurements in patient management? J Clin Densitrom 5(Suppl):S29–S38, 2002.

7. Levis S, Altman R: Bone densitometry: Clinical considerations. Arthritis Rheum 41:577, 1998.

8. Miller PD, Zapalowski C, Kulak CA, Bilezikian JP: Bone densitometry: The best way to detect osteoporosis and to monitor therapy. J Clin Endocrinol Metab 84:1867, 1999.

9. Miller P: Bone mineral density-clinical use and application. Endocrinol Metab Clin North Am 32:159–179, 2003.

10. Shagam J: Bone densitometry: An update. Radiol Technol 74:321–338, 2003.

11. The WHO Study Group: Assessment of Fracture Risk and Its Application to Screening for Postmenopausal Osteoporosis. WHO Tech Rep Ser 843. Geneva, World Health Organization, 1994.

CHAPTER 12

OSTEOMALACIA AND RICKETS

William E. Duncan, M.D., Ph.D.

1. **What are osteomalacia and rickets?**

   Osteomalacia and rickets are terms that describe the clinical, histologic, and radiologic abnormalities of bone that are associated with more than 50 different diseases and conditions. Osteomalacia is a disorder of mature bone, while rickets occurs in growing bone. Mineralization of newly formed osteoid (the bone protein matrix) is inadequate or delayed in both conditions. Thus, in individuals with rickets, defective mineralization occurs both in bones and in cartilage of the epiphyseal growth plates and is associated with growth retardation and skeletal deformities, which are not typically seen in adults with osteomalacia. Although rickets and osteomalacia were initially viewed as distinct clinical entities, the same pathologic processes may result in either disorder, depending on whether a growing or nongrowing skeleton is involved.

2. **Why is it important to know about osteomalacia and rickets?**

   In the United States at the beginning of the 20th century, rickets caused by a deficiency of vitamin D was common in urban areas. In the 1920s, it was virtually eliminated by an appreciation of the antirachitic properties of sunlight and the use of cod liver oil (which contains vitamin D). However, with the development of effective treatments for previously fatal diseases (such as chronic renal failure) that affect vitamin D metabolism and with an improved understanding of both vitamin D and mineral metabolism, many additional syndromes with osteomalacia or rickets as a feature have become recognized. In addition, for a significant number of adult women with osteoporosis in the United States, vitamin D insufficiency may be an unsuspected component of their bone loss.

3. **List the causes of osteomalacia and rickets.**

   The primary abnormality of bone in patients with osteomalacia or rickets is defective mineralization of bone matrix. The major mineral in bone is hydroxyapatite [$Ca_{10}(PO_4)_6(OH)_2$]. Thus, any disease that limits the availability of calcium or phosphorus may result in osteomalacia or rickets (Table 12-1). The causes of osteomalacia and rickets fall into three categories: (1) disorders associated with abnormalities of vitamin D metabolism or action that limit the availability of calcium for mineralization of bone; (2) disorders associated with abnormalities of phosphorus metabolism; and (3) a small group of disorders in which there is normal vitamin D and mineral metabolism.

4. **Describe how vitamin D is metabolized.**

   Serum vitamin D comes from two sources: dietary intake and conversion by ultraviolet (UV) irradiation of 7-dehydrocholesterol to vitamin D in the skin. Vitamin D is then transported through the blood to the liver where it is converted to 25-hydroxyvitamin D by the hepatic 25-hydroxylase enzyme. The 25-hydroxyvitamin D is then converted in the kidney to the active vitamin D hormone, 1,25-dihydroxyvitamin D, by the renal 1-α-hydroxylase. The active vitamin D hormone has effects in many tissues, including the intestine (increases calcium absorption), the kidney (increases calcium reabsorption), and bone (stimulates osteoblast maturation and bone matrix synthesis) (Fig. 12-1). From an understanding of how vitamin D is metabolized, it is apparent that even when dietary intake and UV-mediated vitamin D synthesis are sufficient, malabsorptive, renal, and liver diseases may be associated with vitamin D deficiency.

TABLE 12–1. CONDITIONS ASSOCIATED WITH OSTEOMALACIA AND RICKETS	
Condition	**Primary Mechanism***
Abnormal vitamin D metabolism or action	
▪ Nutritional deficiency	Vitamin D deficiency
▪ Malabsorption	Vitamin D deficiency
▪ Primary biliary cirrhosis	Malabsorption of vitamin D
▪ Chronic renal disease	Impaired 1α-hydroxylation of 25 hydroxyvitamin D
▪ Chronic liver disease	Impaired 25-hydroxylation of vitamin D
▪ VDDR type I	1α-hydroxylase deficiency
▪ VDDR type II	Abnormal vitamin D receptor
▪ Drugs (phenytoin, barbiturates, cholestyramine)	Increased catabolism and/or excretion of vitamin D
Phosphate deficiency or renal phosphate wasting	
▪ Diminished phosphate intake	Phosphate deficiency
▪ Excessive aluminum hydroxide intake	Increasing binding of intestinal phosphate
▪ X-linked hypophosphatemic rickets	Renal phosphate transport defect
▪ Tumor-induced osteomalacia	Renal phosphate transport defect
▪ Miscellaneous renal tubular defects (RTA, FS)	Renal phosphate transport defect
Normal vitamin D and phosphate metabolism	
▪ Hypophosphatasia	Alkaline phosphatase deficiency
▪ Drugs (fluoride, aluminum, high-dose etidronate)	Inhibition of mineralization or stimulation of matrix synthesis
▪ Osteogenesis imperfecta	Abnormal bone collagen
▪ Fibrogenesis imperfecta ossium	Defective bone matrix

VDDR, vitamin D-dependent rickets; RTA, renal tubular acidosis; FS, Fanconi syndrome.
*Although only one mechanism for osteomalacia or rickets is given, other mechanisms also may contribute to the bone disease.

5. **Discuss the disease processes that interfere with the metabolism of vitamin D.**
Clinically apparent vitamin D deficiency is rarely seen in the United States except when exposure to sunlight or intake of vitamin D-fortified milk and dairy products is limited. However, the elderly in America are particularly at risk for occult vitamin D deficiency because an age-related decrease in the dermal synthesis of vitamin D, an impaired hepatic and renal hydroxylation of vitamin D and a diminished intestinal responsiveness to 1,25-dihydroxyvitamin D. People with malabsorption associated with diseases of the small intestine, the hepatobiliary tree, the pancreas, and the kidney are also at risk for vitamin D deficiency. Celiac disease or sprue, regional enteritis, intestinal bypass surgery, partial gastrectomy, chronic liver disease, primary biliary cirrhosis, pancreatic insufficiency, and chronic renal failure have been associated with the development of osteomalacia. Anticonvulsant drugs (e.g., phenytoin, phenobarbital) may interfere with the action of 1,25-dihydroxyvitamin D in the peripheral tissues and accelerate hepatic metabolism of this steroid hormone.

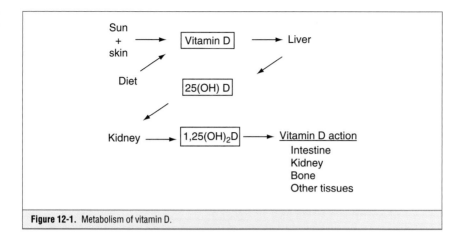

Figure 12-1. Metabolism of vitamin D.

6. **List two genetic disorders that interfere with vitamin D synthesis or action.**
   Two extremely rare genetic syndromes are also associated with rickets. Vitamin D-dependent rickets (VDDR) type I is associated with an almost complete absence of renal 25-hydroxyvitamin D-1α-hydroxylase activity. VDDR type II is caused by a defective vitamin D receptor, which results in an end-organ resistance to 1,25-dihydroxyvitamin D and a lack of vitamin D action.

7. **What conditions associated with abnormalities of phosphate metabolism result in osteomalacia or rickets?**
   Nutritional phosphate deficiency, decreased intestinal absorption of phosphate due to ingestion of phosphate binders, such as aluminum hydroxide, or renal phosphate wasting may result in osteomalacia or rickets. Hypophosphatemic rickets (also called vitamin D-resistant rickets) is a syndrome of renal phosphate wasting and decreased renal synthesis of 1,25-dihydroxyvitamin D and is the most common inherited form of rickets. It is transmitted as an X-linked dominant trait. The abnormal gene for this disorder has been localized to the short arm of the X chromosome. Tumor-induced osteomalacia is an uncommon syndrome, in which usually benign neoplasms (frequently of mesenchymal origin) are found in association with nonfamilial acquired osteomalacia. Such tumors appear to elaborate an as yet unidentified humoral factor that is responsible for renal phosphate wasting.

8. **Does chronic renal failure cause osteomalacia and rickets?**
   Chronic renal failure is associated with several bone diseases: osteomalacia or rickets, adynamic bone, osteitis fibrosa cystica (due to long-standing secondary hyperparathyroidism), and a combination of both osteomalacia and osteitis fibrosa cystica (termed mixed renal osteodystrophy). Rickets or osteomalacia is usually a late finding in the course of the kidney disease and is rarely seen before patients begin dialysis. Rickets and osteomalacia in chronic renal failure are caused by decreased concentrations of circulating 1,25-dihydroxyvitamin D, aluminum intoxication from aluminum-containing antacids used as phosphate binders or an aluminum-contaminated dialysate, and possibly by the chronic metabolic acidosis associated with the renal failure.

9. **What clinical findings are associated with osteomalacia?**
   In adults, osteomalacia may be asymptomatic. When symptomatic, osteomalacia may present with diffuse skeletal pain (often aggravated by physical activity or palpation), proximal muscle weakness, and sometimes muscle wasting. The muscle weakness often involves the proximal muscles of the lower extremities and may result in a waddling gait and difficulties rising from a chair or climbing stairs. The bone pain is described as dull and aching and is usually located in

the back, hips, knees, legs, and at sites of fractures. Fractures may result from only minor trauma.

10. **Describe the clinical findings in children with rickets.**

    Because of the impaired calcification of cartilage at the growth plates in children with rickets, clinical manifestations of rickets are significantly different from those of osteomalacia. Widening of the metaphyses (the growth zones between the epiphysis and diaphysis), slowed growth, and various skeletal deformities are prominent in this condition. The effects of rickets are greatest at sites where the growth of bone is most rapid. Because the rate of growth of the skeleton varies with age, the manifestations of rickets likewise will vary with age. One of the earliest signs of rickets in infants is craniotabes (abnormal softness of the skull). In older infants and young children, thickening of the forearm at the wrist and of the costochondral junctions (also known as the rachitic rosary) and Harrison's groove, a lateral indentation of the chest wall at the site of attachment of the diaphragm, may be present. In older children, bowing of the tibia and fibula may be observed. At any age, if the rickets (or osteomalacia) is associated with hypocalcemia, paresthesias of the hands and around the mouth, muscle cramps, positive Chvostek's and Trousseau's signs, tetany, and seizures may be evident.

11. **What are the calcium and phosphate concentrations associated with osteomalacia and rickets?**

    The laboratory abnormalities associated with osteomalacia or rickets depend on the underlying defect or process causing the bone disease. To understand the biochemical abnormalities observed in conditions associated with the abnormal metabolism of vitamin D, an understanding of the body's response to hypocalcemia and knowledge of the vitamin D metabolic pathway is necessary. Thus, in patients with nutritional vitamin D deficiency or malabsorption, the low vitamin D concentrations result in a low-to-low normal serum calcium concentration, which serves as a stimulus for increased secretion of parathyroid hormone (secondary hyperparathyroidism). This hyperparathyroid state in turn causes increased renal excretion of phosphate, decreased serum phosphate, elevated alkaline phosphatase, and a reduced urinary calcium excretion.

12. **What are the vitamin D metabolite concentrations associated with the diseases that interfere with vitamin D metabolism or action?**

    Depending on the abnormality of vitamin D metabolism, different vitamin D metabolite patterns may be observed. In nutritional vitamin D deficiency, the 25-hydroxyvitamin D concentrations are low. In VDDR type I, in which there is a deficiency of the renal 25-hydroxyvitamin D-1α-hydroxylase enzyme, normal or increased serum 25-hydroxyvitamin D and low or undetectable serum 1,25-dihydroxyvitamin D concentrations are observed. On the other hand, in VDDR type II, which is caused by a mutation of the vitamin D receptor resulting in resistance of target organs to 1,25-dihydroxyvitamin D, the concentrations of both 25-hydroxyvitamin D and 1,25-dihydroxyvitamin D are elevated.

13. **Describe the laboratory finding in disorders associated with the hypophosphatemic osteomalacia syndromes?**

    The hallmarks of the hypophosphatemic osteomalacia syndromes are fasting hypophosphatemia and renal phosphate wasting (as assessed by a decrease in the maximum renal tubular reabsorption of phosphate/glomerular filtration rate [TmP/GFR]). Serum calcium and parathyroid hormone concentrations are usually normal. Inexplicably, serum 1,25-dihydroxyvitamin D concentrations are inappropriately low for the degree of hypophosphatemia, which is normally a stimulus for renal 1α-hydroxylation of 25-hydroxyvitamin D.

14. **What radiographic findings are associated with osteomalacia and rickets?**

    The histologic and biochemical abnormalities associated with rickets and osteomalacia are usually found before radiographic abnormalities are observed. The most common radiographic change in patients with osteomalacia is a reduction in skeletal density (generalized osteopenia or osteoporosis). Pseudofractures (also called Looser zones or Milkman fractures) or complete fractures also may be observed. Pseudofractures are straight transverse radiolucent bands ranging from a few millimeters to several centimeters in length, usually perpendicular to the surface of the bones. They are most often bilateral and are particularly common in the femur, pelvis, and small bones of the hands and feet.

Abnormalities, including fraying of the metaphyses of the long bones, widening of the unmineralized epiphyseal growth plates, and bowing of the legs, are observed in children. The skeletal deformities observed in patients with rickets may persist into adulthood. Patients with osteomalacia may have additional radiographic findings due to secondary hyperparathyroidism. Such findings may include subperiosteal resorption of the phalanges, loss of the lamina dura of the teeth, widening of the spaces at the symphysis pubis and sacroiliac joints, and presence of brown tumors or bone cysts.

KEY POINTS: OSTEOMALACIA AND RICKETS ✓

1. Osteomalacia and rickets are disorders resulting in inadequate or delayed mineralization of bone.

2. Osteomalacia occurs in mature bone while rickets occurs in growing bone. Thus, the clinical and radiographic findings of the two conditions differ.

3. The causes of osteomalacia and rickets fall into three categories: (1) disorders associated with abnormal vitamin D metabolism or action; (2) disorders associated with abnormal phosphate metabolism; and (3) a small group of disorders with normal vitamin D and mineral metabolism.

15. **Discuss the histologic features of osteomalacia.**
The two diagnostic bone biopsy features of osteomalacia are the presence of wide osteoid seams and increased mineralization lag time (the time necessary for newly deposited matrix to mineralize). The mineralization lag time is assessed clinically by administration of two short courses of oral tetracycline several weeks apart. Because the tetracycline is deposited at the mineralization front, the lag time may be determined by measuring the distance between the two fluorescent tetracycline bands in the biopsied bone. Depending on the cause of the osteomalacia, hyperparathyroid bone changes also may be seen. Because of the varied clinical signs and symptoms, radiographic findings, and biochemical abnormalities associated with osteomalacia and rickets, none of these tests or findings is pathognomonic. The bone biopsy remains the gold standard in establishing the diagnosis of rickets and osteomalacia. The evaluation of a bone biopsy must be performed by personnel specially trained in the interpretation of bone histology.

16. **Describe the therapy for vitamin D deficiency.**
The goal of therapy for patients with osteomalacia and rickets caused by an abnormality of vitamin D metabolism is to correct the hypocalcemia and the deficiency of active vitamin D metabolites by administration of calcium salts and vitamin D preparations. In the United States, vitamin D_2 (ergocalciferol), 25-hydroxyvitamin D (calcifediol), 1,25-dihydroxyvitamin D (calcitriol), and dihydrotachysterol are available. Each of these preparations has a different half-life and potency. The choice and dose of vitamin D preparation are determined by the underlying pathologic defect of vitamin D metabolism. For example, for patients with vitamin D deficiency, a daily dose of 5000–10,000 IU of ergocalciferol (along with 1 gm of elemental calcium) is often sufficient to heal the osteomalacia.

17. **What are the treatments for osteomalacia and rickets not caused by vitamin D deficiency?**

In contrast to the treatment for vitamin D deficiency, therapy for osteomalacia associated with VDDR type II, which involves profound resistance to the effects of vitamin D, consists of administration of the most potent vitamin D metabolite, 1,25-dihydroxyvitamin D, in doses up to 60 μg/day (an extraordinarily high dose), along with large doses of oral calcium. In severe cases, high-dose intravenous calcium infusions are required to heal the rickets in patients with VDDR type II. For treatment of hypophosphatemic rickets, both phosphate supplements and calcitriol are required to heal the bone disease. Tumor removal or irradiation is required to treat tumor-induced osteomalacia. In chronic renal failure with aluminum-induced osteomalacia, aluminum is removed from the affected bone by treatment with the chelating agent deferoxamine. The osteomalacia can then be treated by calcium together with 1,25-dihydroxyvitamin D. Osteomalacia associated with renal tubular acidosis is treated with vitamin D and bicarbonate to correct the acidosis.

18. **What are the complications of treatment with vitamin D_2 or other vitamin D metabolites?**

When high doses of vitamin D_2 or one of the potent vitamin D metabolites are used, it is important to monitor carefully for the development of hypercalcemia. Mild hypercalcemia may be asymptomatic. However, severely hypercalcemic patients may complain of anorexia, nausea, vomiting, weight loss, headache, constipation, polyuria, polydipsia, and altered mental status. Impaired renal function, nephrocalcinosis, nephrolithiasis, and even death may eventually ensue. If vitamin D intoxication occurs, all calcium supplements and vitamin D preparations must be discontinued immediately and therapy for hypercalcemia instituted.

BIBLIOGRAPHY

1. Berry JL, Davies M, Mee AP: Vitamin D metabolism, rickets, and osteomalacia. Semin Musculoskelet Radiol 6:173, 2002.

2. Bingham CT, Fitzpatrick LA: Noninvasive testing in the diagnosis of osteomalacia. Am J Med 95:519, 1993.

3. Bliziotes M, Yergey AL, Nanes MS, et al: Absent intestinal response to calciferols in hereditary resistance to 1,25-dihydroxyvitamin D: Documentation and effective therapy with high-dose intravenous calcium infusions. J Clin Endocrinol Metab 66:294, 1988.

4. Drezner MK: Vitamin D-resistant rickets/osteomalacia. Endocrinologist 3:392, 1991.

5. Francis RM, Selby PL: Osteomalacia. Baillieres Clin Endocrinol Metab 11:145, 1997.

6. Glorieux FH: Hypophosphatemic vitamin D-resistant rickets. In Favus MJ (ed): Primer on the Metabolic Bone Diseases and Disorders of Mineral Metabolism, 5th ed. Washington, DC, American Society for Bone and Mineral Research, 2003, p 414.

7. Harvey JN, Gray C, Belchetz PE: Oncogenous osteomalacia and malignancy. Clin Endocrinol 37:379, 1992.

8. Holick MF: Vitamin D: Photobiology, metabolism, mechanism of action and clinical applications. In Favus MJ (ed): Primer in the Metabolic Bone Diseases and Disorders of Mineral Metabolism, 5th ed. Washington, DC, American Society for Bone and Mineral Research, 2003, p 129.

9. Holick MF: Vitamin D: A millennium perspective. J Cell Biochem 88:296, 2003.

10. Jan de Beur SM: Tumor-induced osteomalacia. In Favus MJ (ed): Primer on the Metabolic Bone Diseases and Disorders of Mineral Metabolism, 5th ed. Washington, DC, American Society for Bone and Mineral Research, 2003, p 418.

11. Liberman UA, Marx SJ: Vitamin D-dependent rickets. In Favus MJ (ed): Primer on the Metabolic Bone Diseases and Disorders of Mineral Metabolism, 5th ed. Washington, DC, American Society for Bone and Mineral Research, 2003, p 323.

12. Parfitt AM: Osteomalacia and related disorders. In Avioli LV, Krane SM (eds): Metabolic Bone. Diseases and Clinically Related Disorders, 2nd ed. Philadelphia, W.B. Saunders, 1990, p 329.

13. Pettifor JM: Nutritional and drug-induced rickets and osteomalacia. In Favus MJ (ed): Primer on the Metabolic Bone Diseases and Disorders of Mineral Metabolism, 5th ed. Washington, DC, American Society for Bone and Mineral Research, 2003, p 399.

14. Pitt MJ: Rickets and osteomalacia are still around. Radiol Clin North Am 29:97, 1991.

15. Reichel H, Koeffler HP, Norman AW: The role of the vitamin D endocrine system in health and disease. N Engl J Med 320:980, 1989.

16. Wolinsky-Friedland M: Drug-induced metabolic bone disease. Endocrinol Metab Clin North Am 24:395, 1995.

CHAPTER 13

PAGET'S DISEASE OF BONE

William E. Duncan, M.D., Ph.D.

1. **What is Paget's disease of bone?**

   Paget's disease is characterized by abnormal bone architecture resulting from an imbalance between osteoblastic bone formation and osteoclastic bone resorption. Sir James Paget first described this disease in 1876. Although he called the condition osteitis deformans, we now know that Paget's disease of bone is not an inflammation of bone (osteitis) and only rarely results in deformity.

2. **Discuss how Paget's disease is diagnosed.**

   The diagnosis of Paget's disease is generally based on a combination of clinical manifestations, radiographic signs, and characteristic biochemical changes. Although histologic examination of pagetic bone is diagnostic, a bone biopsy is often unnecessary. Bone biopsy should be performed when the diagnosis of Paget's disease is unclear or when osteogenic sarcoma or metastatic carcinoma must be excluded.

3. **What are the clinical manifestations of Paget's disease?**

   Most patients (70–80%) with Paget's disease are asymptomatic. The diagnosis is often suspected from radiographs done for other reasons or from an unexpected elevation of the serum alkaline phosphatase concentration. The most common symptom of Paget's disease is bone or joint pain. The pain is often described as dull and aching. Other manifestations of Paget's disease, such as headache, bone deformity, skull enlargement, fracture, change in skin temperature over an involved bone, high-output congestive heart failure, and entrapment neuropathies that cause loss of hearing or other neurologic deficits, are much less common (Table 13-1).

TABLE 13-1. COMPLICATIONS ASSOCIATED WITH PAGET'S DISEASE OF BONE

- Bone pain
- Bone deformity and enlargement
- Secondary osteoarthritis adjacent to pagetic bone
- Neurologic abnormalities
    - Spinal stenosis
    - Hearing loss and other cranial nerve palsies
    - Radiculopathy
- Obstructive hydrocephalus
- Cardiovascular complications
    - High output cardiac failure
    - Vascular and aortic valve calcifications
- Fracture
- Malignant transformation
- Immobilization hypercalcemia

Neurologic deficits arise from bony impingement on the brain and cranial nerves exiting from the skull, spinal nerve entrapment, and direct pressure of pagetic vertebrae on the spinal cord. Bony deformity is usually seen in patients with long-standing Paget's disease. Most commonly, the skull, clavicles, and long bones are deformed and exhibit both an increase in size and an abnormal contour. There is speculation that Ludwig Von Beethoven's hearing loss, headaches, and progressive hyperostosis frontalis were the results of long-standing Paget's disease of bone.

4. **What disorders are associated with Paget's disease of bone?**
   Several disorders are statistically more prevalent in patients with Paget's disease than in unaffected individuals. These include arthritis, fractures, primary hyperparathyroidism, osteoporosis, thyroid disease, and kidney stones.

5. **What are the three phases of Paget's disease of bone?**
   Paget's disease progresses through three distinct phases. The initial phase is the osteolytic phase where osteoclastic bone resorption predominates. About 1–2% of patients exhibit this purely lytic phase. The osteolytic phase evolves into one marked by both osteoclastic and osteoblastic overactivity. This mixed phase is followed by a less active period of bone remodeling and marked sclerosis. In the final phase, excessive osteoblastic bone deposition predominates. Most patients who come to medical attention will be in this final phase.

6. **Describe the radiographic findings during the osteolytic phase of the disease.**
   The characteristic radiographic finding found in patients in the initial osteolytic phase of Paget's disease of bone is an advancing wedge-shaped resorption front at either end of the long tubular bones. In the skull, this phase is manifested by large circumscribed osteolytic lesions (termed osteoporosis circumscripta).

7. **What are the radiographic findings most commonly found in the osteoblastic phase of the disease?**
   Evolution of osteolytic lesions into the osteoblastic phase may require years or even decades, during which the affected bone may become sclerotic and enlarged and demonstrate bowing deformities, incomplete transverse fractures (pseudofractures), and even complete fractures. When the skull is involved in the osteoblastic phase, thickening of the calvarium and a patchy increase in bone density may give the skull a "cotton-wool" appearance. In this sclerotic phase, the sclerotic bone changes may be so extensive that they may be confused with metastatic disease. Both metastatic cancer and Paget's disease are common in the elderly and may coexist in the same patient. Thus, the clinician caring for patients with Paget's disease must be alert for evidence of metastatic disease to bone.

8. **What is the best radiographic test to determine the extent of Paget's disease?**
   The metabolic activity of osteoblastic pagetic bone lesions is most easily assessed by radionuclide scanning since active pagetic bone lesions avidly take up the technetium-labeled bisphosphonate. Although bone scans are diagnostically less specific than radiographic studies, they will identify approximately 15–30% of pagetic lesions not visualized in x-rays. Conversely, when radiographs demonstrate pagetic involvement but the serum alkaline phosphatase concentration is normal and the bone scan reveals little isotope uptake at those sites, the diagnosis of relatively inactive or "burned out" Paget's disease is most likely. Predominantly lytic bone lesions (such as osteoporosis circumscripta) may not be detected in bone scan. Computed tomography (CT) and magnetic resonance imaging (MRI) scans add little to the work-up of patients with uncomplicated Paget's disease.

9. **Which bones are involved in Paget's disease?**
   Paget's disease is monostotic in about 20% of patients, and involves only one skeletal site. Polyostotic Paget's disease involves several different areas of the skeleton. Common sites of

pagetic involvement include the pelvis, hip, spine, skull, tibia, and humerus. Less common sites of involvement (<20% of cases) include the forearm, clavicles, scapulae, and ribs.

10. **Discuss the laboratory abnormalities associated with Paget's disease.**
The abnormal laboratory values associated with Paget's disease reflect either increased bone formation or increased bone resorption. Unless a patient with widespread Paget's disease is immobilized, the serum calcium and phosphate concentrations should be normal. An elevated serum alkaline phosphatase concentration reflects increased osteoblastic function. Serum osteocalcin, another marker of bone formation, provides little additional information to that supplied by alkaline phosphatase. The serum bone-specific alkaline phosphatase is a more sensitive marker of bone formation than the total alkaline phosphatase concentration and thus may be a useful parameter to follow in the management of monostotic disease. Urinary pyridinium collagen cross-links (pyridinoline) is a better indicator of increased bone resorption than measurement of urinary hydroxyproline.

11. **Which laboratory test should be used to follow patients with Paget's disease?**
When the Paget's disease is primarily lytic, the alkaline phosphatase concentration may be normal. Otherwise, the serum alkaline phosphatase activity generally parallels the indices of bone resorption. Thus, the total serum alkaline phosphatase concentration is the simplest and least expensive laboratory test to follow the course and response to treatment of most cases of Paget's disease. Of interest, a markedly elevated alkaline phosphatase concentration (e.g., 10 times the upper limit of normal) is usually associated with pagetic involvement of the skull, whereas widespread disease in the rest of the skeleton without involvement of the skull may be associated with a more modest elevation of serum alkaline phosphatase concentration. In patients with increased total alkaline phosphatase concentrations, liver disease should be excluded because this enzyme is abundant in both liver and bone. If liver-specific tests, such as 5′-nucleotidase, γ-glutamyl transferase, or the liver alkaline phosphatase isoenzyme, are normal, it is likely that the elevated alkaline phosphatase originates from bone.

12. **What are the histologic findings in bone affected by Paget's disease?**
The early lesions of Paget's disease are characterized by increased numbers of large multinucleated osteoclasts, some containing up to 100 nuclei. In the mixed osteolytic-osteoblastic phase, large numbers of active osteoblasts are seen forming bone at sites of prior osteoclastic bone resorption. The intense osteoblastic reaction in this phase is characterized by bone deposited in a chaotic fashion (the so-called mosaic or woven pattern) rather than in the orderly lamellar pattern of uninvolved bone. The woven bone of Paget's disease is structurally weaker than normal lamellar bone and explains the propensity for pagetic bone to fracture or deform.

13. **Which patient is most likely to have Paget's disease?**
The incidence of Paget's disease varies with age, gender, and geographic location. Although Paget's disease may present in younger people, it is most common in patients older than 50 years. Men are more commonly affected than women. (The male-to-female ratio is about 3:2.) Although there is no definite hereditary pattern, a significant number of patients with Paget's disease (up to 30%) report affected family members. Analyses of large kindreds with Paget's disease suggest that both sporadic and familial forms of the disease exist. Paget's disease is more common in the populations of eastern and northern Europe and in areas where Europeans have immigrated (such as the United States, Australia, New Zealand, and South Africa). Paget's disease is uncommon in Scandinavia, Asia, Africa, and in African Americans.

14. **What is the cause of Paget's disease?**
Although the cause of Paget's disease is unknown, the primary defect appears to be an abnormality of the osteoclast. Reports of viral nucleocapsid-like structures in the osteoclasts of active pagetic bone suggest a viral etiology. These nuclear inclusions resemble paramyxovirus

nucleocapsids. The measles virus, respiratory syncytial virus, and canine distemper virus have been implicated as etiologic agents although to date, no virus has ever been cultured from pagetic osteoclasts or osteoclast precursors. Nevertheless, it appears most plausible that Paget's disease is the late result of a viral infection of bone.

15. **What medications are available to treat Paget's disease?**
There is no cure for Paget's disease, but several medications are used to decrease the accelerated rate of osteoclastic bone resorption. The medications used for the treatment of Paget's bone disease include bisphosphonates, calcitonin, plicamycin, and gallium nitrate. The last two agents are rarely used for this disorder. The bisphosphonates available for use in the United States for the treatment of Paget's disease include etidronate (Didronel), alendronate (Fosamax), risedronate (Actonel), tiludronate (Skelid), and pamidronate (Aredia). Salmon calcitonin (Calcimar, Miacalcin injection) is a parenteral preparation that requires intramuscular or subcutaneous injection. Salmon calcitonin nasal spray (Miacalcin) is not effective for treating Paget's disease because of low bioavailability.

16. **Does resistance to therapy for Paget's disease of bone occur?**
Resistance to both bisphosphonates and calcitonin does occur. Resistance to treatment of Paget's disease with salmon calcitonin is usually associated with neutralizing antibody formation. Development of resistance after bisphosphonate therapy has also been reported. However, studies suggest that resistance to one bisphosphonate does not preclude a good response to a second bisphosphonate.

17. **Which agent is the treatment of choice for Paget's disease of bone?**
After treatment with bisphosphonates, suppression of disease activity is usually prolonged, sometimes lasting for several years, whereas the response to calcitonin is generally short-lived once treatment is discontinued. Thus, for treatment of uncomplicated Paget's disease, an oral bisphosphonate is the agent of choice. Calcitonin should be reserved for patients with primarily lytic disease, for patients in whom a particularly rapid response is required (e.g., patients with high-output cardiac failure or symptomatic disease of the spine), or before elective surgery on pagetic bone. Treatment of symptomatic patients also should include other therapeutic modalities, such as analgesics, nonsteroidal anti-inflammatory drugs, canes, shoe lifts, hearing aids, and surgery.

18. **Give the indications for treatment of Paget's disease.**
The primary indication for treatment is the presence of symptoms. However, not all symptoms respond to treatment. Bone pain usually responds, as do certain neurologic compression syndromes. In contrast, hearing loss, bony deformities, and mechanically dysfunctional joints are not likely to improve with therapy. Additional indications for treatment of Paget's disease are the prevention of local progression and future complications (Table 13-2), planned surgery at a pagetic site, and widespread pagetic involvement in patients in whom prolonged immobilization is anticipated, as immobilization increases the risk for hypercalcemia.
Treatment of asymptomatic patients with Paget's disease is controversial. However, untreated Paget's disease appears to be progressive with time, and not all asymptomatic patients remain asymptomatic. Thus, many physicians treat patients with osteolytic Paget's disease or asymptomatic patients with active disease involving weight-bearing bones, vertebral bodies, the skull, or areas adjacent to major joints.

19. **In asymptomatic patients with Paget's disease, at what concentration of alkaline phosphatase should treatment begin?**
The answer to this question is controversial. The level of alkaline phosphatase should be viewed in the context of the radiographic picture. A concentration of alkaline phosphatase only two to three times the upper limit of normal with polyostotic involvement may simply reflect the late

TABLE 13-2. INDICATIONS FOR TREATMENT OF PAGET'S DISEASE OF BONE
■ Symptoms (bone pain, headache, some neurologic abnormalities)
■ Osteolytic bone disease
■ Active asymptomatic disease in
Weight-bearing bones
Areas adjacent to major joints
Vertebral bodies
Skull
■ Young patients
■ Before orthopedic surgery on pagetic bone
■ Immobilization hypercalcemia

"burned-out" phase of the disease. Little benefit results from treatment in these cases. However, the same alkaline phosphatase concentration in a patient with monostotic Paget's disease in a weight-bearing bone or in an area adjacent to a major joint would lead most physicians to consider treatment. In addition, patients with lytic pagetic lesions and normal or near-normal alkaline phosphatase values should also be considered for treatment.

20. **What is the most serious complication of Paget's disease of bone?**
The most serious complication of Paget's disease is the development of malignant sarcomas in pagetic bone. Such tumors are usually isolated, but 20% may be multicentric. Fortunately, this is a rare complication of Paget's disease, occurring in less than 1% of patients with clinically apparent disease. The tumors are extremely aggressive. Patients with Paget's sarcoma generally survive less than a year. The pelvis and long bones (humerus, femur, and tibia) are the most common sites for sarcomatous transformation. The tumors are usually osteogenic sarcomas, but fibrosarcomas and chondrosarcomas have also been reported in bone affected by Paget's disease. A biopsy of the involved bone is usually diagnostic. Other bone neoplasms, such as benign giant cell tumors, are also associated with Paget's disease, but these tumors do not carry such a grave prognosis.

21. **When should malignant sarcoma in a pagetic bone lesion be suspected?**
Malignant transformation within pagetic bone is usually heralded by the onset of new or worsening bone pain and/or soft tissue swelling. Usually, progressive destruction of pagetic bone is found on radiographs. Less commonly, increasing sclerosis or masses of dense amorphous deposits in bone are suggestive of malignant change. The concentration of serum alkaline phosphatase may rise rapidly in an otherwise previously stable patient. Bone scans usually demonstrate decreased uptake of radionucleotide in the area of the tumor. However, gallium scans show increased uptake in the involved area(s).

KEY POINTS: PAGET'S DISEASE OF BONE ✓

1. Paget's disease is the second most common metabolic bone disease, affecting up to 5% of the Caucasian population over the age of 50.

2. Paget's disease is characterized by abnormal bone architecture resulting from an imbalance between osteoblastic bone formation and osteoclastic bone resorption.

3. Bisphosphonates are the most effective treatment for Paget's disease of bone.

WEBSITE

The Paget Foundation: http://www.paget.org

BIBLIOGRAPHY

1. Ankrom MA, Shapiro JR: Paget's disease of bone (osteitis deformans). J Am Geriatr Soc 46:1025, 1998.

2. Delmas PD, Meunier PJ: The management of Paget's disease of bone. N Engl J Med 336:558, 1997.

3. Drake WM, Kendler DL, Brown JP: Consensus statement on the modern therapy of Paget's disease of bone from a Western Osteoporosis Alliance Symposium. Clin Ther 23:620, 2001.

4. Hadjipavlou A, Lander P, Srolovitz H, Enker IP: Malignant transformation in Paget's disease of bone. Cancer 70:2802, 1992.

5. Hain SF, Fogelman I: Nuclear medicine studies in metabolic bone disease. Semin Muscoskelet Radiol 6:323, 2002.

6. Hamdy RC: Pharmacologic treatment of Paget's disease. Endocrinol Metab Clin North Am 24:421, 1995.

7. Joshua F, Epstein M, Major G: Bisphosphonate resistance in Paget's disease of bone. Arthritis Rheum 48:2321, 2003.

8. Leach RJ, Singer FR, Roodman GD: The genetics of Paget's disease. J Clin Endocrinol Metab 86:24–28, 2001.

9. Lyles KW, Siris ES, Singer FR, Meunier PH: A clinical approach to diagnosis and management of Paget's disease of bone. J Bone Miner Res 16:1379, 2001.

10. Mills BG: Etiology and pathophysiology of Paget's disease—update. Endocrinologist 7:222, 1997.

11. Papapoulos SE: Paget's disease of bone: Clinical, pathogenetic and therapeutic aspects. Baillieres Clin Endocrinol Metab 11:117, 1997.

12. Proceedings of the Third International Symposium on Paget's Disease. J Bone Mineral Res 14(Suppl 2),1999.

13. Sawin CT: Historical note: Sir James Paget and osteitis deformans. Endocrinologist 7:205, 1997. (also see p 255 in the same issue for a reproduction of one of James Paget's original articles on osteitis deformans).

14. Sellars SL: Beethoven's deafness. S Afr Med J 48:1585, 1974.

15. Siris ES: Clinical review—Paget's disease of bone. J Bone Miner Res 13:1061, 1998.

16. Siris ES: Extensive personal experience—Paget's disease of bone. J Clin Endocrinol Metab 80:35, 1995.

17. Siris ES, Roodman GD: Paget's disease of bone. In Favus MJ (ed.): Primer on the Metabolic Bone Diseases and Disorders of Mineral Metabolism, 5th ed. New York, Raven Press, 2003, p 495.

18. Wimalawansa SJ, Gunasekera RD: Pamidronate is effective for Paget's disease of bone refractory to conventional therapy. Calcif Tissue Int 53:237, 1993.

CHAPTER 14

HYPERCALCEMIA

Leonard R. Sanders, M.D.

1. **What is hypercalcemia? How does protein binding affect the calcium level?**
   Hypercalcemia is a corrected total serum calcium value above the upper limit of the normal range or elevated ionized calcium. Calcium is 50% free (ionized), 40% protein-bound, and 10% complexed to phosphate, citrate, bicarbonate, sulfate, and lactate. Only elevations in the free calcium are associated with symptoms and signs. Of the protein-bound calcium, about 80% is bound to albumin and 20% to globulins. A decrease or increase in serum albumin of 1 gm/dL from 4 gm/dL decreases or increases the serum calcium by 0.8 mg/dL. An increase or decrease in serum globulin by 1 gm/dL increases or decreases serum calcium by 0.16 mg/dL. Such protein changes do not affect free calcium and do not cause calcium-related symptoms.

2. **How common are hypercalcemia and its main associated conditions?**
   Hypercalcemia affects 0.5–1% of the general population. The incidence may increase to 3% among postmenopausal women. Primary hyperparathyroidism causes 70% of outpatient and 20% of inpatient hypercalcemia. Cancer causes 50% of inpatient hypercalcemia. Ten percent of patients with malignancy develop hypercalcemia. Hyperparathyroidism and cancer cause 90% of all hypercalcemia. About 10% of patients with hyperparathyroidism develop nephrolithiasis. Although calcium oxalate stones are common, calcium phosphate stones are most characteristic of hyperparathyroidism.

3. **How would you classify mild, moderate, and severe hypercalcemia?**
   First, consider the patient's general health and hypercalcemic symptoms. For example, a patient with renal failure and serum phosphorus of 8.5 mg/dL may have metastatic calcification with serum calcium of 10.5 mg/dL. Then correct the serum calcium for the albumin concentration:

   $$Ca_{corrected} = Ca_{observed} + [(4.0 - albumin) \times 0.8]$$

   With this in mind, serum calcium of 1.5–3.5 mg/dL above the upper normal limit defines moderate hypercalcemia. Mild hypercalcemia occurs below this range, and severe hypercalcemia, above. Thus, if the upper normal limit for calcium is 10.5 mg/dL, serum calcium of 12–14 mg/dL is moderate hypercalcemia. Serum calcium < 12 mg/dL is mild hypercalcemia and > 14 mg/dL severe hypercalcemia.

4. **Discuss the signs and symptoms of hypercalcemia.**
   No symptoms are usually present with mild hypercalcemia (< 12 mg/dL). Moderate or severe hypercalcemia and rapidly developing mild hypercalcemia may cause symptoms and signs. Common symptoms and signs involve: (1) the central nervous system (lethargy, stupor, coma, mental changes, psychosis); (2) the gastrointestinal tract (anorexia, nausea, constipation, acid peptic disease, pancreatitis); (3) the kidneys (polyuria, nephrolithiasis); (4) the musculoskeletal system (arthralgias, myalgias, weakness); and (5) the vascular system (hypertension). The classic electrocardiographic (ECG) change associated with hypercalcemia is a short Q-T interval. Occasionally, severe hypercalcemia also causes dysrhythmias, ST segment depression, sinus arrest, and disturbances in atrioventricular (AV) conduction.

5. **What are the sources of serum calcium?**
Bone calcium approximates 1 kg and 99% of body calcium. Normal serum calcium is maintained by integrated regulation of calcium absorption, resorption, and reabsorption; these processes occur, respectively, in the gut, bone, and kidney. Of the 1000 mg/day of dietary calcium intake, the gut absorbs 300 mg/day, secretes 100 mg/day, and excretes 800 mg/day. Net absorption averages 200 mg/day. Absorption may vary from 30% to 70% of dietary calcium depending on the amount of $1,25(OH)_2D$ present. The kidney reabsorbs 98% of filtered calcium and excretes 200 mg/day. Bone exchanges about 500 mg of calcium per day with serum (Fig. 14-1).

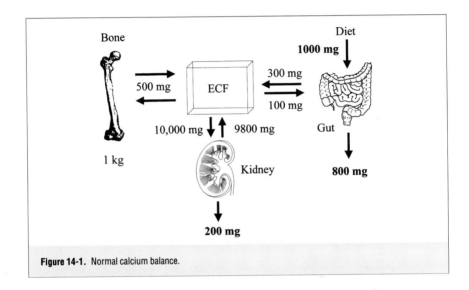

Figure 14-1. Normal calcium balance.

6. **What are the major anatomic and physiologic determinants of vitamin D?**
Diet, skin, liver, and kidney control the synthesis and secretion of vitamin D. Vitamin D is absorbed from the gut and synthesized in the skin. Hepatic 25-hydroxylase converts vitamin D to 25-hydroxyvitamin D (25-OHD). 25-OHD circulates and interacts with two renal mitochondrial hydroxylases. When there is increased parathyroid hormone (PTH) and/or decreased phosphate, 1-α-hydroxylase converts more 25-OHD to $1,25(OH)_2D$, causing bone calcium mobilization and increasing intestinal calcium absorption. When PTH and phosphate are normal, 24-hydroxylase converts 25-OHD to 24,25-dihydroxyvitamin D [$24,25(OH)_2D$], causing antiresorptive effects on bone and positive calcium balance. $1,25(OH)_2D$ is 100 times more potent than 25-OHD and 10,000 times more potent than vitamin D (see Fig. 14-2).

7. **Describe the effects of PTH and vitamin D on bone.**
PTH and $1,25(OH)_2D$ provide the main control of serum calcium. Both PTH and $1,25(OH)_2D$ increase bone resorption by increasing osteoclast activity. Because osteoclasts have no known receptors for either hormone, PTH and $1,25(OH)_2D$ stimulate osteoclast activity indirectly. PTH enhances the activity of osteoblasts, which secrete factors that stimulate osteoclastic bone resorption. $1,25(OH)_2D$ promotes osteoclast differentiation from promonocytes to monocytes to macrophages and finally to osteoclasts. In addition, $1,25(OH)_2D$ increases calcium transport from bone to blood. Both hor-

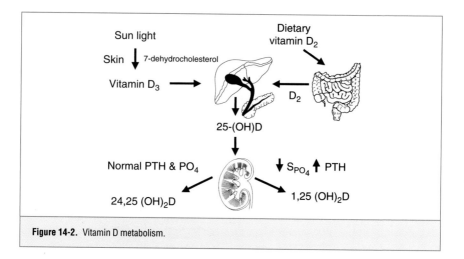

Figure 14-2. Vitamin D metabolism.

mones promote normal bone formation by action on osteoblasts, and $1,25(OH)_2D$ maintains a favorable calcium-phosphate product necessary for normal bone mineralization.

8. **How do calcium and phosphate interact with calcium-regulating hormones?**
   Table 14-1 summarizes the main factors controlling serum calcium. The arrows show direct actions of factors in the left column on factors in the top row, whereas the plus (+) and minus (−) signs show indirect actions. As a rule, the direct effects predominate as the net effect. Table 14-2 outlines the specific effects of each of the above factors.

TABLE 14-1.	INTERACTION OF FACTORS CONTROLLING SERUM CALCIUM				
	PTH	$1,25(OH)_2D$	Calcitonin	Calcium	PO_4
PTH	—	↑+	+	↑+	↓↑+
$1,25(OH)_2D$	↓−	↓−	+	↑	↑
Calcitonin	+	+	—	↓	↓
Calcium	↓	↓	↑	—	↓
PO_4	↑+	↓	—	↓	—

9. **List the main causes of hypercalcemia.**
   The mnemonic VITAMINS TRAP (Pont, 1989) includes most causes of hypercalcemia:
   V = **V**itamins
   I = **I**mmobilization
   T = **T**hyrotoxicosis
   A = **A**ddison's disease
   M = **M**ilk-alkali syndrome
   I = **I**nflammatory disorders
   N = **N**eoplastic-related disease
   S = **S**arcoidosis
   T = **T**hiazide diuretics (drugs)
   R = **R**habdomyolysis
   A = **A**IDS
   P = **P**aget's disease
      Parenteral nutrition
      Pheochromocytoma
      Parathyroid disease

TABLE 14-2. SUMMARY OF CALCIUM AND PHOSPHATE CONTROL	
Variable	**Direct Action**
PTH	Increased bone resorption of calcium and phosphate
	Increased distal renal tubular calcium reabsorption
	Decreased renal tubular phosphate reabsorption
	Increased renal production of $1,25(OH)_2D$
	Net effect: increased serum calcium and decreased phosphate
$1,25(OH)_2D$	Increased bone resorption of calcium and phosphate
	Increased renal reabsorption of calcium and phosphate
	Increased gut absorption of calcium and phosphate
	Decreased parathyroid production of PTH
	Decreased renal production of $1,25(OH)_2D$
	Net effect: increased serum calcium and phosphate
Calcitonin	Decreased bone resorption of calcium and phosphate
	Decreased renal reabsorption of calcium and phosphate
	Decreased gut absorption of phosphate
	Net effect: decreased serum calcium and phosphate
Calcium	Decreases PTH
	Decreases $1,25(OH)_2D$
	Decreases calcitonin
	Decreases phosphate
Phosphate	Decreases $1,25(OH)_2D$
	Decreases calcium

10. **How do various causes of hypercalcemia increase the serum calcium?**
True hypercalcemia results from altered bone resorption, renal tubular reabsorption, and gut absorption of calcium. Although the bone (resorption and formation), kidney (reabsorption and excretion), and gut (absorption and secretion) have two major processes involved with mineral metabolism, only resorption, reabsorption, and absorption play a significant role in hypercalcemia. An exception to this rule occurs when decreased renal function from renal or prerenal disease impairs calcium filtration and excretion. In Figure 14-3, solid arrows represent potential causes of increased calcium and dashed arrows represent potential causes of decreased calcium.

11. **What are the mechanisms and causes of hypercalcemia?**
From the discussions above, one appreciates that mechanisms of hypercalcemia are usually multifactorial. However, most hypercalcemic syndromes have a primary or predominant mechanism, as outlined in Table 14-3. Most resorptive hypercalcemia is humoral (PTH, parathyroid hormone related peptide [PTHrP], transforming growth factor-α [TGFα], tumor necrosis factor [TNF]) or local osteolytic hypercalcemia (PTHrP, interleukins, prostaglandins). Most increased calcium absorption occurs in response to excess $1,25(OH)_2D$ produced by granulomas or tumors. Ninety percent of hypercalcemia results from hyperparathyroidism or cancer.

KEY POINTS: HYPERCALCEMIA ✓

1. Therapy for hypercalcemia should be directed at the underling etiology, including excess bone resorption, renal tubular reabsorption, and gut absorption.

2. Although there are over 30 major causes of hypercalcemia, hyperparathyroidism and hypercalcemia of malignancy account for > 90%.

3. Most patients with severe hypercalcemia require normal saline hydration and multiple drug therapy, but most therapies for hypercalcemia inhibit bone resorption.

4. Zoledronic acid is the most potent bisphosphonate approved for treatment of hypercalcemia and has the advantage over pamidronate of a short infusion time (4 mg IV over 15 minutes).

5. Cinacalcet is a calcimimetic just approved for treatment of secondary HPT and parathyroid carcinoma. Cinacalcet reduces PTH 40–50% and lowers calcium and phosphate in patients with secondary HPT of renal disease. Although not approved for treatment of primary HPT, cinacalcet also lowers PTH in this disorder.

12. **What is the relative frequency of skeletal lesions in patients with advanced cancer?**
The relative frequency is as follows: myeloma 95–100%, breast and prostate 70%, thyroid 60%, bladder 40%, lung 35%, renal 25%, and melanoma 14–45%. Common sites of bone metastases are ribs, spine, pelvis, and proximal extremities.

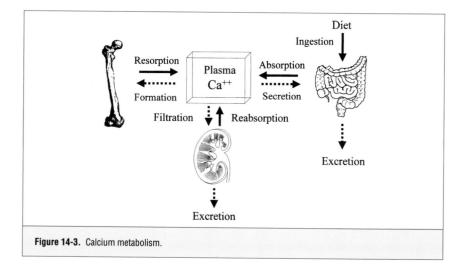

Figure 14-3. Calcium metabolism.

13. **What is the relative incidence of hypercalcemia in patients with advanced cancer?**
The incidence is as follows: lung and breast 25%; myeloma 7%; squamous head and neck cancer 7%; unknown primary 5%; lymphoma, renal, and gastrointestinal 4%.

14. **What are the multiple endocrine neoplasia (MEN) syndromes?**
MEN is associated with three familial syndromes, two of which present with hypercalcemia due to hyperparathyroidism. MEN-I or Wermer's syndrome includes the three P's: pituitary, parathyroid, and pancreatic tumors. Hypercalcemia due to hyperparathyroidism is usually the first feature of this syndrome to appear. MEN-II has two variants. Patients with MEN-IIa or Sipple's syndrome have medullary carcinoma of the thyroid (MCT), pheochromocytoma, and hyperparathyroidism.

TABLE 14-3. MECHANISMS AND CAUSES OF HYPERCALCEMIA	
Primary Mechanism	**Cause of Hypercalcemia**
Increased bone resorption	Hyperparathyroidism
	Local osteolytic hypercalcemia
	Humoral hypercalcemia of malignancy
	Thyrotoxicosis
	Pheochromocytoma
	Excessive vitamin A (usually > 25,000 IU/day)
	Lithium carbonate
	Immobilization
	Addison's (? sensitivity to thyroid hormone)
	Vasoactive intestinal polypeptide-secreting tumor
Increased renal reabsorption	Milk-alkali syndrome
or decreased excretion	Rhabdomyolysis
	Thiazide diuretics
	FHH
	Renal failure
	Lithium carbonate
Increased gut absorption	Excessive vitamin D (usually > 10,000 IU/day)
	Berylliosis
	Candidiasis
	Coccidioidomycosis
	Eosinophilic granuloma
	Histoplasmosis
	Sarcoidosis
	Silicone implants
	Tuberculosis
	Inflammatory disorders
	AIDS
	Lymphomas

Patients with MEN-IIb have MCT, pheochromocytoma, multiple mucosal neuromas, and marfanoid habitus; they usually do not have hyperparathyroidism. Relative to sporadic hyperparathyroidism, parathyroid tumors in the MEN syndromes are more often bilateral, hyperplastic, and malignant.

15. **How would you diagnose familial hypocalciuric hypercalcemia (FHH)?**
    FHH, also called benign familial hypercalcemia, is due to an autosomal-dominant genetic mutation resulting in an inactivating mutation for the calcium-sensing receptor (CaR) on the membranes of parathyroid and renal tubular cells. The most important diagnostic features of FHH are the combination of no symptoms, a family history of benign hypercalcemia, mild hypercalcemia, normal-to-high serum levels of PTH, and decreased renal clearance of calcium (fractional excretion of calcium [FECa] < 1%). The clinical importance of FHH is to distinguish it from primary hyperparathyroidism to avoid needless and ineffective parathyroidectomy. Patients with primary hyperparathyroidism usually have an FECa > 2%.

16. **What is the likely cause of hypercalcemia in the following patient?**
    An 18-year-old man presents with calcium values of 10.5–11.8 for the last 2 years, a normal physical examination, and a family history of hypercalcemia. Current laboratory values are as follows: calcium 11.5 mg/dL, intact PTH 70 pg/mL (NL< 65), serum creatinine (Cr) 1.0 mg/dL, random urine calcium 5 mg/dL, and urine Cr 90 mg/dL. Because circulating proteins bind 40% of the calcium, the kidney filters only 60%. Plasma calcium available for filtration is 0.6×11.5 or 6.9 mg/dL:

    $$FE_{Ca} = [U_{Ca}/P_{Ca}]/ [U_{Cr}/P_{Cr}] = [U_{Ca}/P_{Ca}] \times [P_{Cr}/U_{Cr}]$$

    $$FE_{Ca} = [5 \text{ mg/dL}/6.9 \text{ mg/dL}] \times [1 \text{ mg/dL}/90 \text{ mg/dL}] \times 100\% = 0.8\%$$

    Where U_{Ca} = urine calcium, U_{Cr} = urine creatine, P_{Ca} = plasma calcium, and P_{Cr} = plasma creatine. The history, physical, laboratory, and FE_{Ca} of < 1% support the diagnosis of FHH.

17. **What therapy is useful for hypercalcemia?**
    Most patients with severe hypercalcemia require treatment with multiple drugs. Give the lowest amount and least frequent dose that will achieve and maintain acceptable serum calcium. The usual order of therapy includes normal saline, calcitonin, zoledronic acid, and glucocorticoids if indicated. Give furosemide after good hydration primarily to avoid volume overload and improve urinary volume. Reserve dialysis, plicamycin, and gallium for severe or refractory hypercalcemia and hypercalcemic crisis, usually with expert consultation (see Table 14-4.)

18. **Describe the mechanisms of action of drug therapies for hypercalcemia.**
    See Table 14-5.

19. **How might calcimimetic drugs be useful in therapy of hypercalcemia?**
    Cinacalcet is a new calcimimetic currently in phase 4 clinical trials. Calcimimetics are potentially the most useful drugs for treatment of hypercalcemia caused by hyperparathyroidism. They stimulate or activate the parathyroid CaR. The CaR is located in various tissues, including chief cells of the parathyroid gland, where it senses the extracellular calcium concentration and alters the rate of secretion of PTH. Calcimimetics alter the sensitivity of the parathyroid CaR, which shifts the calcium–PTH curve to the left, decreases the responsiveness of parathyroid cells to the stimulatory effects of low extracellular calcium, and increases the sensitivity of parathyroid cells to the suppressive effects of high calcium. The net effect is marked reduction (> 50%) in PTH secretion and a proportionate decrease in PTH-induced hypercalcemia.

TABLE 14-4. THERAPY FOR HYPERCALCEMIA

Therapy	Dose	Route	Monitor/Comment
Saline	250–1000 mL/h	IV	Cardiopulmonary function with examination, CVP/PCWP and CXR
Furosemide	20–80 mg every 2–4 h or 40 mg/h CI	IV	Serum and urine electrolytes. Replace K, Mg, and PO_4 based on serum levels and urinary losses.
Salmon calcitonin	4–8 IU/kg every 6–12 h	IM, SC	Allergic reaction. Give a skin test of 1 IU intradermally before treatment.
Prednisone/ methylpred- nisolone	20 mg 2–3 times a day	PO/IV	Possible adjunct to calcitonin. Effective in $1,25(OH)_2D$ associated hypercalcemia.
Zoledronic acid	4 mg IV over 15 min every 2–4 weeks PRN	IV	Drug of choice for malignancy-associated hypercalcemia. Caution with CKD and myeloma.
Pamidronate	30–90 mg over 2–24 h every 1–3 weeks PRN	IV	Infuse over at least 4 hours in severe renal failure (GFR <30 mL/minute).
Plicamycin	25 μg/kg/day	IV	Infuse over 4–6 hours as needed every 2–3 days. Monitor CBC, platelets PT/PTT, Cr, and liver enzymes. Avoid in hepatic and renal dysfunction and thrombocytopenia.
Gallium nitrate	200 mg/m^2/day CI over 24 h PRN for 5 days	IV	Avoid in renal failure. Monitor Cr, PO_4, and CBC.
Dialysis	Low or no calcium dialysate	HD/PD CVVHD	Hypercalcemic crisis or refractory hypercalcemia. Useful in renal failure. Nephrologic consultation.

CI, continuous infusion; BSA, body surface area; IV, intravenously; IM, intramuscularly; SC, subcutaneously; PO, orally; HD, hemodialysis; PD, peritoneal dialysis; CVVHD, continuous venovenous hemodialysis; CVP, central venous pressure; PCWP, pulmonary capillary wedge pressure; CXR, chest radiograph; Na, sodium; K, potassium; Mg, magnesium; PO_4, phosphate; CBC, complete blood count; PT, prothrombin time; PTT, partial thromboplastic time; Cr, creatinine; CKD, chronic kidney disease.

TABLE 14-5.   MECHANISM OF ACTION OF HYPERCALCEMIC THERAPY

Drug	Mechanism of Action
Saline	Dilutes serum calcium by volume expansion and increases urinary flow and calcium excretion
Furosemide	Impairs renal sodium and calcium reabsorption in Henle's loop increasing urinary flow and calcium excretion
Calcitonin	Binds to receptors on osteoclasts, inhibiting osteoclast activity and decreasing bone resorption. Also decreases renal reabsorption
Glucocorticoids	Antagonism of vitamin D causing decreased absorption and reabsorption. In tumoral states may be tumor lytic and decrease production of OAFs and vitamin D
Bisphosphonates	Impair osteoclast differentiation, recruitment, motility, and attachment. Incorporate into bone matrix, making the matrix resistant to hydrolysis. Overall effect is decreased bone resorption
Plicamycin	Inhibits RNA synthesis and is cytotoxic to osteoclasts, decreasing bone resorption
Gallium nitrate	Adsorbs to and decreases solubility of hydroxyapatite crystals, decreasing bone resorption
Dialysis	Direct removal of calcium from blood

OAFs, osteoclast-activating factors.
Note: For long-term hypocalcemic effects, drug therapy for hypercalcemia must antagonize one of the three main causes of hypercalcemia: bone resorption, renal reabsorption, or gut absorption. All hypercalcemia results from some abnormality in one of the three. Thus, it is good to think about one of these etiologies when choosing drug therapy. As noted, most drug therapy for hypercalcemia impairs bone resorption.

WEBSITES

1. American Academy of Family Physicians. Available at http://www.aafp.org/afp/20030501/1959.html

2. National Cancer Institute. Available at http://www.meb.uni-bonn.de/cancer.gov/CDR0000062737.html

3. Zometa International: Zoledronic acid review. Available at http://www.zometa.com/monographs.html

BIBLIOGRAPHY

1. Body JJ: Current and future directions in medical therapy: Hypercalcemia. Cancer 88(Suppl 12):3054–3058, 2000.

2. Brown EM: Familial hypocalciuric hypercalcemia and other disorders with resistance to extracellular calcium. Endocrinol Metab Clin North Am 29:503–522, 2000.

3. Carroll, MF, Schade, DS: A practical approach to hypercalcemia. Am Fam Physician 67:1959–1966, 2003.

4. Kaye TB: Hypercalcemia. How to pinpoint the cause and customize treatment. Postgrad Med 97:153–155, 159–160, 1995.

5. Major P: The use of zoledronic acid, a novel, highly potent bisphosphonate, for the treatment of hypercalcemia of malignancy. Oncologist 7(6):481–491, 2002.

6. Popovtzer MM: Disorders of calcium, phosphorus, vitamin D, and parathyroid hormone activity. In Schrier RW (ed): Renal and Electrolytes Disorders. Philadelphia, Lippincott Williams & Wilkins, 2003, pp 216–277.

7. Pont A: Unusual causes of hypercalcemia. Endocrinol Metab Clin North Am 18:753–764, 1989.

8. Rabbani SA: Molecular mechanism of action of parathyroid hormone related peptide in hypercalcemia of malignancy: Therapeutic strategies. Int J Oncol 16(1):197–206, 2000 (review).

9. Shoback DM, Bilezikian JP, Turner SA, et al: The calcimimetic cinacalcet normalizes serum calcium in subjects with primary hyperparathyroidism. J Clin Endocrinol Metab 88(12):5644–5649, 2003.

10. Thakker RV: Multiple endocrine neoplasia type I. Endocrinol Metab Clin North Am 29:541–567, 2000.

CHAPTER 15

HYPERPARATHYROIDISM

Leonard R. Sanders, M.D.

1. **Define hyperparathyroidism.**
   Hyperparathyroidism (HPT) is a clinical syndrome causing specific symptoms and signs that result from elevated parathyroid hormone (PTH), PTH-induced bone resorption, and hypercalcemia. The three types of HPT are primary, secondary, and tertiary.

2. **How common is primary HPT?**
   The prevalence of HPT in the U.S. is 28/100,000; the female-to-male ratio is 2–3:1. The incidence increases with age, and postmenopausal women have an incidence five times higher than the general population.

3. **What causes primary HPT?**
   Primary HPT is characterized by abnormal regulation of PTH secretion by calcium, resulting in excessive PTH secretion. Although the cause of HPT is not known, increased PTH secretion is due in part to an elevation of the set point and a change in the slope of the calcium-PTH curve, causing relative nonsuppressibility of PTH secretion. Expression of the calcium-sensing receptor (CaR) is reduced in parathyroid adenomas and hyperplasia and may be partly responsible for this relative PTH nonsuppressibility.

4. **What anatomic alterations occur in HPT?**
   Most hyperparathyroid patients (85%) have single parathyroid adenomas, 5% have multiple adenomas, 10% have four-gland hyperplasia, and < 1% have parathyroid carcinomas. Normal parathyroid glands weigh < 50 mg each. The average weight of parathyroid adenomas is 0.5–5 gm; however, they may be > 25 gm. The largest reported tumor weighed 120 gm.

5. **Describe how to diagnose HPT.**
   Persistent hypercalcemia with increased serum PTH levels makes the diagnosis of HPT. Suspect HPT whenever the patient has documented hypercalcemia. Because symptoms of HPT are nonspecific or absent (see question 12), one must base the diagnosis primarily on laboratory studies. Furthermore, most patients with mild HPT have no specific symptoms or signs. Most cases are suspected after finding an elevated calcium value on routine laboratory screening.

6. **How does age complicate the diagnosis of HPT?**
   The laboratory normal range for intact PTH (10–65 pg/mL) and calcium (9–10.5 mg/dL) may not apply in the elderly. PTH levels normally decrease with age. A 50-year-old should not have intact PTH levels exceeding 40–50 pg/mL. Thus, normal PTH levels may exist in HPT in older patients. Furthermore, calcium levels decline with age and high normal calcium levels (10 mg/dL) are probably abnormally high over the age 50.

7. **How might you make the diagnosis of primary HPT more certain before recommending parathyroidectomy?**
   Obtain at least three fasting samples for calcium, ideally with no venous occlusion, and two PTH measurements at least several weeks apart. Ensure that the patient has normal renal function. Discontinue any thiazide diuretic for at least 1 week before measurement. Total calcium

measurement is sufficient if albumin and total protein are normal. If not, measure ionized calcium or correct for the protein change. If calcium is elevated and PTH is high or high normal, primary HPT is usually present. If calcium is not elevated and PTH is high, measure 25-hydroxyvitamin D levels. To exclude vitamin D deficiency, levels should be > 20 ng/mL. Use the immunoradiometric (IRMA) or bio-intact immunochemiluminometric (ICMA) assays that are specific for intact PTH.

8. **When lab results are not specific for primary HPT what other classic laboratory changes may help with diagnosis?**
Increased chloride (Cl) and decreased phosphate (PO_4) with a Cl/PO_4 ratio of > 33, elevated urinary pH (> 6.0), and increased alkaline phosphatase concentrations support the diagnosis of primary HPT but are not specific. Assess PTH-related protein (PTHrP) in any patient with suspected malignancy and hypercalcemia. Ectopic PTH is rare and should be considered only if the patient has evidence of malignancy or a negative neck exploration for HPT.

9. **What differentiates familial hypocalciuric hypercalcemia (FHH) from primary HPT?**
If measured PTH is borderline or normal but PTH is inappropriately increased for the level of calcium, consider familial (benign) hypocalciuric hypercalcemia (FHH). Calculate the fractional excretion of calcium (FE_{Ca}) (see Chapter 14). The FE_{Ca} in FHH is < 1%. If the FE_{Ca} is low, test family members to confirm the diagnosis. If positive, FHH is probably present. Avoid neck exploration, which will have no effect on reversing the hypercalcemia.

10. **How does renal failure complicate the diagnosis of HPT?**
Renal failure increases serum phosphate and decreases 1,25-dihydroxyvitamin D (calcitriol) levels. Because phosphate directly stimulates and calcitriol directly inhibits PTH secretion, serum PTH levels increase in renal failure. In addition, increased phosphate and decreased calcitriol decrease serum calcium. The resulting absolute or relative hypocalcemia further increases PTH secretion. Symptoms and signs of renal insufficiency may be identical to those of HPT, including lethargy, depression, anorexia, nausea, constipation, and weakness. Thus, unless overt, the diagnosis of primary HPT may be more difficult in renal failure. Before parathyroidectomy for presumed primary HPT, tissue localization with technetium-99m sestamibi scan may be appropriate.

11. **What changes occur in renal failure that may complicate the PTH assay?**
In renal failure, PTH increases above the normal range due to the stimulatory effects of high phosphate and low calcitriol. In addition, a molecular fragment of PTH (7–84) that does not have biologic activity accumulates in renal failure and cross-reacts with the intact molecule in the intact two-site assays. For this reason, patients with renal failure may have measured levels of intact PTH > 1.5 times that of normal subjects to maintain physiologic PTH (1–84) concentrations. Bio-intact on whole-PTH assays eliminate this cross-reactivity.

12. **Describe the symptoms and signs of primary HPT.**
More than 85% of primary hyperparathyroid patients are asymptomatic. However, neurologic, gastrointestinal, musculoskeletal, and vascular changes all can occur in primary HPT. The classic phrase for many of these features is stones, bones, abdominal groans, and psychic moans. Proximal muscle weakness is also quite characteristic. Other characteristic symptoms and signs and their probable cause are outlined in Table 15-1.

13. **What is band keratopathy?**
Band keratopathy is a classic but unusual sign of HPT characterized by an irregular region of calcium phosphate deposition at the medial and lateral limbic margins of the outer edge of the cornea. The location is believed to be a result of diffusion of carbon dioxide from

air-exposed areas of the cornea, leaving an alkaline environment that favors precipitation of calcium phosphate crystals. Band keratopathy occurs only with a high calcium-phosphate product. Diagnosis is made by ophthalmologic slit-lamp examination. It differs from arcus senilis, an age-related, linear, concentric gray crescent separated from the extreme periphery (limbus corneae) by a rim of clear cornea that with time completely encircles the cornea.

TABLE 15-1. HPT: SYMPTOMS, SIGNS, AND THEIR PROBABLE CAUSES	
Symptoms and Signs	Probable Cause
Renal: hypercalciuria, nephrolithiasis, nephrocalcinosis, polyuria, polydipsia, renal insufficiency	PTH stimulates bone resorption, hypercalcemia, bicarbonaturia, and phosphaturia, causing decreased tubular responsiveness to antidiuretic hormone (ADH), polyuria, calcium oxalate and phosphate crystallization, nephrocalcinosis, and renal insufficiency
Neuromuscular: weakness, myalgia	Prolonged excessive PTH arguably causes direct neuropathy with abnormal nerve conduction velocities (NCVs) and characteristic electromyographic (EMG) changes and myopathic features on muscle biopsy
Neurologic and psychiatric: memory loss, depression, psychoses, neuroses, confusion, lethargy, fatigue, paresthesias	PTH and calcium cause peripheral neuropathy with abnormal NCVs and central nervous system damage with abnormal electroencephalographic (EEG) changes
Skeletal: bone pain, osteitis fibrosa, osteoporosis, and subperiosteal skeletal resorption	PTH increases bone resorption and acidosis with subsequent bone buffering and bone loss of calcium and phosphate
Gastrointestinal: abdominal pain, nausea, peptic ulcer, constipation, and pancreatitis	Hypercalcemia stimulates gastrin secretion, decreases peristalsis, and increases the calcium-phosphate product with calcium-phosphate deposition and obstruction in pancreatic ducts
Hypertension	Hypercalcemia causes vasoconstriction, and parathyroid hypertensive factor (PHF) may increase blood pressure
Arthralgia, synovitis, arthritis	HPT is associated with increased crystal deposition from calcium phosphate (para-articular calcification), calcium pyrophosphate (pseudogout), and uric acid/urate (gout)
Band keratopathy	Calcium-phosphate precipitation in medial and limbic margins of cornea
Anemia	Unknown

14. **Describe the classic radiographic findings in HPT.**
Because most patients are diagnosed early, there are usually no radiographic findings related to HPT. If HPT is prolonged, osteopenia develops. However, the classic radiographic finding is subperiosteal bone resorption along the radial aspect of the middle and distal phalanges and distal clavicles. Salt-and-pepper skull is another classic finding.

15. **What is the differential diagnosis of primary HPT?**
Because the main abnormality in primary HPT is hypercalcemia, the differential diagnosis initially is that of hypercalcemia (see Chapter 14). A history and physical examination focused on symptoms and signs (see question 12) may suggest one of the causes of hypercalcemia. If hypercalcemia is mild and history and physical examination are nonspecific, primary HPT is likely. The two most common causes of hypercalcemia are primary HPT and malignancy. In humoral hypercalcemia of malignancy (HHM), the tumor usually produces a PTH-like hormone called PTHrP.

16. **What lab tests help to distinguish the three types of HPT?**
See Table 15-2.

TABLE 15-2. PTH AND CALCIUM IN HPT		
	PTH	Calcium
Primary	Normal ↑	↑
Secondary	↑	↓ Normal
Tertiary	↑ ↑	↑

17. **What pathophysiologic changes occur in primary HPT?**
Primary HPT is idiopathic and results from excessive secretion of PTH from parathyroid adenomas, hyperplasia, or rarely carcinoma. The increased PTH causes hypercalcemia. PTH is inappropriately normal or high.

18. **What pathophysiologic changes occur in secondary HPT?**
Secondary HPT is excessive PTH secretion as a secondary response to hypocalcemia. Hyperphosphatemia and low levels of calcitriol also stimulate PTH secretion. Renal failure is the most common cause of secondary HPT. Other causes of hypocalcemia are renal calcium leak, dietary calcium malabsorption, and vitamin D deficiency. Hypocalcemia causes parathyroid hyperplasia. Attempting to return the calcium to normal, the enlarged glands secrete excessive PTH.

19. **Describe the pathophysiologic changes in tertiary HPT.**
Tertiary HPT results from progression of secondary HPT. In tertiary HPT, prolonged hypocalcemia causes development of autonomous parathyroid function and hypercalcemia. Spontaneous change from low or normal calcium levels to hypercalcemia marks the transition from secondary to tertiary HPT. In tertiary HPT, PTH levels are usually > 10–20 times normal. This most commonly occurs in chronic renal failure. PTH remains elevated despite vitamin D therapy and correction of hyperphosphatemia. Hypercalcemia remains despite discontinuation of vitamin D and calcium supplements. Tertiary HPT usually requires resection of at least 3 ½ parathyroid glands to correct the hypercalcemia.

20. **How is HHM distinguished from primary HPT?**
The main distinguishing features are the levels of intact PTH, PTHrP, and 1,25(OH)$_2$D. The classic and most common patterns of these hormones are shown in Table 15-3. Primary HPT usually has elevated levels of intact PTH. PTHrP levels, when measured, are low. Malignancy-associated hypercalcemia, in contrast, has low levels of intact PTH, but 80% of cases have increased levels of PTHrP and 20% have both low intact PTH and PTHrP. Thus, measuring the two hormones distinguishes all three disorders.

TABLE 15-3. HYPERCALCEMIA, PRIMARY HPT, AND MALIGNANCY				
	Intact PTH	**PTHrP**	**1,25(OH)$_2$D**	**Calcium**
Primary HPT	↑	↓	↑	↑
PTHrP malignancy	↓	↑	↓	↑
Non-PTHrP malignancy	↓	↓	↓	↑

21. **How do PTHrP and PTH differ?**
PTHrP consists of three protein forms with 139, 141, and 173 amino acids. The first 139 amino acids are the same among the three forms. Eight of the first 13 N-terminal amino acids are identical to intact PTH (1–84), allowing PTHrP to stimulate the same receptors as PTH and to have similar biologic effects. The two hormones have different effects on levels of 1,25(OH)$_2$D, probably because of their differing secretion patterns. Both PTH and PTHrP stimulate receptors that activate renal 1α-hydroxylase. The continuous secretion of PTHrP by malignant tumors probably down-regulates these receptors, inhibiting 1α-hydroxylase activity and decreasing 1,25(OH)$_2$D production. Continuous infusion of PTH causes similar decreases in 1,25(OH)$_2$D.

22. **Summarize the association of PTH with HPT.**
Secretion of PTH in HPT is intermittent; intermittent secretion avoids down-regulation and results in increased 1,25(OH)$_2$D. In addition, serum calcium levels are higher in HHM than in HPT. The higher calcium levels further decrease production of 1,25(OH)$_2$D. Thus, 1,25(OH)$_2$D levels tend to be high in HPT and low in HHM. Traditional associations of primary HPT include mild renal tubular acidosis, hypophosphatemia, hyperchloremia, and an increased ratio of chloride to phosphate. Unfortunately, such associations are nonspecific and too insensitive to be of diagnostic use.

23. **What PTH assay is most useful in the work-up of hypercalcemia?**
Intact PTH has 84 amino acids and a half-life of 2–4 minutes. Although the first 34 amino acids of the N-terminus contain the full biologic activity of the hormone, intact PTH (1–84 pg/mL) is the active hormone in vivo. The preferred assays for measurement are the ICMA and IRMA for intact PTH; both are highly sensitive and specific. Because of availability, the IRMA is more commonly used. At times, a midmolecule assay for PTH will support the clinical diagnosis of HPT when the ICMA and IRMA assays are both negative. The IRMA also measures a 7–84 amino-acid fragment of intact PTH (1–84 pg/mL). The newer scantibodies (whole-PTH) and bio-intact PTH assays measure the true intact PTH molecule. These assays may be more useful in patients with renal failure. This assay has not been more useful than the usual IRMA. A rapid PTH is often measured during surgery.

24. **What methods best localize the parathyroid tumor in HPT?**
Technetium-99m sestamibi single proton emission computed tomography (SPECT) scintigraphy may be > 85–90% sensitive, specific, and accurate and therefore is the procedure of choice. Sestamibi scanning is most accurate for localizing parathyroid adenomas and is much less

useful for parathyroid hyperplasia. Ultrasonography is usually a complementary test for localization. Less commonly used localization studies that may be useful include intraoperative guidance with a γ-probe, cervical computed tomography (CT), magnetic resonance imaging, positron emission tomography (PET), intravenous digital subtraction angiography (IVDSA), arteriography, and selective venous sampling.

KEY POINTS: HPT ✓

1. Primary HPT is associated with hypercalcemia, osteoporosis, nephrolithiasis, and symptoms associated with these conditions.

2. The new recommendations for surgery in patients with asymptomatic HPT are as follows: serum calcium > 1 mg/dL above the upper normal limit, hypercalciuria > 400 mg per 24 hours, decreased creatinine clearance < 70% of age matched normal persons, reduced bone density with T-score < −2.5, age < 50 years, and calcium nephrolithiasis.

3. It is never wrong to recommend surgery for treatment of asymptomatic HPT if the patient has no contraindications to surgery and has access to a skilled parathyroid surgeon.

4. Advantages of parathyroid surgery include cure of HPT and hypercalcemia in most cases with a single operation, no need for regular prolonged follow-up, decreased fracture rate, and increased bone mass in most patients.

5. Most surgeons prefer preoperative localization studies before minimally invasive parathyroidectomy, before reoperative parathyroid surgery, and for suspected bilateral disease.

25. **When should you use preoperative localization of a parathyroid adenoma?**
The following statement by John Doppman in 1986 generally holds true today: "the only localization study indicated in a patient with untreated primary hyperparathyroidism is the localization of an experienced parathyroid surgeon." More than 90–95% of the time, a skilled parathyroid surgeon can localize and remove a parathyroid adenoma without preoperative localization. For this reason, preoperative localization before standard bilateral neck exploration is not usually necessary. However, most surgeons prefer localization studies before minimally invasive parathyroidectomy, before reoperative parathyroid surgery, and for suspected bilateral disease.

26. **Do all asymptomatic patients with HPT require surgical treatment?**
No. Many asymptomatic hyperparathyroid patients do not need surgery (see question 27). However, the only definitive therapy for HPT is parathyroidectomy, and it is never wrong to recommend parathyroidectomy for asymptomatic HPT if you have access to an experienced parathyroid surgeon. Many patients prefer surgery and do not need to meet NIH guidelines for surgical referral. Advantages of parathyroid surgery are cure of HPT and hypercalcemia in most cases with a single operation, no need for regular prolonged follow-up, decreased fracture rate, increased bone mass in most patients, and decreased cardiovascular disease.

27. **List the indications for parathyroidectomy as recommended by the April 2002 NIH-sponsored workshop on asymptomatic HPT.**
    1. Hypercalcemia > 1.0 mg/dL above the upper normal limit.
    2. Hypercalciuria > 400 mg/24 hours.
    3. Decreased creatinine clearance 30% from baseline or < 70% of age-matched normal persons.

4. Reduced bone density by dual-energy x-ray absorptiometry (DEXA) bone densitometry (T-score < −2.5).
5. Age < 50 years with mild hypercalcemia.
6. Calcium nephrolithiasis.
7. When good follow-up is not possible or inadvisable due to medical illness.

28. **How should you monitor patients with asymptomatic HPT who have not had parathyroidectomy?**
Initially measure serum calcium, creatinine, PTH, 24-hour urine calcium, creatinine clearance, FECa, abdominal radiograph (KUB), and DEXA bone densitometry. Measure serum calcium biannually. Obtain three-site bone densitometry (lumbar spine, femur, and forearm) serum creatinine, and estimated creatinine clearance or glomerular filtration rate (GFR) annually. Schedule office visits every 6 months and as needed. Evaluate for symptoms of HPT. Make sure patients maintain adequate hydration, exercise, and a normal calcium diet. Avoid thiazide diuretics, lithium, and excessive calcium input. Alert the primary physician to watch for medical illness predisposing to dehydration.

29. **Estimate the creatinine clearance or GFR without doing a 24-hour urine collection.**
Use either the Cockcroft-Gault formula or the Modification of Diet in Renal Disease (Study Group) (MDRD) equation, noting that the MDRD equation is the best equation for estimating GFR but is difficult to calculate. However, the MDRD calculation of GFR is easy if you have web access at *http://www.nkdep.nih.gov/GFR-cal.htm*.

Cockcroft-Gault formula:

$$C_{Cr} = (140 - age) \times \text{ideal body weight (kg)}/[72 \times \text{serum Cr (mg/dL)}] \times (0.85 \text{ if female})$$

MDRD equation:

$$\text{GFR (mL/minute/1.73 m}^2) = 186 \times (Pcr)^{-1.154} \times (age)^{-0.203} \times (0.742 \text{ if female}) \times (1.210 \text{ if African American})$$

30. **Estimate the GFR for a 60-year-old Caucasian woman with serum creatinine of 0.8 mg/dL and a weight of 60 kg.**
Cockcroft-Gault formula:

$$C_{Cr} = (140-60) \times 60 \text{ kg} \times 0.85/(72 \times 0.8 \text{ mg/dL}) = 83 \text{ mL/minute}$$

MDRD equation:

$$\text{GFR} = 78 \text{ mL/minute/1.73 m}^2$$

31. **Estimate the 24-hour urine calcium excretion without doing a 24-hour urine collection.**
A good estimate of the 24-hour urine calcium excretion is 1.1 times the calcium-to-creatinine ratio on a random urine specimen. An example in the same patient as in question 30 follows:

$$U_{Ca} = 20 \text{ mg/dL and } U_{Cr} = 70 \text{ mg/dL calcium/creatinine} = 20/70 = 0.286 \text{ gm}$$

Estimated 24-hour urinary calcium excretion is 1.1×286 mg/day = 315 mg/day.
Because normal 24-hour urinary calcium is up to 4 mg/kg/day or about 240 mg/day in a 60-kg woman, the urinary calcium is elevated, as would be expected in HPT. However, it is not elevated to a degree that requires surgical recommendation in an asymptomatic patient with normal renal function for age.

32. **What are new medical approaches to asymptomatic HPT?**
Calcimimetics, now in phase 4 trials, bind to the extracellular calcium-sensing receptor on parathyroid cells and alter their sensitivity to extracellular calcium. This shifts the calcium-PTH curve to the left, decreases parathyroid responsiveness to the stimulatory effects of low extracellular calcium, and increases parathyroid sensitivity to the suppressive effects of calcium at all concentrations. The calcimimetic cinacalcet is available for treatment of secondary HPT in end-stage renal disease and parathyroid carcinoma. Cinacalcet reduces PTH by 40–50% and lowers calcium and phosphate. Alendronate inhibits osteoclast-mediated bone resorption and can increase bone mass in HPT by > 6%. Estrogen should not be used routinely for osteopenia in HPT due to increased risk of breast cancer and cardiovascular disease.

WEBSITES

1. National Kidney Disease Education Program. Available at http://www.nkdep.nih.gov/GFR-cal.htm

2. Good review of all aspects of parathyroid disease. Available at http://www.parathyroid.com

BIBLIOGRAPHY

1. Bilezikian JP: Primary hyperparathyroidism: When to observe and when to operate. Endocrinol Metab Clin North Am 29:465–478, 2000.

2. Bilezikian JP, Potts JT, Fuleihan Gel-H, et al: Summary statement from a workshop on asymptomatic primary hyperparathyroidism: A perspective for the 21st century. J Bone Miner Res 17(Suppl 2):N2–N11, 2002.

3. Block GA: The impact of calcimimetics on mineral metabolism and secondary hyperparathyroidism in end-stage renal disease. Kidney Int 64(Suppl 87):131–136, 2003.

4. Civelek AC, Ozalp E, Donovan P, et al: Prospective evaluation of delayed technetium-99m sestamibi SPECT scintigraphy for preoperative localization of primary hyperparathyroidism. Surgery 131(2):149–157, 2002.

5. Goodman WG: Medical management of secondary hyperparathyroidism in chronic renal failure. Nephrol Dial Transplant 18(Suppl 3):iii, 2–8, 2003.

6. Haciyanli M, Lal G, Morita E, Duh QY, et al: Accuracy of preoperative localization studies and intraoperative parathyroid hormone assay in patients with primary hyperparathyroidism and double adenoma. J Am Coll Surg 197:739–746, 2003.

7. Kennedy RJ, Roberts AP, Reece GJ, et al: Minimally invasive parathyroidectomy for recurrent or persistent hyperparathyroidism using carbon track localization. ANZ J Surg 73:853–855, 2003.

8. Marx SJ: Hyperparathyroid and hypoparathyroid disorders. N Engl J Med 343:1863, 2000.

9. Perrier ND, Ituarte PHG, Morita E, et al: Parathyroid surgery: Separating promise from reality. J Clin Endocrinol Metab 87(3):1024–1029, 2002.

10. Strewler GJ: The parathyroid hormone-related protein. Endocrinol Metab Clin North Am 29:629–645, 2000.

11. Vestergaard P, Mosekilde L: Cohort study on effects of parathyroid surgery on multiple outcomes in primary hyperparathyroidism. BMJ 327:530–534, 2003.

CHAPTER 16

HYPERCALCEMIA OF MALIGNANCY

Michael T. McDermott, M.D.

1. **What are the two general categories of hypercalcemia of malignancy?**
   - Humoral hypercalcemia of malignancy (HHM).
   - Local osteolytic hypercalcemia (LOH).

2. **What types of cancer are associated with HHM?**
   Carcinoma of the lung, particularly squamous cell carcinoma, is the most common. Other tumors associated with this disorder include squamous cell carcinomas of the head, neck, and esophagus and adenocarcinomas of the breast, kidney, bladder, pancreas, and ovary.

3. **What is the cause of HHM?**
   HHM results when solid malignancies, both solitary and metastatic, secrete into the circulation one or more substances that cause hypercalcemia. The humoral mediator identified in over 90% of cases is parathyroid hormone-related peptide (PTHrp). Other humoral substances that are occasionally secreted and contribute to the development of hypercalcemia include transforming growth factor-alpha (TGFα), tumor necrosis factor (TNF), and various interleukins and cytokines.

4. **What is PTHrp?**
   PTHrp is a protein that has sequence homology with the first 13 amino acids of parathyroid hormone (PTH). Both PTH and PTHrp bind to a common receptor (PTH/PTHrp receptor), resulting in stimulation of bone resorption and inhibition of renal calcium excretion. PTHrp is found in high concentrations in breast milk and amniotic fluid, but it can be detected in almost every tissue in the body; it is increased in the circulation during pregnancy. Its physiologic endocrine function may be to govern the transfer of calcium from the maternal skeleton and bloodstream into the developing fetus and into breast milk. As a generalized paracrine factor, it also regulates growth and development of many tissues, most prominently the skeleton and breast.

5. **How does PTHrp cause hypercalcemia in patients with cancer?**
   Elevated circulating levels of PTHrp stimulate generalized bone resorption, flooding the bloodstream with excessive calcium; PTHrp also acts on the kidneys, preventing excretion of the increased calcium load. This combination produces an increase in the serum calcium concentration. Hypercalcemia induces polyuria, which leads to dehydration with impaired renal function, further reducing calcium excretion and leading to a cycle of progressive and eventually life-threatening hypercalcemia.

6. **How do you make a diagnosis of HHM?**
   Hypercalcemia in any patient with a known malignancy should make one suspect this diagnosis. Occasionally, however, a raised serum calcium is the first clue to an underlying cancer. The key to the diagnosis is a suppressed serum intact PTH level; this finding reliably excludes hyperparathyroidism, the other leading cause of hypercalcemia. Serum PTHrp levels are nearly always high, but this expensive test is not necessary for diagnosis in most instances. If a patient meeting these diagnostic criteria does not have a known tumor, a careful search for an occult malignancy should be undertaken.

7. **What types of cancer are associated with LOH?**
   Breast cancer with skeletal metastases, multiple myeloma, and lymphoma are the major cancers associated with LOH.

KEY POINTS: HYPERCALCEMIA OF MALIGNANCY ✓

1. Hypercalcemia of malignancy is most often due to tumor production of PTHrp, which binds to PTH and PTH/PTHrp receptors to stimulate bone resorption.

2. The key diagnostic test in hypercalcemic patients is measurement of serum PTH, which is elevated or high normal in primary hyperparathyroidism but low or undetectable in hypercalcemia of malignancy and other hypercalcemic disorders.

3. The development of hypercalcemia of malignancy portends a poor prognosis in most cancer patients, since it tends to occur with advanced tumor stages.

4. Serum calcium levels can be lowered effectively in patients with hypercalcemia of malignancy by the intravenous administration of saline and bisphosphonates.

---

8. **What is the cause of LOH?**
   LOH generally occurs when cancer cells are present in multiple sites throughout the skeleton. The pathogenesis involves the elaboration by malignant cells of osteoclast-stimulating factors directly onto the surface of bone. Such factors include PTHrp, lymphotoxin, interleukins, transforming growth factors, prostaglandins, and procathepsin D.

9. **How do you make a diagnosis of LOH?**
   The diagnosis is fairly straightforward when a patient with one of the above malignancies develops hypercalcemia. Again, the key is demonstration of a suppressed serum intact PTH, indicating that hyperparathyroidism is not the culprit. Patients without a known malignancy should have a complete blood count, serum and urine protein electrophoresis, and bone scan; if these studies are not informative, a bone marrow biopsy should be performed.

10. **Can lymphomas cause hypercalcemia by other mechanisms?**
    Some lymphomas express 1α hydroxylase activity. This enzyme converts 25-hydroxyvitamin D to 1,25-dihydroxyvitamin D, which then stimulates increased intestinal calcium absorption. This may eventually lead to hypercalcemia, particularly in patients who have reduced renal calcium excretion due to dehydration or intrinsic renal disease.

11. **What is the prognosis for patients with hypercalcemia of malignancy?**
    Because hypercalcemia generally correlates with far advanced disease, the overall prognosis is quite poor. In one study, the median survival of patients who developed hypercalcemia was only 30 days. Effective treatments are available to reduce the serum calcium levels, however.

12. **How do you treat hypercalcemia of malignancy?**
    Treatment of the underlying malignancy, when possible, is the most effective solution. For the symptomatic patient, however, rapid reduction of serum calcium is indicated. An intravenous saline infusion to enhance renal calcium excretion is the initial measure in almost all patients. Medication to inhibit bone resorption should be given concomitantly. The most effective of these are the intravenous bisphosphonates. Calcitonin plus prednisone is not effective long term but may be useful to use for 2–3 days with a bisphosphonate for rapid calcium reduction in patients with severe hypercalcemia. Suggested treatment regimens are listed in the following:

Medications	Initial Dose	Maintenance
Zoledronic acid	5 mg IV over 5 minutes	Repeat q 2 weeks
Pamidronate	60–90 mg IV over 4 hours	Repeat q 2 weeks
Etidronate	7.5 mg/kg/day IV over 4 hours for 4–7 days	20 mg/kg/day orally
Calcitonin	100–200 units SQ b.i.d. for 2–3 days only	
± Prednisone	30–60 mg qd for 2–3 days only	
Plicamycin	25 µg/kg IV	Repeat in 48 hours

BIBLIOGRAPHY

1. Bilezikian JP: Management of acute hypercalcemia. N Engl J Med 326:1196–1203, 1992.

2. Grill V, Ho P, Body JJ, et al: Parathyroid hormone related protein: Elevated levels in both humoral hypercalcemia of malignancy and hypercalcemia complicating metastatic breast cancer. J Clin Endocrinol Metab 73:1309–1315, 1991.

3. Hortobagyi GN, Theriault RL, et al: Efficacy of pamidronate in reducing skeletal complications in patients with breast cancer and lytic bone metastases. N Engl J Med 335:1785–1791, 1996.

4. Mundy GR, Guise TA: Hypercalcemia of malignancy. Am J Med 103:134–145, 1997.

5. Nussbaum SR, Younger J, et al: Single dose intravenous therapy with pamidronate for the treatment of hypercalcemia of malignancy. Comparison of 30, 60 and 90 mg doses. Am J Med 95: 297–304, 1993.

6. Ralston SH, Gallacher SJ, Patel U, et al: Cancer associated hypercalcemia: Morbidity and mortality. Clinical experience in 126 treated patients. Ann Intern Med 112:499–504, 1990.

7. Singer FR, Ritch PS, Lad TE, et al: Treatment of hypercalcemia of malignancy with intravenous etidronate. A controlled multicenter study. Arch Intern Med 151:471–476, 1991.

8. Stewart AF, Broadus AE: Parathyroid hormone related proteins: Coming of age in the 1990's. J Clin Endocrinol Metab 71:1410–1414, 1990.

CHAPTER 17

HYPOCALCEMIA

Reed S. Christensen, M.D.

1. **Define hypocalcemia.**
   Hypocalcemia is the state in which the serum ionized calcium level drops below the normal range of 1.0–1.3 mmol/L. This corresponds, under normal conditions, to a total serum calcium level of 2.1–2.5 mmol/L (8.5–10.5 mg/dL).

2. **How are serum calcium and serum albumin levels related?**
   Approximately 50% of serum calcium is bound to albumin, other plasma proteins, and related anions, such as citrate, lactate, and sulfate. Of this, 40% is bound to protein, predominantly albumin, and 10–13% is attached to anions. The remaining 50% is unbound or ionized calcium. The total serum calcium level reflects both the bound and the unbound portions with a normal range of 2.1–2.5 mmol/L (8.5–10.5 mg/dL).

3. **How is the total serum calcium corrected for a low serum albumin level?**
   Total serum calcium levels are corrected for hypoalbuminemia by adding 0.8 mg/dL to the serum calcium level for every 1.0 gm/dL that the albumin level is below 4.0 gm/dL. The adjusted level of total serum calcium correlates with the level of ionized calcium, which is the physiologically active form of serum calcium.

4. **What factors other than albumin influence the levels of serum ionized calcium?**
   Serum pH influences levels of ionized calcium by causing decreased binding of calcium to albumin in acidosis and increased binding in alkalosis. As an example, respiratory alkalosis, seen in hyperventilation, causes a drop in the level of serum ionized calcium. A shift of 0.1 pH unit is associated with an ionized calcium change of 0.04–0.05 mmol/L. Increased levels of chelators, such as citrate, also may lower the levels of ionized calcium, as does heparin.

5. **How is serum calcium regulated?**
   Three hormones maintain calcium homeostasis: parathyroid hormone (PTH), vitamin D, and calcitonin. PTH acts in three ways to raise serum calcium levels: (1) stimulates osteoclastic bone resorption; (2) increases conversion of 25-hydroxyvitamin D to 1,25-dihydroxyvitamin D, increasing intestinal calcium absorption; and (3) increases renal reabsorption of calcium. Calcitonin decreases the level of serum calcium by suppressing osteoclast activity in bone. The interplay of these hormones maintains calcium levels within a very narrow range in a normal individual. Calcium levels are also influenced by the presence or absence of hyperphosphatemia.

6. **What steps in vitamin D metabolism may influence serum calcium levels?**
   Vitamin D is obtained through the diet or is formed in the skin in the presence of ultraviolet light. Vitamin D is converted to 25-hydroxyvitamin D in the liver and finally to 1,25-dihydroxyvitamin D, the most active form of vitamin D, in the kidney. 1,25 dihydroxyvitamin D acts directly on intestinal cells to increase calcium absorption. Deficiency in any of these steps may cause hypocalcemia.

7. **What are the major causes of hypocalcemia?**
   The multiple organ and hormonal regulatory systems involved in calcium homeostasis create the potential for multiple causes of hypocalcemia. The etiology of hypocalcemia must be

considered in relation to the level of serum albumin, the secretion of PTH, and the presence or absence of hyperphosphatemia. Initially, hypocalcemia may be approached by looking for failure in one or more of these systems. The systems primarily involved are the parathyroid glands, bone, kidney, and liver:

Clinical Entity	Mechanism
Hypoparathyroidism	Decreased PTH production
Hypomagnesemia	Decreased PTH release
Pseudohypoparathyroidism	PTH ineffective at target organ
Liver disease	Decreased albumin production
	Decreased 25-hydroxyvitamin D production
	Drugs that stimulate 25-hydroxyvitamin D metabolism
Renal disease	Renal calcium leak
	Decreased 1,25-dihydroxyvitamin D production
	Elevated serum phosphate (PO_4) from decreased PO_4 clearance
	Drugs that increase renal clearance of calcium
Bone disease	Drugs suppressing bone resorption
	"Hungry bone syndrome"—recovery from hyperparathyroidism or hyperthyroidism
Phosphate load	Endogenous: tumor lysis syndrome, hemolysis, and rhabdomyolysis
	Exogenous: phosphate-containing enemas, laxatives, and phosphorus burns
Pancreatitis	Sequestration of calcium in the pancreas
Toxic shock syndrome, other critical illness	Decreased PTH production or PTH resistance

PTH, parathyroid hormone.

8. **What physical signs suggest hypocalcemia?**
Chvostek's and Trousseau's signs are useful in detecting hypocalcemia. Chvostek's sign is a facial twitch elicited by tapping over the zygomatic arch. Trousseau's sign is a forearm spasm induced by inflation of an upper arm blood pressure cuff for up to 3 minutes. It is important to note that 4–25% of normal individuals have a positive response.

9. **What laboratory tests are clinically useful in distinguishing among the causes of hypocalcemia?**
Table 17-1 summarizes the laboratory findings in the conditions listed.

10. **Describe the neurologic and psychological symptoms of hypocalcemia.**
Hypocalcemia may present with numbness, tingling, muscle cramps, and fasciculations. Psychiatric symptoms include irritability, paranoia, depression, psychosis, and organic brain syndrome. Subnormal intelligence also has been reported with hypocalcemia. Of note, individuals

TABLE 17-1. DIFFERENTIAL DIAGNOSIS OF LABORATORY EVALUATION OF HYPOCALCEMIA

	Calcium	Phosphate	PTH	25-Vitamin D	1.25-Vitamin D
Hypoparathyroidism	↓	↑	↓	Normal	↓
Pseudohypoparathyroidism	↓	↑	↑	Normal	↓ or Normal
Liver disease	↓	↓	↑	↓	↓ or Normal
Renal disease	↓	↑	↑	Normal	↓ or Normal

PTH, parathyroid hormone.

may be unaware of symptoms because of gradual onset and may realize an abnormality only when their sense of well-being improves with treatment. Neurologic symptoms may progress to tetany and seizures. Seizures occur because of a lowered seizure threshold revealing underlying epilepsy. "Cerebral tetany" (see question 12), which is not a true seizure, may also be seen in hypocalcemia.

11. **What radiographic findings may be present with hypocalcemia?**
Calcifications of basal ganglia may occur in the small blood vessels of that region. These occasionally may cause extrapyramidal signs but usually are asymptomatic. Of note, 0.7% of routine computed tomographic (CT) scans of the brain show calcification of the basal ganglia.

12. **What is cerebral tetany and how does it differ from a true seizure?**
Cerebral tetany is manifested by generalized tetany without loss of consciousness, tongue biting, incontinence, or postictal confusion. Anticonvulsants may relieve the symptoms but, because they enhance 25-hydroxyvitamin D catabolism, they also may worsen the hypocalcemia.

KEY POINTS: HYPOCALCEMIA ✓

1. Serum calcium levels must be corrected for serum albumin levels in hypocalcemia.

2. Multiple organ systems, minerals, anions, and drugs affect calcium levels and must be considered when evaluating hypocalcemia.

3. Hypocalcemia is a frequent problem in intensive care settings and is often a result of intravenous agents.

4. 1,25-dihydroxyvitamin D is the treatment for hypocalcemia in hypoparathyroidism and renal failure.

5. PTH is not currently a treatment for hypocalcemia.

13. **How does hypocalcemia affect cardiac function?**

Calcium is involved in cardiac automaticity and is required for muscle contraction. Hypocalcemia can therefore result in arrhythmias and reduced myocardial contractility. This decrease in the force of contraction may be refractory to pressor agents, especially those that involve calcium in their mechanism of action. Through this process, beta-blockers and calcium channel blockers can exacerbate cardiac failure. With low serum calcium, the Q-T interval is prolonged and ST changes may mimic myocardial infarction. Although the relationship is variable, the calcium level correlates moderately well with the interval from the Q-wave onset to the peak of the T-wave.

14. **What are the potential ophthalmologic findings in hypocalcemia?**

Papilledema may occur with subacute and chronic hypocalcemia. Patients are most often asymptomatic, and the papilledema usually resolves with normalization of the serum calcium level. If symptoms develop or if papilledema does not resolve when the patient is normocalcemic, a cerebral tumor and benign intracranial hypertension must be excluded. Optic neuritis with unilateral loss of vision occasionally develops in hypocalcemic patients. Lenticular cataracts also may occur with long-standing hypocalcemia but usually do not increase in size once hypocalcemia is corrected.

15. **With what autoimmune disorders is hypocalcemia sometimes associated?**

Hypoparathyroidism may result from autoimmune destruction of the parathyroid glands. This disorder has been associated with adrenal, gonadal, and thyroid failure, as well as with alopecia areata, vitiligo, and chronic mucocutaneous candidiasis. This combination of conditions, each associated with organ-specific autoantibodies, has been termed the autoimmune polyglandular syndrome, type 1.

16. **Hypocalcemia is frequently encountered in intensive care settings. What are the potential causes?**

Low total serum calcium levels are found in 70–90% of intensive care patients and result from multiple causes including:

- Hypoalbuminemia.
- Administration of anionic loads causing chelation (i.e., citrate, lactate, oxalate, bicarbonate, phosphate, ethylenediaminetetraacedic acid [EDTA], and radiographic contrast).
- Rapid blood transfusion with citrate ion as a preservative and anticoagulant therapy.
- Parathyroid failure and decreased vitamin D synthesis in severe illness.
- Sepsis inducing some degree of resistance to the biologic effects of PTH.

Because of all the above factors, it is recommended that ionized serum calcium rather than total serum calcium be measured in patients with severe illness.

17. **Hypercalcemia is not unusual in patients with cancer. What conditions may lead to hypocalcemia in this patient group?**

- Tumor lysis syndrome from hyperphosphatemia and associated formation of intravascular and tissue calcium-phosphate complexes.
- Multiple chemotherapeutic agents and antibiotics (amphotericin B and aminoglycosides) induce hypomagnesemia. Hypomagnesemia impairs secretion of PTH and causes resistance to PTH in skeletal tissue.
- Thyroid surgery and neck irradiation with transient or permanent hypoparathyroidism.
- Medullary carcinoma of the thyroid and pheochromocytoma may secrete calcitonin and on rare occasions cause hypocalcemia.

18. **What drugs may cause hypocalcemia?**

Phenobarbital, phenytoin, primidone, rifampin, and glutethimide increase hepatic metabolism of 25-hydroxyvitamin D and may thereby cause hypocalcemia. Aminoglycosides, diuretics (furosemide), and chemotherapeutic agents that induce renal magnesium wasting, and laxatives or enemas that create a large phosphate load, also may be associated with hypocalcemia. Ketoconazole, isoniazid, heparin, fluoride, bisphosphonates, foscarnet, and glucagon may also induce hypocalcemia by a variety of mechanisms.

19. **Which vitamin D metabolite is best for assessing total body vitamin D stores, 25-hydroxyvitamin D or 1,25-dihydroxyvitamin D?**
The serum level of 25-hydroxyvitamin D best reflects the total body stores of vitamin D. The conversion of 25-hydroxyvitamin D to 1,25-dihydroxyvitamin D is tightly controlled and the level of serum 1,25-dihydroxyvitamin D is maintained despite significant vitamin D depletion. Increases in PTH (secondary hyperparathyroidism) stimulate increased conversion of 25-hydroxyvitamin D to 1,25-dihydroxyvitamin D in this situation.

20. **How is hypocalcemia treated?**
Asymptomatic hypocalcemia requires supplementation with oral calcium and vitamin D derivatives to maintain the serum calcium level at least in the range of 7.5–8.5 mg/dL. When the serum calcium falls acutely to a level where the patient is symptomatic, intravenous administration is recommended. The dose of calcium depends on the amount of elemental calcium present in a given preparation (Table 17-2). Approximately 90 mg of elemental calcium can be given intravenously as a bolus for a hypocalcemic emergency, followed by an infusion of 0.5–2.0 mg/kg/h.

TABLE 17-2. ELEMENTAL CALCIUM CONTENT OF COMMONLY USED PREPARATIONS		
Preparation	**Oral Dose**	**Elemental Calcium (mg)**
Calcium citrate		
Citracal	950 mg	200
Calcium acetate		
PhosLo	667 mg	169
Calcium carbonate		
Tums	500 mg	200
Tums Ex	750 mg	300
Oscal	625 mg	250
Oscal 500	1250 mg	500
Calcium 600	1500 mg	600
Titralac (suspension)	1000 mg/5 mL	400
Intravenous Agent	**Volume**	**Elemental Calcium (mg)**
Calcium chloride	2.5 mL of 10% solution	90
Calcium gluconate	10 mL of 10% solution	90
Calcium gluceptate	5 mL of 22% solution	90

21. **When is treatment with 1,25 dihydroxyvitamin D (calcitriol) indicated?**
Under normal conditions, 25-hydroxyvitamin D is converted to 1,25-dihydroxyvitamin D (calcitriol) in the kidney under the stimulatory influence of PTH. Two conditions can therefore make the body unable to produce adequate amounts of calcitriol: hypoparathyroidism and renal failure. Since calcitriol is essential for normal intestinal calcium absorption, oral calcitriol (Rocaltrol) supplementation is indicated in patients who have either hypoparathyroidism or

chronic renal failure. Of note, since vitamin D has very weak biologic activity, these patients may be given large doses of vitamin D (50,000–100,000 U/day) if calcitriol is unavailable.

22. **Can recombinant human PTH (rhPTH) be used in the treatment of hypocalcemia?**
Subcutaneous injections of PTH have been shown to be effective in normalizing serum calcium levels in hypoparathyroidism. The therapy is not approved, however, and is considered experimental.

BIBLIOGRAPHY

1. Bringhurst FR, Demay MB, Kronenberg HM: Hypocalcemic disorders. In Wilson JD (ed): Williams Textbook of Endocrinology, 10th ed. Philadelphia, W.B. Saunders, 2003, pp 1340–1348.

2. Kastrup EK (ed): Drug Facts and Comparisons. St. Louis, Wolters Kluwer Health, 2003, pp 27–29, 112–113.

3. Lebowitz MR, Moses AM: Hypocalcemia. Semin Nephrol 12:146–158, 1992.

4. Lind L: Hypocalcemia and parathyroid hormone secretion in critically ill patients. Crit Care Med 28:93–98, 2000.

5. McEvoy GK (ed): Calcium salts. In AHFS Drug Information. Bethesda, MD, American Society of Hospital Pharmacists, 2003, pp 2481–2487.

6. Olinger ML: Disorders of calcium and magnesium metabolism. Emerg Med Clin North Am 7:795–822, 1989.

7. Potts JT: Hypocalcemia. In Fauci AS (ed): Principles of Internal Medicine, 14th ed. New York, McGraw-Hill, 1998, pp 2241–2247.

8. Shane E: Hypocalcemia: Pathogenesis, differential diagnosis and management. In Favus MJ (ed): Primer on the Metabolic Bone Diseases and Disorders of Mineral Metabolism, 4th ed. Philadelphia, Lippincott Williams & Wilkins, 1999, pp 223–226.

9. Winer KK, Yanovski JA, Sarani B, Cutler GB: A randomized, cross-over trial of once-daily versus twice-daily parathyroid hormone 1–34 in treatment of hypoparathyroidism, J Clin Endocrinol Metab 83:3480–3486, 1998.

10. Zaloga GP: Hypocalcemia in critically ill patients. Crit Care Med 20:251–262, 1992.

CHAPTER 18

NEPHROLITHIASIS

Leonard R. Sanders, M.D.

1. **Define hypercalciuria, kidney stones, renal calculi, nephrolithiasis, urolithiasis, renal lithiasis, and nephrocalcinosis.**
   Hypercalciuria is urinary excretion of > 300 mg/day of calcium in men and > 250 mg/day in women. A more accurate definition is urinary calcium excretion > 4 mg/kg ideal body weight/day in either sex. Kidney stones, renal calculi, nephrolithiasis, urolithiasis, and renal lithiasis are synonymous terms that define the clinical syndrome of formation and movement of stones in the urinary collecting system. Renal calculi are abnormally hard, insoluble substances that form in the renal collecting system. Nephrocalcinosis is deposition of calcium salts in the renal parenchyma.

2. **Who is at risk of developing kidney stones?**
   Five to ten percent of the United States population is at risk of developing one stone; 50–60% have recurrence within 5–10 years. Stones occur most commonly between ages 18 and 45, in men three times greater than women, and in Caucasians more than other races. Women have had more stones in recent years possibly due to increased calcium and protein intake and increased exercise (dehydration). Risk factors include a family history of stones, autosomal dominant polycystic kidney disease, medullary sponge kidney, renal tubular acidosis, urine volume < 2 L/day, dietary sodium > 2 gm/day, low water intake, and high protein intake (see question 4).

3. **What are the composition and approximate frequency of most kidney stones?**
   There are six major types of stones as outlined in Figure 18-1. The figure also shows approximate frequency of occurrence of each type of stone.

4. **What are the main causes of nephrolithiasis?**
   The most common causes of nephrolithiasis are the various types of idiopathic hypercalciuria (IH): absorptive hypercalciuria (AH) types AH-I to AH-III (renal phosphate leak) and renal hypercalciuria (RH). Other causes include primary hyperparathyroidism, hyperoxaluria, hyperuricosuria, hypocitraturia, hypomagnesuria, infection stones, gouty diathesis, renal tubular acidosis, cystinuria, and possibly nanobacteria. Rarely, kidney stones may form from xanthine, triamterene, monosodium urate, ephedrine, guaifenesin, and indinavir (protease inhibitor). Patients with idiopathic nephrolithiasis make up 10–20% of stone formers and have no identifiable cause after routine work-up.

5. **Describe the conditions associated with both renal stone disease and hypercalciuria.**
   Calcium stones account for 80% of all kidney stones. About 40–50% of calcium stone formers have hypercalciuria. Of those with hypercalciuria 40% have IH, 5% have primary hyperparathyroidism, and 3% have renal tubular acidosis. Other causes of hypercalciuria include excessive dietary vitamin D, excessive calcium and alkali intake, sarcoidosis, Cushing's syndrome, hyperthyroidism, Paget's disease of bone, and immobilization.

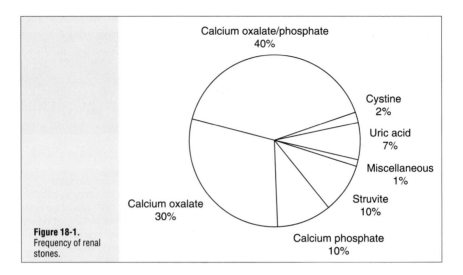

Figure 18-1. Frequency of renal stones.

6. **What are the most important causes of normocalciuric calcium nephrolithiasis?**
   The most important and most common causes of normocalciuric calcium nephrolithiasis are hypocitraturia (50%), hyperuricosuria (25%), hyperoxaluria (10%), and urinary stasis (5%).

7. **Describe the process of renal stone formation.**
   Initially, urinary crystallization or precipitation of sparingly soluble salts and acids occurs. Nucleation follows as the initial crystals and urinary matrix ions form a stable framework for crystal enlargement through growth and aggregation. Once sufficiently large, crystals become trapped in a narrow portion of the urinary collecting system, forming a nidus for further stone growth. Usually stones originate in the renal papilla and may detach, move distally, and cause obstruction. Common sites for obstruction are the ureteropelvic junction, mid-ureter, and ureterovesical junction.

8. **Discuss the pathophysiologic factors that influence formation of renal stones.**
   Renal stones result from hereditary or acquired disorders causing supersaturation of stone pre-cursors, deficiency of stone inhibitors, and possibly excess promoters. Supersaturation causes crystallization with mineral precursors, such as calcium oxalate. Calcium oxalate crystals bind to anionic, sialic acid-containing glycoproteins on the apical surface of renal tubular epithelial cells, allowing further growth. Other factors that increase stone formation include urinary stasis (medullary sponge kidney), decreased flow (obstruction), increased urine ammonium (infec-tion), dehydration (concentrated urine), and increased level of urinary acidity (renal tubular acidosis). Renal tubular acidosis promotes stone formation by causing hypercalciuria, hypoci-traturia, and alkaline urine.

9. **What are the main chemical precursors of renal stones?**
   Relatively high concentrations of salt and acid solutes are the main determinants of crystalluria and stone formation. Calcium oxalate is most common and is supersaturated to four to five times its solubility in normal urine. Other precursors are calcium phosphate (hydroxyapatite) and calcium phosphate monohydrate (brushite). Uric acid, cystine, struvite (magnesium ammo-nium phosphate), and mucoprotein are undersaturated stone precursors. Drugs such as ascor-bic acid (conversion to oxalate) and triamterene (nidus for stone formation) also may promote renal stone formation.

10. **What are the main inhibitors of renal stone formation? How do they work?**
Inhibitors include urinary citrate, pyrophosphate, magnesium, nephrocalcin, uropontin, glycosaminoglycans, and Tamm-Horsfall protein. Most of these bind crystal precursors; for example, citrate binds calcium, making it less available to bind to oxalate. Inhibitors improve solubility and impair precipitation, nucleation, crystal growth, or aggregation. They also compete with stone precursor minerals, such as calcium oxalate, for binding to the apical surface of epithelial cells and inhibit epithelial cell adhesion and internalization of calcium oxalate crystals. Finally, inhibitors impair stone precursor transformation to a focus for crystallization and stone growth.

11. **What is nephrocalcin? What role does it play in formation of renal stones?**
Nephrocalcin is an anionic protein produced by the proximal renal tubule and the loop of Henle. It normally inhibits the nucleation, crystal growth, and aggregation phases of stone formation. However, nephrocalcin isolated from some stone formers has defective structure and function and is found in the matrix of many calcium stones. Thus, nephrocalcin may have a dual role in stone formation. When normal, it acts as an inhibitor of stone formation. When abnormal, it may act as a promoter by binding calcium and forming a nidus for crystallization.

12. **What are promoters of renal stone formation?**
Promoters of renal stone formation are poorly characterized but are believed to be primarily urinary mucoproteins and glycosaminoglycans. Under certain conditions, promoters enhance the formation of renal stones.

13. **Summarize the basic determinants of serum calcium.**
In the serum, calcium is 40% protein-bound, 10% complexed, and 50% ionized. The three sources of serum calcium are intestinal absorption, bone resorption, and renal reabsorption. Intestinal calcium absorption is a variable proportion of the intake (30–70%). Ninety percent of calcium absorption occurs in the small intestines and 10% in the cecum and ascending colon. Renal calcium reabsorption is a variable portion of the filtered load (95–99.5%). The net flux of calcium from bone varies, depending on changes in the intestines and kidney. Under normal physiologic conditions, flux of calcium into and out of bone is the same. Parathyroid hormone (PTH) and vitamin D control normal bone, gastrointestinal, and renal handling of calcium (see Fig. 14-1).

14. **How does the kidney handle calcium?**
About 60% of the serum calcium is ionized or complexed and freely filtered by the glomerulus. The kidney reabsorbs 98% of the filtered calcium passively throughout the nephron. Sixty percent reabsorption occurs in the proximal convoluted tubule, 30% in the loop of Henle, and 10% in the distal tubule. Furosemide impairs calcium reabsorption in the loop of Henle and increases urinary calcium excretion. Thiazide diuretics impair distal tubule reabsorption of sodium, which increases intracellular negativity and calcium reabsorption. PTH increases distal tubular calcium reabsorption by enhancing calcium channel activity.

15. **Calculate the normal filtered and excreted load of calcium per day.**
The serum calcium is normally 10 mg/dL. The kidney filters complexed and free calcium, which makes up 60% of the total or 6 mg/dL. The normal glomerular filtration rate (GFR) = 120 mL/minute. Thus, the filtered load of calcium is 6 mg/100 mL × 120 mL/minute × 1440 minutes/day = 10,368 mg/day. Because the kidney reabsorbs 98% of the filtered calcium, only 2% is excreted. Thus, normally the kidney excretes about 200 mg of calcium/day (10,368 mg/day × 0.02 = 207 mg/day). If the excreted calcium increases to 5%, the urinary calcium increases to 500 mg/day.

KEY POINTS: INCIDENCE AND ETIOLOGY OF NEPHROLITHIASIS ✓

1. Kidney stones are increasingly more common, possibly due to excessive dietary protein and calcium and exercise without adequate hydration.

2. About 10% of the U.S. population has a lifetime risk for at least one kidney stone.

3. Stones form because of supersaturation of urinary stone precursors (such as calcium and oxalate), insufficient stone inhibitors (such as citrate), abnormal urine pH, or insufficient urine volume.

4. Stones are most commonly calcium based and result from hypercalciuria caused by excess absorption of dietary calcium, resorption of bone calcium, and unusually decreased renal calcium reabsorption.

5. Restricting dietary calcium increases oxalate absorption and calcium oxalate stones.

16. **How do serum calcium and dietary sodium affect hypercalciuria?**
To help prevent hypercalcemia, nonrenal elevation in serum calcium causes increased filtered calcium and increased urinary calcium. Increased sodium delivery to the loop of Henle and the distal tubule also increases urinary calcium. In non-stone formers, urinary calcium excretion increases about 40 mg for each 100 mEq sodium excretion. In hypercalciuric stone formers, calcium excretion increases up to 80 mg per each 100 mEq of sodium. Since urinary sodium excretion equals dietary sodium input, restricting dietary sodium decreases urinary calcium excretion. In stone patients, recommended daily dietary sodium is no more than 100 mEq (2300 mg).

17. **Discuss the etiology and pathophysiology of IH.**
Idiopathic hypercalciuria (IH) affects 10% of the general population and 40% of stone formers. The four types of IH are AH-I to AH-III and RH. AH-I and AH-II result from increased intestinal sensitivity to calcitriol with intestinal calcium hyperabsorption and increased numbers of vitamin D receptors in osteoblasts causing increased bone resorption and resorptive hypercalciuria. The latter accounts for decreased bone mass seen in many AH-I and some AH-II patients. AH-III, an unusual disorder, is due to a renal phosphate leak with urinary loss of phosphate, decreased serum phosphate, increased renal calcitriol production, and increased intestinal calcium absorption. RH is characterized by impaired tubular reabsorption of calcium, causing decreased serum calcium, increased PTH and calcitriol, increased bone resorption, and increased intestinal calcium absorption.

18. **Distinguish among the various forms of IH.**
See Table 18-1.

19. **When is it necessary to distinguish among the various forms of IH?**
Only complicated nephrolithiasis unresponsive to usual therapy requires differentiation (see Internet reference on hypercalciuria review).

20. **Explain the differences in serum levels of phosphorus and PTH in AH-III and RH.**
Serum phosphorus is low in AH-III because of a primary renal phosphate leak. Intact PTH is high in RH because the primary defect is decreased renal tubular calcium reabsorption, causing relative hypocalcemia that stimulates PTH.

Lab Value	AH-I	AH-II	AH-III	RH
TABLE 18-1. FORMS OF IH				
Serum calcium	Normal	Normal	Normal	Normal
Serum phosphorus	Normal	Normal	↓	Normal
Serum intact PTH	Normal	Normal	Normal	↑
24-hour urinary calcium (1-gm calcium diet)	↑	↑	↑	↑
Urine Ca/Cr ratio (1-gm calcium load)	↑	↑	↑	↑
24-hour urinary calcium (400-mg calcium diet)	↑	Normal	↑	↑
Fasting urinary calcium (mg/dL GFR)	Normal	Normal	↑	↑

AH, absorptive hypercalciuria; RH, renal hypercalciuria; PTH, parathyroid hormone; Ca/Cr, calcium/creatinine; GFR, glomerular filtration rate.

21. **Explain the differences in 24-hour calcium urine levels on a restricted calcium diet.**
    In AH-II, the 24-hour urine calcium normalizes on a restricted calcium diet (400 mg/day) because the absorptive excess is not as severe. However, the 24-hour urine calcium during calcium restriction remains high in AH-I, AH-III, and RH: AH-I because of marked calcium hyperabsorption; AH-III because hypophosphatemia decreases renal tubular reabsorption of calcium; and RH because decreased renal tubular reabsorption is the primary defect.
    High 24-hour urinary calcium is > 4 mg/kg ideal body weight. Normal 24-hour urinary calcium on a 400-mg/day calcium restriction is < 200 mg/day. Normal fasting urine calcium is < 0.11 mg/100 ml GFR. Normal urine Ca/Cr is < 0.20 after a 1-gm oral load of calcium.

22. **Define low serum phosphorus level on an 800-mg/day phosphorus-restricted diet.**
    Low serum phosphorus is < 2.5 mg/dL on an 800-mg/day-phosphorus diet.

23. **What causes hyperoxaluria?**
    About 14% of urinary oxalate comes from dietary absorption and the remainder from metabolism of glyoxylate and ascorbic acid. Increased oxidation of glyoxylate to oxalate occurs in the rare autosomal recessive hereditary hyperoxaluria. The clinically more important enteric hyperoxaluria occurs with small bowel resection, bypass, or inflammation. Small bowel disease may cause bile salt and fat malabsorption resulting in increased delivery of bile salts and fats to the colon. Bile salts damage colonic mucosa, increasing colonic permeability and oxalate absorption. Intestinal fatty acids are negatively charged and bind calcium and magnesium, decreasing calcium and magnesium available for binding intestinal oxalate and leaving more oxalate free for intestinal absorption. Low calcium diets do the same. Since oxalate is primarily absorbed in the colon, patients with small bowel disease and an ileostomy do not hyperabsorb oxalate. Excessive dietary oxalate or ascorbic acid (> 2 gm/day) also leads to hyperoxaluria.

24. **Why is hyperoxaluria important in nephrolithiasis?**
Because hyperoxaluria causes calcium oxalate supersaturation more potently than hypercalciuria, it is a powerful stimulus for calcium oxalate stone formation.

25. **How does hyperuricosuria contribute to renal stones?**
About 25% of patients with symptomatic tophaceous gout develop uric acid stones. Excessive urinary uric acid (> 600 mg/day) supersaturates the urine, crystallizes, and forms uric acid stones. However, most uric acid stone formers do not have gout, hyperuricemia, or hyperuricosuria. All do have a urinary pH < 5.5, which promotes uric acid stone formation. Approximately 25% of calcium stone formers have hyperuricosuria. Monosodium urate may form a nidus for calcium phosphate and calcium oxalate deposition, or interfere with inhibitors, resulting in increased calcium stone formation. This disorder, called hyperuricosuric calcium nephrolithiasis, is characterized by normal serum calcium, urinary uric acid > 600 mg/day, urine pH > 5.5, and recurrent calcium stones.

26. **How does urinary pH relate to renal stones?**
Because uric acid has a pK_a of 5.5, acid urine shifts the equilibrium so that the concentration of uric acid is greater than the concentration of sodium urate. At urine pH 6.5 only 10% will be in the form of uric acid and about 90% in the form of sodium urate. Because uric acid is 100 times less soluble than urate, uric acid stones are more likely to form in acid urine. This equilibrium is so important that uric acid stones virtually never develop unless the urinary pH is < 5.5. Cystine stones are also more likely in acid urine, whereas calcium phosphate (brushite) stones usually form only in alkaline urine, and calcium oxalate stones may develop in either.

27. **What conditions cause low levels of urinary citrate?**
Patients with hypocitraturia excrete < 320 mg/day. IH occurs in < 5% of patients with calcium stones, and secondary hypocitraturia may occur in 30%. Citrate is freely filtered by the glomerulus, 75% is reabsorbed by the proximal renal tubule, and little citrate is secreted. Most secondary causes of hypocitraturia decrease urinary citrate by increasing proximal renal tubular reabsorption. Secondary causes of low citrate include dehydration, metabolic acidosis, hypokalemia, thiazide diuretics, carbonic anhydrase inhibitors, magnesium depletion, renal tubular acidosis, and diarrhea. Diarrhea also causes direct gastrointestinal loss of citrate and magnesium.

28. **What is the role of diet in the formation of kidney stones?**
The high animal protein (beef, poultry, pork, and fish) intake of the average American diet (1.2–1.5 gm/kg/day) acidifies the urine with phosphoric, sulfuric, and uric acids; decreases urinary citrate; increases urinary calcium; and increases risk for nephrolithiasis. Higher protein diets, such as Atkins', worsen these effects. Increased sulfates and uric acid may act as cofactors in the formation of calcium oxalate and uric acid stones. High sodium intake increases urinary calcium (see question 16). High calcium intakes (> 1200 mg) contribute to hypercalciuria. However, low calcium intakes decrease oxalate binding in the gut, increase oxalate absorption, and increase urinary oxalate. High dietary oxalate (see Table 18-2) increases calcium oxalate crystalluria. Potassium citrate juices (orange and cranberry) help prevent kidney stones by increasing urinary potassium and citrate. An 8-oz glass of orange juice supplies 12 mEq potassium and 38 mEq citrate (more than a 1080-mg tablet of potassium citrate). Orange juice increases urinary oxalate somewhat but overall decreases the stone risk. Cranberry juice decreases urinary oxalate and phosphate. Citric acid juices (lemon and lime) supply little potassium and only one-third as much citrate as orange juice. Although potassium citrate juices are more powerful at stone inhibition, nearly all citrate drinks are useful. An exception is grapefruit juice, which increases stone formation by 30–50%.

TABLE 18-2. SELECTED HIGH-OXALATE FOODS		
Fruits	**Vegetables**	**Others**
Rhubarb	Leafy dark greens	Roasted coffee
Raspberries	Spinach	Ovaltine
Blueberries	Mustard greens	Tea
Blackberries	Collard greens	Cocoa
Gooseberries	Cucumbers	Chocolate
Strawberries	Green beans	Nuts
Fruit cocktail	Beets	Peanuts
Tangerines	Sweet potatoes	Wheat germ
Purple grapes	Summer squash	Baked beans
Citrus peel	Celery	Tofu

Adapted from Renal diseases and disorders. In Nelson JK, Moxness KE, Jensen MD, Gastineau CF (eds): Mayo Clinic Diet Manual, 7th ed. St. Louis, Mosby, 1994.

29. **Summarize the presenting symptoms and signs of renal stones.**
Renal stones may be asymptomatic, found incidentally on radiographic studies, and may present as a dull ache in the posterior flank. However, the classic symptom of renal stones is excruciating pain that waxes and wanes. The pain starts in the posterior lumbar area and then radiates anteroinferiorly into the abdomen, groin, genital region, and medial thigh. Intense pain may last several hours and be followed by dull flank pain. Nausea, vomiting, sweating, fever, chills, and hematuria may occur. Patients with renal colic appear acutely ill and restless and move from side to side, attempting to relieve the pain. Physical examination shows tenderness and guarding of the respective lumbar area. Deep palpation worsens discomfort, but rebound tenderness is absent. Urinary tract infection may be present. Obstruction, if present, is usually unilateral. Clinical evidence of renal failure is usually absent.

30. **What elements of the history and physical examination are important in patients with kidney stones?**
Obtain present, past, and family histories and ask about previous stone disease. Since all of the following may be associated with stones, ask about use of guaifenesin, ephedrine, indinavir, triamterene, and vitamins A, C, and D. Determine fluid intake and sources of excess calcium, salt, oxalate, uric acid, and protein. Physical examination is generally not helpful except during acute disease (see question 29).

31. **What lab tests are appropriate in the diagnosis of kidney stones?**
Evaluate urine for pH, hematuria, pyuria, bacteriuria, and crystalluria. If pH is high or bacteriuria is seen, perform urine culture. Perform appropriate radiographic studies (see question 35). Have the patient strain all urine and save the stone, if passed, for stone analysis. If this is the patient's first stone, the pain subsides, and the stone is < 5 mm, follow-up for several months is acceptable. Ninety percent of stones < 5 mm pass spontaneously. Order a chemistry panel that includes serum sodium, potassium, chloride, carbon dioxide, creatinine, calcium, albumin, phosphorus, magnesium, and uric acid. Consider serum PTH and random urine for determination of the Ca/Cr ratio. If the patient has continued symptoms, if the stone is > 1 cm, or if obvious obstruction is present, consult a urologist and plan for a more extensive evaluation. Include a 24-hour urine for creatinine, sodium, calcium, phosphorus, magnesium, oxalate, citrate, and uric acid.

32. **Summarize the therapeutic approach to patients with kidney stones.**
Unless contraindicated, all patients should increase fluid intake (10–12 eight-ounce glasses) to increase urine output to > 2 L/day; restrict dietary sodium to 2 gm/day; restrict protein to < 1 gm/kg ideal body weight per day; decrease animal protein intake; avoid grapefruit juice; consume 1000–1200 mg/day of dietary calcium; and avoid excessive calcium, oxalate, and vitamin C.

KEY POINTS: TREATMENT OF NEPHROLITHIASIS ✓

1. Therapy of kidney stones includes daily intake of 10–12 eight-ounce glasses of fluid, increased intake of citrate-containing drinks, 1000–1200 mg of dietary calcium, and no more than 2300 mg of sodium and 1 gm/kg of protein.

2. Avoid grapefruit juice and excessive calcium, oxalate, and vitamin C.

3. Although potassium citrate is preferred for urinary alkalization and citrate replacement, orange and cranberry juice contain potassium citrate and may supplement or substitute for potassium citrate medication if cost or intolerance is an issue.

4. Citrus beverages like lemon and lime may also be beneficial.

33. **Describe the clinical significance of urinalysis in patients with renal stones.**
Most stone formers have macroscopic or microscopic hematuria. The remainder of the urinalysis is usually normal. Crystals are normally absent in warm, freshly voided urine and, if present, suggest a diagnosis. However, most urine specimens cool before examination and crystals may form in normal urine with time and cooling. Thus, by the time urine is usually examined most crystalluria has little clinical significance. An exception is the presence of cystine crystals, which are diagnostic of cystinuria. Persistently acidic urine (pH < 5.5) suggests uric acid or cystine stones. Persistently alkaline urine (pH > 7.0–7.5) and recurrent urinary tract infection strongly suggest struvite stones. Struvite stones never form unless the urine pH is alkaline.

34. **What are the characteristics of urinary crystals in patients with renal stones?**
Calcium oxalate monohydrate crystals may be dumbbell-shaped, needle-shaped, or oval, with the latter resembling red blood cells. Calcium oxalate dihydrate crystals are pyramid-shaped and have an envelope appearance. Calcium phosphate and uric acid crystals are too small for standard light microscopic resolution and look like amorphous debris. Uric acid crystals are characteristically yellow-brown. Less commonly, uric acid dihydrate crystals may be rhomboid-shaped or resemble the six-sided diamonds on a deck of cards. Since all of these crystals may be found in normal urine, they are not necessarily diagnostic of disease. However, cystine crystals always mean cystinuria and are flat, hexagonal plates, resembling benzene rings. Struvite (magnesium ammonium phosphate) crystals are rectangular prisms that resemble coffin lids.

35. **How do radiographic tests help to evaluate patients with renal stones?**
A plain radiograph of the abdomen (KUB) should be obtained in all stone formers and shows stones with the following features: calcium (small, dense, and circumscribed); cystine (faint, soft, and waxy); struvite (irregular and dense). Uric acid stones are radiolucent and not seen. Intravenous pyelography (IVP) localizes stones in the urinary tract and shows degree of obstruction. Radiolucent obstruction on IVP suggests a uric acid stone. Ultrasonography reveals size and location of larger stones, is sensitive for diagnosing obstruction, and may be best when radiation should be avoided as in pregnancy. Non–contrast-enhanced helical CT scanning is the most sensitive, specific, and accurate procedure for localizing kidney stones.

36. **Which medications are useful for treating the various stone-forming conditions?**
See Table 18-3.

37. **What are special considerations in the drug therapy of nephrolithiasis?**
Use potassium citrate and not sodium citrate for alkalinization of urine recommended for uric acid and cysteine stones. Sodium citrate increases urinary sodium and calcium; and in alkaline urine, sodium urate may increase calcium stone formation. Potassium citrate often is the only therapy necessary if uricosuria is < 800 mg/day. Use allopurinol with potassium citrate if uric acid stones continue or hyperuricemia is more severe. Use CSP only for refractory stone disease in AH-I. CSP binds calcium and magnesium in the gut, decreases absorption of both, and may worsen osteopenia and increase urinary oxalate. Replace magnesium as required. Monitor bone mass and treat osteopenia as necessary.

TABLE 18-3. ORAL DRUG THERAPY FOR RENAL STONES

Disorder	Drug	Dosage
Absorptive type I	Hydrochlorothiazide	25–50 mg b.i.d.
	Potassium citrate	10–30 mEq t.i.d.
	Cellulose sodium phosphate (CSP)	5 gm 1–3 times/day with meals
	Magnesium gluconate	1–1.5 gm b.i.d. and as needed
Absorptive type II	Hydrochlorothiazide	25–50 mg/day as needed
Renal phosphate leak	Neutral sodium phosphate	500 mg t.i.d.
RH	Hydrochlorothiazide	25–50 mg b.i.d.
Hypocitraturia	Potassium citrate	10–30 mEq t.i.d.
Hyperuricosuria	Potassium citrate	10–30 mEq t.i.d.
	Allopurinol	200–600 mg/day
Enteric hyperoxaluria	Potassium citrate	10–30 mEq t.i.d.
	Magnesium gluconate	1–1.5 gm b.i.d.
	Calcium citrate	950 mg q.i.d.
	Calcium carbonate	250–500 mg q.i.d.
	Cholestyramine	4 gm t.i.d.
	Pyroxidine	100 mg/day
Cystinuria	Potassium citrate	10–30 mEq t.i.d.
	α-Mercaptopropionylglycine	250–500 mg q.i.d.
	D-Penicillamine	250–500 mg q.i.d.
	Pyroxidine	50 mg/day
Struvite stones	Acetohydroxamic acid	250 mg 2–4 times/day

Note: Dosages are estimated ranges and not absolute recommendations. Each drug must be adjusted according to the patient's tolerance. Use the lowest dosage necessary to attain the desired effect and avoid side effects. Always use drug therapy in addition to appropriate dietary changes and fluid input. Potassium citrate is better tolerated in lower dosages taken three times a day. However, twice-daily dosing may improve compliance. Potassium citrate is often required to correct thiazide-induced hypokalemia and hypocitraturia (see question 37).

38. **Why are thiazide diuretics the first-line therapy for hypercalciuria-induced nephrolithiasis?**
Because they increase proximal (indirectly) and distal (directly) tubular reabsorption of calcium. However, thiazides can cause depletion of potassium and citrate, which should be replaced with potassium citrate. Avoid triamterene, which can cause kidney stones. If potassium supplementation is added, use amiloride with caution to avoid hyperkalemia.

39. **How should you treat a symptomatic patient with a renal stone 1–2 cm in size?**
Apply the therapeutic options in question 32. Most urologists treat symptomatic patients with calcium stones 1–2 cm in size in the renal pelvis or a significant proximally obstructing stone (0.6–2 cm) with extracorporeal shock wave lithotripsy (ESWL).

40. **How should you treat an asymptomatic patient with a renal stone of the same size?**
The asymptomatic patient is a toss-up. Each expert has an opinion based on the experience of the local medical community. Specifics of stone location, duration, and overall patient health are important in the decision. Recurrent, enlarging, or multiple asymptomatic stones probably should be treated. Nephrology and urology consultations are appropriate. Other forms of lithotripsy include percutaneous ultrasonic lithotripsy and endoscopic ultrasonic lithotripsy. Intracorporeal lithotripsy uses the holmium:YAG laser and electrohydraulic lithotripsy (EHL).

41. **What treatment should be used if the stone is larger than 3 cm?**
If the stone is > 3 cm, lithotripsy usually fails. The initial approach to patients with stones of this size is percutaneous nephrolithotomy. Open lithotomy is now unusual. Stones 2–3 cm in size are in a gray area, and therapy depends on the patient's overall status and the wishes and experiences of the patient, primary physician, and urologist. Distal ureteral stones are best managed with ureteroscopic stone extraction or in situ ESWL.

WEBSITES 🌐

1. Contemporary Urology® Archive: Excellent Review of Nephrolithiasis. Available at http://www.conturo.com/be_core/content/journals/u/data/2003/0201/urolithiasis.html

2. Food and health communications: Diet and Kidney Stones. Available at http://www.foodandhealth.com/cpecourses/kidney.php?print=yes

3. EMedicine: Hypercalciuria review. Available at http://www.emedicine.com/med/topic1069.htm

4. EMedicine: Hyperuricemia and gout review. Available at http://www.emedicine.com/med/topic3028.htm

5. EMedicine: Hypocitraturia review. Available at http://www.emedicine.com/med/topic3030.htm

6. EMedicine: Intracorporeal lithotripsy. Available at http://www.emedicine.com/med/topic3034.htm

7. National Institute of Diabetes & Digestive & Kidney Diseases (NIDDK), NIH. Available at http://kidney.niddk.nih.gov/kudiseases/topics/stones.asp

BIBLIOGRAPHY

1. Bhandari A, Menon M: Nephrolithiasis: Reducing the risk of recurrence. Contemp Urol 15:36–52, 2003.

2. Borghi L, Schianchi T, Meschi T, et al: Comparison of two diets for the prevention of recurrent stones in idiopathic hypercalciuria. N Engl J Med 346:77–84, 2002.

3. Frick, KK, Bushinsky, DA: Molecular mechanisms of primary hypercalciuria. J Am Soc Nephrol 14:1082–1095, 2003.

4. Goldfarb DS, Coe FL: Prevention of recurrent nephrolithiasis. Am Fam Physician 60(8):2269–2276, 1999.

5. Lindberg JS, Sprague S: Nephrolithiasis: Causes and treatment. J Critical Illness 16:446–459, 2001.

6. Martini LA, Wood RJ: Should dietary calcium and protein be restricted in patients with nephrolithiasis? Nutr Rev 58(4):111–117, 2000.

7. Ramello A, Vitale C, Marangella, M: Epidemiology of nephrolithiasis. J Nephrol 13(Suppl 3): S45–S50, 2000.

8. Reddy ST, Wang CY, Sakhaee K: Effect of low-carbohydrate high-protein diets on acid–base balance, stone-forming propensity, and calcium metabolism. Am J Kidney Dis 40(2):265–274, 2002.

9. Rivers K, Shetty S, Menon M: When and how to evaluate a patient with nephrolithiasis. Urol Clin North Am 27(2):203–213, 2000.

10. Zheng W, Denstedt JD: Intracorporeal lithotripsy. Update on technology. Urol Clin North Am 27(2):301–313, 2000.

PITUITARY INSUFFICIENCY

William J. Georgitis, M.D.

CHAPTER 19

1. **What causes pituitary insufficiency?**
   Pituitary insufficiency (hypopituitarism) results from pituitary, hypothalamic, or parasellar diseases that disrupt normal pituitary function by displacing, infiltrating, or destroying the hypothalamic–pituitary unit. Pituitary insufficiency is present when inadequate amounts of one or more of the following anterior or posterior pituitary hormones is secreted (Fig. 19-1).

Adenohypophysis	Neurohypophysis
Growth hormone (GH)	Antidiuretic hormone (ADH)
Prolactin (PRL)	Oxytocin (OXT)
Adrenocorticotropic hormone (ACTH)	
Thyrotropin (TSH)	
Luteinizing hormone (LH)	
Follicle-stimulating hormone (FSH)	

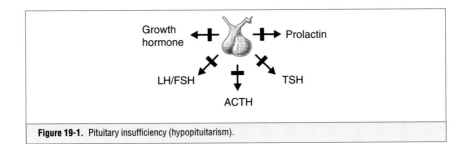

Figure 19-1. Pituitary insufficiency (hypopituitarism).

2. **When the pituitary stalk is severed, what happens to anterior pituitary hormone levels?**
   Serum levels of anterior pituitary hormones secreted in response to hypothalamic releasing hormones decline; this is true for TSH, LH, FSH, GH, and ACTH. In contrast, PRL levels rise. This unique response among the pituitary hormones results from a decline in hypothalamic dopamine, which normally inhibits PRL secretion by lactotropes.

3. **Which parasellar disorders cause pituitary dysfunction?**
   Processes adjacent to the sella that cause hypopituitarism include meningiomas, chordomas, craniopharyngiomas, optic nerve gliomas, carotid aneurysms, sphenoid sinus mucoceles, nasopharyngeal carcinomas, and pineal dysgerminomas.

4. **What is a craniopharyngioma?**

   Craniopharyngioma is a squamous cell tumor that arises from Rathke's pouch remnants. It is the most common tumor in the region of the hypothalamus and pituitary in children but is relatively less common in adults. Two-thirds are suprasellar. One-third extend into or are confined within the sella. Most are cystic, but some contain both cystic and nodular components. The characteristic viscous yellow-brown fluid resembles motor oil. Sometimes the outer border of the tumor becomes calcified and can look like an eggshell on radiographs. Best demonstrated with computed tomography (CT), calcifications are present in 75% of children but in only 35% of adults. Surgery is indicated for both treatment and pathologic confirmation.

5. **How does a pineal dysgerminoma present?**

   Most often this tumor of large undifferentiated germ cells and reactive lymphocytes occurs in males. Dysgerminomas associated with pituitary insufficiency can arise in the suprasellar region or they can grow from the pineal region to involve the hypothalamus and simultaneously disrupt both posterior and anterior pituitary functions, as well as cause hydrocephalus and paralysis of upward gaze (Parinaud's palsy). Patients often present with a combination of secondary hypogonadism and polyuria with polydipsia from neurogenic diabetes insipidus in addition to the neurologic signs associated with the mass or associated hydrocephalus.

6. **What is pituitary apoplexy?**

   Apoplexy means loss of consciousness followed by paralysis. Classic pituitary apoplexy is an acute life-threatening event characterized by severe headache and collapse, with evidence of pituitary hemorrhage. An expanding hemorrhagic mass arising most often from an infarcted pituitary adenoma may compress parasellar structures, including cranial nerves coursing through the adjacent cavernous sinuses. Ocular paralysis and ptosis from involvement of the third, fourth, and sixth cranial nerves, as well as facial nerve involvement, contribute the component of paralysis necessary to fulfill the definition of apoplexy. Following an episode of pituitary apoplexy, anterior pituitary insufficiency is common. Posterior pituitary functions are almost always preserved. Most patients recover spontaneously and often do not require emergent surgical intervention.

   Subacute forms of pituitary necrosis occur in patients with diabetes mellitus and sickle cell disease. Radiologic evidence of pituitary infarction even when unaccompanied by catastrophic symptoms and signs always deserves a comprehensive functional evaluation of the pituitary.

7. **Define empty sella.**

   Empty sella refers to the absence or relative absence of the pituitary gland on radiologic imaging of the sella turcica. The term *sella turcica* (Latin *sella* = saddle and *turcica* = Turkish) stems from the resemblance of the cup-like prominence of the sphenoid bone that contains the pituitary to saddles used by the Turks. These saddles with front and back supports contrasted with the Roman equestrian style of riding on a cloth tied to the horse's back.

8. **What is the distinction between primary and secondary empty sella?**

   Primary empty sella is probably a normal anatomic variant or perhaps results from a congenital defect in the diaphragm sella. The sella is not actually empty but contains cerebrospinal fluid (CSF). The pituitary gland is flattened against the walls of the sella. Hypopituitarism with signs of symptomatic dysfunction occurs in less than 10% of the patients with primary empty sella.

   Secondary empty sella is the end result of infarction, surgical removal, or irradiation of a tumor.

9. **What is Sheehan's syndrome? How common is it?**

   Sheehan's syndrome is an acquired form of empty sella syndrome due to ischemic pituitary necrosis generally following delivery of a child complicated by severe blood loss and hypotension. Thirty percent of women suffering postpartum hemorrhage and vascular collapse eventually may demon-

strate a spectrum of anterior pituitary insufficiency from mild to severe. Failure to lactate sufficiently to nurse a baby followed by persistent amenorrhea postpartum is a feature of this syndrome. If secondary adrenal insufficiency accompanies secondary hypogonadism, loss of adrenal
and ovarian androgenic steroid-dependent axillary and pubic hair may also appear.

10. **Do presenting features of pituitary insufficiency differ between children and
adults?**
In *children*, a signal of hypopituitarism is failure to grow normally. In adolescents, abnormalities
in sexual maturation may be the sentinel features. Failure to achieve puberty or arrest in sexual
maturation may indicate pituitary malfunction. Puberty spans many years and occurs at a time
when patients often change providers from pediatricians to family practitioners and internists.
Signs of pituitary insufficiency can easily be overlooked.
   In *adults*, symptoms and signs of hypogonadism dominate the clinical picture.
Hypogonadism may easily go unsuspected in postmenopausal women or elderly men, since
older patients often fail to complain about declining sexual function or desire. Such complaints
also lack specificity for hypopituitarism because they are so prevalent in the elderly. Features of
hypothyroidism and adrenal insufficiency also may appear insidiously.

11. **Is there an easy way to tell if the sella turcica is enlarged?**
If a dime (diameter = 16 mm) fits within the sella on lateral skull films, enlargement of the sella
turcica is probably present. The most common cause for this finding is a pituitary adenoma.
Pituitary tumors comprise 10–15% of intracranial neoplasms and are present in 6–23% of pituitary glands carefully inspected at autopsy. Carcinoma of the pituitary is extremely rare and
appears mainly as case reports rather than series in the medical literature. Metastases to this
anatomic region from primary tumors elsewhere in the body are also rare and more often
involve the highly vascular hypothalamus, presenting most commonly with features, such as
secondary hypopituitarism and diabetes insipidus.

12. **What tests should be considered for hypopituitary patients?**
The evaluation should include assessment of anterior pituitary hormones, radiographic imaging
by CT or magnetic resonance imaging (MRI) to assess anatomy, and formal visual fields testing.
The tests for anterior pituitary function usually include serum levels of testosterone (men),
estradiol (women), LH, FSH, thyroxine (T_4), TSH, PRL, GH (children), and cortisol (before and
after intravenous ACTH administration). Nocturia, polyuria, or polydipsia suggest the need to
test for adequacy of vasopressin secretion by performing a water deprivation test.

13. **What is the Houssay phenomenon?**
Houssay, an Argentinian Nobel laureate, showed improvement in the diabetes of pancreatec-
tomized dogs following hypophysectomy. He and other investigators subsequently demonstrated the diabetogenic actions of pituitary extracts. The clinical relevance of the Houssay
phenomenon sometimes appears in diabetic patients who demonstrate diminishing insulin
requirements in the presence of hypopituitarism. The diabetic patient with recurrent and serious
hypoglycemic episodes leading to major reductions in medications may have acquired hypopituitarism, with resultant deficiencies of the insulin counter-regulatory factors GH and cortisol. To
further understand the significance of hormones counter-regulatory to insulin in carbohydrate
metabolism, consider that the diabetes secondary to GH excess in acromegaly also may
improve or resolve after pituitary surgery, pituitary apoplexy, or octreotide therapy.

14. **What characteristics of adrenal insufficiency are present in ACTH-deficient
patients?**
Nonspecific symptoms, such as fatigue and weight loss, are often encountered with ACTH deficiency. In women, axillary and pubic hair may diminish or disappear. Serum sodium levels tend

to be low but potassium remains normal. Features of glucocorticoid deficiency are usually not as severe as those seen with primary adrenal failure.

15. **Define primary hypothyroidism.**
Hypothyroidism is primary when the thyroid gland itself fails. Elevation of the serum TSH level is the most sensitive and specific test for the diagnosis of primary hypothyroidism because TSH levels increase as the thyroid's secretion of T_4 declines. In secondary (or central) hypothyroidism, thyroid hormone deficiency is secondary to loss of TSH secretion by the pituitary gland or thyrotropin-releasing hormone (TRH) production by the hypothalamus. Symptoms and signs are similar to those seen in primary hypothyroidism but are generally milder. Even patients with massive pituitary tumors may not have obvious features of hypothyroidism. Laboratory tests abnormalities, like the symptoms and signs, are more subtle than those in primary hypothyroidism. TSH levels are often in the normal range but may be low, whereas serum T_4 levels are decreased.

16. **Why are thyroid hormone levels low in secondary hypothyroidism?**
Several defects explain the decline in thyroid hormone secretion in secondary hypothyroidism. TSH pulsatility in patients with pituitary macroadenomas is often abnormal, as depicted in Figure 19-2. Both, TSH pulse frequency and amplitude, are decreased resulting in loss or diminution of the normal nocturnal surge in TSH secretion. Circulating TSH molecules are also abnormal, having higher molecular weights than TSH molecules produced in normal individuals. Failure to remove sugar moieties during posttranslational processing by the Golgi apparatus appears to be the responsible mechanism. These higher molecular weight forms of TSH show decreased ability to stimulate thyroid hormone secretion by thymocytes in bioassays.

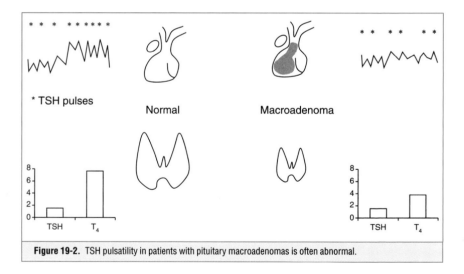

Figure 19-2. TSH pulsatility in patients with pituitary macroadenomas is often abnormal.

17. **What cortisol level is consistent with adrenal insufficiency?**
Morning serum cortisols less than 10 μg/dL or ACTH-stimulated cortisol levels below 20 μg/dL are consistent with adrenal insufficiency. Plasma ACTH levels, when assayed properly, are elevated in primary adrenal insufficiency but are normal or low in secondary (central) adrenal insufficiency.

18. **Is secondary adrenal insufficiency as common as gonadotropin deficiency in patients with pituitary tumor?**
No. The frequency of deficiency among the anterior pituitary hormones at the time of diagnosis of a pituitary tumor presents a spectrum of prevalence with GH > LH/FSH > TSH > ACTH. PRL deficiency rarely is recognized clinically. Posterior pituitary dysfunction with diabetes insipidus is so infrequent that its presence should suggest diseases primarily of hypothalamic or pineal origin, and OXT deficiency is not usually considered at all. Most patients with pituitary adenomas have surprisingly intact anterior pituitary function before treatment and usually acquire hypopituitarism only after surgical or radiation treatment. This is even true for most macroadenomas. The search for medical therapies as alternatives to ablation by surgery and radiation for pituitary tumors continues with a focus on preservation or restoration of normal pituitary function.

19. **Is life expectancy altered by hypopituitarism?**
All-cause mortality in patients with hypopituitarism is significantly increased approximately 1.7-fold. Women tend to fare worse than men, with observed/expected death ratios of 2.3 compared with 1.5, respectively. The increase is suspected to be due to vascular disease events but is probably multifactorial. Age and gonadal status appear to be independent risk factors, with hypogonadal patients having a better prognosis than eugonadal hypopituitary patients.

20. **Are health-related costs greater for patients with hypopituitarism?**
A Swedish endocrine unit reported that hypopituitary patients have almost 2-fold higher direct health-related costs per annum. They also claim disability pensions and take a 1.6-fold greater number of sick days than the general population. None of the studied populations were on somatotropin replacement.

KEY POINTS: PITUITARY INSUFFICIENCY ✓

1. The rise in PRL due to the loss of hypothalamic dopamine inhibitory tone sets it apart from other pituitary hormones that decline secondary to the loss of hypothalamic releasing hormones.

2. The most important hormone deficiency to identify and treat in patients with anterior pituitary disease is cortisol deficiency because acute adrenal insufficiency may be life-threatening.

3. Replacement with thyroid hormone alone in a patient with coexistent adrenal deficiency may precipitate an acute adrenal crisis.

4. Serum TSH can be normal in secondary hypothyroidism.

5. Aldosterone deficiency generally does not occur in hypopituitarism because the principal physiologic regulator of aldosterone secretion is the renin–angiotensin system—not ACTH from the hypothalamic–pituitary system.

21. **What is the most important hormone deficiency to identify and treat in patients with anterior pituitary disease?**
Inadequate cortisol secretion is the most important to identify and treat. Acute adrenal insufficiency may be life-threatening.

22. **Why is aldosterone deficiency generally absent in hypopituitarism?**
   Secretion of aldosterone is regulated primarily by the renin–angiotensin axis, and therefore aldosterone secretion is normal in patients with hypopituitarism. However, hyponatremia may still be a clue to hypopituitarism because it may result from either thyroid hormone or glucocorticoid deficiency and will be corrected with appropriate thyroid hormone and/or glucocorticoid replacement therapy.

23. **Is anterior pituitary hormone deficiency always a commitment to life-long replacement?**
   Yes, in most cases, but there are important exceptions. Primary hypothyroidism sometimes causes significant pituitary hyperplasia with hyperprolactinemia and may present as amenorrhea–galactorrhea in women or as impotence and impaired libido in men. Dramatic reduction of pituitary size, normalization of serum PRL levels, and resolution of the hypogonadism usually occur with thyroid replacement. Hypopituitarism from hemochromatosis, an inherited disorder of iron storage, has also improved with therapy directed at the underlying disorder. Another example is seen in certain patients with pituitary macroadenomas. Mild elevations in serum PRL and deficiencies of other anterior pituitary hormones, especially ACTH, sometimes resolve immediately after surgical excision of the tumor.

24. **When one hormone deficiency in hypopituitarism is diagnosed, why is it important to define whether other hormone deficiencies are present?**
   Replacement with thyroid hormone alone in a patient with coexistent adrenal deficiency may precipitate an acute adrenal crisis. Furthermore, vasopressin deficiency may be masked by adrenal insufficiency. After glucocorticoid replacement, central diabetes insipidus may appear and require specific treatment with a vasopressin analogue.

25. **What is the treatment of pituitary insufficiency?**
   The treatment of pituitary insufficiency consists of replacing the hormones normally made by the pituitary gland or by the endocrine glands regulated by the anterior pituitary hormones. Thus, patients with hypopituitarism are usually treated with replacement doses of thyroid hormone, glucocorticoids, and sex steroids. Patients with diabetes insipidus are treated with a vasopressin preparation.

26. **Who should receive GH treatment?**
   Treatment is indicated for children with short stature, open epiphyses, and documented congenital or acquired GH deficiency. Evidence is also accumulating that adults with GH deficiency may benefit from GH replacement, although the cost effectiveness of this intervention is an unsettled issue.

WEBSITE

Pituitary Foundation. Available at www.pituitary.org.uk

BIBLIOGRAPHY

1. Arafah B: Reversible hypopituitarism in patients with large nonfunctioning pituitary adenomas. J Clin Endocrinol Metab 62:1173–1179, 1986.
2. Bates AS, Van't Hoff W, Jones PJ, Clayton RN: The effect of hypopituitarism on life expectancy. J Clin Endocrinol Metab 81:1169–1172, 1996.

3. Cummings DE, Merriam GR: Age-related changes in growth hormone secretion: Should the somatopause be treated? Semin Reprod Endocrinol 17:311–325, 1999.

4. Ehrnborg C, Hakkaart-Van Roijen L, Jonsson B, et al: Cost of illness in adult patients with hypopituitarism. Pharmacoeconomics 17:621–628, 2000.

5. Gama R, Smith MJ, Wright J, Marks V: Hypopituitarism in primary haemochromatosis; recovery after iron depletion. Postgrad Med J 71:297–298, 1995.

6. Hazouard E, Piquemal R, Dequin PF, et al: Severe non-infectious circulatory shock related to hypopituitarism. Intensive Care Med 25:865–868, 1999.

7. Lurie SN, Doraiswamy PM, Husain MM, et al: In vivo assessment of pituitary gland volume with magnetic resonance imaging: The effect of age. J Clin Endocrinol Metab 71:505–508, 1990.

8. Schmidt DN, Wallace K: How to diagnose hypopituitarism. Learning the features of secondary hormonal deficiencies. Postgrad Med 104:77–87, 1998.

9. Vance ML: Hypopituitarism. N Engl J Med 330:1651–1662, 1994.

10. Webb SM, Rigla M, Wagner A, et al: Recovery of hypopituitarism after neurosurgical treatment of pituitary adenomas. J Clin Endocrinol Metab 84:3696–3700, 1999.

CHAPTER 20

NONFUNCTIONING PITUITARY TUMORS

Michael T. McDermott, M.D.

1. **Name the functioning pituitary tumors.**

   Prolactin-secreting tumors, growth hormone-secreting tumors, corticotropin (adrenocorti-cotropic hormone [ACTH])-secreting tumors, thyrotropin (thyroid-stimulating hormone [TSH])-secreting tumors, and gonadotropin (follicle-stimulating hormone [FSH]/luteinizing hormone [LH])-secreting tumors are the major functioning pituitary neoplasms. Some tumors secrete a mixture of hormones.

2. **What is a nonfunctioning pituitary tumor?**

   A nonfunctioning pituitary tumor arises from cells of the pituitary gland but does not secrete clinically detectable amounts of a pituitary hormone. These tumors are usually benign adenomas.

3. **What is the alpha subunit?**

   The alpha subunit is a component of three pituitary hormones: TSH, LH, and FSH. Each of these hormones consists of the common alpha subunit and a specific beta subunit (TSH beta, LH beta, and FSH beta). The alpha and beta subunits normally combine before the intact hormone is secreted into the circulation. Some nonfunctioning pituitary tumors actually synthesize and secrete measurable amounts of the free alpha subunit, which may therefore serve as a tumor marker.

4. **What other lesions can resemble nonfunctioning pituitary tumors?**

   Tumors that are not of pituitary origin may be found within the sella turcica; examples include metastatic carcinomas, craniopharyngiomas, meningiomas, and neural tumors. Nonneoplastic Rathke's pouch cysts, arterial aneurysms, and infiltrative pituitary diseases, such as sarcoidosis, histiocytosis, tuberculosis, lymphocytic hypophysitis, and hemochromatosis may also be seen in this location.

5. **Differentiate between a microadenoma and a macroadenoma.**

   A pituitary microadenoma is less than 10 mm in its largest dimension, whereas a macroade-noma is 10 mm or larger. A macroadenoma may be contained entirely within the sella turcica or may have extrasellar extension.

6. **Which structures may be damaged by growth of a pituitary tumor outside the sella turcica?**

   Pituitary tumors that grow superiorly may compress the optic chiasm and pituitary stalk. Those that grow laterally can invade the cavernous sinuses and compress cranial nerves III, IV, and V or the internal carotid artery. Inferior growth may erode into the sphenoid sinus. Anterior and posterior growth often erodes the bones of the tuberculum sellae and dorsum sellae, respec-tively (see Fig. 20-1.)

7. **What are the clinical features of nonfunctioning pituitary tumors?**

   Many nonfunctioning pituitary tumors are asymptomatic and are discovered incidentally during cranial imaging procedures done for other reasons. This is true of both microadenomas (< 10 mm) and macroadenomas (≥ 10 mm). Nonfunctioning pituitary tumors that cause symp-toms are usually large space-occupying macroadenomas that compress nearby neurologic

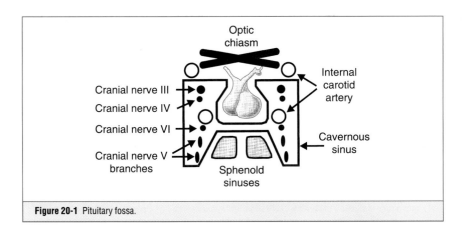

Figure 20-1 Pituitary fossa.

and/or vascular structures. Common clinical manifestations include headaches, visual field defects, visual loss, and extraocular nerve palsies. Pituitary insufficiency also may result from destruction of the remaining normal pituitary tissue.

8. **What anatomic evaluation is necessary for a pituitary tumor?**
Magnetic resonance imaging (MRI) or computed tomography (CT) of the pituitary gland and parasellar regions often allows a precise diagnosis and determines the presence and extent of extrasellar invasion. Visual field testing helps to assess function of the optic chiasm and tracts. Angiography may be needed in some cases to rule out the presence of an aneurysm.

9. **What evaluation is necessary to determine that a pituitary tumor is nonfunctioning?**
A thorough history and physical examination must be performed to detect any signs or symptoms of overproduction of pituitary hormones. Hormone testing should include measurement of serum prolactin, insulin-like growth factor 1 (IGF-1), TSH, free thyroxine (free T_4), LH, FSH, testosterone (men), estradiol (women), and 24-hour urinary free cortisol excretion. Serum alpha subunit, when available, is also helpful.

10. **Does an elevated level of serum prolactin mean that a tumor is functioning?**
No. Secretion of prolactin is negatively regulated by hypothalamic inhibitory factors, such as dopamine, which reach the anterior pituitary gland through the pituitary stalk. Stalk compression from a nonfunctioning tumor can impair dopamine delivery and thus increase the release of prolactin from the normal pituitary gland. The serum prolactin rarely exceeds 100 ng/mL in such cases, whereas it is usually much higher with prolactin-secreting tumors.

11. **What is the primary treatment for a nonfunctioning pituitary tumor?**
Asymptomatic microadenomas can be managed with observation by serial imaging studies. Asymptomatic macroadenomas (≥ 1 cm) should be considered for surgical removal although serial observation is an option if the tumor does not grow and does not cause significant patient anxiety.

The treatment of choice for symptomatic tumors is transsphenoidal surgery, in which access to the pituitary gland is gained through the sphenoid sinus. Radiation therapy may be used if surgery is contraindicated or not desired. Medications, such as bromocriptine, are rarely helpful.

KEY POINTS: NONFUNCTIONING PITUITARY TUMORS ✔

1. Nonfunctioning pituitary tumors cause symptoms primarily by mass effects, resulting in compression of the pituitary stalk and optic chiasm, invasion of the cavernous sinuses, and erosion into the bony sella turcica.

2. Nonfunctioning pituitary tumors do not produce detectable levels of pituitary hormones but may raise serum prolactin levels modestly by pituitary stalk compression, interfering with the flow of dopamine from the hypothalamus.

3. Lesions that can resemble pituitary tumors include metastatic carcinomas, craniopharyngiomas, meningiomas, neural tumors, Rathke's pouch cysts, aneurysms, and infiltrative pituitary diseases.

4. Treatment for nonfunctioning pituitary tumors ≥ 1.0 cm in size is transsphenoidal surgery with subsequent radiation therapy or close monitoring for incompletely resected tumors.

5. Diabetes insipidus and/or secretion of inappropriate ADH (SIADH) may occur in the immediate postoperative period and must be managed appropriately.

6. Anterior pituitary hormone deficiencies (hypopituitarism) can occur months to years after pituitary tumor removal, particularly if radiation therapy was utilized.

12. **Is postoperative radiation therapy recommended for incompletely resected tumors?**

    Older literature, primarily from uncontrolled studies, suggests that postoperative radiation therapy is beneficial. Currently, however, most experts advise radiation only for large tumor remnants that compress vascular or neural structures. Many centers are now utilizing stereotactic rather than conventional radiation therapy in these situations in order to deliver a greater focused radiation dose to neoplastic tissue with less radiation exposure to surrounding structures. Residual disease of lesser severity may be monitored with imaging studies and not treated unless growth occurs.

13. **What endocrine complications occur in the immediate postoperative period?**

    Transient diabetes insipidus (vasopressin deficiency) manifested by high-volume urine output is common in the first few days. It may be followed by a short period (1–2 days) of water intoxication (vasopressin excess) causing hyponatremia. Both conditions result from reversible trauma and/or edema of the neurohypophysis, where vasopressin is stored. Fluid balance and serum electrolytes, therefore, must be closely monitored. Secondary adrenal insufficiency is of little immediate concern because high-dose dexamethasone is often given to prevent cerebral edema, but it may sometimes become apparent after dexamethasone is stopped. Deficiencies of other pituitary hormones do not tend to be an early postoperative problem if they were normal preoperatively.

14. **What is the management of postoperative diabetes insipidus and water intoxication?**

    Mild postoperative diabetes insipidus can be managed with isovolumetric, isotonic fluid replacement. More severe cases should be treated with desmopressin (DDAVP), 0.25–0.5 mL (1–2 µg) two times a day intravenously or subcutaneously or with aqueous vasopressin, 5 units subcutaneously every 4–6 hours, until urine volumes become normal. If hyponatremia develops, vasopressin must be reduced or stopped and free water intake restricted. If diabetes insipidus persists beyond 1 week, patients may be switched to intranasal DDAVP, 0.1–0.2 mL once or twice daily, or oral DDAVP tablets, 0.1–0.4 mg daily.

15. **What endocrine problems may occur during long-term follow-up?**
Deficiency of one or more pituitary hormones may develop weeks, months, or years after treatment, especially if radiation was given. The only major concern in the first month is adrenal insufficiency. During this time one should question the patient about symptoms suggesting this disorder and, if they are present, obtain a morning cortisol level. If the cortisol level is low, hydrocortisone replacement should be initiated and the patient retested in 3–6 months with a Cosyntropin stimulation test. At that time serum free T_4, TSH, IGF-1, LH, FSH, testosterone (men), and estradiol (women) should also be checked and replacement therapy considered for any identified deficiencies. It is recommended that these tests then be monitored at 6 months, 1 year, and annually thereafter.

16. **Summarize the long-term management of pituitary insufficiency.**

Deficiency	Replacement Regimen
Adrenal insufficiency	Hydrocortisone, 20 mg AM, 10 mg PM
Hypothyroidism	Levothyroxine, 1.6 µg/kg/day
Hypogonadism (men)	Androderm patch, 5–7.5 mg patch q.d.
	Androgel, 5–10 gm q.d.
	Testim gel, 5–10 gm q.d.
Hypogonadism (women)	Oral or transdermal contraceptives
	Oral or transdermal postmenopausal hormone replacement
Growth hormone	GH 0.3 mg q.d. subcutaneously
Diabetes insipidus	DDAVP nasal spray, 0.1–0.2 mL q.d. or b.i.d.
	DDAVP tablets, 0.1–0.4 mg q.d. or b.i.d.

17. **Describe the clinical features of pituitary carcinomas.**
Pituitary carcinomas, which are extremely rare, expand rapidly and cause mass effects. Some secrete hormones causing endocrine syndromes similar to those seen with adenomas. Metastatic disease to the central nervous system, cervical lymph nodes, liver, and bone are commonly associated.

18. **What is the treatment for pituitary carcinoma?**
Transsphenoidal surgery is the primary therapy, followed by postoperative radiation. No significant use of chemotherapy has been reported for pituitary carcinoma.

19. **What is the prognosis for pituitary carcinoma?**
The mean survival is approximately 4 years.

20. **Which cancers metastasize to the pituitary gland?**
Metastatic disease to the pituitary gland occurs in approximately 3–5% of patients with widely disseminated carcinoma. The most commonly reported primary tumors are breast, lung, kidney, prostate, liver, pancreas, nasopharynx, plasmacytoma, sarcoma, and adenocarcinoma of unknown primary site.

BIBLIOGRAPHY

1. Arafah BM, Kailani SH, Nekl KE, Gold RS, Selman WR: Immediate recovery of pituitary function after transsphenoidal resection of pituitary macroadenomas. J Clin Endocrinol Metab 79:348–354, 1994.

2. Arafah BM, Prunty D, Ybarra J, et al: The dominant role of increased intrasellar pressure in the pathogenesis of hypopituitarism, hyperprolactinemia, and headaches in patients with pituitary adenomas. J Clin Endocrinol Metab 85:1789–1793, 2000.

3. Branch CL Jr, Laws ER Jr: Metastatic tumors of the sella turcica masquerading as primary pituitary tumors. J Clin Endocrinol Metab 65:469–474, 1987.

4. Gittoes NJL: Review: Current perspectives on the pathogenesis of clinically non-functioning pituitary tumours. J Endocrinol 157:177–186, 1998.

5. Kaltsas GA, Mukherjee JJ, Plowman PN, et al: The role of cytotoxic chemotherapy in the management of aggressive and malignant pituitary tumors. J Clin Endocrinol Metab 83:4233–4238, 1998.

6. Katznelson L, Alexander JM, Klibanski A: Clinically nonfunctioning pituitary adenomas. J Clin Endocrinol Metab 76:1089–1094, 1993.

7. Klibanski A, Zervas NT: Diagnosis and management of hormone-secreting pituitary adenomas. N Engl J Med 324:822–831, 1991.

8. Mountcastle RB, Roof BS, Mayfield RK, et al: Case report: Pituitary adenocarcinoma in an acromegalic patient: Response to bromocriptine and pituitary testing: A review of the literature on 36 cases of pituitary carcinoma. Am J Med Sci 298(2):109–118, 1989.

9. Mukherjee JJ, Islam N, Kaltsas G, Lowe DG, et al: Clinical, radiological and pathological features of patients with Rathke's cleft cysts: Tumors that may recur. J Clin Endocrinol Metab 82:2357–2362, 1997.

10. Pernicone PJ, Scheithauer BW, Sebo TJ, et al: Pituitary carcinoma: A clinicopathological study of 15 cases. Cancer 79:804–812, 1997.

11. Shimon I, Melmed S: Management of pituitary tumors. Ann Intern Med 129:472–483, 1998.

12. Shin JL, Asa SL, Woodhouse LJ, Smyth HS, Ezzat S: Cystic lesions of the pituitary:clinicopathological features distinguishing craniopharyngioma, Rathke's cleft cyst, and arachnoid cyst. J Clin Endocrinol Metab 84:3972–3982, 1999.

13. Wilson CB: Extensive personal experience: Surgical management of pituitary tumors. J Clin Endocrinol Metab 82:2381–2385, 1997.

CHAPTER 21

PROLACTIN-SECRETING PITUITARY TUMORS

Virginia Sarapura, M.D.

1. **Describe the normal control of prolactin secretion. How is it altered in prolactin-secreting tumors?**

   Multiple factors affect prolactin secretion (Fig. 21-1). However, the principal influence on pro-lactin secretion is tonic inhibition by dopamine input from the hypothalamus. Dopamine interaction with receptors of the D2 subtype on pituitary lactotroph membranes activates the inhibitory G-protein, leading to decreased adenylate cyclase activity and decreased levels of cyclic adenosine monophosphate (cAMP). In prolactin-secreting pituitary adenomas, a monoclonal population of cells autonomously produces prolactin, escaping the normal physiologic input of dopamine from the hypothalamus. In almost all cases, responsiveness to a pharmacologic dose of dopamine is maintained.

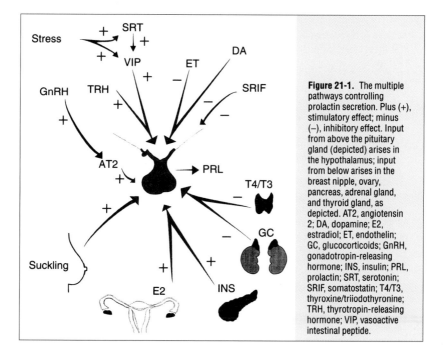

Figure 21-1. The multiple pathways controlling prolactin secretion. Plus (+), stimulatory effect; minus (−), inhibitory effect. Input from above the pituitary gland (depicted) arises in the hypothalamus; input from below arises in the breast nipple, ovary, pancreas, adrenal gland, and thyroid gland, as depicted. AT2, angiotensin 2; DA, dopamine; E2, estradiol; ET, endothelin; GC, glucocorticoids; GnRH, gonadotropin-releasing hormone; INS, insulin; PRL, prolactin; SRT, serotonin; SRIF, somatostatin; T4/T3, thyroxine/triiodothyronine; TRH, thyrotropin-releasing hormone; VIP, vasoactive intestinal peptide.

2. **What are the normal levels of serum prolactin? Are they different in men and women? What levels are seen in patients with prolactin-secreting tumors?**
    The normal serum prolactin level is less than 15 or 30 ng/mL, depending on the laboratory. Women tend to have slightly higher levels than men, probably because of estrogen stimulation of prolactin secretion. In patients with prolactin-secreting tumors, the levels are usually greater than 100 ng/mL but may be as low as 30–50 ng/mL if the tumor is small. A level greater than 200 ng/mL is almost always indicative of a prolactin-secreting tumor. Very high prolactin levels may be found to be falsely normal, due to the high-dose hook effect of the assay; and if clinically indicated, the sample should be assayed again after dilution.

3. **What are the physiologic causes of an elevated prolactin level that need to be considered in the differential diagnosis of prolactin-secreting tumors? What levels can be reached under these circumstances?**
    The most important physiologic states in which prolactin is found to be elevated are pregnancy and lactation. During the third trimester of pregnancy, the prolactin level may reach 200–300 ng/mL. It then gradually decreases during the first months postpartum, despite continued lactation. Prolactin levels are also elevated during sleep, strenuous exercise, stress, and nipple stimulation. In these cases, the elevation is mild, below 50 ng/mL.

4. **List the abnormal causes of an elevated serum prolactin level other than a prolactin-secreting tumor, and state the mechanism underlying the abnormal prolactin production.**
    See Table 21-1.

5. **What are the typical levels of serum prolactin associated with these causes?**
    In all these cases, the prolactin level is usually mildly elevated, 30–50 ng/mL and rarely above 100 ng/mL.

6. **How does prolactin elevation result in gonadal dysfunction? What are the symptoms associated with gonadal dysfunction?**
    Elevated prolactin levels suppress the hypothalamic-pituitary-gonadal axis by interference with the secretion of GnRH in the hypothalamus, resulting in a decrease in circulating levels of estrogen or testosterone. Symptoms in women include infertility, loss of libido, and menstrual irregularity and amenorrhea, and in men, loss of libido and impotence.

7. **What is galactorrhea? Do most patients with prolactin-secreting tumors present with this symptom?**
    Galactorrhea is the discharge of milk from the breast not associated with pregnancy or lactation. Although a typical symptom of prolactin-secreting tumors, it may be absent in up to 50% of women, particularly when estrogen levels are very low. Galactorrhea is uncommon in men, and may be seen in conjunction with gynecomastia when decreased gonadal function results in a low ratio of testosterone to estrogen.

8. **Why do men with prolactin-secreting tumors often present with more advanced disease than do women?**
    The major symptoms of elevated prolactin levels in men are decreased libido and impotence. These symptoms may be ignored or attributed to psychological causes. Many years may go by before an evaluation is sought, often when the patient develops headaches and visual field defects related to the mass effect of the tumor. Women are more likely to seek evaluation early in the disease process, when infertility or menstrual irregularities prompt an evaluation of their hormonal status. In addition, studies have suggested that large (10 mm or bigger) and small (less than 10 mm) tumors may be biologically different from their onset. Also, it was found that

TABLE 21-1.   ABNORMAL CAUSES OF ELEVATED SERUM PROLACTIN LEVEL OTHER THAN PROLACTIN-SECRETING TUMOR AND UNDERLYING MECHANISM OF ABNORMAL PROLACTIN PRODUCTION

Causes	Mechanism

1. Pituitary stalk interruption
    Trauma
    Surgery
    Pituitary, hypothalamic, or
       parasellar tumors
    Infiltrative disorders of the
       hypothalamus
	Interference with the hypothalamic-pituitary pathways: prolactin production increases because the tonic inhibition of prolactin secretion is interrupted; often accompanied by hypopituitarism

2. Pharmacologic agents
    Phenothiazines
    Tricyclic antidepressants
    Alpha-methyldopa
    Metoclopramide
    Cimetidine
    Estrogens
	Specific interference with dopaminergic input to the pituitary gland

3. Hypothyroidism	Increased TRH that stimulates prolactin release
4. Renal failure and liver cirrhosis	Decreased metabolic clearance of prolactin; also increased production in chronic renal failure

5. Intercostal nerve stimulation
    Chest wall lesions
    Herpes zoster
	Mimicking of the stimulation caused by suckling

TRH, thyrotropin-releasing hormone.

there was no difference in the prevalence of large tumors between men and women; however, there was a much higher prevalence of small tumors in women. This suggests that factors in women, possibly estrogen, may promote the appearance of prolactin-secreting tumors, but when these appear they may be smaller and less aggressive.

9. **What is the imaging technique of choice when a prolactin-secreting tumor is suspected? Why?**
Magnetic resonance imaging (MRI) of the pituitary with a contrast agent, such as gadolinium, is the imaging technique of choice in the evaluation of pituitary tumors. In particular, discrimination of small tumors is enhanced. Computed tomographic scanning allows better visualization of bone structures, such as the floor of the sella, in cases of large tumors. However, the relationship of the tumor to other soft tissue structures, such as the cavernous sinuses and carotid arteries, is better visualized with MRI. Skull radiographs and tomograms are not helpful.

10. **Bone metabolism is altered when prolactin levels are elevated. What is the mechanism for this effect? Is it reversible?**

The resulting decrease in circulating levels of estrogen or testosterone causes a corresponding decrease in osteoblastic bone formation and an increase in osteoclastic bone resorption. The consequence is a decrease in bone mineral density and progression to osteoporosis. Studies suggest that normalization of the prolactin level restores bone density in most but not all patients, particularly those affected at an early age prior to reaching the peak bone mass in the third decade of life.

KEY POINTS: PROLACTIN-SECRETING PITUITARY TUMORS ✓

1. When a mild prolactin elevation is found (30–50 ng/mL), physiologic, pathologic, and iatrogenic causes need to be excluded before making the diagnosis of a small prolactin-secreting tumor.

2. A prolactin level over 200 ng/mL is almost always indicative of a prolactin-secreting tumor, except during late pregnancy.

3. Elevated prolactin levels cause galactorrhea and suppress the hypothalamic-pituitary-gonadal axis, which results in hypogonadism and a progressive decrease in the bone mineral density.

4. Untreated prolactin-secreting tumors grow very slowly: less than 5% of small tumors are noticeably larger after 2–5 years.

5. Treatment with dopamine agonists is well tolerated and quickly effective in normalizing the prolactin level and shrinking the tumor mass of even very large prolactin-secreting tumors.

11. **If a prolactinoma is left untreated, what is the risk of tumor enlargement?**

Many longitudinal studies agree that progression of the disease is rare and occurs at a slow pace. This is particularly true of small prolactin-secreting tumors (less than 10 mm), less than 5% of which will enlarge significantly over a 2–5 year period of observation. There is no reliable way to predict which patients will show progression. Spontaneous resolution, attributed to necrosis, has also been described in some patients, particularly after pregnancy.

12. **Is medical treatment available for prolactin-secreting tumors? What is the mode of action?**

Medical treatment with dopamine agonists has been available for about 20 years. The most commonly used drugs are bromocriptine and cabergoline; pergolide and Hydergine are also commercially available but are not approved specifically for treatment of prolactin-secreting tumors. These medications are highly effective in reducing both the prolactin level and tumor size.

13. **Describe the mode of action of commonly used drugs.**

Dopamine agonists bind to the pituitary-specific D2 dopamine receptors on the cell membrane of prolactin-secreting cells, decreasing intracellular levels of cAMP and Ca^{2+}. This results in inhibition of the release and synthesis of prolactin. An increase in cellular lysosomal activity causes involution of the rough endoplasmic reticulum and Golgi apparatus. The action of dopamine agonists on D1 dopamine receptors in the brain causes side effects of nausea and dizziness; dopamine agonists with more D2 specificity, such as cabergoline, are less likely to cause these side effects.

14. **If a woman with a prolactin-secreting tumor becomes pregnant while on medical treatment, should the treatment be continued? Should she be allowed to breast-feed her infant?**

    Even though many studies have found that maternal treatment with dopamine agonists is safe to the fetus, it is recommended that the drug be stopped as soon as pregnancy is diagnosed. The risk of tumor re-expansion is low: < 5% for small prolactin-secreting tumors and 15–35% for large tumors. Assessment of symptoms, particularly headaches, and visual field tests should be done monthly; any evidence of tumor re-expansion should prompt the reinstitution of treatment. Breast-feeding does not appear to add any significant risk for these patients, but close follow-up should be continued.

15. **How long does it take for medical treatment to reduce the serum prolactin level? To reduce the size of the tumor?**

    The onset of action of dopamine agonists is rapid, and because prolactin has a serum half-life of 50 minutes, a decrease in the prolactin level may be noted within 2 hours. However, normalization of the prolactin level may take weeks or months, with the maximal decrease usually seen by 3 months. A reduction in tumor size may be apparent within the first 48 hours and may be demonstrated by improvement in the visual fields, when these are affected by the tumor. Tumor shrinkage of at least 50% is usually evident by 3 months. Maximal tumor shrinkage, however, is not usually observed until after at least 6–12 months of treatment.

16. **How long is medical treatment of prolactin-secreting tumors required? Why?**

    In general, life-long treatment is required, because prolactin levels rise and tumors re-expand when treatment is interrupted, suggesting that the effect is mostly cytostatic. Recent reports, however, suggest that about 20% of cases may be cured after 2–5 years of treatment, and some evidence suggests that dopamine agonists may have a cytolytic effect.

17. **When is surgical removal of a prolactin-secreting tumor indicated?**

    With the availability of dopamine agonists, surgery has become a secondary choice in the treatment of prolactin-secreting tumors, particularly since the long-term surgical cure rate for large tumors is only 25–50%. The principal indications for surgical treatment of a prolactin-secreting tumor are intolerance or resistance to dopamine agonists and acute hemorrhage into the tumor. A cerebrospinal fluid (CSF) leak due to erosion of the floor of the sella turcica is another indication for surgical debulking and repair.

18. **When is radiotherapy indicated to treat a prolactin-secreting tumor?**

    Radiotherapy has been rarely utilized because hypopituitarism is a common side effect. This complication is of critical concern, particularly in patients under treatment for infertility. However, radiotherapy may be a useful adjunct in patients who need additional treatment after surgery and who do not tolerate dopamine agonists. Some experts advocate the use of radiotherapy 3 months before attempting pregnancy in women with large tumors in order to avoid tumor re-expansion during pregnancy. The development of new stereotactic radiosurgical techniques, such as the gamma-knife, may improve outcomes and minimize radiation side effects.

WEBSITES

1. National Institute for Diabetes, Digestive and Kidney Disorders. Available at http://www.niddk.nih.gov/health/endo/pubs/prolact/prolact.htm

2. Pituitary Society. Available at http://pituitarysociety.med.nyu.edu/ [click on "Information for the Public", and then "Prolactinomas in Men"]

BIBLIOGRAPHY

1. Colao A, Di Sarno A, Cappabianca P, et al: Withdrawal of long-term cabergoline therapy for tumoral and nontumoral hyperprolactinemia. N Engl J Med 34:2023–2033, 2003.

2. Colao A, Sarno AD, Cappabianca P, et al: Gender differences in the prevalence, clinical features and response to cabergoline in hyperprolactinemia. Eur J Endocrinol 148:325–331, 2003.

3. Colao A, DiSomma C, Loche S, et al: Prolactinomas in adolescents: Persistent bone loss after 2 years of prolactin normalization. Clin Endocrinol 52:319, 2000.

4. Corsello SM, Ubertini G, Altomare M, et al: Giant prolactinomas in men: Efficacy of cabergoline treatment. Clin Endocrinol (Oxf) 58:662–670, 2003.

5. Losa M, Mortini P, Barzaghi R, et al: Surgical treatment of prolactin-secreting pituitary adenomas: Early results and long-term outcome. J Clin Endocrinol Metab 87:3180–3186, 2002.

6. Molitch ME: Prolactinoma. In Melmed S (ed): The Pituitary, Oxford, Blackwell Scientific Publications, 2002.

7. Passos VQ, Souza JJ, Musolino NR, Bronstein MD: Long-term follow-up of prolactinomas: Normoprolactinemia after bromocriptine withdrawal J Clin Endocrinol Metab 87(8; August):3578–3582, 2002.

8. Pollock BE, Nippoldt TB, Stafford SL, et al: Results of stereotactic radiosurgery in patients with hormone-producing pituitary adenomas: Factors associated with endocrine normalization. J Neurosurg 97:525–530, 2002.

9. Schlechte JA: Clinical practice: Prolactinoma. N Engl J Med 349:2035–2041, 2003.

CHAPTER 22

GROWTH HORMONE–SECRETING PITUITARY TUMORS

Mary H. Samuels, M.D.

1. **What is the normal function of growth hormone (GH) in children and adults?**
   In children, GH is responsible for linear growth. In children and adults, GH has many effects on intermediary metabolism, including protein synthesis and nitrogen balance, carbohydrate metabolism, lipolysis, and calcium homeostasis.

2. **How are levels of GH normally regulated?**
   Pituitary secretion of GH is regulated by two hypothalamic hormones: stimulatory GH-releasing hormone (GH-RH) and inhibitory somatostatin. Secretion of GH is also affected by adrenergic and dopaminergic hormones, as well as by other central nervous system factors.

3. **Does GH directly affect peripheral tissues?**
   No. Many (although not all) effects of GH are mediated by another hormone called somatomedin-C or insulin-like growth factor type 1 (IGF-1). IGF-1 is made by the liver and other organs in response to stimulation by GH. IGF-1 feeds back to the pituitary gland and suppresses GH secretion. Unlike GH, IGF-1 has a long half-life in plasma; and thus plasma levels of IGF-1 are helpful in the diagnosis of GH abnormalities.

4. **What are the clinical features of excessive production of GH in children?**
   In children who have not yet undergone puberty and whose long bones still respond to GH, excessive GH causes accelerated linear growth. The result is gigantism.

5. **Describe the clinical features of excessive production of GH in adults.**
   In adults, excessive GH causes acromegaly. The pathologic and metabolic effects of acromegaly are summarized in Table 22-1.

6. **What is the single best clue in examining a patient suspected of having acromegaly?**
   An old driver's license picture or other old photographs provide the best clues. Patients with acromegaly are often unaware of the gradual disfigurement due to the disease or attribute it to aging. Comparing serial photographs can help to establish the diagnosis, as well as date its onset.

7. **From what do patients with acromegaly die?**
   The mortality from untreated or inadequately treated acromegaly is about double the expected rate in healthy subjects matched for age. Major causes of death include hypertension, cardiovascular disease, diabetes, pulmonary infections, and cancer.

8. **In patients with acromegaly, are skin tags all over the neck and chest a relevant finding?**
   There appears to be an association between multiple skin tags and colonic polyps in acromegaly. Therefore, the patient should undergo careful colonoscopic screening for polyps and colon cancer. However, even patients without active disease or skin tags may be at risk for colonic neoplasia and probably should be screened regularly.

TABLE 22-1. CLINICAL EFFECTS OF ACROMEGALY	
Clinical Effect	Cause
Coarse features	Periosteal formation of new bone
Enlarged hands and feet	Soft tissue hypertrophy
Excess sweating	Hypertrophy of sweat glands
Deepened voice	Hypertrophy of larynx
Skin tags	Hypertrophy of skin
Upper airway obstruction and sleep apnea	Hypertrophy of tongue and upper airway
Osteoarthritis	Hypertrophy of joint cartilage and osseous overgrowth
Carpal tunnel syndrome	Hypertrophy of joint cartilage and osseous overgrowth
Hypertension, congestive heart failure	Cardiac hypertrophy
Hypogonadism	Multifactorial
Diabetes mellitus, glucose intolerance	Insulin antagonism, other factors
Colonic polyps	Colonic hypertrophy

9. **The husband of the patient with acromegaly complains that he cannot sleep because his wife snores so loudly. Is this complaint relevant?**
Sleep apnea occurs in up to 80% of patients with acromegaly. It can be due to soft tissue overgrowth of the upper airway or to altered central respiratory control. Sleep apnea may contribute to morbidity and mortality in acromegaly by producing hypoxia and pulmonary hypertension.

10. **If I suspect that a patient may have acromegaly, what test should I order?**
The single best screening test for acromegaly is the plasma level of IGF-1. Because plasma levels of IGF-1 are independent of food intake, samples can be drawn any time of day. In adults, acromegaly is essentially the only condition that causes elevated IGF-1 levels. In children, IGF-1 levels are more difficult to interpret because growing children normally have higher levels than adults.

11. **The patient's IGF-1 level is not elevated, but I still think that she may have acromegaly. What other test should I do?**
The gold standard test to rule out acromegaly is the measurement of serum GH levels in the fasting state and after glucose suppression. Some patients with acromegaly have extremely elevated fasting levels of GH, and further testing is not necessary. Most patients, however, have GH levels that are only mildly elevated or overlap with levels in healthy subjects. Therefore, the diagnosis is usually made by measuring GH levels after a glucose tolerance test. Healthy subjects suppress GH levels after glucose, whereas patients with acromegaly show no suppression or an increase in GH levels.

12. **Once the biochemical diagnosis of acromegaly or gigantism is made, what is the next step?**
Excessive secretion of GH is almost always due to a benign pituitary tumor. Therefore, the next step is to obtain a radiologic study of the pituitary gland. The optimal study is magnetic resonance imaging (MRI) with special cuts through the pituitary gland. If MRI is not available, the best alternative study is a computed tomography (CT) scan with special cuts through the pituitary gland.

13. **What causes GH-secreting pituitary tumors?**

GH-secreting pituitary tumors have been shown to be monoclonal, suggesting that a sponta-neous somatic mutation is a key event in neoplastic transformation of somatotrophs. Further studies have clarified the nature of the mutation in some GH tumors that appear to have an altered stimulatory subunit (G_S) of the G-proteins that regulate adenylate cyclase activity. In a mutated cell, alterations in the G_S subunit cause autonomous adenylate cyclase activity and ele-vated secretion of GH. However, the mutant G_S is found only in a subset of patients with acromegaly. The mechanism of GH regulation and tumor growth may differ in other patients with acromegaly.

14. **Are other endocrine syndromes possible in patients with acromegaly or gigantism?**

Of course. Otherwise, acromegaly and gigantism would not be endocrine disorders. Three endocrine syndromes include acromegaly (Table 22-2).

TABLE 22-2.   ENDOCRINE SYNDROMES ASSOCIATED WITH ACROMEGALY

Syndrome	Major Involved Organs	Clinical Findings	Other Clues
Multiple endocrine neoplasia type 1 (MEN-1)	Pituitary tumors		Autosomal dominant
	Parathyroid hyperplasia	Hypercalcemia (most)	Check calcium levels in
	Islet-cell tumors	Peptic ulcer disease (if gastrinoma)	patients with acromegaly
		Hypoglycemia (if insulinoma)	
McCune-Albright syndrome	Bones	Polyostotic fibrous dysplasia	Mostly in girls
	Skin	Café-au-lait spots	
	Gonads	Sexual precocity	
	Others		
Carney's complex	Heart	Cardiac myomas	Autosomal dominant
	Skin	Pigmented skin lesions	
	Adrenals	Pigmented nodular adrenal hyperplasia	
	Others	Many other tumors	

15. **Do other tumors besides pituitary tumors make GH and cause acromegaly or gigantism?**

Yes. Rare tumors of the pancreas, lung, ovary, and breast may produce GH. However, only one patient has been reported to develop clinical acromegaly from ectopic GH production (from a pancreatic tumor).

16. **Do tumors ever cause acromegaly or gigantism by making excessive GH-RH?**
    Yes. Over 50 cases of GH-RH production by various tumors have been described. These tumors occur in the lung, gastrointestinal tract, or adrenal glands and cause acromegaly by stimulating pituitary secretion of GH. The clinical and biochemical features of acromegaly in such patients are indistinguishable from those of acromegaly due to a pituitary adenoma. Pituitary enlargement also occurs as a result of hyperplasia of somatotrophs. Some patients have had inadvertent transsphenoidal surgery before the correct diagnosis was made. Therefore, the plasma level of GH-RH should be measured in any acromegalic patient with an extrapituitary abnormality or with hyperplasia on pituitary pathology.

17. **If MRI of the pituitary confirms a tumor in the acromegalic patient, what issues other than the metabolic effects of excessive GH should be considered?**
    1. Is the tumor making any other pituitary hormones besides GH? For example, many GH-secreting tumors also produce prolactin; rare tumors also make thyroid-stimulating hormone or other pituitary hormones. In patients with acromegaly, prolactin levels should be measured, as well as other hormones when clinically indicated.
    2. Is the tumor interfering with the normal function of the pituitary gland? Specifically, what is the patient's thyroid, adrenal, and gonadal function? Does the patient have diabetes insipidus? It is important to diagnose and treat pituitary insufficiency before therapy for the excessive secretion of GH, especially if the patient is scheduled for surgery.
    3. Is the tumor causing effects owing to its size and location? Possible effects include headache, visual field disturbances, and extraocular movement abnormalities. Formal visual fields examination should be carried out in patients with large pituitary tumors.

18. **How big are GH-secreting pituitary tumors?**
    GH-secreting tumors vary considerably in size, but most are larger than 1 cm in diameter when diagnosed (i.e., macroadenomas), and some can be very large. Tumor size is an important issue because it determines success rates of treatment.

KEY POINTS: ACROMEGALY ✓

1. Acromegaly leads to gradual soft tissue enlargement and disfigurement over many years, and the patient may be unaware of the changes.

2. Acromegaly causes damage to bones, joints, the heart, and other organs and is associated with considerable morbidity and excess mortality.

3. The best screening test for acromegaly is an IGF-1 level.

4. The best initial treatment for acromegaly is usually surgery, done by an experienced pituitary surgeon.

5. There are new medical treatments for acromegaly that are effective in controlling the metabolic effects of excess GH secretion.

19. **How should acromegaly or gigantism be treated?**
    The treatment of choice for GH-secreting tumors is transsphenoidal surgery by an experienced neurosurgeon. Most patients with microadenomas are cured, and larger tumors are debulked. Significant reduction in GH levels and improvement in symptoms typically follow surgery, even when further treatment is required.

20. **What if surgery does not cure the patient? Should I recommend radiation therapy?**

Conventional radiation therapy of GH-secreting tumors causes a gradual decline in GH levels over many years, and is not recommended as sole therapy. Stereotactic "radiosurgery" has been applied to pituitary tumors, including acromegaly. Stereotactic radiosurgery consists of applying a highly concentrated high-energy radiation therapy beam to the tumor, and it appears to be more effective and to work more quickly than conventional radiation therapy for pituitary tumors. However, stereotactic radiosurgery still takes months to years to work. Therefore, although it is not a good initial choice, radiation therapy is often used after surgery for additional control of the residual tumor. Many patients eventually develop hypopituitarism from radiation therapy.

21. **Are there any options for medical therapy of acromegaly?**

Two agents are effective: octreotide and pegvisomant.

22. **Discuss the mechanisms of action of octreotide.**

Most GH-secreting tumors have somatostatin receptors and respond to exogenous somatostatin with decreases in GH levels. The development of octreotide, a long-acting analog of somatostatin, was a major advance in the treatment of acromegaly.

23. **How effective is octreotide?**

Given as injections two or three times a day, octreotide leads to markedly decreased levels of GH in most acromegalic patients. It also causes tumor shrinkage in some patients. However, it does not cure acromegaly; stopping the drug usually leads to increases in GH levels and tumor regrowth. Therefore, octreotide must be given indefinitely or while waiting for radiation to take effect. Recently, long-acting depo forms of octreotide have been developed. Now most patients can be treated with an injection every 28 days rather than two to three times a day.

24. **Describe the mechanism of action of pegvisomant. When is it used?**

Pegvisomant, the newest therapeutic option for acromegaly, blocks GH action at peripheral receptors, improving IGF-1 levels, reducing clinical effects, and correcting metabolic defects. It does not appear to affect tumor size. It is currently used for patients who are resistant to or do not tolerate octreotide.

25. **What are the side effects of octreotide and pegvisomant?**

Gastrointestinal side effects are common with octreotide, including abdominal bloating, mild diarrhea, nausea, and flatulence. The incidence of gallstones may be increased with octreotide, and therefore patients should be monitored with serial ultrasonography of the gallbladder. Pegvisomant appears to have few adverse effects.

26. **How can one tell whether a patient has been cured of acromegaly?**

The criteria for cure of acromegaly are somewhat controversial. Older studies defined cure as a random GH level below 5 ng/mL. More recent studies have shown that this criterion is inadequate because patients with low levels of GH may still have acromegaly. Therefore, more rigorous criteria have been developed depending on specific GH assays. At the least, patients should have a normal IGF-1 level and GH levels < 1 ng/mL following oral glucose.

27. **The patient has undergone transsphenoidal surgery for acromegaly and now has normal postoperative fasting levels of GH, suppressed levels of GH following oral glucose, and a normal level of IGF-1. How should the patient be followed?**

It appears that the patient is cured, but GH tumors can slowly regrow over years. At the least, measurements of GH and/or IGF-1 should be repeated every 6–12 months. Some physicians also repeat a pituitary MRI at yearly intervals. The patient also needs monitoring for colonic neoplasia at regular intervals. In addition, one needs to assess whether the surgery damaged normal pituitary function by determining the patient's thyroid, adrenal, gonadal, and posterior pituitary function. Finally, the effects of surgery on visual fields should be assessed, especially if the patient had preoperative defects.

28. **The patient asks which symptoms and physical abnormalities will improve after cure is confirmed. What is the appropriate answer?**
Most soft tissue changes improve, including coarsening of facial features, increased size of hands and feet, upper airway hypertrophy, carpal tunnel syndrome, osteoarthritis, and excessive sweating. Hypertension, cardiovascular disease, and diabetes also improve. Unfortunately, bony overgrowth of the facial bones does not regress after treatment.

29. **For bonus points, name an actor with acromegaly and the movie in which he starred.**
Andre the Giant starred in *The Princess Bride.*

BIBLIOGRAPHY

1. Ben-Shlomo A, Melmed S: Acromegaly. Endocrinol Metab Clin North Am 30:565–583, 2001.
2. Clemmons DR, Chihara K, Freda PU, et al: Optimizing control of acromegaly: Integrating a growth hormone receptor antagonist into the treatment algorithm. J Clin Endocrinol Metab 88:4759–4767, 2003.
3. Freda PU: Somatostatin analogs in acromegaly. J Clin Endocrinol Metab 87:3013–3018, 2002.
4. Melmed S, Casanueva FF, Cavagnini F, et al: Guidelines for acromegaly management. J Clin Endocrinol Metab 87:4054–4058, 2002.
5. Sheppard MC: Primary medical therapy for acromegaly. Clin Endocrinol 58:387–399, 2003.

CHAPTER 23

GLYCOPROTEIN-SECRETING PITUITARY TUMORS

Robert C. Smallridge, M.D.

1. **What are glycoprotein hormones?**
   The glycoprotein hormones are luteinizing hormone (LH), thyrotropin (TSH), follicle-stimulating hormone (FSH), and chorionic gonadotropin (CG). Glycoprotein hormones are composed of two noncovalently bound subunits. The alpha subunit (α-SU) is similar among all four hormones. In contrast, the beta subunit (β-SU) is unique both immunologically and biologically for each hormone; these subunits are identified as LHβ, FSHβ, TSHβ, and βCG.

2. **Name two types of glycoprotein-secreting pituitary tumors.**

Type	Secretory Products
Gonadotropinomas	LH, FSH, LHβ, FSHβ, α-SU
Thyrotropinomas (TSHomas)	TSH, α-SU

3. **Do pituitary tumors secrete only a single hormone?**
   No. Many tumors make two or more hormones or subunits. In some circumstances, sufficient quantities of multiple hormones are secreted to produce clinical symptoms characteristic of several syndromes within the same patient.

4. **Under what circumstances should a TSH-secreting tumor be considered?**
   - Suspected hyperthyroidism
   - Increased serum free thyroxine (T_4) or FT_4 index
     and
   - Detectable serum TSH

5. **Describe the differential diagnosis for patients with a transient increase in serum total T_4 and a detectable or elevated level of serum TSH.**
   Exogenous
   - L-Thyroxine (L-T_4) therapy (noncompliant patient who took L-T_4 the day blood was drawn)
   - Other drugs (amiodarone, ipodate, amphetamines)
   Endogenous (subgroup of nonthyroidal illness)
   - Acute psychiatric illness
   - Acute liver disease

6. **Describe the differential diagnosis for patients with a permanent increase in serum total T_4 and detectable or elevated level of serum TSH.**
   Binding protein disorders
   - Excessive thyroxine-binding globulin (TBG)
   - Abnormal thyroxine-binding prealbumin (TBPA) (transthyretin)
   - Familial dysalbuminemic hyperthyroxinemia (FDH)

- T_4 autoantibody
- TSH heterophile antibody (requires separate cause for T_4 elevation)

Inappropriate TSH secretion

- Resistance to thyroid hormone (generalized, central)
- Pituitary tumor

7. **What tests are useful in the differential diagnosis of the patient with an elevated serum total T_4 and a detectable or elevated serum TSH?**
The history and physical examination usually rule out medications and nonthyroidal illnesses. The most important laboratory test is the free T_4. A normal free T_4 strongly suggests one of the binding protein disorders. An elevated free T_4, in contrast, generally narrows the differential to two disorders: a thyroid hormone resistance syndrome or a TSH-secreting pituitary tumor. Clinical thyrotoxicosis is commonly present in patients with either condition. One should confirm the abnormal test results in a second laboratory prior to initiating a work-up for these uncommon disorders.

8. **How can one distinguish between the hyperthyroid patient with thyroid hormone resistance and the patient with a pituitary tumor?**
TSH tumors secrete α-SU in excess of the whole TSH molecule. The molar ratio of serum α-SU to TSH is increased in most patients with TSH tumors but normal in thyroid hormone resistance. A thyrotropin-releasing hormone (TRH; protirelin) test is also helpful. Fewer than 20% of patients with a tumor have a 2-fold increase in serum TSH after TRH, whereas those with resistance respond briskly. If tumor is suspected after both tests, a magnetic resonance imaging (MRI) scan of the pituitary should be obtained. Most TSH tumors (about 90%) are macroadenomas (i.e., ≥ 10 mm). Most microadenomas (< 10 mm) are also visualized, but rarely sampling of inferior petrosal sinus blood has helped localize the tumor. Dynamic MRI scan or somatostatin receptor scintigraphy (OctreoScan) is also useful.

9. **Describe how to calculate an α/TSH molar ratio.**
TSH values are expressed as μU/mL (or mU/L). One must know the bioactivity and convert these units to ng/ml, the units of α-SU. Furthermore, the molecular weight of the subunit is only half the molecular weight of the whole TSH molecule; this fact also must be considered in calculating the molar ratio. From a practical standpoint, the following formula can be used:

$$\text{molar ratio} = [\alpha\text{-SU (ng/mL)/TSH (}\mu\text{U/mL)}] \times 10$$

10. **Name the treatment of choice for TSH-secreting tumors and its likelihood of success.**
Pituitary surgery is the treatment of choice, but it is curative in only one-third patients. Results are somewhat better if surgery is followed by radiation therapy. Since more microadenomas are being identified, results are improving.

11. **How effective is radiation as the sole therapy?**
Because so few cases have been reported, results are uncertain.

12. **List the medical therapies used for TSH-secreting tumors.**
- Octreotide (somatostatin analog) decreases TSH in > 90% and normalizes free T_4 in 75% of cases. Tumor size decreases, and vision improves. Long-acting (monthly) analogs are effective.
- Bromocriptine (limited success).
- Dexamethasone reduces TSH, but its side effects exclude long-term use.

13. **Summarize the role of thyroid gland ablation in the treatment of TSH-secreting tumors.**
Thyroidectomy and [131]iodine are contraindicated. Thyroid ablation does not control TSH secretion and may enhance pituitary activity and growth.

14. **Do all patients with an enlarged pituitary gland and an elevated level of serum TSH have thyrotropinomas?**
No. Patients with long-standing hypothyroidism may develop pituitary hyperplasia, producing a pseudotumor (Fig. 23-1). The pituitary mass can extend into the suprasellar region and cause visual field defects. Serum T_4 is always low, and shrinkage of the enlarged gland usually occurs with L-T_4 replacement therapy. No patient should undergo pituitary gland surgery without a preoperative measurement of serum T_4 and TSH.

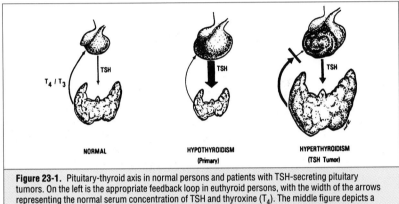

Figure 23-1. Pituitary-thyroid axis in normal persons and patients with TSH-secreting pituitary tumors. On the left is the appropriate feedback loop in euthyroid persons, with the width of the arrows representing the normal serum concentration of TSH and thyroxine (T_4). The middle figure depicts a small thyroid gland due to primary hypothyroidism. The low T_4 levels result in markedly increased secretion of TSH and, in some patients, a generalized hyperplasia of the anterior pituitary gland. On the right is an autonomous pituitary tumor secreting TSH. Serum TSH levels may vary greatly but in all cases are sufficiently biologically active to increase levels of T_4 above normal. The elevated T_4 level has little, if any, ability to suppress tumor function.

15. **What clinical features raise suspicion of a TSH-secreting pseudotumor?**
Almost all patients have symptoms of hypothyroidism, and the serum T_4 concentration is always low. The underlying abnormality is usually autoimmune thyroiditis, predominantly a disease of women. Approximately 80% of reported cases of pituitary enlargement with hypothyroidism were in women, while only 55% of true TSH tumors have occurred in women. In children, precocious puberty may occur. Thyroid antibodies are present in more than 75% of cases with pseudotumor, compared with about 10% of patients with TSH tumors that produce hyperthyroidism.

16. **Does the presence of abnormal visual fields help to distinguish between patients with pituitary hyperplasia due to primary hypothyroidism and patients with TSH-secreting tumors?**
No. Abnormal visual fields have been reported in 28% of patients with pituitary hyperplasia compared with 42% of patients with tumors. In contrast, patients with thyroid hormone resistance have normal vision.

17. **Does family history provide any clues in distinguishing these disorders?**
    In pseudotumor from thyrotroph hyperplasia, the family history may be positive for the presence of autoimmune diseases (e.g., thyroiditis, Graves' disease, type 1 diabetes mellitus, rheumatoid arthritis, lupus erythematosus, Sjögren's syndrome, vitiligo, Addison's disease, pernicious anemia). In TSH tumors, family history is of no use. Most cases of generalized thyroid hormone resistance are familial with autosomal dominant inheritance (i.e., 50% of the family have the biochemical abnormalities).

18. **Which hormones are elevated in the serum of patients with gonadotroph adenomas?**
    Serum FSH is increased much more often than LH. An increase in α-SU is not specific for gonadotrophs because it may also derive from thyrotrophs. Furthermore, an α/LH (or FSH) molar ratio has not been clinically useful.

KEY POINTS: GLYCOPROTEIN-SECRETING PITUITARY TUMORS ✓

1. Glycoprotein-secreting pituitary tumors include gonadotropinomas (LH- or FSH-secreting) and TSHomas.

2. Hyperthyroid patients with detectable serum TSH should always be evaluated for inappropriate TSH secretion (either a TSH-tumor or thyroid hormone resistance).

3. TSH tumors are best managed by transsphenoidal surgery and possibly long-term use of octreotide analog.

4. Gonadotropinomas often present with neurologic symptoms due to mass effect and require pituitary surgery.

5. Hypothyroidism can produce thyrotroph hyperplasia and pituitary pseudotumors.

19. **List the presenting symptoms of patients with gonadotropinomas.**
    Mass effect (common)
    - Large tumors with extrasellar growth
    - Visual impairment/diplopia
    - Headaches
    - Apoplexy
    - Hypopituitarism
    Endocrine excesses (uncommon)
    - Ovarian hyperstimulation
    - Testicular enlargement
    - Precocious puberty

20. **When gonadotropin levels are elevated, how can one distinguish clinically between a gonadotroph adenoma and primary hypogonadism?**
    This distinction can be difficult, especially in women, because their levels of LH and FSH increase after menopause. This is probably why most gonadotroph adenomas have been recognized in men. Historically, men with such tumors experienced a normal puberty and may have fathered children.
    On examination, testicular size may be normal. In contrast, men with hypogonadism may have had abnormal pubertal development or a history of testicular injury; the testes are small.

21. **What laboratory tests are helpful?**

In primary hypogonadism, both FSH and LH are increased, whereas FSH is elevated but LH is usually normal in patients with gonadotropinomas. When LH is high in men with gonadotropinomas, testosterone also is high rather than low, as in hypogonadism. For unexplained reasons, about one-third of patients with a tumor have an anomalous rise in serum FSH or LHβ when given a TRH injection. An MRI scan of the pituitary reveals a large tumor. Occasionally, a patient with long-standing hypogonadism may have some degree of pituitary enlargement.

22. **How are gonadotropinomas treated?**

Pituitary surgery is the treatment of choice. Although complete cure is often impossible, substantial reduction in tumor size and hormone secretion is common. Reduced hormone secretion provides a convenient marker for monitoring recurrence of tumor; an abrupt increase in FSH or α-SU should prompt a repeat imaging study. Radiation therapy is often given after surgery in the hope of delaying tumor recurrence.

23. **Is medical therapy effective?**

Agonist analogs of gonadotropin-releasing hormone (GnRH) reduce secretion from normal gonadotrophs. Unfortunately, they usually have the opposite effect on gonadotropinomas. An antagonist analog (Nal-Glu-GnRH) has effectively reduced serum FSH in a small group of men with gonadotropinomas but did not reduce tumor size. Bromocriptine has reduced hormone levels in an occasional patient, whereas octreotide has reduced α-SU and improved visual fields in certain patients.

24. **Are pituitary tumors malignant?**

Carcinomas are rare but occasionally have been reported for:
- ACTH
- GH
- PRL
- TSH ($n = 1$)

25. **What causes pituitary tumors?**
- Oncogene overexpression (e.g., pituitary tumor transforming gene [PTTG], others).
- Silencing of tumor suppressor genes (e.g., hypermethylation).
- Corticotropin-releasing factor (CRF_2) expression.

WEBSITE

http://www.thyroidmanager.org

BIBLIOGRAPHY

1. Beck-Peccoz P, Brucker-Davis F, Persani L, et al: Thyrotropin-secreting pituitary tumors. Endocr Rev 17:610–638, 1996.
2. Burch HB: Abnormal thyroid function test results in euthyroid persons. In Becker KL (ed): Principles and Practice of Endocrinology and Metabolism, 3rd ed. Philadelphia, Lippincott Williams & Wilkins, 2001, pp 351–360.
3. Caron P, Arlot S, Bauters C, et al: Efficacy of the long-acting octreotide formulation (octreotide-LAR) in patients with thyrotropin-secreting pituitary adenomas. J Clin Endocrinol Metab 86:2849–2853, 2001.
4. Chaidarun SS, Klibanski A: Gonadotropinomas. Semin Reprod Med 20:339–348, 2002.
5. Lamberts SW, Krenning EP, Reubi JC: The role of somatostatin and its analogs in the diagnosis and treatment of tumors. Endocr Rev 12:450–482, 1991.

6. McGrath GA, Goncalves RJ, Udupa JK, et al: New technique for quantitation of pituitary adenoma size: Use in evaluating treatment of gonadotroph adenomas with a gonadotropin-releasing hormone antagonist. J Clin Endocrinol Metab 76:1363–1368, 1993.

7. Refetoff S, Weiss RE, Usala SJ: The syndromes of resistance to thyroid hormone. Endocr Rev 14:348–399, 1993.

8. Reubi JC, Waser B, Vale W, et al: Expression of CRF1 and CRF2 receptors in human cancers. J Clin Endocrinol Metab 88:3312–3320, 2003.

9. Simard MF: Pituitary tumor endocrinopathies and their endocrine evaluation. Neurosurg Clin N Am 14:41–54, 2003.

10. Smallridge RC: Thyrotropin-secreting tumors. In Mazzaferri EL, Samaan NA (eds): Endocrine Tumors. Boston, Blackwell Scientific Publications, 1993, pp 136–151.

11. Smallridge RC: Thyrotropin- and gonadotropin-producing tumors. In Korenman SG, Molitch ME (eds): Atlas of Clinical Endocrinology. Neuroendocrinology and Pituitary Disease. Philadelphia, Blackwell Science, 2000, pp 95–113.

12. Smallridge RC: Thyroid function tests. In Becker KL (ed): Principles and Practice of Endocrinology and Metabolism, 3rd ed. Philadelphia, Lippincott Williams & Wilkins, 2001, pp 329–336.

13. Smallridge RC, Czervionke LF, Fellows DW, et al: Corticotropin- and thyrotropin-secreting pituitary microadenomas: Detection by dynamic magnetic resonance imaging. Mayo Clin Proc 75:521–528, 2000.

14. Smallridge RC: Thyrotropin-secreting pituitary tumors: Clinical presentation, investigation, and management. Curr Opin Endocrinol Diabetes 8:253–258, 2001.

15. Snyder PJ: Extensive personal experience: Gonadotroph adenomas. J Clin Endocrinol Metab 80:1059–1061, 1995.

16. Young WF Jr, Scheithauer BW, Kovacs KT, et al: Gonadotroph adenoma of the pituitary gland: A clinicopathologic analysis of 100 cases. Mayo Clin Proc 71:649–656, 1996.

CHAPTER 24

CUSHING'S SYNDROME

Mary H. Samuels, M.D.

1. **Describe the normal function of cortisol in healthy people.**
   Cortisol and other glucocorticoids have many effects as physiologic regulators. They increase glucose production, inhibit protein synthesis and increase protein breakdown, stimulate lipolysis, and affect immunologic and inflammatory responses. Glucocorticoids are important for maintenance of blood pressure and form an essential part of the body's response to stress.

2. **How are cortisol levels normally regulated?**
   Adrenal production of cortisol is stimulated by the pituitary hormone adrenocorticotropin (ACTH). ACTH production is stimulated by the hypothalamic hormones corticotropin-releasing hormone (CRH) and vasopressin (ADH). Cortisol feeds back to the pituitary and hypothalamus to suppress levels of ACTH and CRH. Under nonstress conditions, cortisol is secreted with a pronounced circadian rhythm, with higher levels early in the morning and lower levels late in the evening. Under stressful conditions, secretion of CRH, ACTH, and cortisol increases and the circadian variation is blunted. Because of the wide variation in cortisol levels over 24 hours and appropriate elevations during stressful conditions, it may be difficult to distinguish normal secretion from abnormal secretion. For this reason, the evaluation of a patient with suspected Cushing's disease is often complex and confusing.

3. **What are the clinical symptoms of excessive levels of cortisol?**
   1. Obesity, especially central (truncal) obesity, with wasting of the extremities, moon facies, supraclavicular fat pads, and buffalo hump.
   2. Thinning of the skin, with facial plethora, easy bruising, and violaceous striae.
   3. Muscular weakness, especially proximal muscle weakness, and atrophy.
   4. Hypertension, atherosclerosis, congestive heart failure, and edema.
   5. Gonadal dysfunction and menstrual irregularities.
   6. Psychologic disturbances (e.g., depression, emotional lability, irritability, sleep disturbances).
   7. Osteoporosis and fractures.
   8. Increased rate of infections and poor wound healing.

4. **All of my clinic patients look like they have Cushing's syndrome. Are some clinical findings more specific for Cushing's syndrome than others?**
   Some manifestations of Cushing's syndrome are common but nonspecific, whereas others are less common but quite specific. The clinical findings are listed in Table 24-1, with the more specific findings listed first. The sensitivity and specificity for the diagnosis are listed separately.

5. **A patient presents with a history of obesity, hypertension, irregular menses, and depression. Does she have excessive production of cortisol?**
   Excessive cortisol is highly unlikely. Although the listed findings are consistent with glucocorticoid excess, they are nonspecific; most patients with such findings do *not* have Cushing's syndrome (see Table 24-1).

TABLE 24-1. SYMPTOMS AND SIGNS OF CUSHING'S SYNDROME		
Sign/Symptom	Sensitivity (%)	Specificity (%)
Hypokalemia (K$^+$ < 3.6)	25	96
Ecchymoses	53	94
Osteoporosis	26	94
Weakness	65	93
Diastolic blood pressure (> 105 mmHg)	39	83
Red or violaceous striae	46	78
Acne	52	76
Central obesity	90	71
Hirsutism	50	71
Plethora	82	69
Oligomenorrhea	72	49
Generalized obesity	3	38
Abnormal glucose tolerance	88	23

6. **The patient also complains of excessive hair growth and has increased terminal hair on the chin, along the upper lip, and on the upper back. Is this finding relevant?**
Hirsutism is a common, nonspecific finding in many female patients. However, it is also consistent with Cushing's syndrome. If it is due to Cushing's syndrome, hirsutism is a complication not of excessive glucocorticoids but of excessive production of androgen by the adrenal glands under ACTH stimulation. Thus, hirsutism in a patient with Cushing's syndrome is a clue that the disorder is due to excessive production of ACTH. (The only other condition associated with excessive production of glucocorticoids and androgen is a malignant adrenal tumor, which is usually obvious on presentation.)

7. **The patient also has increased pigmentation of the areolae, palmar creases, and an old surgical scar. Are these findings relevant?**
Hyperpigmentation is a sign of elevated production of ACTH and related peptides by the pituitary gland. It is uncommon (but possible) in Cushing's syndrome due to benign pituitary tumors because levels of ACTH do not usually rise high enough to cause hyperpigmentation. It is more common in the ectopic ACTH syndrome because ectopic tumors produce more ACTH and other peptides. The combination of Cushing's syndrome and hyperpigmentation may be bad news.

8. **What is the cause of death in patients with Cushing's syndrome?**
Patients with Cushing's syndrome have a markedly increased mortality rate, usually from cardiovascular disease or infections.

9. **What causes Cushing's syndrome?**
Cushing's syndrome is a nonspecific name for any source of excessive glucocorticoids. There are four main causes, which are further detailed in Table 24-2:
1. Exogenous glucocorticoids (ACTH-independent)
2. Pituitary Cushing's syndrome (ACTH-dependent)
3. Ectopic production of ACTH (ACTH-dependent)
4. Adrenal tumors (ACTH-independent)

TABLE 24-2.	CAUSES OF CUSHING'S SYNDROME AND THEIR RELATIVE FREQUENCY	
ACTH-Dependent (80%)	**ACTH-Independent (20%)**
Pituitary (85%)	Adrenal tumors
Corticotroph adenoma	Adrenal adenoma (> 50%)
Corticotroph hyperplasia (rare)	Adrenal carcinoma (< 50%)
Ectopic ACTH syndrome (15%)	Micronodular hyperplasia (rare)
Oat-cell carcinoma (50%)	Macronodular hyperplasia (rare)
Foregut tumors (35%)	Exogenous glucocorticoids (common)
Bronchial carcinoid	Therapeutic (common)
Thymic carcinoid	Factitious (rare)
Medullary thyroid carcinoma	
Islet-cell tumors	
Pheochromocytoma	
Other tumors (10%)	
Ectopic CRH (< 1%)	

10. **Of the various types of Cushing's syndrome, which is the most common?**
Overall, exogenous Cushing's syndrome is most common. It rarely presents a diagnostic dilemma, because the physician usually knows that the patient is receiving glucocorticoids. Of the endogenous causes of Cushing's syndrome, pituitary Cushing's disease accounts for at least 70% of cases. Ectopic secretion of ACTH and adrenal tumors cause approximately 15% of cases each (see Table 24-1 for frequencies).

11. **Do age and gender matter in the differential diagnosis of Cushing's syndrome?**
Of patients with Cushing's disease (pituitary tumors) 80% are women, whereas the ectopic ACTH syndrome is more common in men. Therefore, in a male patient with Cushing's syndrome, the risk of an extrapituitary tumor is increased. The age range in Cushing's disease is most frequently 20–40 years, whereas ectopic ACTH syndrome has a peak incidence at 40–60 years. Therefore, the risk of an extrapituitary tumor in an older patient with Cushing's syndrome is increased. Children with Cushing's syndrome have a higher risk of malignant adrenal tumors.

12. **The patient with obesity, hypertension, irregular menses, depression, and hirsutism looks like she may have Cushing's syndrome. What should I do?**
A widely used screening test for Cushing's syndrome is the overnight low-dose dexamethasone suppression test. The patient takes 1 mg of dexamethasone at 11 PM and measures her serum cortisol level at 8 AM the next morning. In healthy unstressed subjects, dexamethasone (a potent glucocorticoid that does not react with the cortisol assay) suppresses production of CRH, ACTH, and cortisol. Patients with Cushing's syndrome of any cause should not suppress cortisol production (serum cortisol remains > 5 mg/dL) when given 1 mg of dexamethasone.

13. **The patient had a cortisol level drawn after a 1-mg dose of dexamethasone. The level is 12 (μg/dL. Does she have Cushing's syndrome?**
Unfortunately, the overnight dexamethasone suppression test is not foolproof. Occasional patients with Cushing's disease suppress cortisol levels with dexamethasone, and many patients without Cushing's syndrome do not. Acute or chronic illnesses, depression, and alcohol abuse

all activate the hypothalamic-pituitary-adrenal axis because of stress and make the patient resistant to dexamethasone suppression. In fact, because Cushing's syndrome is so rare, a nonsuppressed cortisol level after dexamethasone is more likely to be a false-positive result, rather than truly indicating the presence of Cushing's syndrome. A more accurate screening test is a 24-hour urine sample for free cortisol levels, which should be ordered in this case.

14. **The patient has an elevated 24-hour urinary level of free cortisol, and serum cortisol levels are not suppressed after overnight 1-mg dexamethasone administration. What should I do?**
It looks like the patient has Cushing's syndrome. However, it is still possible that the patient has other reasons for her symptoms and elevated cortisol levels. It can be very difficult to distinguish mild or moderate Cushing's syndrome from stress-induced hypercortisolism, especially in patients who have active medical or psychiatric illnesses. The distinction between true Cushing's syndrome and pseudo-Cushing's syndrome (stress-induced hypercortisolemia) depends on the clinical suspicion and degree of elevation of the cortisol levels. In general, a 24-hour urine free cortisol level of greater than three times normal levels is diagnostic of true Cushing's syndrome in the absence of severe stress. Lesser elevations of urine free cortisol may require confirmatory tests for the presence of Cushing's syndrome.

15. **I am not convinced that the patient has Cushing's syndrome. How can I confirm it?**
The best confirmatory test is controversial, but two commonly used tests are loss of diurnal variation in plasma cortisol levels and the dexamethasone-CRH test (Fig. 24-1). These tests are best administered and interpreted by experienced endocrinologists, since the results can be skewed if the tests are not performed properly.

16. **The patient has elevated cortisol levels at night and an abnormal dexamethasone-CRH test. Now I am convinced that she has Cushing's syndrome. What should I do next?**
Once you have made the biochemical diagnosis of Cushing's syndrome, the next step is to determine whether she has ACTH-dependent or ACTH-independent disease (Fig. 24-2). This

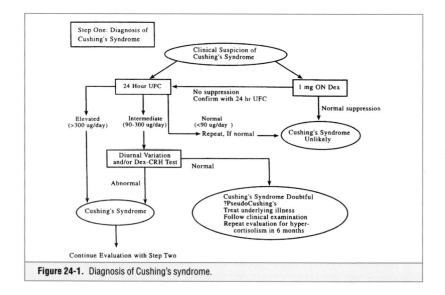

Figure 24-1. Diagnosis of Cushing's syndrome.

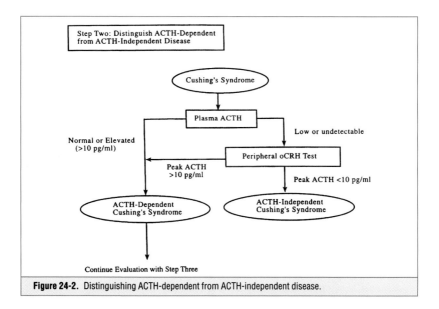

Figure 24-2. Distinguishing ACTH-dependent from ACTH-independent disease.

distinction is made by measuring plasma levels of ACTH. Measurements should be repeated a number of times because secretion of ACTH is variable.

17. **The patient's ACTH level is "normal." Was the original suspicion of Cushing's syndrome incorrect?**
No. Normal levels of ACTH are a common finding in pituitary-dependent Cushing's disease. A normal or slightly elevated ACTH level is the usual finding in ACTH-secreting pituitary adenomas. More marked elevations of ACTH levels suggest ectopic secretion of ACTH, although small carcinoid tumors also have normal or mildly elevated levels of ACTH. Suppressed ACTH levels, in contrast, suggest an adrenal tumor.

18. **What happened to the 2-day low-dose and high-dose dexamethasone tests for the differential diagnosis of Cushing's syndrome?**
The 2-day low-dose and high-dose dexamethasone suppression tests were once widely used in attempts to distinguish pituitary, ectopic, and adrenal causes of Cushing's syndrome. Although they are still performed, the results are often confusing, and rates of both false-positive and false-negative results are high. Therefore, these tests have been abandoned by many endocrinologists and supplanted by more accurate ACTH assays, the overnight high-dose dexamethasone test, CRH stimulation tests, and inferior petrosal sinus sampling (IPSS).

19. **After diagnosis of ACTH-dependent Cushing's syndrome, what is the next step?**
Because the most common site of excessive secretion of ACTH is a pituitary tumor, radiologic imaging of the pituitary gland is the next step. The best study is high-resolution magnetic resonance imaging (MRI) with thin cuts through the pituitary gland. A chest radiograph should also be obtained at this point in case the patient has a carcinoid tumor large enough to be seen on plain film.

20. **The pituitary MRI in the patient with ACTH-dependent Cushing's syndrome is normal. Is the next step a search for carcinoid tumor, under the assumption that the pituitary is not the source of excessive ACTH?**
Not so fast. At least one-half of pituitary MRI or computed tomography (CT) scans are negative in proven pituitary-dependent Cushing's syndrome because most corticotroph adenomas are tiny and may not be visible on MRI or CT.

21. **The pituitary MRI shows a 3-mm hypodense area in the lateral aspect of the pituitary gland. Is it time to call the neurosurgeon?**
Again, not so fast. This finding is nonspecific and occurs in many healthy people. It may or may not be related to Cushing's syndrome. The odds are good that the patient has a pituitary tumor, but the MRI does not prove so. The MRI is diagnostic in Cushing's syndrome only if it shows a large tumor.

22. **So what is the next step?**
One option is to proceed directly to pituitary surgery because a patient with an abnormal MRI has a 90% chance of having an ACTH-secreting pituitary tumor. To achieve more diagnostic certainty, one has to perform bilateral simultaneous IPSS for ACTH levels (Fig. 24-3). Catheters are advanced through the femoral veins into the inferior petrosal sinuses, which drain the pituitary gland. Blood samples are obtained through the catheters for ACTH levels. If ACTH levels in the petrosal sinuses are significantly higher than those in peripheral samples, the pituitary gland is the source of excessive ACTH. If there is no gradient between petrosal sinus and peripheral levels of ACTH, the patient probably has a carcinoid tumor somewhere. The accuracy of the test is further increased if ACTH responses to injection of exogenous CRH are measured. Bilateral IPSS should be performed by experienced radiologists at referral centers.

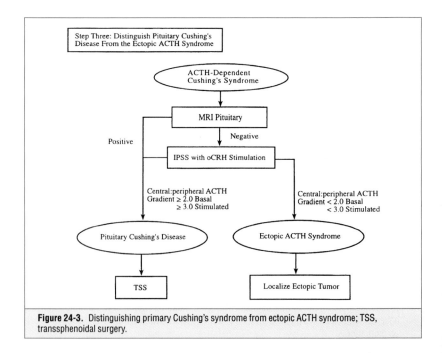

Figure 24-3. Distinguishing primary Cushing's syndrome from ectopic ACTH syndrome; TSS, transsphenoidal surgery.

23. **IPSS shows no gradient in ACTH levels. Now what?**
Start the search for a carcinoid tumor. Because the most likely location is the lung, a CT scan of the lungs should be ordered. If the results are negative, a CT scan of the abdomen should be ordered because carcinoids also occur in the pancreas, intestinal tract, and adrenal glands.

24. **IPSS shows a marked central-to-peripheral gradient in ACTH levels. Now what?**
TSS should be scheduled with an experienced neurosurgeon who is comfortable examining the pituitary for small adenomas. ACTH levels from the right and left petrosal sinuses obtained during the sampling study may tell the neurosurgeon in which side of the pituitary gland the tumor is likely to be found, but this information is not 100% accurate.

25. **What if surgery is unsuccessful?**
If TSS does not cure a patient with Cushing's disease, alternative therapies must be tried because patients with inadequately treated hypercortisolism have increased morbidity and mortality rates. Of the various options after failed surgery, none is ideal. Patients may need repeat pituitary surgery, radiation therapy, medical therapy to block cortisol secretion, and/or bilateral adrenalectomy. These decisions should be made in consultation with an experienced endocrinologist.

KEY POINTS: CUSHING'S SYNDROME ✓

1. The clinical manifestations of Cushing's syndrome can be subtle and/or nonspecific.

2. Most patients who look like they might have Cushing's syndrome do not.

3. Screening biochemical tests for Cushing's syndrome can be misleading, and repeated testing or more extensive confirmatory testing is often needed.

4. Most patients with Cushing's syndrome have a small pituitary tumor producing ACTH.

5. Patients with pituitary tumors causing Cushing's syndrome should undergo pituitary surgery by an experienced neurosurgeon because none of the other treatment options are ideal.

26. **Why not just take out the patient's adrenal glands?**
One drawback is the extensive nature of the surgery. This problem has been addressed recently by performing adrenalectomy via a laparoscopic approach, which is easier on the patient. Another drawback is lifelong adrenal insufficiency and dependence on exogenous glucocorticoids and mineralocorticoids. However, the main drawback is the development of Nelson's syndrome in up to 30% of patients after adrenalectomy. Nelson's syndrome is the appearance, sometimes years after adrenalectomy, of an aggressive corticotroph pituitary tumor.

27. **What are the correct diagnostic and treatment options for patients with ACTH-independent (adrenal) Cushing's syndrome?**
Such patients usually have either an adrenal adenoma or an adrenal carcinoma. Once consistent suppression of ACTH levels is confirmed, an adrenal CT scan should be ordered. A mass is almost always present, and surgery should be planned. If the mass is obviously cancer, surgery may still help in debulking the tumor and improving the metabolic consequences of hypercortisolemia. If there are multiple adrenal nodules, the patient may have a rare form of Cushing's syndrome and should be evaluated by an experienced endocrinologist.

28. **What happens to the hypothalamic-pituitary-adrenal axis after a patient undergoes successful removal of an ACTH-secreting pituitary adenoma or a cortisol-secreting adrenal adenoma?**
The axis is suppressed, and the patient develops clinical adrenal insufficiency, unless he or she is given gradually decreasing doses of exogenous glucocorticoids for a time after surgery.

29. **What would be the most likely diagnosis if the original patient had all the signs of Cushing's syndrome but *low* urinary and serum levels of cortisol?**
The most likely scenario is that the patient is surreptitiously or accidentally ingesting a glucocorticoid that gives all the findings of glucocorticoid excess but is not measured in the cortisol assay. The patient and family members should be questioned about possible access to medications, and special assays can measure the different synthetic glucocorticoids.

30. **Do tumors ever cause Cushing's syndrome by making excessive CRH?**
Yes. Occasionally patients who undergo TSS for a presumed corticotroph adenoma have corticotroph hyperplasia instead. At least some of these cases are secondary to ectopic production of CRH from a carcinoid tumor in the lung, abdomen, or other location. Therefore, levels of serum CRH should be measured in patients with Cushing's syndrome and corticotroph hyperplasia. If the levels are elevated, a careful search should be performed for possible ectopic sources of CRH.

BIBLIOGRAPHY

1. Arnaldi G, Angeli A, Atkinson AB, et al: Diagnosis and complications of Cushing's syndrome: A consensus statement. J Clin Endocrinol Metab 88:5593–5602, 2003.
2. Findling JW, Raff H: Diagnosis and differential diagnosis of Cushing's syndrome. Endocrinol Metab Clin N Am 30:729–747, 2001.
3. Graham KE, Samuels MH: Recent advances in the evaluation of Cushing's syndrome. Endocrinologist 8:425–345, 1998.
4. Morris D, Grossman A: The medical management of Cushing's syndrome. Ann N Y Acad Sci 970:119–133, 2002.
5. Nieman LK: Diagnostic tests for Cushing's syndrome. Ann N Y Acad Sci 970:112–118, 2002.
6. Raff H, Findling JW: A physiologic approach to diagnosis of the Cushing syndrome. Ann Intern Med 138:980–991, 2003.

CHAPTER 25

WATER METABOLISM

Leonard R. Sanders, M.D.

1. **What is the water composition of the human body?**
   Water composition of the body depends on age, sex, muscle mass, body habitus, and fat content. Various body tissues have the following water percentages: lungs, heart, and kidneys (80%); skeletal muscle and brain (75%); skin and liver (70%); bone (20%); and adipose tissue (10%). Clearly, people with more muscle than fat will have more water. Generally, thin people have less fat and more water. Men are 60% and women 50% water by weight. Older people have more fat and less muscle. The average man and woman older than 60 years are made up of 50% and 45% water, respectively (see Table 25-1). Most discussions of total body water (TBW) consider a man who is 60% water, weighs 70 kg, and is 69 in. (175 cm) tall.

TABLE 25-1.	WATER AS A PERCENT OF BODY WEIGHT		
Body Habitus	**Infant**	**Man**	**Woman**
Thin	80	65	55
Medium	70	60	50
Obese	65	55	45

2. **Where is water located within the body?**
   TBW equals water located inside the cells (intracellular fluid [ICF]) and outside the cells (extracellular fluid [ECF]). TBW is 60% of body weight; ICF and ECF water are 40% and 20%, respectively, of body weight. ECF contains both interstitial (15%) and intravascular water (5%). Thus, in a 70-kg man, TBW = 42 L, ICF water = 28 L, and ECF water = 14 L. The interstitial fluid (ISF) is 10.5 L, and intravascular (plasma) fluid (IVF) is 3.5 L. Therefore, of the TBW, ⅔ is ICF and ⅓ is ECF. Of the ECF, about ¼ is IVF and ¾ is ISF. Tight regulation of the relatively small volume of IVF (plasma) maintains blood pressure and avoids symptomatic hypovolemia and congestive heart failure. Normal plasma is 93% water and 7% proteins and lipids. Total blood volume (TBV) is only a small portion of the ECF, and arterial volume is only 15% of TBV. Although arterial volume is small, its integrity is most important for maintaining the effective circulation and preventing abnormalities of water balance (see Fig. 25-1).

3. **What is transcellular water (TCW)? What is its importance?**
   TCW is water formed by cellular transport activities and located in various ducts and spaces throughout the body. This water includes cerebrospinal fluid (CSF) and aqueous humor; secretions in the sweat, salivary, and lacrimal glands; secretions in pancreas, liver, biliary, gastrointestinal, and respiratory tracts; and peritoneal, pleural, and synovial fluids.

4. **Explain the significance of TCW.**
   TCW carries secretions to specific sites for enzymatic and lubricant activity and is normally quite small, =1.5% of body weight. In disease states, excess or deficiency of TCW can cause dysfunction. Marked excess TCW formation—third spacing—may decrease effective circulating

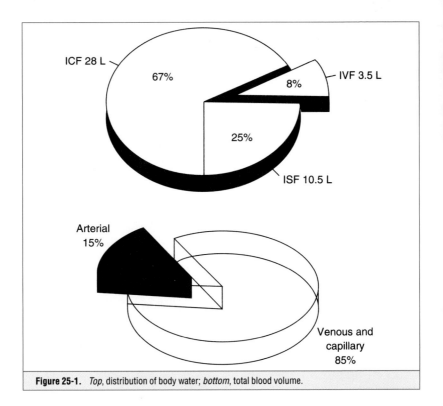

Figure 25-1. *Top,* distribution of body water; *bottom,* total blood volume.

volume (ECV), stimulate antidiuretic hormone (ADH) and aldosterone release, increase retention of salt and water, and cause hyponatremia.

5. **What controls distribution of body water?**
   With few exceptions (e.g., ascending loop of Henle [LOH] and distal nephron), water moves freely across cell membranes, depending on tonicity. Because tonicity depends on impermeable solutes, such as sodium (Na), disorders of water metabolism are reflected by changes in solute concentrations. In addition to changes in water distribution, changes in TBW, blood volume, and ECV also affect overall water balance. A thorough understanding of disorders of water metabolism requires a clear understanding of changes in plasma Na concentration (P_{Na}), plasma osmolality (P_{osm}), and ECV.

6. **What is ECV?**
   ECV is the arterial volume required to maintain *normal baroreceptor pressure* that is appropriate for a given level of vascular resistance. ECV is also called effective arterial blood volume (EABV). By inducing changes in baroreceptor tone, alterations in ECV have a major impact on water balance. Low ECV causes renal salt and water retention, whereas high ECV causes renal salt and water loss. Depending on the patient's water intake, these changes may produce significant hyponatremia. Maintaining normal ECV preserves circulatory homeostasis.

7. **How do baroreceptors affect ECV?**
   Baroreceptors are the major sensors of changes in ECV (Fig. 25-2). However, their main role is to maintain normal pressure (not volume) at the level of the baroreceptor sensors located

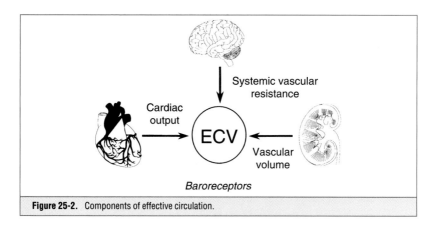

Figure 25-2. Components of effective circulation.

primarily in the carotid sinus, aortic arch, atria, pulmonary veins, and afferent renal arterioles. These anatomic locations are important because perfusion to these areas affects the three main effectors of circulatory homeostasis and ECV: brain, heart, and kidneys.

8. **How does vascular pressure as sensed by the baroreceptors relate to ECV and hyponatremia?**
   Baroreceptors normally have tonic inhibition of vasoconstrictor nerves and natriuretic hormone release but tonic stimulation of vagal cardiac nerves. A drop in ECV decreases effective vascular pressure (EVP), baroreceptor tone, tonic inhibition, and tonic stimulation. This causes vasoconstriction; increases heart rate; and increases renin, aldosterone, angiotensin II, and ADH secretion. It decreases atrial natriuretic peptide (ANP), brain natriuretic peptide (BNP; atrial and ventricle), and urodilatin (kidney). These alterations enhance renal Na and water retention. If the patient receives free water, these changes may lead to hyponatremia. Hyponatremia cannot develop unless the patient retains more water than is excreted. Decreased ECV/EVP predisposes to water retention, but the patient must receive free water to develop hyponatremia. The venous system, via atrial stretch receptors, has similar effects but responds to changes in ECV earlier than the arterial system.

9. **Define osmolality and tonicity and outline their effects on water movement.**
   Osmolality is the concentration of the substance in 1 L of water divided by its molecular weight. Tonicity is effective osmolality—the osmotic pressure caused by dissolved particles restricted to one side of the cell membrane. Because Na and glucose are partially restricted to the ECF, they are effective osmols and account for normal tonicity. Mannitol, sorbitol, glycerol, and glycine are also effective osmols. Urea freely crosses cell membranes and distributes evenly in TBW, and therefore changes osmolality but not tonicity. Thus, except during early and rapid solute and water changes, urea is an ineffective osmol. Ethanol and methanol are other ineffective osmols. Water always moves across cell membranes from lower osmolality to higher osmolality until osmolality on both sides is equal. At equilibrium, the following is always true:

$$\text{ICF osmolality} = \text{ECF osmolality} = P_{osm}$$

10. **What formulas are useful in evaluating osmolality and tonicity?**

$$\text{ECF osmolality} = 2P_{Na} + \text{glucose}/18 + \text{blood urea nitrogen (BUN)}/2.8$$

$$\text{normal osmolality} = 2(140) + 90/18 + 14/2.8 = 280 + 5 + 5 = 290 \text{ mOsm/kg}$$

$$\text{ECF tonicity (effective osmolality)} = 2P_{Na} + \text{glucose}/18$$

$$\text{normal tonicity} = 2(140) + 90/18 = 280 + 5 = 285 \text{ mOsm/kg}$$

The normal range for P_{osm} of 275–295 mOsm/kg varies with the normal ranges for plasma Na, urea, and glucose. Correction factors for other effective solutes (osmols) are mannitol/18, sorbitol/18, and glycerol/9. Correction factors for other ineffective solutes (osmols) are ethanol/4.6 and methanol/3.2.

11. **How does P_{Na} relate to TBW?**
    The following formulas are useful in understanding the relationship of P_{Na}, plasma potassium (P_K), total body sodium and potassium [$Na^+ + K^+$], and TBW. [$Na^+ + K^+$] estimates total body solute:
    1. $P_{Na} \cong \text{total body } [Na^+ + K^+]/\text{TBW}$
    2. $\text{TBW} \cong [Na^+ + K^+]/P_{Na}$
    3. $P_{Na} \cong P_{osm} \cong [\text{total body osmolality}] \cong [\text{total body solutes}] \cong 1/\text{TBW}$
    Thus, P_{Na} is proportional to [$Na^+ + K^+$] and inversely proportional to TBW. An increase or decrease in total plasma Na particles can proportionately change the P_{Na}. However, in clinical medicine, *changes in P_{Na} usually reflect changes in plasma water.* When P_{Na} is high, plasma water is low. When P_{Na} is low, plasma water is high.

12. **How does P_K relate to P_{Na} and TBW?**
    Although 98% of K^+ is intracellular, a K^+ infusion increases P_{Na}. This occurs as follows. In hypokalemia, infused K^+ enters cells. To preserve electroneutrality, Na^+ leaves cells or chloride (Cl^-) enters. ECF water follows K^+ and Cl^- into cells due to increased ICF osmolality. Both mechanisms increase P_{Na}. Hypokalemic patients infused with equal amounts of KCl or NaCl will have equal increases in P_{Na}. Thus, addition of KCl to isotonic saline makes hypertonic saline, and infusion of saline with KCl may correct hyponatremia too rapidly (see questions 36 and 44).

13. **Describe the input and output of water.**
    TBW is a balance of input (including endogenous production) and output. In an average adult, input approximates 1600 mL (liquids), 700 mL (foods), and 200 mL (metabolic oxidation of carbohydrate and fat) for a total of 2500 mL/day. Average water losses are 1500 mL (kidneys), 500 mL (skin [400 mL evaporation and 100 mL perspiration]), 300 mL (lung—respiration), and 200 mL from the gastrointestinal tract (stool) for a total of 2500 mL/day. Large losses of water (increased output) occur with excessive sweating, respiration (exercise), burns, diarrhea, vomiting, and diuresis. Decreased water input occurs when defects in thirst and altered mental or physical function (especially in the elderly) prevent access to water.

14. **What are the normal limits of urine output?**
    Water intake and osmotic products of metabolism determine the usual daily output of urine. On a normal diet, a normal adult must excrete 800–1000 mOsm of solute per day. The range of normal renal concentrating function is 50–1200 mOsm/kg. Based on this fact, the obligate water excretion varies from 0.8 to 20 L/day. The calculations are as follows:

    $$1000 \text{ mOsm}/1200 \text{ mOsm/kg} = 0.8 \text{ L/day at maximal concentration}$$

    $$1000 \text{ mOsm}/50 \text{ mOsm/kg} = 20 \text{ L/day at maximal dilution}$$

    Note that higher solute loads (e.g., dietary) require more water excretion. Thus, low solute intake (starvation) with high water intake predisposes to water retention and water intoxication. This combination exists in binge beer drinkers, in whom the solute load may be only 300 mOsm/day. The range of urine output would drop to 0.25–6 L/day in such patients.

15. **What are the main factors controlling water metabolism?**
    Thirst, hormonal, and renal mechanisms are tightly integrated for control of water metabolism.

16. **What are the stimuli of thirst?**

Osmoreceptors in the organum vasculosum of the anterior hypothalamus control thirst. Increasing plasma tonicity stimulates thirst at a threshold about 5 mOsm/kg higher than that which stimulates ADH release. However, oropharyngeal receptors are also important in thirst regulation. A dry mouth increases thirst. Drinking and swallowing water decrease thirst even without changing P_{osm}. Volume depletion changes afferent baroreceptor input and increases angiotensin II—both changes increase thirst. An unusual idiosyncratic effect of angiotensin-converting enzyme (ACE) inhibitors causes central polydipsia, increased ADH release, and propensity to hyponatremia.

17. **What hormonal mechanisms are involved in control of body water?**

Although natriuretic peptides, aldosterone, prostaglandins, angiotensin II, and neurohumoral changes affect renal retention and excretion water, ADH is most important. Supraoptic and paraventricular nuclei in the hypothalamus secrete ADH in response to increased osmolality and decreased volume. ADH attaches to vasopressin 2 (V_2) receptors on the basolateral membrane of collecting tubular cells. This activates cyclic adenosine monophosphate (cAMP) and protein kinase, causing intracellular water channels called aquaporins (AQPs) to insert into the luminal membrane. Water moves down osmotic gradients from tubular lumen through AQP channels into the cell and interstitium. At least six AQP isoforms are present in the kidney. The collecting duct has high concentrations of AQP2 that serve as the major target for ADH-mediated water reabsorption. Abnormalities of the V_2 receptor cause most cases of nephrogenic diabetes insipidus (DI), but some are caused by abnormalities of AQP2. Increased AQP2 may cause water retention in conditions, such as pregnancy and congestive heart failure. Twenty percent of ADH receptors in the collecting tubular cells are vasopressin 1 (V_1) receptors. ADH activates V_1 receptors only at very high ADH levels. This increases prostaglandin E_2 (PGE_2) and prostacyclin that opposes the antidiuretic effects of excessive ADH.

18. **What are the major conditions that influence ADH secretion?**

ADH functions to maintain osmotic and volume homeostasis. Secretion starts at an osmotic threshold of 280 mOsm/kg and increases proportionately to further rises in tonicity. A 1–2% increase in osmolality stimulates ADH secretion, whereas a 10% drop in vascular volume is required for the same effect. By action on baroreceptors, increased ECV raises the osmotic threshold for ADH secretion and decreased ECV lowers this threshold. Severe volume depletion and hypotension may completely override the hypo-osmotic inhibition of ADH secretion. This finding has been called the *law of circulating volume*. In severe volume depletion and hypotension, ADH secretion continues despite low osmolality, thereby worsening the hyponatremia. Nausea, pain, and stress (as seen postoperatively) are also potent stimuli of ADH release and may produce life-threatening hyponatremia if hypotonic fluid is given. This is particularly true if associated with drugs that potentiate release or action of ADH.

19. **What are the major causes of ADH secretion?**

Major causes of ADH secretion include hyperosmolality, hypovolemia, nausea, pain, stress, human chorionic gonadotropin as in pregnancy, hypoglycemia, corticotropin-releasing hormone (CRH)/ADH release, central nervous system (CNS) infections, CNS tumors, vascular catastrophes (thrombosis, hemorrhage), and ectopic ADH of malignancy (carcinomas of lung [primarily small cell], duodenum, pancreas, ureter, bladder, and prostate, and lymphoma). ADH secretion may be increased by any major pulmonary disorder, including pneumonia, tuberculosis, asthma, atelectasis, cystic fibrosis, positive pressure ventilation, and adult respiratory distress syndrome. HIV infection may have the multifactorial role of causing CNS dysfunction, pulmonary disease, and malignancy. Excessive exogenous ADH or desmopressin acetate (DDAVP) in patients with DI directly increases ADH effect. Oxytocin also has significant ADH activity in the large doses used to induce labor. Other drugs that affect ADH secretion and action are listed in Table 25-2.

TABLE 25-2.   DRUGS THAT AFFECT ADH SECRETION AND ACTION[*]

Increase ADH Secretion	Increase ADH Effect	Decrease ADH Secretion	Decrease ADH Effect	SIADH Unknown
Bromocriptine	Acetaminophen	Ethanol	Demeclocycline	Amitriptyline
Carbamazepine	Carbamazepine	Phenytoin	Lithium	Fluphenazine
Chlorpropamide	Chlorpropamide		Acetohexamide	Haloperidol
Clofibrate	Cyclophosphamide		Tolazamide	SSRIs[†]
Cyclophosphamide	NSAIDs[‡]		Glyburide	Fluoxetine
Ifosfamide	Tolbutamide		Methoxyflurane	MAOIs[§]
Morphine			Propoxyphene	Phenothiazines
Nicotine			Colchicine	Butyrophenones
Thioridazine			Amphotericin	Ecstasy
Vincristine			Vinblastine	
			PGE_2	
			Prostacyclin	

[*]Because psychosis itself may cause syndrome of inappropriate secretion of ADH (SIADH), one must question the true ADH stimulatory effect of the antipsychotic drugs. Changes in ADH secretion may be direct or indirect.
[†]Selective serotonin reuptake inhibitors.
[‡]Nonsteroidal antiinflammatory drugs.
[§]Monoamine oxidase inhibitors.

20. **How does the kidney handle salt and water?**
To control excess or deficiency of water intake, there must be adequate glomerular filtration rate (GFR) and delivery of filtrate to the LOH and distal nephron. Solute is separated from water in the ascending limb of the LOH, distal convoluted tubule (DCT), and cortical connecting segment; normal action of ADH allows controlled reabsorption of water in the cortical and medullary collecting tubules (CCT and MCT). The proximal convoluted tubule (PCT) reabsorbs 65% and the descending limb of the LOH 25% of filtered solute and water isotonically. The ascending limb is impermeable to water but removes solute that dilutes the luminal filtrate, concentrates the interstitium (important for ADH action), and delivers 10% of the filtrate to the CCT with osmolality of 100 mOsm/kg. In the absence of ADH, this fluid (about 18 L/day) would be lost in the urine and cause marked dehydration. In the presence of ADH, the collecting duct becomes permeable to water and reabsorbs all but 1% of the filtrate. Thus, the final urine volume is only 1.5–2.0 L/day. Because normal GFR is 125 mL/minute, the normal kidneys filter 180 L of plasma each day and reabsorb 99%.

21. **What are the consequences and causes of decreased renal excretion of water?**
Any reduction in water excretion predisposes to hyponatremia and hypo-osmolality. Conditions that impair GFR, delivery of tubular fluid to the distal nephron, ability of the distal nephron to separate solute from water, or that increase the permeability of the collecting tubule to water will impair water excretion. Such conditions include renal failure, decreased ECV, diuretics (thiazides loop), and excessive ADH or ADH action.

22. **How do hypothyroidism and adrenal insufficiency cause hyponatremia?**
Hypothyroidism and adrenal insufficiency decrease cardiac output. Adrenal insufficiency also causes volume depletion and decreased blood pressure. The resulting decreased ECV lowers GFR, which reduces delivery of filtrate to the distal nephron and enhances proximal tubular water reabsorption. Decreased ECV also stimulates secretion of ADH, further promoting water reabsorption. Normally, CRH and ADH are cosecreted from the same neurons in the paraventricular nuclei of the hypothalamus, and both hormones work synergistically to release ACTH from the anterior pituitary. Cortisol then feeds back negatively at the hypothalamus and pituitary to inhibit the release of both CRH and ADH. Cortisol deficiency decreases this negative feedback and increases ADH levels to enhance further water reabsorption. Although hyponatremia may occur with both primary and secondary adrenal insufficiency, it occurs more commonly in primary adrenal insufficiency. This emphasizes the importance of aldosterone deficiency in the pathogenesis of the hyponatremia. Aldosterone deficiency directly causes salt wasting and volume depletion and thus indirectly increases ADH secretion. All of these events combined with continued water intake strongly contribute to the resulting hyponatremia.

KEY POINTS: WATER METABOLISM ✓

1. Rapid changes in body water or distribution can cause severe neurologic dysfunction and are reflected clinically by hyponatremia or hypernatremia.

2. Treatment requires a clear understanding of changes in plasma sodium, plasma osmolality, and effective circulating volume.

3. Water always moves across cell membranes from lower to higher osmolality.

4. This movement is determined by the concentration of effective osmotic solute in the intracellular or extracellular fluid and is responsible for neurologic symptoms and signs.

5. Water content of the body is a balance of input and output.

6. Balance is controlled by thirst, access to water, solute intake, ADH, cortisol, aldosterone, natriuretic peptides, renal receptors for hormone action, renal water channels called AQPs, level of kidney function, and drugs.

23. **What P_{Na} concentrations are causes for concern?**
The severity of hyponatremia or hypernatremia depends on the rapidity of development. Normal P_{Na} ranges from 136 to 145 mEq/L. Patients with a P_{Na} of 115 or 165 mEq/L may not show any clinical abnormalities if they develop the problem over days to weeks. However, both conditions may produce major neurologic dysfunction if they develop over hours to days. As a rule, however, Na concentrations of 120–155 mEq/L are not usually associated with symptoms. P_{Na} outside these limits and occasionally rapidly developing disturbances within these limits may be of major concern. With appropriate care, patients with P_{Na} as low as 85 mEq/L and as high as 274 mEq/L have survived without permanent sequelae.

24. **What causes the symptoms and signs of increased or decreased TBW?**
The main symptoms and signs of too much (decreased P_{Na}) or too little (increased P_{Na}) TBW result from brain swelling or contraction. If changes in TBW occur more rapidly than the brain can adapt, symptoms and signs will occur. The severity of the symptoms and signs depends on the degree and rapidity of the TBW change. Once adaptation occurs, correcting the disturbance in body water too rapidly may be more deleterious than the initial disturbance.

25. **What are the symptoms and signs of hyponatremia and hypernatremia?**
Hyponatremia: Headache, confusion, muscle cramps, weakness, lethargy, confusion, apathy, agitation, nausea, vomiting, anorexia, altered levels of consciousness, seizures, depressed deep tendon reflexes, hypothermia, Cheyne-Stokes respiration, respiratory depression, coma, and death.
    Hypernatremia: Weakness, irritability, lethargy, confusion, somnolence, muscle twitching, seizures, respiratory depression, paralysis, and death.

26. **How does the brain adapt to hyponatremia?**
Because ICF and ECF osmolality must always be equal, developing hyponatremia immediately shifts water into the brain, increasing intracranial pressure (ICP). The increased ICP causes loss of NaCl into the CSF. Over the next several hours, there is also loss of intracellular K and over the next few days, loss of organic solute. These changes return the brain volume to normal. However, if severe hyponatremia occurs too rapidly, there is not enough time for cerebral adaptation. Brain edema occurs, further increasing ICP; the brain herniates and the patient dies.

27. **How does the brain adapt to hypernatremia?**
With acute hypernatremia and increased P_{osm}, water immediately shifts out of the brain and decreases ICP. The decreased ICP promotes movement of CSF with NaCl into the brain ICF, partially correcting volume. Within hours, further brain adaptation occurs, increasing brain ICF K^+, Na^+, and Cl^-. The resulting increase in osmolality pulls water from the ECF and restores about 60% of the brain volume. Over the next several days, the brain accumulates organic solutes (osmolites), previously called idiogenic osmoles, that return the brain volume to a near-normal level. These solutes include glutamine, taurine, glutamate, myoinositol, and phosphocreatine. If the brain has no time to adapt to rapidly developing hypernatremia, it will shrink, retract from the dura, and tear vessels, causing intracranial hemorrhage, increased ICP, compressive injury, herniation, and death.

28. **How should you approach the patient with hyponatremia?**
Hyponatremia occurs in > 3% of hospitalized patients and always means too much ECF water relative to Na. Because total body volume is proportional to total body Na, a thorough assessment of the patient's volume status helps rational selection of therapy. Patients with flat neck veins and postural changes in blood pressure and pulse (standing blood pressure decreases > 20/10 mmHg and pulse increases > 20 beats/minute) are invariably saline (isotonic NaCl) depleted. Patients with distended neck veins and edema are saline overloaded. Always direct treatment at correcting the underlying disorder (Table 25-3). If patients have lost saline, give them saline. If they have retained too much water, restrict their water. If they have retained too much salt and water but more water than salt, restrict their salt and water but water more than salt. It sounds simple, and it is.

29. **Explain the importance of an initial thorough volume assessment.**
The difficulty is remembering the importance of and performing an initial thorough volume assessment. Assess the patient's volume by looking at neck veins, postural signs, and edema. At times, the best clinician cannot get a good assessment of ECV, but central monitoring with a Swan-Ganz catheter is rarely necessary. Urinary Na and edema are clues to ECV. Get an initial weight and assess weight daily. Continue assessment of postural signs as needed. Initially, obtain P_{osm}, general chemistry panel (Na, K, Cl, CO_2, Cr, BUN, glucose, albumin, Ca, Mg), and urinary Na, Cl, Cr, and fractional excretion of Na. Approach therapy as outlined in Table 25-4.

30. **How should you characterize and diagnose the patient with SIADH?**
Hyponatremia is the tip-off to SIADH. Approach the patient as in question 28. It is important to establish normovolemia by physical examination. Then measure P_{osm}, U_{osm}, P_{Na}, U_{Na}, and U_K. Finally, exclude pituitary, adrenal, and thyroid dysfunction before diagnosis. Confirmatory

TABLE 25-3. CAUSES OF HYPONATREMIA

Pathophysiology	Associated Conditions
Renal saline loss	Diuretics
	Primary adrenal insufficiency
	Renal tubular acidosis
	Salt-losing nephritis
Nonrenal saline loss	Vomiting
	Diarrhea
	Pancreatitis, rhabdomyolysis, burns
Water excess	SIADH
	Secondary adrenal insufficiency
	Hypothyroidism
Saline excess with decreased ECV	Congestive heart failure
	Cirrhosis
	Nephrotic syndrome
Saline excess without decreased ECV	Acute renal failure
	Chronic renal failure

Hyponatremia always means too much plasma water relative to Na. Volume assessment is crucial. Volume loss = saline loss. Water excess usually means normal saline volume, but an excess in water sufficient to produce a mild excess of volume that stimulates baroreceptor activity.

TABLE 25-4. APPROACH TO HYPONATREMIA

Condition	Postural Signs	Edema	U_{Na}	Treatment
Renal saline loss	Yes	No	> 20	Give isotonic saline
Nonrenal saline loss	Yes	No	< 10	Give isotonic saline
Water excess	No	No	> 20	Restrict water
Na and water excess	No	Yes	< 10	Restrict water > salt
Na and water excess	No	Yes	> 20	Restrict water > salt

Because P_{Na} is usually measured with ion-selective electrodes, artifactual lowering of the P_{Na} is now unusual. If your lab does not use ion-selective electrodes, marked hyperlipidemia or hyperproteinemia may produce pseudohyponatremia. Notwithstanding, measured P_{osm} will differentiate these disorders. Because P_{osm} measures the osmotic activity of plasma water and because plasma water excludes lipids and proteins contribute little to P_{osm}, the measured P_{osm} will be essentially normal in pseudohyponatremia.

criteria of SIADH include P_{Na} (< 135 mEq/L), low P_{osm} (< 280 mOsm/kg), U_{osm} > 100 mOsm/kg, U_{Na} > 40 mEq/L, and $[U_{Na} + U_K] > P_{Na}$. Patients with SIADH are usually said to have normal volume status. However, they actually have excessive TBW. Unlike excessive saline, which is limited to ECF, excessive water distributes two-thirds to the ICF and one-third to the ECF. Thus, the ECF excess is minor and not usually perceptible by clinical examination. Nonetheless, patients with SIADH have mildly increased ECV, which is sensed by the kidney. The kidney increases GFR, which causes a low uric acid, BUN, and creatinine. The increased ECV also increases ANP and along with increased GFR promotes natriuresis. These are the classic findings in SIADH. Obviously, SIADH does not protect against dehydration and other conditions that can obscure the classic presentation. For example, a patient with ectopic ADH from lung cancer may present with dehydration from diarrhea and lack of water intake from debilitation. In this instance, the U_{Na} and U_{Cl} may be less than 10 mEq/L.

31. **How do you treat the patient with SIADH?**

Initially, treat SIADH with water restriction. If the patient has marked symptoms, treat for symptomatic hyponatremia (see question 40). Also, attempt to correct the underlying abnormality (see questions 18 and 19). If the patient has unresectable cancer and water restriction (500–1500 mL/day) is not tolerated, give demeclocycline, 600–1200 mg/day, or lithium carbonate, 600–1200 mg/day, in two to four divided doses. Because lithium carbonate can cause neurologic, cardiovascular, and other toxicities, avoid it unless there are no other therapeutic options. Demeclocycline may cause severe renal failure in patients with cirrhosis. Thus, it is contraindicated in patients with cirrhosis and severe liver disease. A high Na diet (4–8 gm) may be necessary in addition to water restriction to correct the hyponatremia.

32. **What are the four patterns of SIADH?**

The four patterns of SIADH are distinguished according to responses of ADH to P_{osm}:

Type I	Erratic ADH secretion with no predictable response to Posm (20% of cases)
Type II	Reset osmostat with normal relationship of ADH to P_{osm} but a lower threshold for ADS release (e.g., 250–260 mOsm/kg) (35% of cases)
Type III	ADH leak with selective loss of ADH suppression and continued secretion when P_{osm} is low but normal suppression and secretion when P_{osm} is normal (35% of cases)
Type 1V	ADH-dissociated antidiuresis at low P_{osm} with appropriately low or undetectable ADH (possibly from increased renal sensitivity to ADH or unknown ADH-like substance) (10% of cases)

33. **Define polyuria and list the main causes.**

Polyuria is a urine output > 3.0 L/day. Four main disorders cause polyuria: psychogenic polydipsia (psychosis), dipsogenic DI (defect in thirst center), central neurogenic DI (defect in ADH secretion), and nephrogenic DI (defect in ADH action on the kidney). All forms of DI may be partial or complete. Polyuria also may occur from osmotic diuresis in such conditions as diabetes mellitus (glucose), recovery from renal failure (urea), and IV infusions (saline, mannitol). See Table 25-2 for drugs and conditions that decrease ADH secretion and action. Causes of acquired nephrogenic DI include chronic renal disease, electrolyte abnormalities (hypokalemia and hypercalcemia), drugs (lithium, demeclocycline), sickle-cell disease (damaged medullary interstitium), diet (increased water and decreased solute—beer, starvation), inflammatory or infiltrative renal disease (multiple myeloma, amyloidosis, sarcoidosis), and others.

34. **How do you distinguish polyuric patients with the various forms of DI from excessive water drinking?**

In excessive water drinking the P_{Na}, BUN, and uric acid are relatively low. In DI, the P_{Na} and uric acid are relatively high and the BUN is relatively low. Central DI often has an abrupt onset due to loss of a critical amount of arginine vasopressin (AVP) resulting from destruction of > 80–90% of the ADH-secreting hypothalamic neurons at a critical point in time. However, the diagnosis of polyuria is not always clear from the history and lab tests. In that case, perform a water restriction test (WRT). Other names for the WRT are dehydration test and water deprivation test. The test may take 6–18 hours depending on the initial state of hydration.

35. **How is the WRT performed?**
    1. Office testing is acceptable unless the patient cannot be watched closely—then hospitalization may be required.
    2. Measure *baseline* weight, P_{osm}, P_{Na}, P_{BUN}, $P_{glucose}$, U_{volume}, U_{osm}, U_{Na}, and U_K. Measure *hourly* weight and U_{osm}.
    3. Allow no food or water.
    4. Watch the patient closely for signs of dehydration and surreptitious water drinking.
    5. End the WRT when U_{osm} has not increased more than 30 mOsm/kg for three consecutive hours, P_{osm} has reached 295–300 mOsm/kg, or the patient has lost 3–5% of body weight. If weight loss exceeds 3–5% of body weight, further dehydration is unsafe.
    6. At P_{osm} of 295–300 mOsm/kg, endogenous ADH levels should be $= 5$ pg/mL, and the kidney should respond with maximal urinary concentration.
    7. Repeat all baseline tests toward and at the end of the WRT.
    8. Give 5 units of aqueous AVP or 2 µg of DDAVP subcutaneously.
    9. Repeat the baseline tests at 30, 60, and 120 minutes.
    10. Calculate U_{osm}/P_{osm} and $[U_{Na} + U_K]/P_{Na}$ as a check on measured U_{osm}/P_{osm}.

36. **How do you interpret the results of the WRT?**
    Table 25-5 summarizes the expected results of the WRT. The WRT stimulates maximal endogenous release of ADH by increasing P_{osm} and evaluates the concentrating ability of the kidney by measuring U_{osm}. Giving exogenous ADH allows evaluation of the renal concentrating response to ADH if dehydration-induced ADH production was impaired. Save frozen baseline and end-test plasma to measure ADH if results are equivocal. Expected normal values for P_{ADH} are $= 0.5$ pg/mL for $P_{osm} \leq 280$ mOsm/kg and ≥ 5 pg/mL for $P_{osm} = 295$ mOsm/kg.

TABLE 25-5. VALUES BEFORE AND AFTER WATER RESTRICTION

	Pre P_{osm}	Pre P_{Na}	Post U_{osm}/P_{osm}	Post U_{osm}/P_{osm} + ADH	Post P_{ADH}
Normals	NL	NL	>1	>1 (<10%)	↑
PPD/DDI	↓	↓	>1	>1 (<10%)	↑ on NL
CCDI	↑	↑	<1	>1 (>50%)	–
PCDI	↑	↑	>1	>1 (10–50%)	↓
CNDI	↑	↑	<1	<1 (<10%)	↑↑
PNDI	↑	↑	>1	>1 (<10%)	↑↑

PPD/DDI, psychogenic polydipsia/dipsogenic DI; CCDI, complete central DI; PCDI, partial central DI; CNDI, complete nephrogenic DI; PNDI, partial nephrogenic DI. Relative to the normal range, the down and up arrows, respectively, mean low or low normal and high or high normal values for P_{osm}, P_{Na}, and P_{ADH}. Recall that when $U_{osm} > P_{osm}$, there is antidiuresis and the kidney is retaining free water. The same is true when $[U_{Na} + U_K] > P_{Na}$, and these tests are more easily obtainable. When $U_{osm} < P_{osm}$ or $[U_{Na} + U_K] < P_{Na}$, there is net loss of free water with little net clinical ADH effect. The value in parentheses indicates the percentage change in U_{osm} (not the U_{osm}/P_{osm} ratio) after 5 units of subcutaneous aqueous vasopressin or 2 µg of DDAVP.

37. **What are the expected plasma ADH concentrations and urinary osmolality in polyuric patients after water restriction?**
    See Table 25-6.

TABLE 25-6.	EXPECTED VALUES FOR ADH AND U_{osm} AFTER WATER RESTRICTION	
Cause of Polyuria	ADH (pg/mL)	U_{osm} (mOsm/kg)
Normal	> 2	> 800
Primary polydipsia	< 5	> 500
Complete central DI	Undetectable	< 300
Partial central DI	< 1.5	300–800
Nephrogenic DI	> 5	300–500

38. How should you approach the patient with hypernatremia?

Problems of hypernatremia are uncommon compared with hyponatremia and occur in < 1% of hospitalized patients. Loss of water, not gain of Na, usually causes hypernatremia (Table 25-7). However, unless patients have an abnormality of thirst or do not have access to water, they usually maintain near-normal P_{Na} by drinking water in proportion to losses. As in questions 28 and 29, assess the patient's volume status. Once lab studies are obtained, approach the patient according to Table 25-8. If the patient has polyuria, also include the approach in questions 33 and 34.

39. How should you diagnose and manage the patient with DI?

DI is a syndrome of excessive water loss by the kidney due to decreased ADH (central DI) or renal unresponsiveness to ADH (nephrogenic DI). Therefore, the hallmark of DI is polyuria. Mild hypernatremia, a low BUN, and a relatively high uric acid are suggestive of DI. In idiopathic central DI, magnetic resonance imaging (MRI) of the pituitary shows absence of the normal pituitary bright spot. However, the pituitary bright spot decreases with age and may be absent in a majority of the elderly without DI. An abrupt onset of polyuria is also suggestive of central DI since 80–90% of the ADH-secreting neurons must be lost prior to polyuria and very little ADH is needed to have some urinary concentration. As in questions 33 and 34, first distinguish primary polydipsia from DI and identify the DI as central or nephrogenic. Then give water to prevent dehydration until the evaluation suggests definitive therapy. A patient with DI will probably self-treat with water unless there is a thirst deficit or the patient has no access to water.

40. How quickly should you correct states of water excess or deficiency?

The main concern of therapy for abnormal TBW is to prevent devastating neurologic complications. Understanding brain adaptation to changes in TBW, as outlined in questions 25 and 26, emphasizes the need for urgent therapy only in the symptomatic patient. There are three useful rules in treating disturbances of water (measured by changes in P_{Na}):

1. Return the P_{Na} to normal at the relative speed that it became abnormal. If the change in P_{Na} was slow (days), correct it slowly (days). If the change was rapid (minutes to hours), correct it rapidly (minutes to hours).
2. If there are no symptoms of water or Na imbalance (see question 24), there is no immediate urgency. If there are symptoms, there is urgency. Questions 25 and 26 outline the brain adaptations to altered tonicity that may cause devastating changes in brain volume. These adaptations also cause the patient's symptoms. Thus, symptoms should drive the clinician to correct the altered tonicity rapidly.
3. The degree of rapid P_{Na} correction should be *toward normal* (until symptoms abate) not *to* normal.

The above concepts of speed, symptoms, and degree of P_{Na} correction apply for both hyponatremia and hypernatremia.

TABLE 25-7. CAUSES OF HYPERNATREMIA

Pathophysiology	Associated Condition
Low total body Na and H_2O with H_2O loss > Na loss	Renal Na and H_2O loss
	Osmotic diuretics
	Loop diuretics
	Renal disease
	Postobstructive diuresis
	Osmotic diarrhea
	Vomiting
	Nonrenal Na and H_2O loss
	Sweating
	Diarrhea
	Burns
High total body Na	Hyperaldosteronism
	Cushing's syndrome
	Excessive intake of NaCl or $NaHCO_3$
	Hypertonic saline and bicarbonate
	Hypertonic dialysis
Normal total body Na with excessive H_2O loss	Renal water losses
	Central DI
	Nephrogenic DI
	Nonrenal Na and H_2O loss
	Increased sensible loss
	No access to H_2O

Hypernatremia always means too little plasma water relative to Na. With access to water, hypernatremia usually does not occur or is mild. However, unattended patients who are too old, too young, or too sick may not have adequate access to water, and hypernatremia may be severe.

TABLE 25-8. APPROACH TO HYPERNATREMIA

Condition	Postural Signs	Edema	U_{Na}	U_{osm}	Treatment
Renal Na and H_2O loss	Yes	No	> 20	↓–	Give isotonic saline
Nonrenal Na and H_2O loss	Yes	No	< 10	↑	Give isotonic saline
Na excess	No	No	> 20	↑–	Restrict water
Renal H_2O excess	No	No	VAR	↓↑–	Restrict water > salt
Nonrenal H_2O loss	No	No	VAR	↑	Restrict water > salt

VAR, variable; ↑, hypertonic; ↓, hypotonic; –, isosmotic.

KEY POINTS: SYNDROMES AND TREATMENT OF WATER DYSFUNCTION ✓

1. Clinical syndromes of water dysfunction include SIADH, DI, and changes in effective circulating volume that can cause marked retention of salt and water, pulmonary and peripheral edema, and severe neurologic dysfunction.

2. Effective correction of water problems requires a thorough assessment of volume and neurologic symptoms.

3. If symptoms are present, correction must be rapid; if absent, there is no urgency and correction should occur more slowly.

4. Depending on the water disturbance, treatment includes water restriction or administration; hypertonic, isotonic, or hypotonic saline; sodium; diuretics; antidiuretic hormone; and other medications.

41. **How do frequent measurements of urinary Na and K help with hyponatremia therapy?**

    Initial assessments for Na repletion, as outlined in question 47, do not account for urinary water and electrolyte losses that may alter the expected P_{Na} response to therapy. Therefore, replace urinary losses for more accurate correction of P_{Na}. Initially, measure the U_{Na} and U_K and urine volume every 1–2 hours, and replace urine volume with saline of appropriate strength. For example, if the urinary volume was 100 mL/h, the U_{Na} = 43 mEq/L and the U_K = 35 mEq/L, the sum of $U_{Na} + U_K$ = 78 mEq/L at 100 mL/h. In this case, replacing urinary losses with 0.45% saline (77 mEq/L NaCl) IV at 100 mL/h will prevent major deviations in P_{Na} from the value calculated. Give this replacement fluid in addition to that calculated to correct the P_{Na}. KCl replacement depends on serum K. Replace K to correct the serum K to normal, remembering that K replacement will increase P_{Na}. Therefore, decrease the replacement Na by the amount of K given. Some evidence also suggests that hypokalemia may predispose to osmotic demyelination. Therefore, correcting serum K may decrease this risk.

42. **What are vasopressin receptor antagonists? How might they change the future of hyponatremia therapy?**

    The conventional treatment of hyponatremia is water restriction or saline administration. In the future, vasopressin receptor antagonists that are selective for the V_2 (antidiuretic) receptor will provide more effective therapy for hyponatremia. These agents are now being tested in humans and produce a selective water diuresis with no effect on Na and K excretion. The term *aquaretic drugs* (aquaretics) has been coined for these medications to highlight their different mechanisms of action compared with the saluretic diuretic furosemide. They will prove beneficial in SIADH and in hyponatremic patients with congestive heart failure and cirrhosis. By blocking ADH effect, rapid correction of hyponatremia may occur; therefore, judicious monitoring of P_{Na} changes is important to prevent excessively rapid correction of the serum Na concentration.

43. **What is the appropriate P_{Na} correction factor for hyperglycemia?**

    The standard correction factor is a 1.6-mEq/L decrease in P_{Na} for each 100-mg/dL increase in plasma glucose concentration above 100 mg/dL. For glucose values greater than 400 mg/dL, recent data suggest a correction factor as high as a 4.0-mEq/L decrease in P_{Na} for each 100 mg/dL increase in plasma glucose and an average correction factor of 2.4 mEq/L.

CLINICAL PROBLEMS IN WATER METABOLISM

44. **A 75-year-old woman presents with confusion but no focal neurologic signs. She has type 2 diabetes mellitus. Blood pressure is 110/54 mmHg. Pulse is 96 beats/minute. Neck veins are not visualized in the supine position. $P_{glucose}$ = 900 mg/dL, P_{Na} = 135 mEq/L, plasma creatinine = 3.0 mg/dL, BUN = 50 mg/dL, U_{Na} = 40 mEq/L, urine glucose is 4+ and ketones 3+. Describe her fluid and volume status and treatment.**

Glucose remains in the ECF because of insulin deficiency and increases ECF tonicity. Increased tonicity pulls water from the ICF to the ECF, concentrating the ICF and diluting the ECF until ICF and ECF osmolalities are equal. The osmotic pressure of 900 mg/dL glucose (900/18 = 50 mOsm/kg) is the driving force for water movement from ICF to ECF. Water movement from ICF to ECF dilutes the ECF and decreases P_{Na}. Each 100-mg/dL rise in $P_{glucose}$ above 100 mg/dL decreases the P_{Na} by 1.6 mEq/L. In this patient, the predicted decrease in P_{Na} = (900 – 100)/100 × 1.6 = 13 mEq/L. The predicted P_{Na} would be 140 – 13 = 127 mEq/L. P_{Na} of 135 suggests further water loss from osmotic diuresis. The P_{osm} of 2(135) + 900/18 + 56/2.8 = 340 mOsm/kg is compatible with hyperosmolar coma. Because this woman has decreased TBW and volume, you might expect her to be prerenal, the U_{Na} to be low, and the U_{osm} high. However, osmotic diuresis caused by urine glucose, ketones, and urea increases urinary Na and water, making U_{Na} and U_{osm} less useful markers of dehydration. Flat neck veins in the supine position are usually due to intravascular volume depletion. Rapid lowering of her glucose to 100 mg/dL will rapidly decrease P_{osm}, shift water to the ICF, increase P_{Na} by 13 mEq/L, and potentially cause cardiovascular collapse and cerebral edema. Thus, therapy is normal saline to replace volume, and judicious lowering of $P_{glucose}$ with IV insulin.

45. **You admit a 35-year-old schizophrenic because of a change in mental function and excessive urine output. U_{osm} = 70 mOsm/kg. P_{osm} = 280 mOsm/kg. 24-hour urine output = 12 L/day. How much free water is being excreted each day?**

Free water clearance (C_{H_2O}) is the amount of solute free water excreted per day. Osmolar clearance is the amount of urine excreted per day that contains all the solute that is isosmotic to plasma. When the urine is hypotonic to plasma, the total urine volume consists of two components: one part free of solute (C_{H_2O}) and the other, all of the solution that is isosmotic to plasma (C_{osm}). To measure how much of the urine is pure (free) water, calculate the free water clearance. To do so, you need to know the osmolar clearance (C_{osm}) and the urine volume (V). The formula for clearance of any substance (including osmols) is always the same:

$$C = UV/P$$

where C is the volume of plasma cleared of the substance per unit time, U is the urinary concentration of the substance, P is the plasma concentration of the substance, and V is the total urinary volume per unit time. The calculations for this patient follow:

1. $V = C_{osm} + C_{H_2O}$
2. $C_{H_2O} = V - C_{osm}$
3. $C_{osm} = U_{osm} V / P_{osm}$
4. C_{osm} = (70 mOsm/kg × 12 L/day)/280 mOsm/kg = 3.0 L/day
5. $C_{H_2O} = V - C_{osm}$ = 12 L/day – 3 L/day = 9 L/day

By manipulating formula (2), another means of calculating free water clearance follows:

1. $C_{H_2O} = V(1 - U_{osm}/P_{osm})$
2. C_{H_2O} = 12 L/day(1 – 70/280) = 9 L/day

Thus, the patient's daily urine output contains 9 L/day of pure (free) water and 3 L/day that is isotonic to plasma. This information does not distinguish *primary polydipsia* from DI. However, the low P_{osm} of 280 suggests primary polydipsia.

46. **A 45-year-old-man with a 30 pack-year history of smoking presents with cough, dyspnea, fatigue, and a 15-lb weight loss. Chest x-ray shows mediastinal adenopathy and right atelectasis with pleural effusion. P_{osm} = 270 mOsm/kg, P_{Na} = 125 mEq/L, U_{osm} = 470 mOsm/kg, U_{Na} = 130 mmol/L, U_K = 60 mmol/L, and urine volume = 1 L/day. How much free water is being excreted each day? What is the likely pulmonary lesion?**

Urine is hypertonic to plasma if the $U_{osm} > P_{osm}$ or the $U_{[Na+K]} > P_{Na}$. Urine hypertonic to plasma contains two parts: the volume that would be required to contain all solute and remain isosmotic to plasma is the osmolar clearance (C_{osm}); the volume of free water that was removed from the isotonic glomerular filtrate to make $U_{osm} > P_{osm}$ or the $U_{Na+K} > P_{Na}$ is the negative free water clearance ($T^{C}H_2O$). There are two ways to calculate free water clearance: one method uses osmolality as in question 14; the other uses electrolytes (Na and K). Electrolyte free water clearance more accurately estimates free water clearance and negative free water clearance, especially when urine contains large numbers of nonelectrolyte osmolites, such as urea, that increase osmolality unrelated to free water clearance. To calculate electrolyte free water clearance, use the urinary concentrations of Na and K and the plasma Na. Because $[U_{Na} + U_K] > P_{Na} [(130 + 60) > 130]$, the *net* urinary excretion of free water is negative, and therefore free water clearance is negative. Calculations for osmolar and electrolyte free water clearance in the above patient follow:

Calculations for classic osmolar (negative) free water clearance:

1. $V = C_{osm} - T^{C}H_2O$
2. $T^{C}H_2O = C_{osm} - V$
3. $C_{osm} = 1$ L/day $[470/270] = 1.74$ L/day
4. $T^{C}H_2O = 1.74$ L/day $- 1$ L/day $= 0.74$ L/day

By manipulating formula (2), another means of calculating negative free water clearance follows:

1. $T^{C}H_2O = V[U_{osm}/P_{osm} - 1]$
2. $T^{C}H_2O = 1$ L/day $[470/270 - 1] = 0.74$ L/day

Calculations for electrolyte (negative) free water clearance:

1. $T^{C}H_2O = C_{[Na + K]} - V$
2. $C_{[Na + K]} = [U_{[Na + K]}/P_{Na} \times V]$
3. $C_{[Na + K]} = [190$ mEq/L/125 mEq/L $\times 1$ L/day$] = 1.52$ L/day
4. $T^{C}H_2O = 1.52$ L/day $- 1$ L/day $= 0.52$ L/day

Thus, the patient's kidneys add (by water reabsorption) a net of 520–740 mL of free water to plasma each day. With a low P_{osm}, it is usually inappropriate to retain water in excess of output. This finding suggests SIADH. You must exclude volume depletion, adrenal insufficiency, and hypothyroidism before making the diagnosis of SIADH. This patient had small cell carcinoma of the lung with ectopic ADH secretion. Fifteen percent of patients with small cell carcinoma of the lung develop SIADH. This tumor is highly associated with smoking and accounts for 15–25% of lung cancer. Other lung cancers rarely secrete ADH.

47. **A 34-year-old, 60-kg woman presents 12 hours after discharge following cholecystectomy. She has headache, confusion, muscle cramps, weakness, lethargy, agitation, nausea, and vomiting. She had no symptoms at discharge. P_{Na} was 110 mEq/L. What has caused the hyponatremia? How quickly should you treat it?**

By this history, hyponatremia developed rapidly and was symptomatic. Treatment is intensive care unit admission and administration of 3% saline and furosemide at rates sufficient to increase P_{Na} 1.5–2.0 mEq/L/h for 2–4 hours based on symptom resolution. Measure hourly P_{Na}, U_{Na}, and U_K to follow progress and guide therapy. Once serious signs and symptoms improve, decrease the rate of correction to 0.5–1.0 mEq/h until symptoms further improve or the P_{Na} is 120 mEq/L. Avoid a net increase in P_{Na} > 12 mEq/L in the first 24 hours and 18–20 mEq/L over 48 hours. For chronic hyponatremia without symptoms, the appropriate rate of correction is 0.5 mEq/L/h with similar net daily increases in P_{Na}. Acute symptomatic hyponatremia requires expeditious correction of the P_{Na} because the symptomatic patient has cerebral edema caused by "normal" brain-cell solute content that pulls water into the brain. Acutely raising P_{Na} increases ECF tonicity, pulls water out of the swollen brain, and reduces the brain volume toward normal. The brain has no room in the skull to swell more than 8–10% prior to herniation. Therefore, there is no benefit to acutely correcting the Na more than 8%— in this case to a P_{Na} > 119 mEq/L. Conversely, the patient with chronic asymptomatic hyponatremia has adapted by loss of brain solute and has near-normal brain volume. Increasing this patient's P_{Na} too rapidly (> 0.5 mEq/L/h) will shrink the brain and predispose to the osmotic demyelination syndrome (previously called central pontine myelinolysis). The risks of not correcting acute symptomatic hyponatremia include increased cerebral edema, seizures, coma, and death. Outlined below are the calculations of water excess. Calculations for 3% saline needed to correct the P_{Na} to 120 mEq/L are also shown.

$$\text{Water excess} = [(\text{normal } P_{Na} - \text{observed } P_{Na})/\text{normal } P_{Na}] \times TBW$$
$$= [(140 - 110)/140] \times 0.5 \times 60 \text{ kg}$$
$$= 0.21 \times 30 \text{ L}$$
$$= 6.3 \text{ L excess in TBW}$$

$$Na^+ \text{ deficit} = (\text{desired } P_{Na} - \text{observed } P_{Na}) \times TBW$$
$$= (120 - 110) \times 0.5 \times 60 \text{ kg}$$
$$= 10 \text{ mEq/L} \times 30 \text{ L}$$
$$= 300 \text{ mEq Na}$$

Knowing the Na deficit is useful clinically because it can be replaced at a controlled rate to improve the hyponatremia. The Na^+ in 3% saline is 513 mEq/L:

$$300 \text{ mEq } Na^+/513 \text{ mEq/L} = 0.585 \text{ L}$$

Thus, assuming no Na or water loss, giving 585 mL of 3% saline will correct the P_{Na} to 120 mEq/L. Make a similar calculation for 3% saline to infuse over 3–4 hours to increase the P_{Na} by 6 mEq/L. The answer is 350 mL. However, you must also measure P_{Na}, U_{Na}, and U_K frequently to estimate loss and gain of Na and water during therapy and replace those losses. Empiric rate of 3% saline infusion for rapid treatment of symptomatic hyponatremia is 2 mL/kg/h. Use ideal body weight unless the patient is below ideal body weight and in that case use actual weight. In this patient, 3% saline infusion would be 60 kg × 2 mL/kg/h or 120 mL/h × 4 h = 480 mL.

48. **An 80-year-old woman who rarely leaves her home is brought to the hospital after being found confused. Three weeks ago she saw her physician who started a diuretic for systolic hypertension. On arrival, her P_{Na} is 110 mmol/L. What is the cause of her hyponatremia?**

As a consequence of aging, elderly patients lose GFR, concentrating ability, and diluting ability. Thus, an 80-year-old woman may have a normal (for age) renal-concentrating range of 100–700 mOsm/kg. However, maximal U_{osm} in the elderly may be as low as 350 mOsm/kg. This woman's average diet may generate only 600 mOsm/day. Her normal range of urine output would then be 0.9–6.0 L/day. If her dietary intake fell to 300 mOsm/day, her maximal urine output would fall to 3 L/day:

$$300 \text{ mOsm/day} \div 100 \text{ mOsm/kg} = 3 \text{ L/day}$$

Given free access to water and a thiazide diuretic, which impairs urinary dilution, she could easily become water intoxicated and hyponatremic. The mechanism of hyponatremia in beer potomania and the "tea and toast diet" is low total osmolar intake and relatively increased water intake. The decreased osmotic load for excretion limits the amount of water excreted.

49. **A 35-year-old female marathon runner collapses, unable to finish a 42-km race averaging 5 mph. She water-loaded before the race and drank as much as possible to maintain hydration during the race. She is brought to you confused, afebrile and tachypneic. Physical examination shows BP 120/60, pulse 110 beats/minute and regular, lungs with bilateral crackles, continued confusion, and involuntary twitching during your examination. Laboratory studies show a P_{Na} of 112 mEq/L, and the remainder of the screening laboratory test results is normal. What is the cause of exercise-induced hyponatremia and how would you treat it?**

Exertional hyponatremia may occur in 20% of ultra-endurance sports participants and be symptomatic in 20–30% of these athletes. Excess water intake is the primary cause, and this is suggested by the clinical history. Loss of sweat with Na concentrations of 40–80 mEq/L and replacement with hypotonic fluids also contributes to the hyponatremia. In addition, the pain and stress of exercise are known stimulants to ADH secretion. This patient with symptoms and signs of pulmonary and cerebral edema requires urgent treatment as outlined in question 47.

WESITES

1. American Academy of Family Physicians: Hyponatremia and Hypernatremia in the Elderly Available at http://www.aafp.org/afp/20000615/3623.html

2. Annals of Pharmacotherapy: Hyponatremia review. Available at http://www.theannals.com/cgi/reprint/37/11/1694.pdf

3. British Medical Journal: Exercise-induced hyponatremia. Available at http://bmj.bmjjournals.com/cgi/content/full/327/7407/113#REF3

4. EMedcine: SIADH review. Available at http://www.emedicine.com/ped/topic2190.htm

5. EMedicine: Lithium nephropathy review. Available at http://www.emedicine.com/med/topic1313.htm

6. EMedicine: Diabetes insipidus review. Available at http://master.emedicine.com/ped/topic580.htm

7. EMedcine: Hyponatremia review. Available at http://www.emedicine.com/med/topic1130.htm

8. Quarterly Journal of Medicine: Primary polydipisia review. Available at http://qjmed.oupjournals.org/cgi/content/full/96/7/531

BIBLIOGRAPHY

1. Adrogue HJ, Madias NE: Hypernatremia. N Engl J Med 342:1493–1499, 2000.

2. Adrogue HJ, Madias NE: Hyponatremia. N Engl J Med 342:1581–1589, 2000.

3. Ayus JC, Varon J, Arieff AI: Hyponatremia, cerebral edema, and noncardiogenic pulmonary edema in marathon runners. Ann Intern Med 132:711–714, 2000.

4. Berl T, Schrier RW: Disorders of water metabolism. In Schrier RW (ed): Renal and Electrolyte Disorders, 6th edition, Philadelphia, Lippincott Williams & Wilkins, 2003, pp 1–63.

5. Fall PJ: Hyponatremia and hypernatremia: A systematic approach to causes and their correction. Postgrad Med 107:75–82, 179, 2000.

6. Hillier TA, Abbott RD, Barrett EJ: Hyponatremia: Evaluating the correction factor for hyperglycemia. Am J Med 106:399–403, 1999.

7. Kugler JP, Hustead T: Hyponatremia and hypernatremia in the elderly. Am Fam Physician 61:3623–3630, 2000.

8. Mayinger B, Hensen J: Nonpeptide vasopressin antagonists: A new group of hormone blockers entering the scene. Exp Clin Endocrinol Diabetes 107(3):157–165,1999.

9. Moritz ML, Ayus JC: Prevention of hospital-acquired hyponatremia: A case for using isotonic saline. Pediatrics 111:227–230, 2003.

10. Nielsen S, Kwon TH, Christensen BM, et al: Physiology and pathophysiology of renal aquaporins. J Am Soc Nephrol 10:647–663, 1999.

11. Oster JR, Singer I: Hyponatremia, hypo-osmolality, and hypotonicity: Tables and fables. Arch Intern Med 159:333–336,1999.

12. Palmer BF, Gates JR, Malcolm L: Causes and management of hyponatremia. Ann Pharmacother 37:1694–1702, 2003.

13. Singer I, Oster JR, Fishman LM: The management of diabetes insipidus in adults. Arch Intern Med 157(12):1293–1301, 1997.

CHAPTER 26

DISORDERS OF GROWTH

Philip Zeitler, M.D., Ph.D.

1. **Summarize normal growth velocity for children until the pubertal growth spurt.**
   - First 6 months: 16–17 cm
   - Second 6 months: approximately 8 cm
   - Second year: just over 10 cm
   - Third year: approximately 8 cm
   - Fourth year: 7 cm
   - Later childhood until puberty (5–10 years): growth averages 5–6 cm/year

2. **Summarize growth velocity during the pubertal growth spurt.**
   - Maximum growth rate of 11–13 cm/year.
   - In girls, growth spurt occurs early in puberty (breast Tanner stage II).
   - Growth spurt is later in boys (pubic hair Tanner stage III–IV, testicular volume 12–15 mL).
   - Some children may experience a transient period of slow growth just prior to the onset of puberty.

3. **How is height measured accurately?**
   The most essential tool for the detection of growth abnormalities is the ability to obtain accurate and reproducible measurements. This ability requires the availability of appropriate equipment, as well as proper positioning of the patient.
   - At all ages, children should be measured at *full stretch* with a straight spine, since this is the only position that will be reproducible.
   - Children should be shoeless, and hair decorations or braids may need to be removed.
   - Scales with floppy arms are unreliable.

4. **What technique is used for infants up to 2 years of age?**
   The supine length of infants. Accurate measurement requires a supine stadiometer, a box-like structure with a headboard and movable footplate. Two people are needed, with one holding the infant's head against the headboard while the other straightens the legs and places the ankles at 90 degrees against the movable footplate. The length is read from the attached measuring device or marks are made for measurement by tape measure.

5. **Describe the technique for children 2 years of age and older.**
   Standing height is measured. Accurate measurement requires a stadiometer with a rigid headboard, footplate, and backboard.
   - The child stands against the backboard, with heels, buttocks, thoracic spine, and head touching.
   - The measurer exerts upward pressure on the patient at the angle of the jaw to bring the spine into full stretch, and the headboard is lowered until it touches the top of the head. A counter reads the measurement.
   - If a stadiometer is not available, the child should stand against a wall in the same position as used for a stadiometer. A rigid right angle is moved downward to touch the top of the head, and a mark is made and measured.
   - Weight and head circumference (when appropriate) should be recorded.

6. **How is height recorded?**
   The second critical tool for evaluation of growth is the standardized growth curve, and all measurements should be plotted rather than just recorded in the chart. A carefully constructed and up-to-date growth curve is critical to the recognition of growth abnormalities. Furthermore, the more points that are plotted on the curve, the greater the understanding of the child's growth. Thus, efforts should be made to obtain growth measurements at all patient contacts, including illness visits, since well-child visits are infrequent during the middle childhood years when growth abnormalities are most common.

7. **List the common errors in plotting growth charts.**
   Errors in plotting of growth points are a frequent cause of apparent growth abnormalities. Common errors include:
   - Plotting the wrong height.
   - Not plotting the patient's height at the *exact* chronologic age. Height should be plotted to the nearest month or decimal age.
   - Use of an inappropriate growth chart.

8. **What is meant by appropriate growth chart?**
   A number of growth charts are available, and careful consideration should be given to the appropriate chart for a particular patient at a particular time. Commonly available growth charts include:
   - Charts for plotting supine length (the 0 to 36-month charts in common use).
   - Charts for plotting stature (i.e., standing height) (2 to 18-year charts).
   Other specific growth charts include:
   - Ethnic-specific charts.
   - Growth charts specific for common syndromes (e.g., Turner's syndrome, Down syndrome, achondroplasia) should be used when appropriate.

9. **How do age and position affect growth measurements?**
   - A patient measured supine is slightly longer than the same patient measured standing up.
   - Charting of a standing patient on a supine chart gives the erroneous impression of decreased growth velocity. This is a common cause of apparent growth abnormality in children aged 2–3 years who are measured standing up for the first time.

10. **What historic information is necessary for interpreting a growth chart?**
    - Birth history and birth weight
    - Developmental milestones
    - History of chronic illnesses
    - Long-term medication use
    - History of surgery or trauma
    - Current symptoms
    - Height of biologic parents and family history of significant short stature
    - Timing of parental puberty and family history of significant pubertal delay

11. **What physical examination findings help interpret a growth chart?**
    - Signs of chronic illness
    - Stigmata of a syndrome
    - Specific signs of hormonal abnormality (thyroid deficiency, growth hormone [GH] deficiency, glucocorticoid excess)

KEY POINTS: GENERAL GROWTH ✓

1. Proper evaluation of growth depends on accurate measurement of height and correct plotting of measurements on the appropriate growth curve.

2. Common errors in plotting include plotting the wrong height, not plotting the patient's height at the *exact* chronologic age, and use of an inappropriate growth chart.

3. An abnormal growth velocity for age generally distinguishes growth abnormalities from normal growth variants.

4. Apparent abnormalities in growth are most frequently due to normal growth variants. Poor growth secondary to chronic medical illness is the next most frequent cause. Hormonal causes are less frequent.

12. **How does radiologic imaging help interpret a growth chart?**
    - A bone-age film can provide important information about skeletal maturity.
    - A radiograph of the left hand and wrist is obtained in children over 2 years of age, and maturation of epiphyseal centers is compared with available standards.

13. **Explain the significance of parental target height or "midparental height."**
    Parental height helps determine genetic potential. Add the parents' heights in centimeters; add 13 cm if the child is male, or subtract 13 cm if the child is female; and then divide by two. The resulting midparental height ± 5 cm gives an approximate target range for adult height.

14. **What is the most important factor in identifying an abnormal growth curve?**
    An abnormal growth velocity for age generally distinguishes growth abnormalities from normal growth variants. Although there are many causes of short stature, including genetic and ethnic inheritance, short normal children grow normally, whereas children with a problem have an abnormal growth velocity. For example, a fifth percentile child growing with a normal growth velocity is less worrisome than the child who has fallen from the 90th to the 75th percentile, even though the latter is taller than the former. Growth velocity abnormalities may, however, be subtle.

15. **What causes abnormal growth in children?**
    Abnormalities in growth are most frequently due either to normal growth variants (familial short stature or constitutional delay of growth and puberty) or underlying chronic medical illness, either recognized or unrecognized. Hormonal causes are less frequent.

16. **Which syndromes are associated with abnormal growth?**
    - Down syndrome
    - Prader-Willi syndrome
    - Turner's syndrome
    - Noonan's syndrome
    - Other chromosomal abnormalities

17. **List nonendocrine diseases and treatments that may be associated with poor growth.**
    - Malnutrition
    - Pulmonary disease (cystic fibrosis, asthma)
    - Cardiac disease
    - Rheumatologic disease
    - Gastrointestinal disease (Crohn's disease, inflammatory bowel disease)
    - Neurologic disease (ketogenic diet, stimulant medications)

- Renal disease
- Anemia
- Neoplasia
- Chronic glucocorticoid use

18. **Using the tools of growth curve, bone age, and height, how does one distinguish between familial (genetic) short stature and other causes?**
Children with familial short stature grow at a normal velocity for age but with stature below the normal curve. They also grow within the expected target height percentile (i.e., they are as tall as expected for their genetic potential). If the child's projected height (by extrapolation of the growth curve) falls within the target range, the likelihood is high that current height is explained by genetic factors. Children with familial short stature also have a bone age approximately equal to chronologic age.

19. **Give an example of familial short stature versus other causes of short stature.**
A 5-year-old whose height is below the third percentile, whose growth has traced a line parallel to the third percentile, whose height projects within the parental target range, and whose bone age is also 5 years is likely to have familial short stature. However, if the growth velocity is abnormal or projected height falls below the predicted range, other factors *may* be involved in the short stature (see Figs. 26-1 and 26-2).

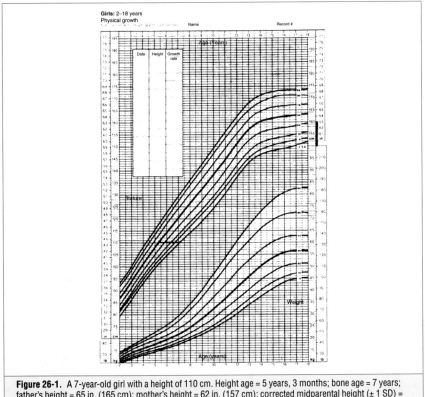

Figure 26-1. A 7-year-old girl with a height of 110 cm. Height age = 5 years, 3 months; bone age = 7 years; father's height = 65 in. (165 cm); mother's height = 62 in. (157 cm); corrected midparental height (± 1 SD) = 155 ± 5 cm; predicted adult height = 60 in. The child has a predicted adult height within genetic potential and a bone age equal to chronologic age. She has genetic or familial short stature.

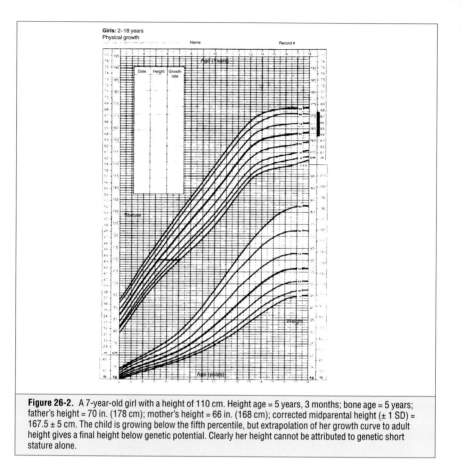

Figure 26-2. A 7-year-old girl with a height of 110 cm. Height age = 5 years, 3 months; bone age = 5 years; father's height = 70 in. (178 cm); mother's height = 66 in. (168 cm); corrected midparental height (± 1 SD) = 167.5 ± 5 cm. The child is growing below the fifth percentile, but extrapolation of her growth curve to adult height gives a final height below genetic potential. Clearly her height cannot be attributed to genetic short stature alone.

20. **Other than familial short stature, what is the most common cause of short stature?**
    Constitutional delay of growth (constitutional short stature), which affects up to 2% of children, is characterized by short stature and delayed bone age and represents a normal growth pattern simply shifted to a later age. Affected children typically have a period of subnormal growth between 18 and 30 months of age followed by normal growth velocity throughout the remainder of childhood. In accord with the delayed developmental pattern, bone age is delayed. The continuing growth delay also results in a delay in pubertal development and physical maturity. Such children (usually boys) often have a family history of a similar growth pattern and may have a more dramatic deceleration of growth velocity before entering puberty than normal children. They complete their growth at a later age, reaching an adult height within the expected genetic potential (Fig. 26-3).

21. **How is the diagnosis of constitutional delay of growth made?**
    The diagnosis of constitutional delay of growth based on the following criteria does not need further laboratory support:
    - Period of slowed growth in the second year of life with downward crossing of percentiles.
    - Normal growth velocity during childhood but with stature below the normal curve.

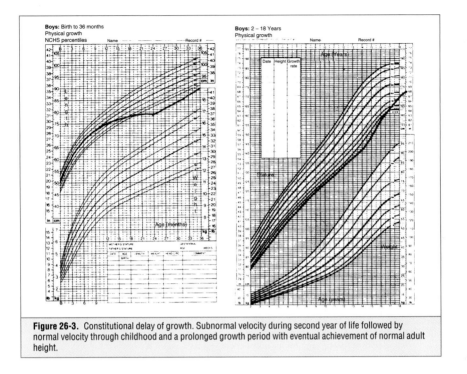

Figure 26-3. Constitutional delay of growth. Subnormal velocity during second year of life followed by normal velocity through childhood and a prolonged growth period with eventual achievement of normal adult height.

- Delayed bone age.
- Height prediction appropriate for family. (Plot the current height at the patient's bone age and follow the resulting percentile to adult height. In constitutional delay, this generally leads to a projected height within the parental target range.)
- Positive family history, delayed dentition, and delayed puberty in adolescence.

22. **What is the effect of testosterone therapy on boys with constitutional delay of growth?**
Short-term testosterone therapy for boys with constitutional delay (75–100 mg/month of long-acting testosterone esters given for 6 months, starting at bone age 12.5 years) accelerates growth and stimulates pubertal development without compromising final adult height or advancing bone age. Clinically the boys experience pubertal changes, including genital enlargement (but not testicular growth), growth of pubic and axillary hair, deepening of voice, body odor, and acne. There may be personality changes characteristic of early puberty as well.

23. **List the endocrine causes for short stature in children in order of prevalence.**
- Hypothyroiditis: congenital or acquired
- GH deficiency
- Glucocorticoid excess: iatrogenic or endogenous (less common)
- Pseudohypoparathyroidism

24. **What laboratory measures should be considered in evaluating a patient for short stature?**
Laboratory tests should be designed to achieve two goals: (1) exclusion of undiagnosed chronic illness and (2) exclusion of specific disorders associated with poor growth.

25. **Which laboratory tests help to exclude undiagnosed chronic illness?**
    - Electrolytes
    - Blood urea nitrogen/creatinine
    - Liver transaminases
    - Complete blood count
    - Erythrocyte sedimentation rate

26. **Which laboratory tests help to exclude gastrointestinal disorders associated with poor growth?**
    Because symptoms may be limited, the following tests are recommended:
    - Celiac antibody (antiendomysial, antitissue transglutaminase)
    - Inflammatory bowel disease screen

KEY POINTS: GROWTH VARIANTS ✓

1. Children with familial short stature grow at a normal velocity for age and within their expected target height percentile and have a bone age approximately equal to chronologic age.

2. Children with constitutional delay of growth have a period of slow growth in the second year of life but then grow with a normal growth velocity.

3. Children with constitutional delay of growth also have delayed bone age, height prediction appropriate for family, and delayed entry into puberty.

4. The diagnosis of a growth variant does not require laboratory confirmation, but growth should be followed over time to confirm the initial impression.

27. **List the laboratory tests for genetic disorders associated with poor growth.**
    - Karyotype (Turner's syndrome): consider in all short girls
    - High-resolution chromosomal analysis (when examination suggests the presence of anomalies)

28. **Which hormonal disorders should be excluded by laboratory results?**
    - Thyroid deficiency (thyroid-stimulating hormone [TSH] and free T_4)
    - GH deficiency (see question 31)

29. **Describe the causes of GH deficiency.**
    Most cases of GH deficiency are isolated and idiopathic. Idiopathic GH deficiency affects as many as 1:10000 to 1:15000 children. It is sporadic in the great majority of cases, but an increasing number of specific gene mutations involved in the synthesis of GH or the regulation of its secretion are being reported. The other important underlying causes are listed in the following.

30. **How is GH deficiency diagnosed?**
    The diagnosis of GH deficiency is primarily a clinical one, aided by laboratory support, rather than a diagnosis based on definitive testing. Most important is choosing the appropriate patient. Children with subnormal growth should be evaluated for GH deficiency only *after a thorough search fails to reveal any other cause for growth delay.*

31. **List the components of the laboratory evaluation for GH deficiency.**
    1. Serum levels of insulin-like growth factor 1 (IGF-1)
    2. Other GH-dependent proteins of occasional clinical utility:
        - IGF-binding protein 3 (minimal variation with age, less affected by nutritional state)
        - IGF-binding protein 2 (rises in the presence of GH deficiency)

- acid labile subunit (ALS)
3. GH testing.

32. **Why are serum levels of IGF-1 important?**
IGF-1 is a GH-dependent protein that is produced in target tissues in response to GH. Serum levels of IGF-1 reflect production of the protein by the liver and give an indirect indication of GH secretion. The following characteristics of IGF-1 should be kept in mind when serum levels are assessed:
- Concentrations of IGF-1 remain constant during the day, unlike levels of GH.
- Concentrations of IGF-1 vary with age, and values must be compared with appropriate age-specific and pubertal stage–specific norms available from performing laboratories.
- Low serum levels of IGF-1 (> 2 SD below the mean for age) are 70–80% predictive of failing more rigorous tests of GH secretion.

33. **Do normal levels of IGF-1 exclude GH deficiency?**
Normal levels of IGF-1 are reassuring but do not rule out partial GH deficiency in the appropriate clinical context.

34. **Do low serum levels of IGF-1 confirm the diagnosis of GH deficiency?**
No. Poor nutrition, chronic disease, and hypothyroidism may suppress IGF-1 concentrations. In addition, below the age of 6 years values are quite low, and the overlap between normal and GH-deficient levels renders the test highly insensitive.

35. **How is GH testing done?**
Because secretion of GH is episodic, random levels are not helpful for the diagnosis of GH deficiency. GH must be formally measured in response to a series of stimuli. Various pharmacologic agents are used, but there is no consensus about which agents are optimal. The child must have fasted overnight, be euthyroid, and have no underlying chronic disease or psychosocial deviation. In addition, at least two tests are generally performed using different stimulating agents.

36. **How are the results of GH testing interpreted?**
Normal children respond to stimulation with GH concentrations above 10 ng/mL. Failure to respond to all tests with a value greater than 10 ng/mL is consistent with the diagnosis of classic GH deficiency.
    Criteria for the diagnosis of partial GH deficiency and neurosecretory dysfunction (normal pituitary response to stimuli, but low IGF-1, suggesting that endogenous GH secretion is impaired) are less well established.

37. **How is idiopathic GH deficiency diagnosed?**
GH deficiency can be isolated or associated with other pituitary hormone deficiencies. It can be congenital or result from trauma or an intracranial neoplasm. All patients diagnosed with GH deficiency should have cranial imaging, unless the cause of the deficiency is previously known. Isolated GH deficiency without identifiable etiology is considered idiopathic.

KEY POINTS: GROWTH HORMONE DEFICIENCY ✓

1. Growth hormone deficiency is a clinical diagnosis.

2. Other causes of poor growth should be excluded.

3. Laboratory testing is supportive and confirmatory.

4. Laboratory measures include measurement of serum IGF-1 and growth hormone stimulation testing.

38. How is idiopathic GH deficiency treated?

GH is available through recombinant DNA technology, and the majority of children are treated with 6–7 daily shots/week at a total weekly dose of approximately 0.30 mg/kg administered subcutaneously. Because the effect of GH wanes after several years of therapy, it is common to see dramatic catch-up growth (~10–12 cm/year) in the first or second year of therapy, followed by velocities ranging from normal to 1.5 times normal in subsequent years.

39. What is the prognosis for adult height in treated children with idiopathic GH deficiency?

Although nearly all treated children reach an adult height significantly better than predicted before therapy is initiated, many do not reach their predicted genetic potential. Children diagnosed and treated at an earlier age have a better height prognosis than those whose therapy is initiated later. Similarly, the more mature the skeleton at diagnosis, the poorer the final outcome.

40. When is GH therapy discontinued?

In children with idiopathic GH deficiency, the point of diminishing benefit of therapy correlates with skeletal maturity rather than chronologic age or duration of therapy. Therapy often is discontinued at a bone age of 15 years (96% of growth) to 16 years (98% of growth) in boys and 14 years (98% of growth) in girls. However, given what is now known about the effects of GH deficiency in adulthood, some patients with severe deficiencies may require lifelong hormonal replacement.

41. What other syndromes are considered indications for GH therapy?

GH is now FDA-approved for the treatment of short stature in a number of conditions in addition to GH deficiency:
1. Chronic renal insufficiency prior to transplant
2. Turner's syndrome (45 XO or mosaic variants)
3. AIDS wasting syndrome
4. Prader-Willi syndrome
5. Short stature due to intrauterine growth retardation (IUGR) in the absence of "catch-up" growth
6. Idiopathic short stature in boys with predicted adult height < 63 in. and girls with predicted height < 59 in. (normal GH secretion)

Indications 2–6 do not require demonstration of GH deficiency. The use of GH for treatment of idiopathic short stature remains controversial among pediatric endocrinologists.

42. What is the prognosis for girls with Turner's syndrome treated with GH?

Girls with Turner's syndrome generally demonstrate a significant increase in predicted adult height, with an average increase of 8.8 cm. The overall effectiveness of therapy, like that in GH deficiency, depends on chronologic age at initiation, bone age at initiation, and duration of treatment. Since GH therapy in Turner's syndrome normalizes height in younger girls, estrogen replacement therapy can be initiated at an age similar to the age of puberty of the patient's peers.

43. What are the potential risks of human GH therapy?

The side effects of GH therapy can be divided into three categories: (1) common but clinically unimportant; (2) uncommon with potential clinical importance; (3) rare or theoretical.

44. List the common but clinically unimportant side effects of GH therapy.

- Acute correction of body water deficit after initiation of GH in deficient patients (may lead to transient peripheral edema, headache, and joint aches and stiffness)
- Increased average glucose concentration
- Increased systolic blood pressure

45. **List the uncommon side effects with potential clinical importance.**
    - Pseudotumor cerebri
    - Slipped capital femoral epiphysis
    - Glucose intolerance
    - Worsening of underlying scoliosis

46. **What rare or theoretical side effects may be associated with GH therapy?**
    - Increased recurrence of brain tumors: no study to date has documented this phenomenon and it is not currently considered a significant concern.
    - Increased incidence of leukemia: generally reported in children at risk for development of leukemia because of previous chemotherapy and/or radiation; unclear whether rate is higher than the background rate in such children.
    - Increased risk for development of a secondary neoplasm: recent reports suggest a small increase in the long-term risk of a secondary neoplasm in childhood cancer survivors treated with GH. This report remains to be confirmed, and the clinical relevance is unclear.

47. **Should children with idiopathic short stature (without GH deficiency) be treated with GH?**
    The FDA has recently approved the use of GH in children with idiopathic short stature with a predicted adult height < 63 in. for boys and < 59 in. for girls. However, the use of GH in children in whom no secretory abnormality can be demonstrated continues to be intensely controversial among pediatric endocrinologists. Short-term studies involving small cohorts have demonstrated a consistent increase in growth velocity with GH therapy in such children. Several studies that followed children to final height disagreed about the overall effectiveness of therapy. However, most studies agree that the increase in final adult height is limited and can be obtained only at significant financial cost. The decision to use GH in such children should be carefully considered and requires a thoughtful dialogue among child, family, and an experienced pediatric endocrinologist who knows the child well.

48. **How does the pattern of growth in children with excessive glucocorticoids differ from the pattern in children with exogenous obesity?**
    Glucocorticoid excess, whether iatrogenic (common) or intrinsic (rare), results in impairment of linear growth. The mechanism relates to direct glucocorticoid metabolic actions, including increased protein catabolism, increased lipolysis, and a decline in collagen synthesis. Glucocorticoids also suppress the pulsatile release of GH from the pituitary gland and the production of IGF-1 at the target organ. The net result is that children with steroid excess are frequently short. They also have an increased weight/height ratio and appear obese. Children with exogenous obesity, on the other hand, generally show accelerated linear growth; thus they are not only obese but also tall for age.

49. **What conditions are associated with excessive growth in childhood?**
    Relatively few conditions result in overgrowth during childhood. These include familial tall stature (stature appropriate for parental target), constitutional advanced growth, hormonal causes, and genetic syndromes.

50. **Explain constitutional advanced growth.**
    Constitutional advanced growth is associated with advanced bone age, accelerated growth, and early puberty, with predicted adult height appropriate for parental target (see question 21). Obesity and familial factors may be involved.

51. **List the hormonal causes of excessive growth.**
    - Hyperthyroidism
    - GH excess (pituitary gigantism)
    - Androgen excess
    - Estrogen excess

52. **Summarize the characteristics of GH excess in childhood.**

GH excess is rare in children, in whom it causes tall stature rather than the bony overgrowth seen in adults (acromegaly). Diagnosis is based on the following laboratory results:
- Elevated random levels of GH
- Lack of suppression of GH during a standard glucose tolerance test
- Extremely high levels of IGF-1

53. **With what findings is androgen excess associated?**
- Precocious puberty
- Congenital adrenal hyperplasia
- Androgen-producing tumor

54. **With what findings is estrogen excess associated?**
- Precocious puberty
- Estrogen-producing tumor

55. **List the genetic syndromes associated with excessive growth.**
1. Klinefelter's syndrome (47 XXY): tall stature, small testes, delay of puberty
2. Connective tissue disorders:
   - Marfan's syndrome: tall stature, arachnodactyly, joint laxity, lens displacement
   - Stickler's syndrome
3. Sotos' syndrome (cerebral gigantism): macrocephaly, progressive macrosomia, dilated ventricles, retardation, advanced bone age
4. Beckwith-Wiedemann syndrome: macroglossia, umbilical hernia, hypoglycemia, macrosomia in infancy
5. Homocystinuria: arachnodactyly, retardation, homocystine in urine

BIBLIOGRAPHY

1. Binder G, Schwarze CP, Ranke MB: Identification of short stature caused by SHOX defects and therapeutic effect of recombinant human growth hormone. J Clin Endocrinol Metab 85:245–249, 2000.
2. Cohen MM Jr: Overgrowth syndromes: An update. Adv Pediatr 46:441–491, 1999.
3. Juul A, Bernasconi S, Chatelain P, et al: Diagnosis of growth hormone (GH) deficiency and the use of GH in children with growth disorders. Horm Res 51:284–299, 1999.
4. Kelnar CJ, Albertsson-Wikland K, Hintz RL, et al: Should we treat children with idiopathic short stature? Horm Res 52:150–157, 1999.
5. Myers SE, Carrel AL, Whitman BY, Allen DB: Sustained benefit after 2 years of growth hormone on body composition, fat utilization, physical strength and agility, and growth in Prader-Willi syndrome. J Pediatr 137:42–49, 2000.
6. Pasquino AM, Pucarelli I, Roggini M, Segni M: Adult height in short normal girls treated with gonadotropin-releasing hormone analogs and growth hormone. J Clin Endocrinol Metab 85: 619–622, 2000.
7. Rosenfeld RG: Disorders of growth hormone and insulin-like growth factor secretion and action. In Sperling MA (ed): Pediatric Endocrinology. Philadelphia, W.B. Saunders, 1996, pp 117–169.
8. Sas TC, de Muinck Keizer-Schrama SM, Stijnen T, et al: Normalization of height in girls with Turner syndrome after long-term growth hormone treatment: Results of a randomized dose-response trial. J Clin Endocrinol Metab 84:4607–4612, 1999.
9. Zachmann SS, Prader A: Short-term testosterone treatment at bone age of 12 to 13 years does not reduce adult height in boys with constitutional delay of growth and adolescence. Helv Pediatr Acta 42:21, 1987.

CHAPTER 27

GROWTH HORMONE USE AND ABUSE

Jonathan R. Parks, M.D., and Homer J. LeMar, Jr., M.D.

1. **What is growth hormone?**

   Growth hormone (GH) is a single-chain peptide hormone produced and secreted by somatotroph cells in the anterior pituitary gland. It is the most abundant hormone in the human pituitary. GH production increases at puberty and decreases with aging at an average rate of 14% per decade beyond age 40.

2. **How is the release of GH regulated?**

   GH secretion is stimulated by GH-releasing hormone (GH-RH) and inhibited by somatostatin, both from the hypothalamus. Another major regulator of GH production is insulin-like growth factor-1 (IGF-1), which acts at the pituitary to directly inhibit GH production and at the hypothalamus to inhibit the production of GH-RH and to stimulate somatostatin.

3. **List the actions of GH.**

   As the name implies, GH stimulates both linear growth and growth of internal organs (Table 27-1).

4. **Does GH exert all of its effects directly?**

   No. Many of the effects are mediated by IGF-1, which is also called somatomedin C. GH stimulates the production of IGF-1 in peripheral tissues, particularly the liver.

5. **What causes excessive GH secretion and what are the consequences?**

   The only significant cause of excessive GH secretion is a GH-producing pituitary tumor. GH excess during childhood results in gigantism. Robert Wadlow, "the Alton giant," reached a

TABLE 27-1. ACTIONS OF GROWTH HORMONE AT SPECIFIC SITES	
Target System	**Actions**
Liver and muscle	Increases nitrogen retention, amino acid uptake, and protein synthesis
Cardiovascular	Increases cardiac muscle mass and increases cardiac output at rest and during maximal exercise
Hematologic	Increases plasma volume and red cell mass
Skeletal tissue	Increases bone mineral density and bone turnover
Connective tissue	Increases collagen turnover at nonskeletal sites, including tendons
Metabolism	Increases rates of sweating and thermal dispersion during exercise
Endocrine	
Acute action	Increases the uptake and utilization of glucose by muscle; antagonizes the lipolytic effect of catecholamines on adipose tissue
Chronic action	Reduces glucose utilization, enhances lipolysis, and increases lean body mass

height of just over 8 ft 11 in. and wore size 37AA shoes. GH excess after epiphyseal closure results in acromegaly.

6. **What conditions are associated with a deficiency of GH?**
GH deficiency can be congenital (genetic mutations) or may result from damage to the pituitary gland from intracranial tumors, surgery, radiation therapy, trauma, and a variety of infiltrative and infectious diseases. GH deficiency in adults, frequently overlooked in the past, has been more thoroughly studied and more frequently diagnosed in recent years.

7. **What are some common signs and symptoms of GH deficiency?**
Deficient GH production in childhood results in short stature. GH deficiency in adults can result in increased adiposity, decreased lean body mass, decreased bone density, decreased extracellular water, reduced cardiac function, decreased muscle force and strength, and diminished exercise performance. Patients have reduced aerobic capacity and strength levels and often complain of lethargy and fatigue. Their quality of life is diminished, manifested by depression, anxiety, mental fatigue, and decreased self-esteem and life fulfillment. Excessive intra-abdominal fat is associated with an increased risk of cardiovascular disease, which is the predominant cause of mortality in these patients.

8. **Where do we get the GH used therapeutically?**
From 1958 to 1985, GH was available only from the pituitaries of human cadavers. Since 1985, biosynthetic GH preparations have allowed production of much larger quantities of GH and markedly improved availability. A requirement for bioassays has become an FDA requisite to substantiate biologic activity among different preparations. The bioassays could soon be replaced by in vitro binding assays using GH receptors derived from molecular techniques.

9. **Besides availability, what problem was associated with GH derived from human cadavers?**
Creutzfeldt-Jakob disease, an uncommon, rapidly progressive, and fatal spongiform encephalopathy, has been reported to result from iatrogenic transmission through human cadaver pituitary tissue. More than 30 young adults who had received human cadaver pituitary products have died of this disease, and at least 60–70 cases of Creutzfeldt-Jakob disease have been identified in recipients.

10. **List the FDA-approved uses of GH.**
For several years, the only approved indication for GH therapy was treatment of short stature in children with GH deficiency. Currently, GH is also approved for treatment of short stature associated with Turner's syndrome, Prader-Willi syndrome and progressive chronic renal insufficiency in children, for wasting in patients with AIDS, and for replacement therapy in GH-deficient adults.

11. **List the potential uses of GH.**
GH has other potential uses: (1) Noonan's syndrome; (2) Russell-Silver syndrome; (3) intrauterine growth retardation (IUGR); (4) chondrodysplasla in children; (5) steroid-induced growth suppression; (6) short stature associated with myelomeningocele; (7) any severe wasting state (e.g., wounds, burns, cancer); (8) normal aging; (9) nonislet-cell tumor hypoglycemia; (10) gonadal dysgenesis; (11) Down syndrome; (12) short stature associated with neurofibromatosis; (13) osteoporosis; (14) congestive heart failure.

12. **How does GH help GH-deficient adults?**
The reported beneficial effects in GH-deficient adults are an increase in muscle mass and function, reduction of total body fat mass, and increased plasma volume and improved peripheral blood flow. Reductions in serum total and low-density lipoprotein (LDL) cholesterol,

reduction in diastolic blood pressure, a trend toward reduction in systolic blood pressure, and beneficial effects on bone metabolism and skeletal mass have also been documented. In addition, an improvement in psychological well-being and quality of life can occur with GH replacement.

13. **What are the therapeutic doses of GH? How is it administered?**
The recommended doses in North America for children are 0.175–0.35 mg/k/week in GH deficiency, 0.35 mg/k/week for impaired growth of chronic renal insufficiency, and 0.375 mg/k/week for Turner's syndrome. The dose can be divided into twice-weekly, thrice-weekly, or daily regimens. Daily injections appear to give greater growth velocity than less frequent administration. Currently, the appropriate adult replacement dose appears to be 0.006 mg/k/day with a maximal dose of 0.0125 mg/k/day. GH is administered by subcutaneous injection.

14. **Why is GH used as an ergogenic aid by athletes?**
Athletes have used GH in an effort to improve performance. Supraphysiologic doses of GH have been reported to increase lean body mass and to reduce body fat in trained athletes. However, most data available suggest that GH administration has no beneficial effects on muscle strength, growth, or exercise performance in non-GH-deficient adults. In addition, some athletes using GH have reportedly been disappointed with the results.

15. **How is abuse detected?**
To date, there is no reliable way to detect GH use by athletes. During the 2000 Summer Olympics in Sydney, Australia, commentators discussed the use of drugs among athletes and noted the difficulty in detecting GH.

KEY POINTS: GROWTH HORMONE USE AND ABUSE ✓

1. Common side effects of therapeutic growth hormone use are fluid retention, carpal tunnel syndrome, arthralgias, myalgias, paresthesias, and worsening glucose tolerance.

2. To date, there is no reliable way to detect growth hormone use by athletes due to the pulsatile manner of its release and the inability of current assays to distinguish exogenous hormone from endogenous hormone.

3. Chronic abuse of supraphysiologic doses of growth hormone may lead to features of acromegaly; osteoarthritis; irreversible bone and joint deformities; increased vascular, respiratory, and cardiac abnormalities; hypogonadism; diabetes mellitus; and abnormal lipid metabolism.

4. Athletes use growth hormone in an effort to improve performance; however, most available data suggest that the use of growth hormone does not have any effect on muscle strength, growth, or exercise performance in non–growth hormone-deficient adults.

16. **Why is GH abuse so difficult to detect?**
Detection presents a number of unique problems. Endogenous GH is secreted naturally in a pulsatile manner; therefore, an increased level detected on random testing could simply reflect a spontaneous peak, especially since GH secretion is stimulated by acute exercise. Furthermore, GH release can also be affected by the nutritional supplements frequently used by athletes. Finally, exogenous GH is not distinguishable from endogenous GH by biochemical testing.

17. **What is currently being tried to detect GH?**

The International Olympic Committee and the European Union have established a collaborative study group to examine the possibility of developing a test to differentiate exogenous GH from endogenous GH secretion in athletes. Currently, these studies are evaluating the use of serum bone turnover markers, changes in GH-related peptides, and measurements of serum concentrations of mixed GH isomers.

18. **How prevalent is GH use among athletes?**

The prevalence is not known because abuse is currently undetectable, but there has been an increase in reported GH abuse by athletes over the last decade. There have been several reported recent seizures of GH found in athletes' luggage. The well-publicized seizures of recombinant GH from Tour de France cyclists in 1998 suggest use at an elite level. Use is probably not as extensive as with anabolic-androgenic steroids. One limiting factor is the expense. Even a 1 month supply may cost several thousand dollars, depending on doses.

19. **What are the adverse effects of the therapeutic use of GH in adults?**

Fluid retention causing edema and carpal tunnel syndrome are common in adults but not in children. Arthralgias, myalgias, paresthesias, and worsening glucose tolerance are also common and may be present in up to one-third of patients taking GH. Other potential side effects include gynecomastia, pancreatitis, behavioral changes, worsening of neurofibromatosis, scoliosis and kyphosis, and hypertrophy of tonsils and adenoids.

20. **What are the adverse effects of GH in children?**

Pseudotumor cerebri has been reported in children; this is most common in children with renal disease, although it has also been observed in children with GH deficiency and in girls with Turner's syndrome. GH therapy is associated with an increased risk of slipped capital femoral epiphysis in the same three groups of children. Children with GH deficiency due to deletion of the GH gene may develop antibodies to GH with secondary growth deceleration. This phenomenon is rare in other children.

21. **What malignancy has been linked to GH use?**

None. More than 50 cases of leukemia have been reported in GH-treated patients; however, all such patients had risk factors or syndromes associated with the development of leukemia. No data support an increased risk of nonleukemic extracranial neoplasms with therapeutic GH use. Nevertheless, GH must be used cautiously in patients with known malignancy and/or benign tumors given the theoretical risk of potential growth in these lesions.

22. **What adverse effects occur in athletes using GH?**

Little is known about side effects of GH use in athletes. Chronic abuse of supraphysiologic GH doses may lead to features of acromegaly, osteoarthritis, irreversible bone and joint deformities, increased vascular, respiratory and cardiac abnormalities, hypertrophy of other organs, hypogonadism, diabetes mellitus, abnormal lipid metabolism, increased risk of breast and colon cancer, and muscle weakness due to myopathy. Current studies also suggest that GH use in combination with anabolic androgenic steroids may increase left ventricular mass and cause concentric myocardial remodeling. Clearly, in this scenario, the risk to athletes is potentially high.

23. **GH is the proverbial fountain of youth. True or false?**

False. However, alternative medicine companies promote products alleged to stimulate increased production of GH in hopes of reversing normal aging. This theory has been sustained through the years due to a study that suggested diminished secretion of GH is responsible for the effects of aging, including increased adipose tissue, decreased lean body mass, and thinning of the skin. Although GH replacement has a role in deficient individuals, no data prove that supplemental GH can reverse physiologic aging. Nevertheless, many "antiaging" compounds that reportedly stimulate GH release are being marketed to the public with increasing popularity.

WEBSITE ⊕

Human Growth Foundation. Available at http://www.hgfound.org/index.htm

BIBLIOGRAPHY

1. Bildlingmaier M, Wu Z, Strasburger C: Doping with growth hormone. J Pediatr Endocrinol Metab14:1077–1083, 2001.

2. Blackman M, Sorkin J, Munzer T, et al: Growth hormone and sex steroid administration in healthy aged women and men: A randomized controlled trial. JAMA 288:2282–2292, 2002.

3. Blethen SL: Monitoring growth hormone NE treatment: Safety considerations. Endocrinologist 6:369–374, 1996.

4. Bouillanne O, Raenfray M, Tissandier O, et al: Growth hormone therapy in elderly people: An age delaying drug? Fundam Clin Pharmacol 10:416–430, 1996.

5. Consensus guidelines for the diagnosis and treatment of adults with GROWTH HORMONE deficiency: Summary statement of the Growth Hormone Research Society Workshop on Adult Growth Hormone Deficiency. J Clin Endocrinol Metab 83:379, 1998.

6. Cummings DE, Merriam GR: Growth hormone therapy in adults. Annu Rev Med 54:513–533, 2003.

7. Dean H: Does exogenous growth hormone improve athletic performance? Clin J Sport Med 12:250–253, 2002.

8. Hurel SJ, Koppiker N, Newkirk J, et al: Relationship of physical exercise and ageing to growth hormone production. Clin Endocrinol 51:687–691, 1999.

9. Jenkins PJ: Growth hormone and exercise. Clin Endocrinol 50:683–689, 1999.

10. Karila TA, Karjalainen JE, Mantysarri MJ, et al: Anabolic androgenic steroids produce dose-dependent increase in left ventricular mass in power athletes, and this effect is potentiated by concomitant use of growth hormone. Int J Sports Med 24(5):337–343, 2003.

11. Murray RD, Skillicorn CJ, Howell SJ, et al: Influences on quality of life in growth hormone-deficient adults and their effect on response to treatment. Clin Endocrinol 51:565–573, 1999.

12. Reiter EO, Rosenfeld RG: Normal and aberrant growth. In Wilson JD, Foster DW, eds: Williams Textbook of Endocrinology, 10th ed. Philadelphia, W.B. Saunders, 2003, pp 1427–1507.

13. Rodrigues-Arnao J, Jabbar J, Fulcher K, et al: Effects of growth hormone replacement on physical performance and body composition in growth hormone-deficient adults. Clin Endocrinol 51:53–60, 1999.

14. Rudman D, Feller A, Nagraj H, et al: Effects of growth hormone in men 60 years old. N Engl J Med. 323:1–6, 1990.

15. Melmed S, Kleinberg D: Anterior pituitary. In Wilson JD, Foster DW, eds: Williams Textbook of Endocrinology, 10th ed. Philadelphia, W.B. Saunders, 2003, pp 219–242.

16. Wallace JD, Cuneo RC: Growth hormone abuse in athletes: A review. Endocrinologist 10:175–184, 2000.

17. Weber MM: Effects of growth hormone on skeletal muscle. Hormone Res 58(Suppl 3):43–48, 2002.

18. Zachwieja JJ, Yarasheski EK: Does growth hormone therapy in conjunction with resistance exercise increase muscle force production and muscle mass in men and women aged 60 years or older? Phys Ther 79:76–81, 1999.

PRIMARY ALDOSTERONISM

Arnold A. Asp, M.D.

CHAPTER 28

1. **Define primary aldosteronism.**
   Primary aldosteronism is a generic term for a group of disorders, in which excessive production of aldosterone by the zona glomerulosa of the adrenal cortex occurs independently of normal renin-angiotensin stimulation. These primary disorders of the adrenal system are distinct from forms of secondary hyperaldosteronism due to excessive renin, such as renal artery stenosis. The five clinical entities comprising primary aldosteronism include solitary aldosterone-producing adenoma (APA), bilateral hyperplasia of the zona glomerulosa (also known as idiopathic hyperaldosteronism [IHA]), primary adrenal hyperplasia (PAH), adrenal carcinoma, and glucocorticoid-remediable aldosteronism.

2. **How common are these disorders?**
   The most common manifestation of hyperaldosteronism is hypertension. It is estimated that 0.05–12% of the hypertensive population may have primary aldosteronism.

3. **What are the common clinical manifestations of primary aldosteronism?**
   Aldosterone normally acts at the renal distal convoluted tubule to stimulate reabsorption of sodium ions (Na^+), as well as secretion of potassium (K^+) and hydrogen ions (H^+), and at the cortical and medullary collecting ducts to cause direct secretion of H^+. Excess secretion of aldosterone in primary aldosteronism results in hypertension, hypokalemia, and metabolic alkalosis; hypomagnesemia may occur (Fig. 28-1). Spontaneous hypokalemia (K < 3.5 mEq/L) occurs in 80% of cases of primary aldosteronism; the remaining patients develop hypokalemia within 3–5 days of initiation of liberal sodium intake (150 mEq/day). Most symptoms are manifestations of hypokalemia: weakness, muscle cramping, paresthesias, headaches, palpitations, polyuria, and polydipsia. Hyperglycemia due to insulinopenia occurs in approximately 25% of patients.

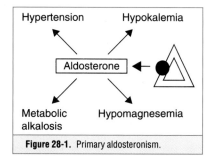

Figure 28-1. Primary aldosteronism.

4. **When and in whom is primary aldosteronism most common?**
   This group of disorders affects more women than men and occurs most commonly in the third through fifth decades of life.

5. **What is the most common form of primary aldosteronism?**
   Of the five causes mentioned in question 1, IHA is most common, accounting for up to 70% of cases in most series. IHA, also known as bilateral adrenal glomerulosa hyperplasia, is characterized by bilateral hyperplasia (diffuse and focal) of the zona glomerulosa layer of both adrenal glands. The most likely cause is supranormal sensitivity of the zona glomerulosa in

affected adrenal glands to physiologic concentrations of angiotensin II. APAs comprise 30% of primary aldosterone cases.

6. **How do adenomas produce symptoms of hyperaldosteronism?**
Adenomas produce greater amounts of aldosterone than do other forms of aldosteronism; consequently, the degree of hypertension and the extent of biochemical abnormalities tend to be more severe. APAs also secrete excess 18-hydroxycorticosterone (18-OHB), an immediate precursor of aldosterone produced by hydroxylation of corticosterone; this facilitates the biochemical diagnosis. APAs demonstrate partial autonomy of function, secreting aldosterone in response to stimulation by corticotropin (adrenocorticotropic hormone [ACTH]) but not by angiotensin II. Aldosterone synthesis by these tumors, therefore, parallels the normal circadian rhythm of ACTH secretion, with the highest serum aldosterone concentrations occurring in the mornings and the lowest in the evenings.

7. **What is the second most common cause of primary aldosteronism?**
APAs are small (< 2 cm), occur more commonly in the left adrenal gland, and are composed of zona glomerulosa cells, zona reticularis cells, and hybrid cells with characteristics of both layers. APAs are also known as Conn's syndrome.

8. **How do symptoms of IHA differ from symptoms of APAs?**
Aldosterone is produced in smaller amounts in IHA than in APA; therefore, the degree of hypertension, hypokalemia, hypomagnesemia, and metabolic alkalosis is less dramatic. Serum aldosterone levels tend to increase during upright posture, perhaps owing to increased sensitivity to angiotensin II.

9. **How commonly does adrenal cancer cause primary aldosteronism?**
Adrenal carcinoma as a cause of aldosteronism is extremely rare. The tumors are very large (> 6 cm) and metastatic at the time of diagnosis.

10. **What is PAH?**
The zona glomerulosa of one adrenal gland becomes hyperplastic and histopathologically resembles unilateral IHA. Biochemically, however, such cases more closely resemble APA and respond to surgical resection.

11. **What is glucocorticoid-remediable aldosteronism?**
In this rare cause of aldosteronism, production of mineralocorticoid is stimulated solely by ACTH. The disorder is inherited in an autosomal-dominant fashion.

12. **How is aldosterone synthesis regulated in the human body?**
Humans possess two mitochondrial 11 β-hydroxylase isoenzymes that are responsible for cortisol and aldosterone synthesis (designated CYP11B1 and CYP11B2). Both are encoded on chromosome 8. CYP11B1, which is responsible for conversion of 11-deoxycortisol to cortisol, is expressed only in the zona reticularis. CYP11B2, which is responsible for the conversion of corticosterone to aldosterone, is expressed only in the zona glomerulosa. CYP11B1 activity is stimulated by ACTH, whereas CYP11B2 is stimulated by angiotensin II or hypokalemia.

13. **Explain the genetic basis of glucocorticoid-remediable aldosteronism.**
Glucocorticoid-remediable aldosteronism results from a heritable mutation that causes the fusion of the promoter region of the CYP11B1 gene with the structural region of the CYP11B2 gene. The resulting chimeric gene responds to ACTH with overproduction of aldosterone, as well as precursors 18-hydroxycortisol and 18-oxocortisol. These metabolites of the cortisol C-18 oxidation pathway are biochemical markers that facilitate identification of affected kindreds. Excessive secretion of aldosterone may be inhibited by administration of glucocorticoids that suppress secretion of ACTH by the pituitary.

14. **How is primary aldosteronism diagnosed?**
The diagnosis of primary aldosteronism is based on the demonstration of inappropriately elevated levels of plasma aldosterone (PA) with concomitantly suppressed plasma renin activity (PRA). Hypokalemia (K < 3.5 mEq/L) is often the first clue.

15. **How are patients screened for primary aldosteronism?**
Unfortunately, there is no single specific and sensitive screening test. One method of screening the hypertensive, hypokalemic patient is to obtain concomitant PA and PRA values. A PA/PRA ratio (PA in ng/dL; PRA in ng/mL/h) that exceeds 20 raises the possibility of primary aldosteronism. Most antihypertensive agents do not affect the PA/PRA ratio; spironolactone, however, must be discontinued for 6 weeks before screening. A 24-hour urine collection for aldosterone should also be collected. Because 12% of patients may have PA/PRA ratios lower than 20, review of the urinary aldosterone value is helpful. Urinary excretion of aldosterone (18-monogluconide) that exceeds 12 mg/day is also suggestive of primary aldosteronism.

16. **How is the diagnosis of primary aldosteronism confirmed?**
Several schemas may be used to confirm the diagnosis of primary aldosteronism. The following test also aids in identification of the specific underlying disorder.
   The patient is instructed to consume at least 150 mEq of sodium each day of the week before testing. Ample potassium supplements are given to ensure a serum potassium level greater than 3.5 mEq/L. The patient is then admitted in the evening and remains recumbent overnight. At 8:00 AM, levels of PA, PRA, and 18-OHB are determined while the patient is supine. The patient then assumes an upright posture and/or ambulates for 4 hours, after which levels of PA and PRA are again determined.

17. **How are the results of the test interpreted?**
In normal and essential hypertensive patients, a high sodium diet suppresses PA, whereas upright posture for 4 hours stimulates PRA. In patients with primary aldosteronism, excessive sodium does not suppress synthesis of aldosterone; supine levels of PA at 8:00 AM exceed 15 ng/dL. Because excessive aldosterone in such patients causes intravascular expansion, PRA is undetectable (< 1 ng/mL/h) and remains suppressed despite 4 hours of upright posture. An unsuppressed PA with a concomitant unstimulated PRA confirms the diagnosis of primary aldosteronism.

18. **Explain the saline-loading procedure for diagnosis of primary aldosteronism.**
Some centers rely on a saline-loading procedure rather than a high-salt diet to assess suppression of aldosterone. In this test, 2 L of saline solution are administered IV over 4 hours. PRA, PA, and 18-OHB are determined at the beginning and PRA and PA at the conclusion of the test. As in the previous test, patients with primary aldosteronism should demonstrate undetectable levels of PRA, whereas PA should exceed 15 ng/dL before and after saline loading.

19. **How are APA and IHA differentiated on the basis of test results?**
APAs produce greater amounts of aldosterone and can be stimulated by ACTH. Patients with APA, therefore, have greater PA levels at 8:00 AM, and these levels decrease over the ensuing 4 hours as normal secretion of ACTH diminishes. Patients with IHA, on the other hand, have somewhat lower levels of PA at 8:00 AM, and they experience an increase with upright ambulation. Finally, APAs produce large amounts of 18-OHB; levels > 100 ng/dL occur only in APA and PAH.

20. **Why is it important to differentiate APA from IHA?**
APA is amenable to surgical resection of the involved adrenal gland, whereas IHA is usually treated medically.

21. **Does computed tomography (CT) or magnetic resonance imaging (MRI) aid in differentiation?**
    To a limited extent, both localizing procedures may aid in identifying the cause of primary aldosteronism. A large APA may be discernible on high-resolution CT, which at some institutions can identify adenomas as small as 5 mm. MRI at present performs, as well as CT, in identifying APA but involves higher cost and longer scan time. The diagnostic accuracy of MRI or CT in preoperatively localizing an APA is approximately 70–85%. Neither modality is able to differentiate IHA from a small APA. Adrenal carcinoma, a rare cause of excessive aldosterone, is easily identified with either modality.

22. **Are other localizing tests of help if CT or MRI fails to identify an APA when biochemical data indicate the presence of an adenoma?**
    Yes. A more invasive localizing procedure to differentiate a normal adrenal gland from one containing an adenoma is adrenal venous sampling. Catheters are introduced into the left and right adrenal veins and the inferior vena cava. Levels of PA are determined from these sites, along with concomitant levels of cortisol following infusion of cosyntropin (synthetic ACTH). PA/cortisol is referred to as "cortisol-corrected" aldosterone. APAs produce large amounts of aldosterone; the normal adrenal vein concentration of PA is 100–400 ng/dL, whereas APAs may generate concentrations of 1000–10,000 ng/dL. The ratio of PA/cortisol produced on the affected side versus the unaffected side always exceeds 14:1. Cortisol levels are determined to ensure that the adrenal veins are properly catheterized.

23. **Explain the difficulty with adrenal venous sampling.**
    Collection of aldosterone and cortisol from the left adrenal gland is relatively simple, because the venous effluent drains directly into the left renal vein. The venous flow from the right adrenal, however, flows directly into the inferior vena cava. Catheterization of the right adrenal vein is difficult because of the few angiographic landmarks. Contrast material used to localize the right adrenal gland can cause corticomedullary hemorrhage during the procedure.

24. **How accurate is adrenal venous sampling?**
    Overall, the procedure is 90% accurate in localizing APA.

25. **How is the patient with APA managed?**
    The patient undergoes screening tests, as described in question 15. The diagnosis of primary aldosteronism is confirmed with salt loading, as described in questions 17 and 18. Levels of aldosterone are elevated but decline during the course of ambulation. 18-OHB exceeds 100 mg/dL. All such findings indicate the probability of APA. If the patient is fortunate, CT scan reveals a unilateral adenoma. If an APA is not visible on CT or if the physician is concerned about a concomitant incidental nonfunctioning adenoma, adrenal venous sampling may be performed.

26. **What should be done after the APA is localized?**
    After the APA is localized, unilateral adrenalectomy is performed. Laparoscopic resection is now widely available and is preferable to the "standard" posterior approach. One year postoperatively, 70% of patients are normotensive. By the fifth postoperative year, only 53% remain normotensive. Normal potassium balance tends to be permanent.

27. **Do all patients with APA require surgery?**
    No. Although surgical resection is preferred, patients who have other comorbid conditions that preclude surgery may be successfully treated medically as described in question 28.

28. **How is a patient with IHA managed?**
    The patient undergoes screening and confirmatory tests, as described in questions 15 and 17. Concentrations of aldosterone are elevated but continue to rise with ambulation over 4 hours.

KEY POINTS: PRIMARY ALDOSTERONISM ✔

1. Spontaneous hypokalemia in a hypertensive patient should suggest the possibility of primary or secondary hyperaldosteronism.

2. Primary hyperaldosteronism may be due to bilateral hyperplasia or small adenomas.

3. The best screen for primary hyperaldosteronism is a PA/PRA ratio > 20.

4. Because CT and MRI are often unable to distinguish adenomas from hyperplasia, adrenal venous sampling may be necessary to localize the lesion.

5. Adenomas are treated surgically; bilateral hyperplasia is treated pharmacologically.

Levels of 18-OHB are less than 100 mg/dL. CT fails to reveal unilateral enlargement of the adrenals. Adrenal venous sampling fails to lateralize. After the diagnosis of IHA is made, the patient is scrupulously sequestered from surgical colleagues.

29. **What is the agent of choice for pharmacologic treatment of IHA?**
Pharmacologic therapy is quite effective. The agent of choice is spironolactone (50–200 mg b.i.d.), a competitive inhibitor of aldosterone. Hypokalemia corrects dramatically, whereas hypertension responds after 4–8 weeks. Unfortunately, spironolactone also inhibits synthesis of testosterone and peripheral action of androgens, causing decreased libido, impotence, and gynecomastia in men. Eplerenone (50 mg b.i.d.) is a recently developed aldosterone antagonist without many of the side effects of spironolactone.

30. **What other pharmacologic options are available?**
In patients intolerant of spironolactone, amiloride (5–15 mg b.i.d.) corrects hypokalemia within several days. A concomitant antihypertensive agent is usually necessary to reduce blood pressure. Success also has been reported in cases of IHA treated with calcium channel blockers (calcium is involved in the final common pathway for production of aldosterone) and angiotensin-converting enzyme (ACE) inhibitors (IHA appears to be sensitive to low concentrations of angiotensin II).

31. **Describe the management of a patient with PAH.**
During evaluation, these rare cases appear to be APA. Screening and confirmatory tests, as described in questions 15 and 17, seemingly indicate an APA. Levels of 18-OHB exceed 100 mg/dL. Localizing tests are consistent with APA, and patients usually undergo surgical resection of a nodular hyperplastic gland. The diagnosis is made retrospectively, but surgery is curative.

32. **How is a patient with glucocorticoid-remediable aldosteronism managed?**
This disorder is discussed in questions 11 and 13. Therapy with low doses of dexamethasone (0.75 mg/day) or any of the agents used for therapy of IHA (see questions 29 and 30) may be effective.

BIBLIOGRAPHY

1. Artega E, Klein R, Biglieri EG: Use of the saline infusion test to diagnose the cause of primary aldosteronism. Am J Med 79:722–728, 1985.

2. Blumenfeld JD, Sealey JE, Schlussel Y, et al: Diagnosis and treatment of primary hyperaldosteronism. Ann Intern Med 121:877–885, 1994.

3. Bornstein SR (moderator): Adrenocortical tumors: Recent advances in basic concepts and clinical management. Ann Intern Med 130:759–771, 1999.

4. Dluhy RG, Lifton RP: Glucocorticoid-remediable aldosteronism. J Clin Endocrinol Metab 84:4341–4344, 1999.

5. Fardella CE, Mosso L, Gomez-Sanchez C, et al: Primary hyperaldosteronism in essential hypertensives: Prevalence, biochemical profile, and molecular biology. J Clin Endocrinol Metab 85:1863–1867, 2000.

6. Ghose RP, Hall PM, Bravo EL: Medical management of aldosterone-producing adenomas. Ann Intern Med 131:105–108, 1999.

7. Harper R, Ferrett CG, McKnight JA, et al: Accuracy of CT scanning and adrenal vein sampling in the pre-operative localization of aldosterone-secreting adrenal adenomas. Q J Med 92:643–650, 1999.

8. Jossart GH, Burpee SE, Gagner M: Surgery of the adrenal glands. Endocrinol Metab North Am 29:57–68, 2000.

9. Liftin RP, Dluhy RG, Powers M, et al: A chimaeric 11-hydroxylase/aldosterone synthetase gene causes glucocorticoid-remediable aldosteronism and human hypertension. Nature 355:262–265, 1992.

10. Magill SB, Raff H, Shaker JL, et al: Comparison of adrenal vein sampling and computed tomography in the differentiation of primary aldosteronism. J Clin Endocrinol Metab 86:1066–1071, 2001.

11. Melby JC: Diagnosis of hyperaldosteronism. Endocrinol Metab Clin North Am 20:247–255, 1991.

12. Mulatero P, Stowasser M, Loh K, et al: Increased diagnoses of primary aldosteronism, including surgically correctable forms, in centers from five continents. J Clin Endocrinol Metab 89:1045-1050, 2004.

13. Sohaib SA, Peppercorn PD, Allen C, et al: Primary hyperaldosteronism (Conn syndrome): MR imaging findings. Radiology 214:527–531, 2000.

14. Tanabe A, Naruse M, Takagi S, et al: Variability in the renin/aldosterone profile under random and standardized sampling conditions in primary aldosteronism. J Clin Endocrinol Metab 88:2489–2492, 2003.

15. Vallotton MB: Primary aldosteronism. Part I: Diagnosis of primary hyperaldosteronism. Clin Endocrinol 45:47–52, 1996.

16. Vallotton MB: Primary aldosteronism. Part II: Differential diagnosis of primary hyperaldosteronism and pseudoaldosteronism. Clin Endocrinol 45:53–60, 1996.

17. White PC: Disorders of aldosterone biosynthesis and action. N Engl J Med 331:250–258, 1994.

18. White PC, Curnow KM, Pascoe L: Disorders of steroid 11-hydroxylase isoenzymes. Endocrine Rev 15:421–438, 1994.

19. Young WF: Pheochromocytoma and primary aldosteronism: Diagnostic approaches. Endocrinol Metab N Am 26:801–827, 1997.

CHAPTER 29

PHEOCHROMOCYTOMA

Arnold A. Asp, M.D.

1. **What is a pheochromocytoma?**
   A pheochromocytoma is an adrenal medullary tumor composed of chromaffin cells and capable of secreting biogenic amines and peptides, including epinephrine (EPI), norepinephrine (NE), and dopamine. These tumors arise from neural crest–derived cells, which also give rise to portions of the central nervous system and the sympathetic (paraganglion) system. Because of this common origin, neoplasms of the sympathetic ganglia, such as neuroblastomas, paragangliomas, and ganglioneuromas, may produce similar amines and peptides.

2. **How common are pheochromocytomas?**
   Pheochromocytomas are relatively rare. Data from the Mayo Clinic indicate that pheochromocytomas occur in 2–8/million people/year; autopsy data from the same institution reflect an incidence of 0.3% (3/1000 autopsies), indicating that many pheochromocytomas go undetected during life. The incidence of pheochromocytoma from other countries, such as Japan, is lower: 0.4 cases/million people/year.

3. **Where are pheochromocytomas located?**
   Nearly 90% of tumors arise within the adrenal glands, whereas approximately 10% are extra-adrenal and therefore classified as paragangliomas. Sporadic, solitary pheochromocytomas are located more commonly in the right adrenal gland, whereas familial forms (10% of all pheochromocytomas) are bilateral and multicentric. Bilateral adrenal tumors raise the possibility of multiple endocrine neoplasia 2A or 2B (MEN-2A or MEN-2B) syndromes (see Chapter 53).

4. **Where are paragangliomas found?**
   Paragangliomas occur most commonly within the abdomen but also have been described along the entire sympathetic paraganglia chain from the base of the brain to the testicles. The most common locations for paragangliomas are the organ of Zuckerkandl, the aortic bifurcation, and the bladder wall; the mediastinum, heart, carotid arteries, and glomus jugulare bodies are less common locations.

5. **Can pheochromocytomas metastasize?**
   Yes. Demonstration of a metastatic focus in tissue normally devoid of chromaffin cells is the only accepted indication that a pheochromocytoma is malignant. Metastasis occurs in 3–14% of cases. The most common sites of metastases include regional lymph nodes, liver, bone, lung, and muscle.

6. **What is the rule of 10s for pheochromocytomas?**
   Approximately 10% are extra-adrenal, 10% bilateral, 10% familial, and 10% malignant.

7. **What are the common clinical features of a pheochromocytoma?**
   The signs and symptoms of a pheochromocytoma are variable. The classic triad of sudden severe headaches, diaphoresis, and palpitations carries a high degree of specificity (94%) and sensitivity (91%) for pheochromocytoma in a hypertensive population. The absence of all three symptoms reliably excludes the condition. Hypertension occurs in 90–95% of cases and is

paroxysmal in 25–50% of these (Fig. 29-1). Orthostatic hypotension occurs in 40% because of hypovolemia and impaired arterial and venous constriction responses. Tremor, pallor, and anxiety also may be accompanying signs, whereas flushing is uncommon.

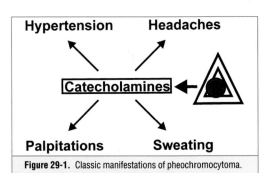

Figure 29-1. Classic manifestations of pheochromocytoma.

8. **What are some of the nonclassic manifestations of pheochromocytomas?**
    Signs and symptoms of other endocrine disorders may dominate the presentation of a pheochromocytoma. Tumors may elaborate corticotropin (adrenocorticotropic hormone [ACTH]) with resultant manifestations of Cushing's syndrome and hypokalemic alkalosis. Vasoactive intestinal peptide may be produced, resulting in severe diarrhea. Hyperglycemia, resulting from catecholamine-associated antagonism of insulin release, and hypercalcemia, resulting from adrenergic stimulation of the parathyroid glands or elaboration of parathyroid hormone-related peptide (PTHrP), also have been encountered. Lactic acidosis may occur as a result of catecholamine-associated decrements in tissue oxygen delivery.

9. **Discuss the cardiovascular manifestations of pheochromocytomas.**
    Cardiovascular manifestations of pheochromocytomas include arrhythmias and catecholamine-induced congestive cardiomyopathy. Atrial and ventricular fibrillations commonly result from precipitous release of catecholamines during surgery or from therapy with tricyclic antidepressants, phenothiazines, metoclopramide, and naloxone. Although cardiogenic pulmonary edema may result from cardiomyopathy, noncardiogenic pulmonary edema also may occur as a result of transient pulmonary vasoconstriction and increased capillary permeability.

10. **Describe the intracerebral symptoms related to pheochromocytoma.**
    Seizures, altered mental status, and cerebral infarctions may occur as a result of intracerebral hemorrhage or embolization.

11. **What do pheochromocytomas elaborate?**
    Most pheochromocytomas secrete NE. Tumors that produce EPI are more commonly intra-adrenal, because the extra-adrenal sympathetic ganglia do not contain phenylethanolamine-N methyltransferase (PNMT), which converts NE to EPI. Dopamine is most commonly associated with malignant tumors.

12. **Why is the blood pressure response among patients with pheochromocytomas so variable?**
    1. The tumors elaborate different biogenic amines. EPI, a beta-adrenergic stimulatory vasodilator that causes hypotension, is secreted by some intra-adrenal tumors, whereas NE, an alpha stimulatory vasoconstrictor that causes hypertension, is produced by most intra-adrenal and all extra-adrenal tumors.
    2. Tumor size indirectly correlates with concentrations of plasma catecholamines. Large tumors (> 50 gm) manifest slow turnover rates and release catecholamine degradation products, whereas small tumors (< 50 gm) with rapid turnover rates elaborate active catecholamines.
    3. Tissue responsiveness to ambient concentrations of catecholamines does not remain constant. Prolonged exposure of tissue to increased plasma catecholamines causes downregulation of alpha$_1$-receptors and tachyphylaxis. Plasma catecholamine levels, therefore, do not correlate with mean arterial pressure.

13. **How is a pheochromocytoma diagnosed?**
The diagnosis depends on the demonstration of excessive amounts of catecholamines in plasma or urine or degradation products in urine. The best screening test is measurement of plasma-free metanephrines (MNs). Plasma-free MNs may be drawn with the patient supine for 15 minutes following an overnight fast. Acetaminophen or labetalol may alter results and should be withdrawn prior to assessment.

14. **How is pheochromocytoma differentiated from essential hypertension?**
Confirmation of elevated plasma-free MNs involves measurement of urinary MN, normetanephrine (NMN), vanillylmandelic acid (VMA), and free catecholamines produced in a 24-hour period. The ability of such tests to differentiate pheochromocytomas from essential hypertension varies among institutions: for VMA, sensitivity is 28–56% and specificity is 98%; for MN and NMN, sensitivity is 67–91% and specificity is 100%; and for free catecholamines, sensitivity is 100% and specificity is 98%. Many groups advocate 24-hour urinary levels of MN and catecholamines as good screening tests. Yield is improved when urine is collected after a paroxysmal episode of symptoms.

15. **What conditions may alter the above diagnostic tests?**
Older assays for VMA were sensitive to dietary vanillin and phenolic acids, requiring patients to restrict their intake of such substances. High-pressure liquid chromatography assays have eliminated most false-positive results due to diet and drugs that alter the metabolism of catecholamines.

16. **Which drugs alter the metabolism of catecholamines?**
   - Drugs that reduce plasma and urine concentrations: alpha$_2$ agonists, calcium channel blockers (chronic), angiotensin-converting enzyme (ACE) inhibitors, bromocriptine.
   - Drugs that decrease VMA and increase catecholamines and MN: methyldopa, monoamine oxidase inhibitors.
   - Drugs that increase plasma or urine catecholamines: alpha$_1$ blockers, beta blockers, labetalol.
   - Drugs that produce variable changes in any test: phenothiazines, tricyclic antidepressants, levodopa.

17. **What other medications may interfere with test results?**
   - Methylglucamine in radiocontrast agents (decreases MN)
   - Methenamine mandelate (decreases urinary catecholamines)
   - Clofibrate (decreases VMA)
   - Nalidixic acid (increases VMA)

18. **List two other conditions that may interfere with test results.**
   - Stimulation of endogenous catecholamines: physiologic stress (ischemia, exercise), drug withdrawal (alcohol, clonidine), vasodilator therapy (nitroglycerin, acute administration of calcium channel blockers).
   - Administration of exogenous catecholamines: appetite suppressants, decongestants.

19. **What other biochemical tests are available?**
Cases in which screening tests are equivocal may warrant a clonidine suppression test. This test employs a centrally acting alpha$_2$ agonist that, in patients without a pheochromocytoma, suppresses neurogenically mediated release of catecholamines through the sympathetic nervous system. Blood samples to assess plasma catecholamines (NE and EPI) are drawn through an indwelling venous catheter; clonidine, 0.3 mg, is administered orally; and plasma catecholamines are sampled again at 1, 2, and 3 hours. Plasma catecholamines decrease to less than 500 pg/mL in patients with essential hypertension but exceed this level in patients with pheochromocytomas.

20. **Compare computed tomography (CT) and magnetic resonance imaging (MRI) for localization of pheochromocytomas.**
The majority of tumors are larger than 3 cm, rendering them detectable by CT or MRI. CT, with special attention to the adrenal glands and pelvis, is advocated as the initial localizing procedure (97% are intra-abdominal). Many also recommend MRI as an adjunctive localizing modality. Advantages of MRI include the lack of radiation exposure and the characteristic hyperintense image on T_2-weighted scans. The hyperintense image allows definition of tumor size, differentiation from vascular structures, and identification of unsuspected metastases.

KEY POINTS: PHEOCHROMOCYTOMA ✓

1. Episodic headache, diaphoresis, and palpitations in a hypertensive patient suggest pheochromocytoma.

2. 10% of pheochromocytomas are bilateral, 10% extra-adrenal, 10% familial, and 10% malignant.

3. The best screening assay for pheochromocytoma is plasma-free metanephrines.

4. Confirmation of the diagnosis of pheochromocytoma is elevated 24-hour urine levels of metanephrines and catecholamines.

5. Localization of tumor is accomplished with MRI (T_2-weighted phase) or CT.

6. Therapy is surgical resection after administration of alpha blockade followed by beta blockade.

21. **What other modalities are useful for localization of pheochromocytomas?**
Scintigraphic localization with m-(^{131}I) iodobenzylguanidine (MIBG) may also reveal unsuspected metastases. MIBG is actively concentrated by sympathomedullary tissue and is subject to interference by drugs that block reuptake of catecholamines (tricyclic antidepressants, guanethidine, labetalol).

22. **Summarize the performance criteria of each localizing procedure.**

	CT (%)	MRI (%)	MIBG (%)
Sensitivity	98	100	78
Specificity	70	67	100
Positive predictive value	69	83	100
Negative predictive value	98	100	87

23. **How are pheochromocytomas treated?**
Surgical resection is the only definitive therapy.

24. **Why is preoperative preparation with alpha blockade recommended?**
Alpha blockade reduces the incidence of intraoperative hypertensive crisis and postoperative hypotension. The most commonly used agent is phenoxybenzamine, a long-acting, noncompetitive antagonist (10–20 mg 2–3 times/day, advanced to 80–100 mg/day), or

prazosin, a short-acting antagonist (1 mg t.i.d., advanced to 5 mg t.i.d.). Therapy may be limited by hypotension, tachycardia, and dizziness. Goals of therapy include blood pressure < 160/90, an electrocardiogram (ECG) free of ST- or T-wave changes over 2 weeks before surgery, and no more than one premature ventricular contraction/15 minutes. Opinions about the duration of preparation vary between 7 and 28 days before surgery.

25. **Discuss the role of beta blocker and other agents in the preoperative period.**
Beta blockade to control tachycardia is added only after alpha-adrenergic blockade has been instituted to prevent unopposed alpha stimulation. Other agents used in the preoperative period include labetalol or calcium channel blockers. Intraoperative hypertension associated with tumor manipulation may be controlled with either phentolamine or nitroprusside. Postoperative hypotension may be minimized by preoperative volume expansion with crystalloid.

26. **How are malignant pheochromocytomas treated?**
Although evidence of malignancy may be discovered at the time of surgery, metastases from slow-growing pheochromocytomas may remain inapparent for several years. Therapy is rarely curative, because the tumors respond poorly to radiation therapy and chemotherapy; treatment is therefore palliative. Surgical debulking is the therapy of choice, followed by use of alpha-methyltyrosine. This drug is a "false" catecholamine precursor that inhibits tyrosine hydroxylase (the rate-limiting enzyme in catecholamine synthesis) and reduces excessive production of catecholamines.

27. **Discuss the role of combination chemotherapy and MIBG ablation.**
Combination chemotherapy with cyclophosphamide, vincristine, and adriamycin may slow tumor growth, as may ablation with MIBG. Unfortunately, neither of these therapeutic measures has resulted in prolonged survival.

28. **What is the prognosis for patients with malignant pheochromocytoma?**
Prognosis is not dismal. Cases of 20-year survival have been reported, and the 5-year survival rate with malignant pheochromocytomas is 44%.

29. **Which medical conditions are associated with pheochromocytomas?**
   - MEN-2A: hyperparathyroidism, medullary carcinoma of the thyroid, pheochromocytoma.
   - MEN-2B: medullary carcinoma of the thyroid, marfanoid habitus, pheochromocytoma.
   - Carney's triad: paragangliomas, gastric epithelial leiomyosarcomas, benign pulmonarychondromas (females), and Leydig's cell tumors (males).
   - Neurofibromatosis: café-au-lait spots in 5% of patients with pheochromocytoma; 1% of patients with neurofibromatosis have pheochromocytomas.
   - von Hippel-Lindau syndrome: retinal and cerebellar hemangioblastomas; as many as 10% may have pheochromocytomas.

BIBLIOGRAPHY

1. Bravo EL: Evolving concepts in the pathophysiology, diagnosis and treatment of pheochromocytoma. Endocrine Rev 15:356–368, 1994.
2. Eisenhofer G: Editorial: Biochemical diagnosis of pheochromocytoma—Is it time to switch to plasma-free metanephrines? J Clin Endocrinol Metab 88:550–552, 2003.
3. Francis IR, Gross MD, Shapiro B, et al: Integrated imaging of adrenal disease. Radiology 187:1–13, 1992.
4. Golub MS, Tuck ML: Diagnostic and therapeutic strategies in pheochromocytoma. Endocrinologist 2:101–105, 1992.
5. Jossart GH, Burpee SE, Gagner M: Surgery of the adrenal glands. Endocrinol Metab Clin North Am 29:57–68, 2000.

6. Krane NK: Clinically unsuspected pheochromocytomas: Experience at Henry Ford Hospital and a review of the literature. Arch Intern Med 146:54–57, 1986.

7. Kudva YC, Sawka AM, Young WF: The laboratory diagnosis of adrenal pheochromocytoma: The Mayo Clinic experience. J Clin Endocrinol Metab 88:4533–4539, 2003.

8. Prys-Roberts C: Phaeochromocytoma—recent progress in management. Br J Anaesth 85:44–57, 2000.

9. Sawka AM, Jaeschke R, Singh RJ, et al: A comparison of biochemical tests for pheochromocytoma: Measurement of fractionated plasma metanephrines compared with the combination of 24-hour urinary metanephrines and catecholamines. J Clin Endocrinol Metab 88:553–558, 2003.

10. Sheps SG, Jiang N, Klee GG, van Heerden JA: Recent developments in the diagnosis and treatment of pheochromocytoma. Mayo Clin Proc 65:88–95, 1990.

11. Ulchaker JC, Goldfarb DA, Bravo EL, et al: Successful outcomes in pheochromocytoma surgery in the modern era. J Urol 161:764–767, 1999.

12. Wittles RM, Kaplan EL, Roizen MF: Sensitivity of diagnostic and localization tests for pheochromocytoma in clinical practice. Arch Intern Med 160:2521–2524, 2000.

13. Young WF: Pheochromocytoma and primary aldosteronism: Diagnostic approaches. Endocrinol Metab Clin N Am 26:801–827, 1997.

CHAPTER 30

ADRENAL MALIGNANCIES

Michael T. McDermott, M.D.

1. **What types of cancer occur in the adrenal glands?**
   Carcinomas may arise in the adrenal cortex (adrenocortical carcinomas) or the adrenal medulla (malignant pheochromocytomas). They also may metastasize to the adrenals from other primary sites.

2. **Do adrenocortical carcinomas produce hormones?**
   Approximately 50–70% secrete steroid hormones, whereas 30–50% are nonfunctioning.

3. **What are the clinical features of functioning adrenocortical carcinomas?**
   Functioning adrenocortical carcinomas secrete aldosterone, cortisol, or androgens—alone or in combination. Excessive aldosterone (Conn's syndrome) causes hypertension and hypokalemia. Cortisol overproduction results in Cushing's syndrome. Excessive androgen secretion causes hirsutism and virilization in women and precocious puberty in children but is often asymptomatic in men (Fig. 30-1).

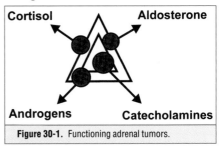

Figure 30-1. Functioning adrenal tumors.

4. **What are the clinical features of nonfunctioning adrenocortical carcinomas?**
   Nonfunctioning adrenocortical carcinomas present clinically as abdominal or flank pain or as an adrenal mass discovered incidentally during an imaging procedure.

5. **What clues are most suggestive that an adrenocortical tumor is malignant?**
   Malignancy is strongly suggested by tumor size > 6 cm, evidence of locally invasive or metastatic disease to the liver or lungs, and elevated urinary 17-ketosteroid excretion. The diagnosis of malignancy is often not suspected, however, until histologic examination after tumor removal.

6. **Describe the treatment for an adrenocortical carcinoma.**
   The treatment of choice is surgery. Mitotane, an adrenal cytotoxic agent, has produced partial or complete tumor regression, reduced production of adrenal hormones, and improved survival in nonrandomized, noncontrolled trials. The combination of mitotane with etoposide, cisplatin, and doxorubicin has shown some promise, but responses to chemotherapy have, in general, been disappointing. Radiation therapy has not been shown to be effective with these tumors.

7. **What is the prognosis for patients with adrenocortical carcinoma?**
   The mean survival is 15 months. The 5-year survival rate is about 20–35%. Prognosis is improved by young age, small tumor size, localized disease, complete tumor resection, and in nonfunctioning tumors.

8. **How often are pheochromocytomas malignant?**
   Approximately 10–15% of pheochromocytomas are malignant.

9. **What are the clinical features of a malignant pheochromocytoma?**
   Most pheochromocytomas, whether benign or malignant, cause hypertension, headaches, sweating, and palpitations. They are diagnosed biochemically by the finding of increased levels of metanephrine or catecholamines in the plasma or urine. Malignant pheochromocytomas usually do not differ clinically at presentation from those that are benign.

10. **What clues suggest that a pheochromocytoma is malignant?**
    Malignancy is most strongly suggested by tumor size > 6 cm, evidence of extra-adrenal spread (usually to the lymph nodes, liver, lungs, or bones) and by disproportionately increased plasma or urine levels of dopamine and/or homovanillic acid (HVA). The malignant character of some tumors may be missed, even histologically, and not become apparent until metastatic disease appears.

KEY POINTS: ADRENAL MALIGNANCIES ✓

1. Adrenal cortical carcinomas present with features of cortisol, aldosterone or androgen excess, with abdominal or flank pain, or as an incidentally discovered adrenal mass.

2. Malignant pheochromocytomas often present with features similar to those of benign pheochromocytomas (hypertension, headaches, palpitations, sweating).

3. Features suggesting that an adrenal tumor is malignant are size > 6 cm, evidence of local invasion or metastases to the liver or lung, and high levels of urinary 17 ketosteroids, HVA, or plasma dopamine.

4. Surgery is the treatment of choice for malignant adrenal tumors; chemotherapy has primarily a palliative role and radiation therapy is largely ineffective.

5. Incidentally discovered adrenal masses should be evaluated for evidence of malignancy (size > 6 cm or progressive growth) and excess hormone secretion (cortisol, aldosterone, androgens, catecholamines).

11. **What is the treatment for a malignant pheochromocytoma?**
    Surgery is the treatment of choice. Alpha-adrenergic blocking agents (phenoxybenzamine, prazosin) are given preoperatively to control blood pressure and replete intravascular volume. Beta blockers may then be added for reflex tachycardia or persistent hypertension. These drugs and alpha-methyltyrosine, an inhibitor of catecholamine synthesis, are also effective chronic therapy for patients with unresectable tumors. Cyclophosphamide, vincristine, dacarbazine, and MIBG may cause partial regression of residual tumors.

12. **What is the prognosis for malignant pheochromocytoma?**
    The 5-year survival rate for malignant pheochromocytoma is 40–45%.

13. **What tumors metastasize to the adrenal glands?**
    The vascular adrenal glands are a frequent site of bilateral metastatic spread from cancers of the lung, breast, stomach, pancreas, colon, and kidney, and from melanomas and lymphomas.

14. **What is the clinical significance of metastatic disease to the adrenal glands?**
Acute adrenal crises are rare. However, up to 33% of patients may have subtle adrenal insufficiency manifested by nonspecific symptoms and an inadequate response (peak cortisol level < 20 (µg/dL) to a cosyntropin stimulation test. These patients may experience improvement in well-being when given physiologic glucocorticoid replacement.

15. **How should the incidentally discovered adrenal mass be managed?**
Incidental adrenal masses should be assessed for evidence of malignancy and excess hormone secretion. Size is the best predictor of cancer; 25% of masses > 6 cm in size are malignant whereas < 2% of those that are < 4 cm in size are malignant. The most common hormonal disorder is subclinical Cushing's syndrome; the most risky is pheochromocytoma. Accordingly, the recommended hormone evaluation is a 1-mg overnight dexamethasone suppression test and plasma-free metanephrine measurement; patients with hypertension should also have plasma aldosterone and renin levels measured. Surgery is indicated for tumors > 6 cm in size, for those 4–6 cm in size with other radiologic features suggesting cancer or rapid growth on follow-up, for pheochromocytomas and for other overt hormonal syndromes.

16. **How should the incidentally discovered adrenal mass be managed?**
Nonfunctioning masses > 6 cm and all hormone-secreting tumors should be removed surgically. Some experts recommend a size cutoff of 4.5 cm for surgery. Smaller masses should be reassessed in 3–6 months, then annually, and removed if growth occurs or if excess hormone secretion develops.

BIBLIOGRAPHY

1. Berruti A, Terzolo M, Pia A, et al: Mitotane associated with etoposide, doxorubicin, and cisplatin in the treatment of advanced adrenocortical carcinoma. Cancer 83:2194–2200, 1998.
2. Beuschlein F, Looyenga BD, Reincke M, et al: Clinical impact of recent advances in the biology of adrenal cortical cancer. Endocrinologist 13:470–478, 2003.
3. Bornstein SR, Stratakis CA, Chrousos GP: Adrenocortical tumors: Recent advances in basic concepts and clinical management. Ann Intern Med 130:759–771, 1999.
4. Demeure MJ, Somberg LB: Functioning and nonfunctioning adrenocortical carcinoma: Clinical presentation and therapeutic strategies. Surg Oncol Clin N Am 7:791–805, 1998.
5. Freeman DA: Adrenal carcinoma. Curr Ther Endocrinol Metab 6:173–175, 1997.
6. Grinspon SK, Biller BMK: Laboratory assessment of adrenal insufficiency. J Clin Endocrinol Metab 79:923–931, 1994.
7. Gross MD, Shapiro B: Clinically silent adrenal masses. J Clin Endocrinol Metab 77:885–888, 1993.
8. Grumbach MM, Biller BK, Braunstein GD, et al: Management of the clinically inapparent adrenal mass ("incidentaloma"). Ann Intern Med 138:424–429, 2003.
9. Harrison LE, Gaudin PB, Brennan MF: Pathologic features of prognostic significance for adrenocortical carcinoma after curative resection. Arch Surg 134:181–185, 1999.
10. Luton J-P, Cerdas S, Billaud L, et al: Clinical features of adrenocortical carcinoma, prognostic factors, and the effect of mitotane therapy. N Engl J Med 322:1195–1201, 1990.
11. Oelkers W: Adrenal insufficiency. N Engl J Med 335:1206–1212, 1996.
12. Reincke M, Nieke J, Krestin GP, et al: Preclinical Cushing's syndrome in adrenal "incidentalomas": Comparison with adrenal Cushing's syndrome. J Clin Endocrinol Metab 75:826–832, 1992.
13. Ross NS, Aron DC: Hormonal evaluation of the patient with an incidentally discovered adrenal mass. N Engl J Med 323:1401–1405, 1990.
14. Schulick RD, Brennan MF: Long-term survival after complete resection and repeat resection in patients with adrenocortical carcinoma. Ann Surg Oncol 6:719–726, 1999.
15. Tritos NA, Cushing GW, Heatley G, Libertino JA: Clinical features and prognostic factors associated with adrenocortical carcinoma: Lahey Clinic Medical Center experience. Am Surg 66:73–79, 2000.

16. Wajchenberg BL, Albergaria Pereira MA, Mendonca BB, et al: Adrenocortical carcinoma: Clinical and laboratory observations. Cancer 88:711–736, 2000.

17. Williamson SK, Lew D, Miller GJ, et al: Phase II evaluation of cisplatin and etoposide followed by mitotane at disease progression in patients with locally advanced or metastatic adrenocortical carcinoma: A Southwest Oncology Group Study. Cancer 88:1159–1165, 2000.

CHAPTER 31

ADRENAL INSUFFICIENCY

Robert E. Jones, M.D., and Cecilia C.L. Wang, M.D.

1. **How is adrenal insufficiency classified?**
   The clinical classification of adrenal insufficiency follows the functional organization of the hypothalamic-pituitary-adrenal axis. Primary adrenal insufficiency is defined as the loss of adrenocortical hormones due to destruction or impairment of the adrenal cortex. Secondary adrenal insufficiency is due to reduced secretion by the pituitary gland of adrenocorticotropin hormone (ACTH), whereas tertiary adrenal insufficiency is caused by failure of the hypothalamus to produce corticotropin-releasing hormone (CRH).

2. **What is the most common cause of primary adrenal insufficiency?**
   Autoimmune adrenalitis, which may be either confined to the adrenal gland or part of a polyglandular autoimmune syndrome.

3. **List the other causes of primary adrenal insufficiency.**
   - Infectious adrenalitis due to tuberculosis or disseminated fungal infections. In patients infected with human immunodeficiency virus (HIV), adrenalitis due to cytomegalovirus or HIV itself occasionally results in adrenal failure.
   - Bilateral adrenal hemorrhage may lead to acute, fulminant adrenal insufficiency in the setting of sepsis or anticoagulant therapy.
   - Adrenomyeloneuropathy, an X-linked recessive disorder, has become more frequently recognized as a cause of adrenal insufficiency in younger men.
   - Bilateral metastatic disease from lung, breast, or enteric carcinomas is common.
   - Certain medications may reduce circulating levels of adrenal steroids, either by inhibiting one or more steroidogenic enzymes (e.g., ketoconazole, aminoglutethimide) or by enhancing the metabolic clearance rate of steroids (e.g., rifampin).

4. **Why do metastatic disease and medications typically not lead to adrenal insufficiency?**
   Metastases rarely result in adrenal insufficiency because greater than 90% of the glandular tissue must be replaced by tumor before clinical insufficiency is seen. Adrenal insufficiency typically does not result from medications unless they are given in high doses or the patient has an underlying adrenal condition that limits adrenal secretory reserve.

5. **What causes secondary adrenal insufficiency?**
   Secondary adrenal insufficiency typically results from either a loss of anterior pituitary corticotrophs or disruption of the pituitary stalk. It usually occurs in association with panhypopituitarism, but selective ACTH deficiency, either inherited or due to autoimmunity, also has been reported.

6. **What is the most common cause of panhypopituitarism?**
   Space-occupying lesions of the sella turcica. Primary pituitary tumors, craniopharyngiomas, or, on rare occasions, metastatic lesions from breast, prostate, or lung carcinomas may infiltrate and destroy corticotrophs.

7. **What other conditions may lead to secondary adrenal insufficiency?**
Aneurysms of the internal carotid artery may erode into the sella, and infiltrative diseases, such as histiocytosis X or sarcoidosis, have been associated with secondary adrenal insufficiency. Severe head trauma that disrupts the pituitary stalk, and either excessive blood loss that causes shock during delivery (Sheehan's syndrome) or hemorrhage into a pituitary adenoma (pituitary apoplexy) may result in panhypopituitarism. Infections due to tuberculosis and histoplasmosis have resulted in a loss of anterior pituitary function. Lymphocytic hypophysitis, another autoimmune disorder, also causes secondary adrenal insufficiency. Loss of corticotrophs also may occur after pituitary surgery or 5–10 years after the delivery of 4800–5200 R to the pituitary fossa as radiation therapy for a pituitary tumor.

8. **What are the causes of tertiary adrenal insufficiency?**
The most common cause of tertiary adrenal insufficiency is the long-term use of suppressive doses of glucocorticoids; for example, the use of prednisone in the treatment of rheumatic disease or inflammatory disease. Suppression of CRH with resultant adrenal insufficiency is a paradoxical concomitant of successful therapy for Cushing's syndrome. Loss of hypothalamic function also may result from various tumors, infiltrative diseases, and cranial radiation therapy.

9. **Which symptoms are frequently encountered in adrenal insufficiency?**
Most of the symptoms of adrenal insufficiency are relatively nonspecific. Weakness, fatigue, and anorexia are almost universal complaints. Most patients also report minor gastrointestinal symptoms, such as nausea, vomiting, ill-defined abdominal pain, or constipation. On occasion, the gastrointestinal symptoms may be the predominant complaint and, as a result, may divert the physician into a long and fruitless evaluation. Symptoms of orthostatic hypotension, arthralgias, myalgias, and salt-craving are also encountered. Psychiatric symptoms may range from mild memory impairment to overt psychosis.

10. **Describe the common signs of adrenal insufficiency.**
Weight loss occurs in all patients with adrenal insufficiency. Hyperpigmentation, presumably caused by elevated levels of ACTH or related peptide fragments, is noted in over 90% of patients with primary adrenal insufficiency. Hyperpigmentation may be generalized or localized to regions subjected to repeated trauma, such as elbows, knees, knuckles, and buccal mucosa. New scars are also frequently hyperpigmented, and preexisting freckles may increase in number. Vitiligo, areas of cutaneous pigment loss, may coexist in 10–20% of patients with autoimmune adrenalitis. Hypotension is also common in both primary and secondary adrenal insufficiency.

11. **Which sign of adrenal insufficiency is more pronounced in women?**
Loss of axillary and pubic hair is more pronounced in women because of the loss of adrenal androgen secretion.

12. **What peculiar finding may be seen in long-standing adrenal insufficiency from any cause?**
Auricular cartilage calcification.

13. **Discuss the laboratory abnormalities associated with adrenal insufficiency.**
Hyponatremia and hyperkalemia are the most common abnormalities. Patients also may have a mild normocytic, normochromic anemia and may demonstrate eosinophilia and lymphocytosis on a peripheral blood smear. Prerenal azotemia secondary to volume depletion is more common in secondary insufficiency. Modest hypercalcemia is present in less than 10% of patients. Moderate elevations of thyroid-stimulating hormone (TSH) (usually < 15 µU/mL) are also common. Whether the elevation is due to underlying autoimmune thyroid disease, to loss of TSH suppression by endogenous steroids, or to the euthyroid sick syndrome is unclear.

14. **How do the presentations of primary and secondary adrenal insufficiency differ?**
The features of primary and secondary adrenal insufficiency have many similarities and two major differences: hyperpigmentation and hyperkalemia are not seen in secondary adrenal insufficiency. Due to the loss of ACTH secretion, hyperpigmentation does not occur in secondary adrenal insufficiency. Similarly, the adrenal zona glomerulosa remains responsive to the renin angiotensin system in secondary adrenal insufficiency, and secretion of aldosterone is not compromised. Consequently, severe volume depletion is uncommon, and hyperkalemia is not encountered with the loss of ACTH. Cortisol is important in clearance of free water; thus, deficiency of cortisol from any cause may result in hyponatremia.

15. **What other autoimmune disease may be associated with autoimmune adrenalitis?**
Both type I and type II polyglandular autoimmune syndromes are associated with primary adrenal insufficiency. In type II, the more common syndrome, adrenal insufficiency, is universally present. Both syndromes are discussed in greater detail in Chapter 53. On rare occasions, patients with other autoimmune endocrinopathies, such as chronic lymphocytic thyroiditis or insulin-dependent diabetes mellitus, may develop adrenal insufficiency.

16. **How is the diagnosis of adrenal insufficiency confirmed?**
A low plasma cortisol level (< 5 µg/dL) in the face of severe physiologic stress provides reasonably solid evidence for adrenal insufficiency. Conversely, a random plasma cortisol level > 20 µg/dL virtually excludes the diagnosis. In the basal or nonstressed state, a morning cortisol level > 10 µg/dL generally correlates well with an intact hypothalamic-pituitary-adrenal axis, but cortisol values in this range also may be seen in patients with limited functional reserve of the axis. Screening patients with an ACTH (Cosyntropin) stimulation test may provide misleading information. A plasma cortisol level > 20 µg/dL during a short ACTH stimulation test excludes the diagnosis of primary adrenal insufficiency, but it does not rule out a subtle ACTH deficiency; additional testing is frequently required (see questions 17–20).

17. **Which tests are useful in distinguishing primary from secondary (or tertiary) adrenal insufficiency?**
Simultaneous measurements of ACTH and cortisol levels clearly differentiate primary adrenal failure from a central cause. In primary adrenal failure, ACTH levels are elevated, while they are low normal to frankly low in secondary or tertiary hypoadrenalism.

18. **Is the ACTH stimulation test helpful in differentiating a partial ACTH deficiency from normal adrenal function?**
Differentiating a partial ACTH deficiency from normal adrenal function is a more challenging problem. A short ACTH (Cosyntropin) stimulation test is always abnormal in primary adrenal insufficiency and may be blunted in central adrenal insufficiency. In order for the short ACTH stimulation test to be abnormal in central adrenal insufficiency, the deficiency of ACTH must be both profound and protracted, resulting in adrenal atrophy due to the loss of the trophic effect of ACTH. Some investigators have advocated using smaller doses of ACTH (1 µg) as opposed to the standard or high-dose (250 µg) test to ferret out milder cases of central adrenal insufficiency.

19. **Discuss the problems associated with the low-dose test.**
There may be some overlap in the cortisol responses between normal people and those with partial deficiency of ACTH. In addition, since the low-dose (1 µg) test is not routinely performed in most settings, technical problems, such as preparation of an accurately diluted ACTH solution and adhesion to tubing, required for ACTH infusion can cause test-to-test variability and false positives. Others question whether sufficient data show an abnormal response to a low-dose test is clinically relevant. A recent review and meta-analysis showed that the sensitivity and

KEY POINTS: CLASSIFICATION AND DIAGNOSIS OF ADRENAL INSUFFICIENCY ✔

1. Adrenal insufficiency is classified as primary (failure of adrenals to produce cortisol), secondary (failure of pituitary to produce ACTH), or tertiary (failure of hypothalamus to produce CRH).

2. Adrenal insufficiency should be suspected in outpatients who have received supraphysiologic doses of glucocorticoids for > 1 month, intensive care unit (ICU) patients who are hemodynamically unstable despite aggressive fluid resuscitation or have septic shock, and any patient with signs or symptoms suggesting adrenal insufficiency.

3. Adrenal insufficiency is diagnosed using a 30- or 60-minute cortisol level of < 20 μg/dL in a standard-dose cosyntropin stimulation test or an increment of < 9 μg/dL in an ICU patient with septic shock.

specificity of low-dose and standard-dose ACTH testing are similar but found no evidence for replacing standard testing with low-dose testing. Associated difficulties with low-dose testing included the need for precise timing of blood sampling and intravenous administration, while standard-dose ACTH can be given intramuscularly and does not require exact timing.

20. **What other tests are used to differentiate a partial ACTH deficiency from normal adrenal function?**
Other tests include insulin-induced hypoglycemia (the gold standard) and the metyrapone test, but metyrapone is currently unavailable in the U.S. On occasion, the patient may be overlooked during the diagnostic evaluation. Do not forget to give replacement glucocorticoids during metabolic testing, and do not forget that exogenous steroids may suppress ACTH, thereby invalidating some testing. Dexamethasone is the recommended supplement because it can be used in low doses and does not interfere with the measurement of cortisol.

21. **Explain how adrenal crisis is managed.**
The five S's of management are salt, sugar, steroids, support, and search for a precipitating illness. Volume should be restored with several liters of 0.9% saline with 5% dextrose. After a sample of blood has been obtained for measurement of cortisol and ACTH, 100 mg of hydrocortisone (cortisol) should be immediately administered intravenously. When hydrocortisone is given in the recommended dose of 100 mg every 8 hours, additional mineralocorticoid is unnecessary. Some authors also advocate the administration of a single dose of dexamethasone (4 mg) during the initial resuscitation of the patient. If the precipitating event or complicating illness has been controlled, the glucocorticoids should be tapered to maintenance levels after 1–3 days.

22. **How urgently should a patient with suspected adrenal crisis be treated?**
Left untreated, adrenal crisis is fatal. If adrenal crisis is suspected, it must be aggressively treated; stress doses of glucocorticoids carry virtually no morbidity when used in the short term. A formal diagnostic evaluation can be performed at a later time, after the patient has been stabilized.

23. **How is chronic adrenal insufficiency best managed?**
Maintenance therapy for adrenal insufficiency involves replacement of both glucocorticoid and, if necessary, mineralocorticoid. Hydrocortisone and cortisone acetate are the most frequently used replacement glucocorticoids; however, prednisone also may be used. The usual dose of

hydrocortisone is 15–20 mg given in the morning and 5–10 mg in the afternoon, whereas the dose for cortisone acetate is usually 25 mg in the morning and 12.5 mg in the afternoon. The total daily dose for prednisone generally ranges from 2.5 to 7.5 mg and may be given either as a single dose in the evening or divided into morning and afternoon doses with the morning dose the larger of the two.

24. **Explain the role of fludrocortisone in maintenance therapy for adrenal insufficiency.**
Fludrocortisone (Florinef), given as a daily dose of 0.05–0.2 mg, is used as a replacement for aldosterone and is generally required to manage the electrolyte abnormalities encountered in primary adrenal insufficiency.

25. **How is the response to treatment monitored?**
The response to replacement therapy may be monitored simply and inexpensively by careful attention to serial weights, blood pressure, electrolytes, and a directed history to assess general health status and well-being. Some authors suggest serial measurements of urinary cortisol excretion to assess the adequacy of cortisol replacement. Care should be taken to avoid excessive doses of glucocorticoids, which may result in osteoporosis or excessive weight gain. The intent of long-term management of adrenal insufficiency is to use the smallest dose of glucocorticoids that provides the maximal benefit in the relief of symptoms.

26. **Do patients with adrenal insufficiency require additional hormone supplementation during times of stress?**
Any stress, including febrile illnesses, trauma, or diagnostic/surgical procedures, may precipitate an acute adrenal crisis. Therefore, the judicious use of supplemental steroids prevents possible tragedy. Doubling or tripling the glucocorticoid dose is sufficient for mild-to-moderate infections. If vomiting is a feature of the illness or if symptoms consistent with acute adrenal crisis supervene, the patient should be hospitalized for therapy.

27. **When should intravenous supplementation be considered?**
More severe infections or surgical procedures involving general anesthesia usually require the intravenous administration of hydrocortisone or an equivalent glucocorticoid.

28. **What are the recommended stress doses of hydrocortisone?**
Stress doses of hydrocortisone should be tailored to the degree of stress. The dosage for moderate surgical stress should be 50–75 mg/day for 1–2 days, whereas major surgical stress should be managed with 100–150 mg/day for 2–3 days. The total dose should be divided into thirds and given every 8 hours. If hypotension ensues, the dose of hydrocortisone may be increased to 100 mg every 8 hours. The stress dose of glucocorticoids may be tapered over 1–2 days, and the previous dose of glucocorticoid may be resumed after resolution of the underlying stress. Additional steroid coverage should also be given in the presence of moderate-to-severe trauma.

29. **Describe the nonpharmacologic interventions necessary for effective management of patients with adrenal insufficiency.**
Education of the patient is paramount. The patient must know what to do during an intercurrent illness. An injectable glucocorticoid, such as dexamethasone, should always be readily available for emergency use. Likewise, a warning tag may prove to be providential in alerting a health care team to the presence of adrenal insufficiency if the patient is incapable of providing an appropriate history.

30. **Discuss the relative potencies of available steroids.**
The biologic potency of steroids depends on various factors, including absorption, affinity to corticosteroid-binding globulin (CBG), hepatic metabolism, and affinity to intracellular

TABLE 31-1.	RELATIVE POTENCIES OF STEROID HORMONES		
Compound	Glucocorticoid Activity	Mineralocorticoid Activity	Duration
Hydrocortisone	1.0	1.0	Short
Cortisone	0.7	0.7	Short
Prednisone	4.0	0.7	Short
Methylprednisolone	5.0	0.5	Short
Dexamethasone	30.0	0.0	Long
Fludrocortisone	10.0	400.0	Long

glucocorticoid receptor. As a general rule, synthetic steroids are poorly bound to CBG and more slowly metabolized; they also have a greater affinity for the glucocorticoid receptor than cortisol. Table 31-1 gives the approximate potencies of available preparations.

31. **When is diagnostic imaging helpful in the evaluation of adrenal insufficiency?**
Pituitary and hypothalamic imaging is absolutely essential to assess the regional anatomy in all patients with newly diagnosed secondary or tertiary adrenal insufficiency. By contrast, adrenal imaging in patients with primary adrenal insufficiency is rarely helpful. The only exception is when the diagnosis of bilateral adrenal hemorrhage is entertained. In this circumstance, an adrenal computed tomography (CT) scan is virtually diagnostic. Imaging of the adrenals and/or pituitary is not appropriate to make the diagnosis of adrenal insufficiency due of the high incidence of incidentally discovered lesions (incidentalomas) that do not account for the observed clinical findings. Imaging should be performed only after the biochemical diagnosis of adrenal insufficiency has been made.

32. **What is the prognosis for patients with adrenal insufficiency?**
Before isolation of glucocorticoids, the life expectancy of patients with adrenal insufficiency was less than 6 months. With prompt diagnosis and appropriate replacement therapy, patients with autoimmune adrenalitis now enjoy a normal life span. The prognosis of adrenal insufficiency due to other causes depends on the underlying disorder.

33. **When patients are given pharmacologic doses of corticosteroids for nonadrenal diseases, how should tapering from steroids be handled?**
There are as many suggested regimens of steroid tapering as there are authors who write on the subject. However, certain universal concepts are common to all approaches. The initial tapering of glucocorticoids from pharmacologic to physiologic doses is limited by the behavior of the treated illness. If the illness flares, the higher dose of steroids should be reinstituted and continued until the symptoms stabilize. Later, a more gradual tapering should be reinitiated.

34. **What should be done when near-physiologic doses of glucocorticoids are reached?**
The patient may be switched either to hydrocortisone or to alternate-day therapy, with tapering continued. Reestablishment of a normal hypothalamic-pituitary-adrenal axis is heralded by the return of the plasma cortisol to > 10 μg/dL 24 hours after the last dose of steroid and normal adrenal responsiveness to exogenous ACTH (short ACTH stimulation). Full recovery of the complete axis may take 6–9 months; the adrenal responsiveness to ACTH is the last limb of the axis to recover.

35. **What is steroid withdrawal syndrome?**

Some patients may develop steroid withdrawal syndrome during rapid tapering, or after steroids have been discontinued. This syndrome is characterized by the typical features of adrenal insufficiency; however, arthralgias, myalgias, and, on rare occasions, desquamation may be the predominating symptoms.

36. **When should a patient on exogenous glucocorticoids be considered functionally suppressed?**

Any patient who has received more than 20 mg of daily prednisone (or glucocorticoid equivalent) for more than 1 month in the preceding year or greater-than-replacement doses of glucocorticoids for more than 1 year should be considered to have a potentially suppressed axis and therefore should be given stress doses of glucocorticoids during intercurrent illness.

KEY POINTS: TREATMENT OF ADRENAL INSUFFICIENCY ✓

1. Treatment of adrenal insufficiency depends on the condition of the patient.

2. Nonstressed outpatients should be treated with replacement doses of hydrocortisone or prednisone with or without fludrocortisone, depending on the type of adrenal insufficiency.

3. Stressed patients should receive supplemental glucocorticoids tailored to the degree of stress.

4. ICU patients may need intravenous glucocorticoids at stress doses until their condition improves.

5. Adrenal crisis should be treated aggressively using normal saline with 5% dextrose, intravenous glucocorticoids (dexamethasone if treating before drawing random cortisol and ACTH, hydrocortisone afterwards), other supportive care, and a search for the precipitating illness.

37. **What role do adrenal androgens play in the replacement therapy of adrenal insufficiency?**

Dehydroepiandrosterone (DHEA) and its sulfated form (DHEA-S) are the major adrenal androgens. Both are weak androgens at best, but in women, they are converted in peripheral tissues to the more potent androgens testosterone and 5α-dihydrotestosterone. This peripheral conversion is a very significant source of circulating testosterone levels in females, and women who have adrenal insufficiency have very low circulating levels of DHEA. This has prompted several groups to investigate the effects of DHEA replacement in women with adrenal insufficiency. Oral DHEA (50 mg/day) essentially normalized circulating levels of androgens in these women and dramatically improved feelings of well-being, as well as mental and physical aspects of sexuality.

38. **When should glucocorticoids be used in the ICU?**

There should be a low threshold for testing for adrenal insufficiency in patients in the ICU with hemodynamic instability despite adequate fluid resuscitation, signs or symptoms suggesting the presence of adrenal insufficiency, or septic shock. A random cortisol level should be drawn since the diurnal rhythm of cortisol secretion is lost in severe stress, and a corticotropin stimulation test should be performed. Hydrocortisone, 50 mg IV every 6 hours or 100 mg IV every 8 hours, can be used empirically until the results of testing are available. If treatment is considered emergent, dexamethasone should be used initially until after the Cortrosyn stimulation test is performed, since dexamethasone is not measured in the cortisol assay and will not interfere with the results. Some data support the use of glucocorticoids in patients with nonresolving acute respiratory distress syndrome and early bacterial meningitis (using dexamethasone).

39. **Explain "functional" adrenal insufficiency.**
Serum cortisol correlates roughly with severity of stress. Functional adrenal insufficiency has been difficult to define biochemically, but it is basically the presence of subnormal adrenal glucocorticoid production in the setting of acute severe illness without obvious structural defects in the hypothalamic-pituitary-adrenal axis. There are some advocates of using 25 μg/dL as the threshold for diagnosing functional adrenal insufficiency in severely ill patients (hypotension, hypoxemia, burns, high fever, multiple trauma). Unfortunately, the data for improved outcomes using glucocorticoid therapy in this setting have not been consistent, except in patients with septic shock with a cortisol increment of < 9 μg/dL during the corticotropin stimulation test.

40. **Explain "relative" adrenal insufficiency.**
The related concept of "relative" adrenal insufficiency refers to ICU patients who have high absolute cortisol levels but continue to have a marked inflammatory response. Few data support the use of glucocorticoid therapy in relative adrenal insufficiency.

BIBLIOGRAPHY

1. Arlt W, Callies F, van Vlijmen JC, et al.: Dehydroepiandrosterone replacement in women with adrenal insufficiency. N Engl J Med 341:1013–1020, 1999.

2. Cooper MS, Stewart PM: Corticosteroid insufficiency in acutely ill patients. N Engl J Med 348:727–734, 2003.

3. Dahlberg PJ, Goellner MH, Pehling GB: Adrenal insufficiency secondary to adrenal hemorrhage: Two case reports and a review of cases confirmed by computed tomography. Arch Intern Med 150:905–909, 1990.

4. Dickstein G, Shechner C, Nicholson WE, et al: Adrenocorticotropin stimulation test: Effects of basal cortisol level, time of day, and suggested new sensitive low dose test. J Clin Endocrinol Metab 72:773–778, 1991.

5. Dorin RI, Qualls CR, Crapo LM: Diagnosis of adrenal insufficiency. Ann Intern Med 139(3):194–204, 2003.

6. Grinspoon SK, Bilezikian JP: Current concepts: HIV disease and the endocrine system. N Engl J Med 327:1360–1365, 1992.

7. Huang TS, Jiang YD: Repetitive graded ACTH stimulation test for adrenal insufficiency. J Endocrinol Invest 23:163–169, 2000.

8. Kamilaris TC, Chrousos GP: Adrenal diseases. In Moore WT, Eastman RC (eds): Diagnostic Endocrinology. Philadelphia, B.C. Dekker, 1990, pp 79–109.

9. Khosa S, Wolfson JS, Demerjian Z, Godine JE: Adrenal crisis in the setting of high-dose ketoconazole therapy. Arch Intern Med 149:802–804, 1989.

10. Marik PE, Zaloga GP: Adrenal insufficiency in the critically ill: A new look at an old problem. Chest 122:1784–1796, 2002.

11. Merenich JA, McDermott MT, Asp AA, et al: Evidence of endocrine involvement early in the course of human immunodeficiency virus infection. J Clin Endocrinol Metab 70:572–577, 1990.

12. Nerup J: Addison's disease—clinical studies: A report of 108 cases. Acta Endocrinol 76:572–577, 1990.

13. Oelkers W: Adrenal insufficiency. N Engl J Med 335:1206–1212, 1996.

14. Oelkers W, Diedrich S, Bähr V: Diagnosis and therapy surveillance in Addison's disease: Rapid adrenocorticotropin (ACTH) test and measurement of plasma ACTH, renin activity and aldosterone. J Clin Endocrinol Metab 75:259–264, 1992.

15. Peacey SR, Guo C-Y, Robinson AM, et al: Glucocorticoid replacement therapy: Are patients overtreated and does it matter? Clin Endocrinol 46:255–261, 1997.

16. Salem M, Tainsh RE Jr, Bromberg J, et al: Preoperative glucocorticoid coverage—a reassessment 42 years after emergence of a problem. Ann Surg 219:416–425, 1994.

17. Seidenwurm DJ, Elmer EB, Kaplan LM, et al: Metastases to the adrenal glands and the development of Addison's disease. Cancer 54:522–527, 1984.

18. Webel SS, Ober KP: Acute adrenal insufficiency. Endocrinol Metab Clin North Am 22:303–328, 1993.

CHAPTER 32

CONGENITAL ADRENAL HYPERPLASIA

Jeannie A. Baquero, M.D., and Robert A. Vigersky, M.D.

1. **Define congenital adrenal hyperplasia.**
   Congenital adrenal hyperplasia (CAH) is a family of inherited disorders that result from a decrease in the activity of one of the various enzymes required for the biosynthesis of cortisol. These defects are inherited as autosomal recessive traits and are manifested during both prenatal and postnatal life.

2. **What enzyme defects can lead to CAH?**
   Defects in any of the enzymes required for the synthesis of cortisol from cholesterol can lead to CAH, including steroidogenic acute regulatory (StAR) protein, which is essential in transporting cholesterol to the mitochondria; 3 β-hydroxysteroid dehydrogenase, which is responsible for cholesterol side-chain cleavage; and three hydroxylases, *CYP 17* (17 α-hydroxylase), *CYP21A2* (21-hydroxylase), and *CYP11B1* (11 β-hydroxylase).

3. **Describe the functions of the three hydroxylases.**
   - *CYP 17* (17 α-hydroxylase) is essential in converting progesterone to 17-hydroxyprogesterone (17-OHP) and pregnenolone to 17-hydroxypregnenolone.
   - *CYP21A2* (21-hydroxylase) converts progesterone to deoxycorticosterone (DOC) and 17-OHP to 11 deoxycortisol.
   - *CYP11B1* (11 β-hydroxylase) converts DOC to corticosterone (which then goes on to aldosterone) and 11 deoxycortisol to cortisol.

4. **How is CAH inherited?**
   All of the enzyme defects leading to CAH are autosomal recessive disorders, that is, both copies of the involved gene must be abnormal for the condition to occur.

5. **What is the most common form of CAH?**
   By far the most common form is 21-hydroxylase deficiency, which accounts for 90% of cases and leads to deficiencies of the salt-retaining hormones DOC and aldosterone in both sexes, and/or virilization of genetic females.

6. **Which genes encode for 21-hydroxylase?**
   Two genes encode for 21-hydroxylase: *CYP21A1* (pseudogene) and *CYP21A2*, both of which are located in a 35-kb region on the long arm of chromosome 6 (6p21.3). Both genes are located downstream of the gene coding for complement factor 4 (C4A and C4B). *CYP21A1* and *CYP21A2* genes are about 90% similar, but the pseudogene lacks eight bases from codons 110 to 112, resulting in a stop codon and production of a truncated enzyme with no activity. *CYP21A1* is thus an inactive pseudogene, while the *CYP21A2* gene codes for the active 21-hydroxylase enzyme.

7. **What causes most of the genetic events responsible for *CYP21A2* deficiencies?**
   Most of the genetic events responsible for *CYP21A2* deficiencies result from the similarity between *CYP21A1* and *CYP21A2*, which leads to recombination events during meiosis. Gene conversions account for approximately 30% of the mutations, followed by gene deletions and then point mutations.

8. **What determines the patient's phenotype?**

The patient's phenotype is generally based on the specific genetic alteration of the *CYP21A2* gene:
- Patients with no enzyme activity typically have large deletions and predominantly have the salt-wasting form of the disorder.
- Patients with low but detectable enzyme activity have point mutations and typically have the simple virilizing form of the disease.
- Patients with 20–60% of normal enzyme activity have conservative amino acid substitutions and most often have the nonclassic form of the disease.
- Patients who are heterozygotes have mild abnormalities but no clinically important endocrine disorder.

9. **What is the second most common cause of CAH?**

The second most common cause of CAH (7% of all cases) is deficiency of the 11 β-hydroxylase enzyme (*CYP11B*), which is also an autosomal recessive defect caused by a mutation on the short arm of chromosome 8 (8q24.3). The result of this deficiency is an increased level of DOC, which causes hypertension, and increased androgen and androgen precursors, which cause ambiguous genitalia in genetic females.

10. **Summarize the rarer forms of CAH.**

The rarer forms of CAH are 17 α-hydroxylase and 3 β-hydroxysteroid dehydrogenase deficiency. There have been fewer than 200 cases of 17 α-hydroxylase with 40 described mutations of *CYP17* that span an 8.7-kb region on the short arm of chromosome 10 (10q24.3). The consequence of this deficiency is hypertension and hypokalemia due to DOC excess (associated with suppressed renin and aldosterone) along with deficiency of androgens and androgen precursors, which causes pseudohermaphroditism in genetic males and delayed puberty in both sexes (see questions 16 and 21).

11. **How common is CAH?**

CAH is one of the most common inherited diseases. The most common form of CAH, 21-hydroxylase deficiency, occurs in about 1/10,000 to 1/15,000 births in most populations. The prevalence of this disorder varies greatly among different ethnic groups and is highest among the Ashkenazi Jewish population of Eastern Europe. The nonclassic 21-hydroxylase deficiency may be as common as 1/100 to 1/1000 in persons of European Jewish heritage; the prevalence is similarly high in Yugoslavians and Hispanics.

12. **What percentage of the population at large are heterozygote carriers of the 12-hydroxylase defect?**

Fewer than 2% of the population at large are heterozygote carriers of the 21-hydroxylase defect; that is, one of the two copies of the 21-hydroxylase gene is abnormal. Such heterozygote carriers appear normal in all respects but may have elevated 17-OHP with adrenocorticotropic hormone (ACTH) stimulation testing.

13. **How common is 11-hydroxylase deficiency?**

The 11-hydroxylase deficiency, the second most frequent form of CAH, occurs in 1/100,000 births in the general population but in 1/5000 births in Jews of Moroccan decent. CAH due to defects of the other enzymes listed here is extremely rare.

14. **Explain why adrenal hyperplasia develops.**

The process of adrenal hyperplasia begins in utero. Reduced production of cortisol in the fetus, due to decreased activity of one of the enzymes needed for cortisol synthesis, results in lowered levels of serum cortisol. Cortisol normally acts through a negative feedback loop to inhibit the secretion of ACTH by the pituitary gland and corticotropin-releasing hormone (CRH) by the hypothalamus. Thus, the low serum cortisol levels that occur in a person with CAH increase the secretion of ACTH and CRH in an attempt to stimulate the adrenal glands to overcome the enzyme block and to return the serum cortisol level to normal. As this process continues over time, the elevated levels of serum ACTH stimulate growth of the adrenal glands, leading to hyperplasia.

15. **What is the most serious clinical consequence of CAH?**
Adrenal crisis in the newborn period is the most serious consequence of CAH. It usually occurs with genetic defects that result in severe reductions in enzyme activity. It is especially insidious in genetic males who do not have ambiguous genitalia as a clue to the diagnosis. Overall, about two-thirds of patients with 21-hydroxylase deficiency have the salt-wasting form. These patients have decreased production of DOC and aldosterone, which results in hypotension, volume depletion, hyponatremia, hyperkalemia, and increased renin activity. The degree of residual activity of the defective enzyme varies greatly from one affected family to another, depending on the specific genetic alteration.

16. **What are other clinical consequences of CAH in females?**
Many of the precursors and metabolites that build up behind the blocked enzymes 21-hydroxylase, 11 β-hydroxylase, or 3β-hydroxysteroid dehydrogenase are androgens. They may cause the following:
- Masculinization of the external genitalia of a genetic female fetus, leading to ambiguous genitalia at birth (female pseudohermaphroditism).
- Behaviors more typical of boys during childhood in terms of toy preference, rough play, and aggressiveness. (However, most females are heterosexual and their sexual identity is invariably female.)
- Rapid growth during early childhood with ultimate short stature as an adult due to early closure of epiphyses.

17. **How do patients with 17 α-hydroxylase deficiency present?**
In 17 α-hydroxylase deficiency, the enzyme defect blocks synthesis of androgens, thus precluding masculinization or ambiguity of the external genitalia. Patients present at puberty with the following:
- Primary (or rarely secondary) amenorrhea
- Hypertension
- Hypokalemia (because of increased mineralocorticoid production)

18. **How do patients with nonclassic CAH present?**
Children with nonclassic CAH (also called late-onset CAH) usually are asymptomatic and have normal external genitalia but later present with the following:
- Premature puberty
- Severe cystic acne
- Hirsutism
- Oligomenorrhea
- Infertility

19. **Summarize the relationship between adrenal "incidentalomas" and CAH.**
Adrenal incidentalomas are more common in patients with CAH and in heterozygotes. Conversely, 60% of patients with incidentalomas have exaggerated 17-OH progesterone responses to ACTH.

20. **How do the manifestations of CAH differ in males?**
Newborn males with CAH due to deficiency of 21-hydroxylase or 11 β-hydroxylase do not have ambiguous genitalia. Due to typical normal physical appearance, it is often difficult to detect an

affected male, especially when symptoms of salt-wasting occur after the first week of life. Later in childhood or early adulthood, males can present with the following:

- Premature puberty
- Advanced height in early childhood with ultimate short stature
- Acne
- Testicular enlargement due to adrenal rests
- Infertility (rare)

21. **Describe the presentation of males with CAD due to deficiency of other enzyme activity.**

Males with CAH due to deficient activity of 3 β-hydroxysteroid dehydrogenase, 17 α-hydroxylase, or cholesterol side-chain cleavage enzymes are unable to produce androgens during fetal development that are necessary for the formation of male external genitalia. As a consequence, they may have the following:

- External genitalia at birth are only partially masculinized.
- Normal female appearance (male pseudohermaphroditism).

22. **Describe the clinical features that suggest the possibility of CAH.**

Adrenal crisis or severe salt-wasting in the newborn period suggests the possibility of CAH. CAH also must be considered prominently in the differential diagnosis of any newborn with ambiguous genitalia. Because adrenal crisis and salt loss in CAH may be fatal if not treated, the finding of ambiguous genitalia in a newborn should trigger a rapid attempt to confirm or exclude CAH. Most males with CAH do not have ambiguous genitalia; consequently, many cases go unrecognized at birth, unless there is a documented family history of the disorder.

23. **What clinical clues help to support or refute the diagnosis of CAH in a newborn with ambiguous genitalia?**

The overwhelming majority of genetic males with CAH have unambiguous external genitalia at birth; conversely, CAH is an uncommon cause of ambiguous genitalia in a genetic male. Thus, determination that the infant with ambiguous genitalia is a genetic male makes CAH unlikely and decreases the diagnostic urgency because the disorders giving rise to ambiguous genitalia in genetic males are rarely associated with a fatal outcome. For example, the finding of palpable gonads in the scrotal or inguinal area suggests that the infant is a genetic male because such palpable gonads are almost always testes. Conversely, the detection of a uterus in an infant with ambiguous genitalia, either by physical examination or by ultrasound, strongly suggests that the infant is a genetic female, thus heightening the possibility of CAH.

24. **Discuss the role of molecular biology techniques in the diagnosis of CAH.**

Molecular biology techniques can rapidly confirm the genetic sex of a newborn without the prolonged wait for a traditional chromosome analysis. Because of the potentially severe consequences of CAH, it is probably prudent to assume that any genetic female with ambiguous genitalia has CAH until proved otherwise. Furthermore, it is probably best to wait to assign gender until molecular testing is done, as gender misassignment may cause long-term psychological problems for the families of such children. Early diagnosis and appropriate therapy also allow one to avoid the progressive effects of excess adrenal androgens, which will cause short stature, gender confusion in girls, and psychosexual disturbances in both boys and girls.

25. **How is the diagnosis of CAH confirmed?**

Because one does not know which enzyme is deficient in a newborn with suspected CAH (unless the family has a documented history of a particular enzyme defect), serum levels of all steroids that may be in the affected biosynthetic pathway can be measured before and after the administration of 250 μg of ACTH. Urinary measurement of these steroids by gas chromatography/mass spectroscopy has recently become economically feasible. Plasma renin activity and aldosterone levels should also be measured to assess the adequacy of aldosterone synthesis. Determination of which steroid levels are supranormal and which are low facilitates localization of the exact enzyme block.

KEY POINTS: CAH ✓

1. CAH, the most common inherited disease, is a group of autosomal recessive disorders, the most frequent of which is 21-hydroxylase deficiency.

2. The most serious consequences of CAH are ambiguous genitalia at birth, neonatal salt-wasting, short stature, and premature puberty.

3. CAH is diagnosed through measurement of cortisol precursors before and 1 hour after the intravenous administration of 250 μg of synthetic ACTH.

4. Predicted adult height can be achieved through early diagnosis, lower doses of corticosteroids in the first year of life, and the use of fludrocortisone even in those who are salt-wasters genetically but not clinically.

5. CAH is a rare cause of ambiguous genitalia in a genetic male.

26. **How are specific genetic defects confirmed?**
Specific genetic defects may be confirmed with molecular genetic testing. Polymerase chain reaction (PCR) amplification for the rapid simultaneous detection of the 10 mutations that are found in approximately 95% of 21-hydroxylase deficiency alleles is used for rapid results.

27. **What should be done when nonclassic CAH is suspected in older patients?**
When nonclassic CAH is suspected in the preteen, teenage, or adult patient, ACTH stimulation testing should be done with 250 μg (not 1 μg) of ACTH; measurement of 17-OHP, 17-OH pregnenolone, and cortisol should be done before and 60 minutes after ACTH injection. Hyperandrogenism can be assessed in women by measuring serum levels of testosterone, androstenedione, or 3 α-androstanediol glucuronide.

28. **Describe the classic test used for newborn screening.**
Newborn screening programs for CAH focus on the rapid detection of classic 21-hydroxylase deficiency on Guthrie cards (filter paper on which blood samples are collected, dried, and transported). This screening method measures 17-hydoxyprogesterone, which, if elevated, can be used for *CYP21A2* genotyping. As stated previously, genotyping can be helpful to determine severity of the disease. In the United States, testing for 21-hydroxylase deficiency is mandatory in only some states.

29. **What other tests may be used?**
If CAH is suspected and newborn filter paper screening is not available, ACTH stimulation with steroid precursor measurements should be done after the first 24 hours of life. Adrenal ultrasonography can also be used as a potential screening test for CAH neonates with ambiguous genitalia and/or salt-losing crisis by detecting > 4 mm adrenal limb width.

30. **How is CAH treated in neonates?**
The most important goal of treatment is to prevent salt loss and adrenal crisis in the newborn period. This goal requires the prompt administration of glucocorticoids and, in many cases,

mineralocorticoids, as well as careful monitoring of salt intake. This treatment not only replaces the deficient hormones but also suppresses elevated serum ACTH levels, thereby reducing adrenal production of androgenic precursors and metabolites. Such treatment may be given presumptively while awaiting the results of definitive laboratory tests and then discontinued if the tests are not confirmatory.

31. **When is surgical correction of ambiguous genitalia carried out?**
Surgical correction of ambiguous genitalia, such as repair of labioscrotal fusion, usually is carried out at a later time. Single-stage surgery is now implemented between 2 and 6 months of life.

32. **Describe the treatment of CAH in children.**
The preferred glucocorticoid for chronic replacement is hydrocortisone because of its short half-life, which minimizes growth suppression. It is sometimes extremely difficult or impossible to find a dosage of glucocorticoid that normalizes production of androgen without impairing growth. In such situations, mineralocorticoids (fludrocortisone) and/or spironolactone/flutamide (androgen receptor blockers that prevent virilization) in combination with the aromatase inhibitor testolactone (which prevents estrogen-induced epiphyseal fusion) may be useful adjunctive therapy in combination with nonsuppressive replacement doses of glucocorticoids. Rarely, adrenalectomy has been used for difficult-to-control patients since treatment of adrenal insufficiency is relatively much simpler.

33. **How is CAH treated in adolescents and adults?**
Prednisone or dexamethasone may be used once growth has been completed.

34. **What factors favor the achievement of predicted adult height?**
   - Early diagnosis.
   - Lower doses of hydrocortisone in the first year of life.
   - Mineralocorticoid treatment in all patients who are genetically determined to be salt-wasters even if they are not so clinically.

35. **What changes in therapy are necessary as a result of medically significant stress?**
Patients with CAH who have been on steroid therapy should wear a medical alert bracelet or necklace and should be provided with an emergency kit of hydrocortisone or dexamethasone for intramuscular use. For medically significant stress, the following measures are recommended:
   - Triple the oral dose of glucocorticoids.
   - Use intramuscular (or intravenous) steroid if the patient is unable to consume oral medications.
   - Sodium chloride, 1–3 gm/day, may be necessary in infants.
   - Fludrocortisone acetate (Florinef) should be used in patients with salt-wasting (infants: 70 $\mu g/m^2$/day; adults: 0.05–0.3 mg/day).

36. **What changes in therapy are necessary during pregnancy?**
   - Use hydrocortisone or prednisone instead of dexamethasone, which passes through the placenta unmetabolized.
   - Adjust steroid dose according to the clinical status.
   - Keep testosterone and free testosterone in the normal range for pregnancy.
   - Use stress doses of steroids during labor and delivery.

37. **How is treatment monitored?**
The goals of treatment are to prevent symptoms of adrenal insufficiency and to suppress ACTH and adrenal androgen production. For the second goal, it is most appropriate to monitor the

levels of the key precursor immediately behind the blocked enzyme (e.g., 17-OHP in the case of 21-hydroxylase deficiency), with the ultimate aim of normalizing its level by adjusting the dosage of glucocorticoid. However, such suppression of 17-OHP and adrenal androgen production often can be achieved only with hydrocortisone doses of 10–20 mg/m^2/day, which are significantly higher than the average replacement doses (6–7 mg/m^2/day). If glucocorticoid dosages are too high, the children become fatter and their growth and development may be irreversibly impaired.

38. **What other monitoring tools may be beneficial?**
Measurement of 24-hour urinary pregnanetriol (a metabolite of 17-OHP) excretion may also be a useful monitoring tool because of its ability to assess the integrated exposure to increased androgen precursors over a 24-hour period. Androgen levels that should also be monitored include testosterone, androstenedione, and 3-α-androstanediol glucuronide. In addition, plasma renin activity should be monitored in patients with salt-wasting CAH. Children must have annual bone age determinations, and their height should be carefully monitored.

39. **What genetic counseling is appropriate for a couple who previously had a child with CAH?**
Because all forms of CAH are autosomal recessive disorders, both parents of a child with CAH are obligate heterozygote carriers of the gene defect. Consequently, the chance that another child of the same couple will have CAH is one in four; 50% of the children will be heterozygote carriers. Modern genetic techniques and chorionic villus sampling of fetal DNA at 9 weeks of gestation allow the diagnosis of CAH during the first trimester of pregnancy. The other use for genotypic identification includes the prediction of the phenotype (i.e., severity of the disease). There appears to be a good relationship between genotype and phenotype in classic but not in nonclassic CAH.

40. **Are any prenatal treatments available for the fetus with CAH?**
Preliminary evidence suggests that prenatal treatment of female fetuses with 21-hydroxylase deficiency in the 5th–7th week of gestation by giving relatively high doses of dexamethasone (0.5–2.0 mg/day) to the mother may ameliorate the masculinization of genitalia. By contrast, male fetuses with 21-hydroxylase deficiencies do not develop ambiguous genitalia and do not require steroid treatment until after birth.

WEBSITES

1. http://www.hormone.org/resources/ext_page.php3?url=http://www.endo-society.org/pubrelations/patientInfo/cah.cfm.

2. http://www3.ncbi.nlm.nih.gov/htbin-post/Omim/dispmim?201710.

3. http://www3.ncbi.nlm.nih.gov/htbin-post/Omim/dispmim?201810.

4. http://www3.ncbi.nlm.nih.gov/htbin-post/Omim/dispmim?201910.

5. http://www3.ncbi.nlm.nih.gov/htbin-post/Omim/dispmim?202010.

6. http://www3.ncbi.nlm.nih.gov/htbin-post/Omim/dispmim?202110.

BIBLIOGRAPHY

1. Balsamo, A, Cicognani, A, Baldazzi, L et al: *CYP21* genotype, adult height, and pubertal development in 55 patients treated for 21-hydroxylase deficiency. J Clin Endocrinol Metab 88:5680–5688, 2003.

2. Cassorla FG, Chrousos GP: Congenital adrenal hyperplasia. In Becker KL (ed): Principles and Practice of Endocrinology and Metabolism. Philadelphia, J.B. Lippincott, 1990, p 604.

3. Chrousos GP, Loriaux DL, Mann DL, et al: Late-onset 21-hydroxylase deficiency mimicking idiopathic hirsutism or polycystic ovarian disease: An allelic variant of congenital virilizing adrenal hyperplasia with a milder enzymatic defect. Ann Intern Med 96:1–43, 1982.

4. Deneux C, Veronique T, Dib A, et al: Phenotype–genotype correlation in 56 women with nonclassical congenital adrenal hyperplasia due to 21-hydroxylase deficiency. J Clin Endocrinol Metab 86:207–213, 2001.

5. Forest MG, Betuel H, David M: Prenatal treatment in congenital adrenal hyperplasia due to 21-hydroxylase deficiency: Update 88 of the French multicenter study. Endocr Res 15:277, 1989.

6. Levine LS: Congenital adrenal hyperplasia. Pediatric Rev 21:159–171, 2000.

7. Linder B, Esteban NV, Yergey AL, et al: Cortisol production rate in childhood and adolescence. J Pediatr 117:892, 1991.

8. Lo JC, Schwitzgebel VM, Tyrrell JB, et al: Normal female infants born of mothers with classic congenital adrenal hyperplasia due to 21-hydroxylase deficiency. J Clin Endocrinol Metab 84:930–936, 1999.

9. Merke DP, Keil MF, Jones JV, et al: Flutamide, testolactone, and reduced hydrocortisone dose maintain normal growth velocity and bone maturation despite elevated androgen levels in children with congenital adrenal hyperplasia. J Clin Endocrinol Metab 85:1114–1120, 2000.

10. Miller WL: Congenital adrenal hyperplasia. Endocrinol Metab Clin N Am 20:721, 1991.

11. Miller WL, Levine LS: Molecular and clinical advances in congenital adrenal hyperplasia. J Pediatr 111:1, 1987.

12. Morel Y, Miller WL: Clinical and molecular genetics of congenital adrenal hyperplasia due to 21-hydroxylase deficiency. Adv Hum Genet 20:1, 1991.

13. Mulaikal RM, Migeon CJ, Rock JA: Fertility rates in female patients with congenital adrenal hyperplasia due to 21-hydroxylase deficiency. N Engl J Med 316:178, 1987.

14. Nordenström, A, Servin A, Bohlin G et al: Sex-typed toy play behavior correlates with the degree of prenatal androgen exposure assessed by *CYP21* genotype in girls with congenital adrenal hyperplasia. J Clin Endocrinol Metab 87:5119–5124, 2002.

15. Pang S: Congenital adrenal hyperplasia. Endocrinol Metab Clin N Am 26:853–891, 1997.

16. Pang S, Pollack MS, Marshall RN, et al: Prenatal treatment of congenital adrenal hyperplasia due to 21-hydroxylase deficiency. N Engl J Med 322:111, 1990.

17. Sherman SL, Aston CE, Morton NE, et al: A segregation and linkage study of classical and nonclassical 21-hydroxylase deficiency. Am J Hum Genet 42:830, 1988.

18. Speiser PW, White PC: Congenital adrenal hyperplasia due to steroid 21-hydroxylase deficiency. Clin Endocrinol 49:411–417, 1998.

19. Speiser PW, White PC: Congenital adrenal hyperplasia. N Engl J Med 349:776, 2003.

20. Therrell BL Jr, Berenbaum SA, Manter-Kapanke V, Simmank J: Results of screening 1.9 million Texas newborns for 21-hydroxylase-deficient congenital adrenal hyperplasia. Pediatrics 101:583, 1998.

21. Urban MD, Lee PA, Migeon CJ: Adult height and fertility in men with congenital virilizing adrenal hyperplasia. N Engl J Med 299:1392, 1978.

22. Van Wyk JJ, Ritzen EM: The role of bilateral adrenalectomy in the treatment of congenital adrenal hyperplasia. J Clin Endocrinol Metab 88: 2993–2998, 2003.

23. Wedell A: Molecular genetics of congenital adrenal hyperplasia (21-hydroxylase deficiency): implications for diagnosis, prognosis and treatment. Acta Paediatr 87:159–164, 1998.

24. White PC, New MI, Dupont B: Structure of the human 21-hydroxylase gene. Proc Natl Acad Sci USA 83:5111, 1986.

25. White PC, New MI, Dupont B: Congenital adrenal hyperplasia (Part 1). N Engl J Med 316:1519, 1987.

26. White PC, New MI, Dupont B: Congenital adrenal hyperplasia (Part 2). N Engl J Med 316:1580, 1987.

27. White PC, Spieser PW: Congenital adrenal hyperplasia due to 21-hydroxylase deficiency. Endocr Rev 21(3):245–291, 2000.

28. Winter JSD, Couch RM: Modern medical therapy of congenital adrenal hyperplasia. Ann N Y Acad Sci 458:165, 1985.

V. THYROID DISORDERS

THYROID TESTING

Michael T. McDermott, M.D.

CHAPTER 33

1. **What is the single best test to screen for abnormal function of the thyroid gland?**
   The serum thyroid-stimulating hormone (TSH) level, using a sensitive TSH assay, is the best test for assessing thyroid function. This is true because the vast majority of thyroid dysfunction is due to primary thyroid disease. The TSH measurement is misleading, however, when thyroid dysfunction is secondary to hypothalamic or pituitary disease that results in abnormal TSH secretion.

2. **How do you interpret the serum TSH level in the evaluation of suspected thyroid disease?**
   When the TSH level is elevated, the patient has primary hypothyroidism. When TSH is low or undetectable, the patient has primary hyperthyroidism. Exceptions to these rules are uncommon, except in patients with pituitary-hypothalamic disorders and patients with significant nonthyroidal illnesses. The serum TSH value can detect mild hypothyroidism or mild hyperthyroidism long before serum thyroid hormone levels are outside their normal ranges. Measurement of free thyroxin (T_4) or a free T_4 index (total $T_4 \times$ triiodothyronine resin uptake [T_3RU]) and sometimes T_3, should be performed whenever the TSH is abnormal.

3. **Explain how the serum TSH is used to manage patients on thyroid hormone therapy.**
   Thyroid hormone therapy is usually given to patients for one of two purposes: replacement therapy for hypothyroidism or suppression therapy for thyroid cancer. When replacement is the goal, the dosage should be adjusted to maintain the serum TSH level within the reference range. When suppression is the goal, the dosage should be adjusted to maintain the serum TSH level in the low normal or slightly low range for most patients and in the undetectable range for those with aggressive or metastatic cancer.

4. **Discuss the advantages of free thyroid hormone assays.**
   Free T_4 and T_3 assays determine the amounts of unbound, bioactive thyroid hormones in the circulation. Free thyroid hormone tests fall into two main categories: equilibrium dialysis and analog assays. Equilibrium dialysis methods are not affected by abnormalities of serum thyroid hormone binding proteins. Analog methods are variably affected by protein binding but still give a more accurate assessment of biologically active thyroid hormone levels than do total T_4 and T_3 assays. Analog assays are used by most commercial laboratories.

5. **What do total T_4 and T_3 assays measure?**
   These assays measure the total T_4 and T_3 concentrations in the circulation. Over 99% of circulating T_4 and approximately 98% of T_3 are bound to proteins, such as thyroxine-binding globulin (TBG), thyroxine-binding prealbumin (TBPA or transthyretin) and albumin. Consequently, serum total T_4 and T_3 levels can be altered by protein binding disorders just as they can by thyroid disease.

6. **Name the major disorders of thyroid hormone-binding proteins.**
Pregnancy, estrogen use, congenital TBG excess, and familial dysalbuminemic hyperthyroxinemia (FDH) are the most common. FDH is an inherited disorder, in which albumin has enhanced affinity for T_4, resulting in increased serum levels of total T_4 but not T_3. Protein binding of thyroid hormones is reduced by androgens and congenital TBG deficiency.

A T_3RU measurement helps clinicians distinguish protein-binding disorders from true thyroid diseases. The T_3RU is inversely proportional to the protein-bound T_4; accordingly, T_3RU is low when T_4 protein binding is increased and high when protein binding is reduced. Table 33-1 indicates how these tests are used to make the correct diagnosis.

TABLE 33-1. DIAGNOSIS OF DISORDERS OF THYROID HORMONE-BINDING PROTEINS			
	Total T_4	Total T_3	T_3RU
Hyperthyroidism	↑	↑	↑
Increased protein-binding state	↑	↑	↓
Hypothyroidism	↓	↓	↓
Decreased protein-binding state	↓	↓	↑

T_4, thyroxin; T_3, triiodothyronine, T_3RU, triiodothyronine resin uptake.

7. **What antithyroid antibody measurements are clinically useful?**
Antibodies against thyroid peroxidase (TPO) and thyroglobulin are present in the serum of most patients with Hashimoto's thyroiditis. Either test can establish a diagnosis of Hashimoto's disease, but the TPO antibodies are more sensitive. Thyroid-stimulating immunoglobulins (TSI) and TSH receptor antibodies (TRAb) are present in the serum of most patients with Graves' disease; their measurement is not necessary in patients with obvious Graves' disease but may be helpful when the diagnosis is in question.

8. **How useful are thyroglobulin (TG) measurements?**
Thyroglobulin (TG) is the major iodoprotein constituent of thyroid follicles. Serum TG levels are mildly increased in many thyroid diseases but marked elevations suggest the presence of destructive thyroiditis (subacute, postpartum, or silent thyroiditis), in which TG leaks from the damaged thyroid gland into the circulation. TG measurements are also useful in monitoring patients with thyroid cancer. When a patient has been thyroidectomized and is cancer-free, the serum TG should be undetectable. Normal or elevated serum TG levels in such patients suggest the presence of residual or metastatic thyroid cancer. Most TG assays are not reliable in patients who have positive anti-TG antibodies, since these antibodies interfere with the method of TG measurement.

9. **Under what circumstances should a serum calcitonin level be measured?**
Calcitonin is made by thyroid parafollicular C cells rather than by follicular cells. Serum calcitonin is elevated in medullary carcinoma of the thyroid (MCT) and in its familial precursor lesion, C-cell hyperplasia. Since MCT is an uncommon thyroid neoplasm, serum calcitonin measurements should not be used in the routine evaluation of most thyroid nodules. They are indicated, however, if a patient exhibits a feature, such as familial occurrence or associated diarrhea, that is characteristic of MCT.

10. **Discuss the utility and interpretation of the radioactive iodine uptake (RAIU) test.**

Thyroid follicular cells have iodine symporters or pumps that bring iodine into the cells for thyroid hormone synthesis. The activity of these iodine pumps can be assessed by measuring the RAIU. The normal 24-hour RAIU is approximately 10–25% in the United States, but this value varies somewhat according to location because of geographic differences in dietary iodine intake. The RAIU is most useful in the differential diagnosis of thyrotoxicosis by separating cases into two distinct categories:

High-RAIU Thyrotoxicosis	Low-RAIU Thyrotoxicosis
Graves' disease	Factitious thyrotoxicosis
Toxic multinodular goiter	Iodine-induced thyrotoxicosis
Solitary toxic adenoma	Destructive thyroiditis
hCG-induced thyrotoxicosis	Subacute thyroiditis
TSH-secreting	Postpartum thyroiditis
tumor	Silent thyroiditis

RAIU, radioactive iodine uptake.

KEY POINTS: THYROID TESTING ✓

1. Serum TSH measurement is the best overall test to screen and evaluate patients for thyroid disease and to monitor thyroid hormone replacement therapy.

2. Serum free T_4 should be measured in all patients whose TSH is elevated, while serum free T_4 and total T_3 or free T_3 should be measured in patients whose TSH is suppressed.

3. Antithyroperoxidase (TPO) antibodies are the most accurate test to establish a diagnosis of chronic lymphocytic thyroiditis (Hashimoto's disease).

4. Serum thyroglobulin (TG) is useful for assisting in the diagnosis of destructive thyroiditis and for monitoring for recurrence of differentiated thyroid cancer.

5. RAIU is used primarily to determine whether patients with thyrotoxicosis have a high RAIU or a low RAIU disorder.

6. A thyroid scan is used mainly to distinguish among the three types of high-RAIU thyrotoxicosis and to determine whether thyroid nodules are nonfunctioning (cold), eufunctioning (warm), or hyperfunctioning (hot).

11. **When and why should a thyroid scan be ordered?**

The thyroid scan helps to distinguish among the three types of high-RAIU thyrotoxicosis. Graves' disease (diffuse toxic goiter) is characterized by diffuse tracer uptake; toxic multinodular goiter, by multiple discrete areas of increased uptake; and the solitary toxic adenoma, by a single area of intense uptake. The scan is not helpful in low-RAIU thyrotoxicosis.

The thyroid scan is also sometimes used in the evaluation of thyroid nodules, although its cost efficiency in this work-up is doubtful. According to the scan, thyroid nodules may be divided into those that are hot (hyperfunctioning), warm (eufunctioning), and cold (nonfunctioning). Cold nodules have a 20% risk of being a carcinoma, whereas malignancy is rare in hot nodules.

12. **What is Thyrogen? How is it used?**

Thyrogen is recombinant human TSH. It can be used to stimulate neoplastic thyroid tissue to absorb radioiodine for an imaging procedure. Thyroid cancer tissue ordinarily traps iodine poorly and can be imaged only if the serum TSH is elevated. This can be accomplished either by stopping levothyroxine treatment for 6 weeks or by giving Thyrogen injections. Once the serum TSH level has been increased by either method, serum TG is measured and radioiodine (I–131 or I–123) is given for whole body scanning. A positive scan or detectable TG level indicates the presence of residual or metastatic thyroid cancer. A Thyrogen stimulated scan and TG measurement has the same accuracy as a levothyroxine withdrawal scan and has the advantage of not causing symptoms of hypothyroidism.

13. **Discuss the role of thyrotropin-releasing hormone (TRH) test in the evaluation of thyroid disease.**

An intravenous bolus of TRH normally elicits a brisk increase in serum TSH and prolactin levels. The TSH rise is exaggerated in patients with primary hypothyroidism and absent in those with hyperthyroidism. The increment may be sluggish or delayed in patients with hypothalamic or pituitary disease. Because of the development of highly sensitive serum TSH assays and free thyroid hormone measurements, this test is rarely needed for the diagnosis of primary thyroid disease and is insufficiently accurate for the diagnosis of secondary thyroid disease. Nevertheless, it is occasionally of supportive value when other tests fail to yield a definitive diagnosis.

BIBLIOGRAPHY

1. Cavaleri R: Thyroid radioiodine uptake: Indications and interpretation. Endocrinologist 2:341, 1992.
2. Haugen BR, Pacini F, Reiners C, et al: A comparison of recombinant human thyrotropin and thyroid hormone withdrawal for the detection of thyroid remnant or cancer. J Clin Endocrinol Metab 84:3877–3885, 1999.
3. Ladenson PW, Braverman LE, Mazzaferri EL, et al: Comparison of administration of recombinant human thyrotropin with withdrawal of thyroid hormone for radioactive iodine scanning in patients with thyroid carcinoma. N Engl J Med 337:888–896, 1997.
4. Nicoloff JT, Spencer CA: The use and misuse of the sensitive thyrotropin assays. J Clin Endocrinol Metab 71:553–558, 1990.
5. Smith SA: Commonly asked questions about thyroid function. Mayo Clin Proc 70:573–577, 1995.
6. Spencer CA, Schwarzbein D, Gutler RB, et al: Thyrotropin (TSH) releasing hormone stimulation test responses employing third and fourth generation TSH assays. J Clin Endocrinol Metab 76:494–498, 1993.
7. Wang R, Nelson JC, Weiss RM, Wilcox RB: Accuracy of free thyroxine measurements across natural ranges of thyroxine binding to serum proteins. Thyroid 10:31–39, 2000.

CHAPTER 34

HYPERTHYROIDISM

Susan T. Wingo, M.D., and Henry B. Burch, M.D.

1. **What is the difference between thyrotoxicosis and hyperthyroidism?**
   Thyrotoxicosis is the general term for the presence of increased levels of thyroxine (T_4) and/or triiodothyronine (T_3) due to any cause. It does not imply that a patient is markedly symptomatic or "toxic." Hyperthyroidism refers to causes of thyrotoxicosis in which the thyroid overproduces thyroid hormone.

2. **Define the term *autonomy* as it applies to thyroid hyperfunction.**
   Thyroid autonomy refers to the spontaneous synthesis and release of thyroid hormone independent of thyroid-stimulating hormone (TSH).

3. **What is subclinical thyrotoxicosis?**
   Subclinical thyrotoxicosis refers to elevation of T_4 and/or T_3 within the normal range, leading to suppression of pituitary TSH secretion into the subnormal range. Clinical symptoms and signs are frequently absent or nonspecific.

4. **What are the long-term consequences of subclinical thyrotoxicosis?**
   Some studies have linked subclinical thyrotoxicosis to accelerated bone loss in postmenopausal women and a higher incidence of atrial dysrhythmia, including atrial fibrillation. A TSH, which is below the lower limit of normal but above 0.1 mIU/L, is less likely to result in such complications.

5. **List the three most common causes of hyperthyroidism.**
   - Graves' disease
   - Toxic multinodular goiter (TMNG)
   - Toxic adenomas or autonomously functioning thyroid nodules (AFTNs)

6. **Define Graves' disease**
   Graves' disease is an autoimmune disorder, in which antibodies directed against the TSH receptor result in continuous stimulation of the thyroid gland to produce and secrete thyroid hormone. Extrathyroidal manifestations of Graves' disease include ophthalmopathy, pretibial myxedema, and thyroid acropachy.

7. **Explain TMNG.**
   Toxic multinodular goiter (TMNG) generally arises in the setting of a long-standing multinodular goiter, in which certain individual nodules have developed autonomous function. Patients with mild or overt TMNG are also at risk for developing iodine-induced thyrotoxicosis (the Jod-Basedow effect) after exposure to intravenous contrast or treatment with the iodine-containing drug amiodarone.

8. **What are AFTNs?**
   Autonomously functioning thyroid nodules (AFTNs) are benign tumors that have excessive constitutive activation of the TSH receptor or its signal-transduction apparatus. These tumors frequently produce subclinical thyrotoxicosis and have a predilection for spontaneous

hemorrhage. AFTNs generally must be larger than 3 cm in diameter before attaining sufficient secretory capacity to produce overt hyperthyroidism. Often inefficient iodine processing leads to an excess of T_3 relative to T_4 in AFTNs.

9. **What are the rarer causes of hyperthyroidism?**
Rarer causes of hyperthyroidism include TSH-secreting pituitary adenomas; stimulation of the TSH receptor by extremely high levels of human chorionic gonadotropin (hCG), such as those found in choriocarcinomas in women or germ cell tumors in men; struma ovarii (ectopic thyroid hormone production in thyroid tissue containing ovarian teratomas); and pituitary-specific thyroid hormone resistance. Thyroiditis and ingestion of excessive exogenous thyroid hormone (iatrogenic, inadvertent, or surreptitious) are causes of thyrotoxicosis but not hyperthyroidism (see question 1).

10. **How do thyrotoxic patients present clinically?**
Common symptoms include palpitations, shakiness, insomnia, difficulty with concentrating, irritability or emotional lability, weight loss, heat intolerance, exertional dyspnea, fatigue, hyperdefecation, menses with lighter flow or shorter duration, and brittle hair. Occasionally patients may experience weight gain rather than loss during thyrotoxicosis, presumably owing to polyphagia beyond that needed to support their increased metabolism.

11. **What is apathetic hyperthyroidism?**
Older patients with hyperthyroidism may lack typical adrenergic features and present instead with depression or apathy, weight loss, atrial fibrillation, worsening angina pectoris, or congestive heart failure.

12. **Describe the physical signs of thyrotoxicosis.**
Tremors, tachycardia, flow murmurs, warm moist skin, hyperreflexia with rapid relaxation phases, and a goiter (with a bruit in patients with Graves' disease) may be found in hyperthyroid patients. Eye findings in thyrotoxicosis are discussed in question 13.

13. **How does hyperthyroidism cause eye disease?**
Lid retraction and stare can be seen with any cause of thyrotoxicosis and are due to increased adrenergic tone. True ophthalmopathy is unique to Graves' disease and is thought to be caused by thyroid autoantibodies that cross-react with antigens in fibroblasts, adipocytes, and myocytes behind the eyes. Common manifestations of ophthalmopathy include proptosis, diplopia, and inflammatory changes, such as conjunctival injection and periorbital edema.

14. **What laboratory testing should be performed to confirm thyrotoxicosis?**
Measurement of serum TSH with a second- or third-generation assay is the most sensitive test for detecting thyrotoxicosis. Because a low TSH also may be seen in central hypothyroidism, a free T_4 level should be measured to confirm thyrotoxicosis. If the free T_4 level is normal, a T_3 level should be determined to rule out T_3 toxicosis. Other associated laboratory findings may include mild leukopenia, normocytic anemia, elevations of hepatic transaminases and bone alkaline phosphatase, mild hypercalcemia, and low levels of albumin and cholesterol.

15. **When is thyroid antibody testing needed for the diagnosis of hyperthyroidism?**
The cause of hyperthyroidism usually can be determined with history, physical examination, and radionuclide studies. Testing for TSH receptor antibodies is useful in pregnant women with Graves' disease to determine the risk of neonatal thyroid dysfunction due to transplacental passage of stimulating or blocking antibodies. It is also useful in euthyroid patients suspected of having euthyroid Graves' ophthalmopathy and in patients with alternating periods of hyperthyroidism and hypothyroidism as a result of fluctuations in blocking and stimulating TSH receptor antibodies.

KEY POINTS: CAUSE AND DIAGNOSIS OF HYPERTHYROIDISM ✓

1. The three most common causes of hyperthyroidism are Graves' disease, TMNG, and toxic adenoma.

2. Older patients may not have classic hyperadrenergic symptoms and may present with weight loss, depression, or heart disease (worsening angina pectoris, atrial fibrillation, and congestive heart failure).

3. Routine diagnostic testing for hyperthyroidism includes TSH, free T_4 with or without free T_3, radioactive iodine uptake (RAIU), and thyroid scanning with radioiodine (I^{123}) or technetium (Tc) 99m.

16. **What is the difference between a thyroid scan and an uptake?**
A RAIU uses I^{131} or I^{123} to assess quantitatively the functional status of the thyroid gland. A small dose of radioactive iodine is given orally followed by measurement of radioactivity in the area of the thyroid in 6–24 hours. Often two measurements are taken, at 4–6 hours and at 24 hours. A high uptake confirms hyperthyroidism. A scan provides a two-dimensional image depicting the distribution of iodine trapping within the thyroid gland. Uniform distribution in a hyperthyroid patient suggests Graves' disease, patchy distribution suggests TMNG, and unifocal activity corresponding to a nodule, with suppression of the rest of the thyroid, suggests a toxic adenoma.

17. **How should hyperthyroidism be treated?**
The three main treatment options are antithyroid drugs (ATDs), including methimazole (MMI) and propylthiouracil (PTU); I^{131} ablation; and surgery. Unless contraindicated, most patients should receive beta blockers for heart rate control and symptomatic relief. Most thyroidologists in the United States prefer I^{131} over surgery or prolonged courses of ATDs. Patients scheduled to receive I^{131} should be advised to avoid pregnancy and should be cautioned that oral contraceptives may not be fully protective in the hyperthyroid state because of increased levels of sex hormone-binding globulin and increased clearance of the contraceptive.

18. **When is surgery indicated for hyperthyroidism?**
Surgery is generally not the treatment of choice for hyperthyroidism. It is most often used when a cold nodule is present in a patient with Graves' disease, in pregnant patients allergic to ATDs (I^{131} is contraindicated in pregnancy), or in patients with extremely large goiters who are less likely to respond to ATDs or I^{131}. Surgery may also be the preferred modality when patients have other serious medical problems that make the rapid attainment of normal thyroid levels crucial or significant eye involvement with Graves' disease. Patients should be euthyroid before surgery to decrease the risk of arrhythmias during induction of anesthesia and the risk of postoperative thyroid storm.

19. **Discuss the role of inorganic iodine in lowering thyroid hormone levels.**
Inorganic iodine acutely reduces the synthesis and release of T_4 and T_3. The inhibition of thyroid hormone synthesis by iodine is known as the Wolff-Chaikoff effect. However, because escape from this effect generally occurs after 10–14 days, iodine is used only to prepare a patient rapidly for surgery or as an adjunctive measure in patients with thyroid storm after ATDs are on board. Typical doses are Lugol's solution, 3–5 drops three times a day, or saturated solution of potassium iodide (SSKI), one drop three times a day.

20. **Are other agents available to lower thyroid hormone levels?**
Iopanoic acid, an oral radiographic contrast agent, has been shown to cause dramatic reductions in serum T_3 and T_4 levels through inhibition of T_4-5′-deiodinase activity and the effect of the iodine contained in the drug. A typical dose of iopanoic acid is 500–1000 mg/day. The closely related drug, ipodate is no longer commercially available, and iopanoic acid may soon unfortunately share a similar fate. Other agents occasionally used to treat hyperthyroidism include lithium, which decreases thyroid hormone release, and potassium perchlorate, which inhibits thyroid uptake of iodine.

21. **Which medications block peripheral conversion of T_4 to T_3?**
Propylthiouracil (PTU), propranolol, glucocorticoids, iopanoic acid, and amiodarone.

22. **How effective are ATDs?**
Ninety percent of patients taking ATDs become euthyroid without significant side effects. Approximately one-half of patients attain a remission from Graves' disease after a treatment course of 12–18 months. However, only 30% maintain long-term remission; the remainder experience recurrence within 1–2 years after the drugs are withdrawn. The usual starting doses are MMI, 30 mg/day, or PTU, 100 mg three times a day.

23. **What side effects are associated with ATDs?**
   - Agranulocytosis
   - Hepatotoxicity and cholestatic jaundice
   - Rashes

24. **How common is agranulocytosis? Describe its symptoms.**
Agranulocytosis, a rare but life-threatening complication of ATD therapy, occurs in approximately 1 in every 200–500 patients treated with ATDs. Patients should be instructed to report promptly for fever, sore throat, or minor infections that do not resolve quickly. Agranulocytosis appears to be dose-related with MMI but not with PTU. Patients developing agranulocytosis on one antithyroid drug should not be exposed to another.

25. **Describe the signs and symptoms of hepatotoxicity and cholestatic jaundice.**
Hepatotoxicity can progress to fulminant hepatitis with necrosis with PTU, and cholestatic jaundice has been reported with MMI. Patients should report right upper quadrant pain, anorexia, nausea, and new pruritus.

26. **What kind of rashes can ATDs produce?**
Rashes can range from limited erythema to an exfoliative dermatitis. Dermatologic reaction to one ATD does not preclude the use of another, although cross-sensitivity occurs in approximately 50% of cases.

27. **What lab tests should be monitored in patients taking ATDs?**
Thyroid hormone levels should be monitored to determine when ATD doses can be reduced from the initial high doses to maintenance doses (usually 25–50% of initial doses). TSH may remain suppressed for several months; in this situation, free T_4 levels are more reliable for assessing thyroid hormone status. Hepatic enzymes and complete blood count with differential should be checked every 1–3 months. Because transaminase elevation and mild granulocytopenia can be seen in untreated Graves' disease, it is important to check these parameters before initiating ATD therapy. Many cases of agranulocytosis appear to arise without preceding granulocytopenia; thus, a high index of suspicion is required even if recent testing is normal.

KEY POINTS: TREATMENT OF HYPERTHYROIDISM ✔

1. The major treatment choices for hyperthyroidism are radioiodine, ATDs (MMI, PTU), and thyroidectomy; beta blockers can significantly improve adrenergic symptoms of thyrotoxicosis, and do not interfere with testing or later treatment.

2. Treatment is generally indicated when TSH is less than 0.1 mIU/L. Patients with a suppressed TSH higher than 0.1 mIU/L should be followed closely.

3. In patients with significant proptosis or periorbital inflammation due to Graves' ophthalmopathy, radioiodine treatment may worsen eye disease. If radioiodine is used, patients should stop smoking and should take a course of oral corticosteroids immediately after the radioiodine treatment.

28. **How does radioactive iodine work?**
Thyroid cells trap and concentrate iodine and use it to make thyroid hormone. I^{131} is organified in the same manner as natural iodine. Because I^{131} emits locally destructive beta particles, cellular damage and death occur over a period of several months after treatment. Doses of I^{131} should be high enough to result in permanent hypothyroidism in order to decrease the recurrence rate. Typical doses for Graves' disease are 8–15 mCi; for TMNG, higher doses of 25–30 mCi are given. These doses are effective in 90–95% of patients.

29. **When is pretreatment with ATDs indicated before I^{131} ablation?**
Elderly patients and patients with underlying systemic illnesses are often pretreated with ATDs in an effort to deplete the thyroid of preformed hormones and thereby theoretically reduce the risk of I^{131}-induced thyroid storm. When pretreatment with ATDs is used, the drugs are generally stopped 4–7 days before I^{131} is given. However, pretreatment with ATDs is associated with a rapid increase in thyroid hormone levels upon ATD discontinuation. Most nonpretreated patients experience a rapid decrease in thyroid hormone levels after radioiodine. Therefore, most patients do not require or benefit from ATD pretreatment. Pretreatment also has the disadvantage of lowering the success rate of radioiodine through residual inhibition of organification of the I^{131}.

30. **How long after I^{131} treatment should women wait before becoming pregnant or resuming breast-feeding?**
Pregnancy should be deferred for at least 6 months after I^{131} ablation. In addition, patients should be on a stable dose of replacement thyroid hormone and free of active ophthalmopathy. Breast milk radioactivity, measured in one study after an 8.3-mCi therapeutic dose of I^{131}, remained unacceptably high for 45 days. If Tc 99m is used for diagnostic studies, breast-feeding may be resumed in 2–3 days.

31. **Does I^{131} cause or worsen ophthalmopathy in Graves' disease?**
This is an area of ongoing controversy. The natural history of Graves' disease is such that 15–20% of patients develop significant ophthalmopathy. The majority of cases arise in the period from 18 months before to 18 months after the onset of thyrotoxicosis. Thus, a fair number of new cases can be expected to coincide with the timing of I^{131} ablation. Two prospective randomized trials have shown that I^{131} is more likely than other treatment modalities to worsen ophthalmopathy. Patients with preexisting eye disease and those who smoke cigarettes are more likely to experience worsening. As a result, it is prudent to avoid I^{131} in patients with active moderate-to-severe Graves' ophthalmopathy, or to treat these patients with a course of oral corticosteroids immediately after the dose of I^{131}.

32. **How is thyrotoxicosis managed in pregnancy?**
    Caution must be used in interpreting thyroid laboratory results during pregnancy because low TSH values are not uncommon in the first trimester, and total T_4 levels are elevated by increased thyroxine-binding globulin (TBG) levels. Free T_4 levels are the best indicator of thyroid function during pregnancy. Nuclear medicine testing with RAIU or thyroid scanning is contraindicated in pregnancy because of concerns about fetal exposure to isotopes. Because I^{131} therapy is also contraindicated during pregnancy, treatment options are limited to ATDs or surgery in the second trimester. PTU is generally the preferred ATD during pregnancy because it crosses the placenta to a lesser extent than MMI, and the use of MMI has been associated with a rare neonatal scalp disorder known as aplasia cutis. Pregnant patients with Graves' disease require close follow-up to ensure adequate control and to prevent hypothyroidism because the disorder frequently remits during the course of pregnancy. TSH receptor antibodies, which are able to cross the placenta after 26 weeks, should be measured in the third trimester to assess the risk of neonatal thyroid dysfunction.

WEBSITES

1. American Association of Clinical Endocrinologists. Available at www.aace.com.

2. American Thyroid Association. Available at www.thyroid.org.

BIBLIOGRAPHY

1. Bartalena L, Marcocci C, Bogazzi F, et al.: Relation between therapy for hyperthyroidism and the course of Graves' ophthalmopathy. N Engl J Med 338:73–78, 1998.

2. Burch HB, Wartofsky L: Graves' ophthalmopathy: Current concepts regarding pathogenesis and management. Endocr Rev 14:747–793, 1993.

3. Burch HB, Shakir F, Fitzsimmons TR, et al: Diagnosis and management of the autonomously functioning thyroid nodule: The Walter Reed Army Medical Center experience, 1975–1996. Thyroid 8:871–880, 1998.

4. Burch HB, Solomon BL, Wartofsky L, Burman KD: Discontinuing antithyroid drug therapy before ablation with radioiodine in Graves' disease. Ann Intern Med 121:553–559, 1994.

5. Burrow GN: Thyroid function and hyperfunction during gestation. Endocr Rev 14:194–202, 1993.

6. Col NF, Surks MI, Daniels GH: Subclinical thyroid disease: Clinical applications. JAMA 291:239–243, 2004.

7. Cooper DS: Antithyroid drugs for the treatment of hyperthyroidism caused by Graves' disease. Endocrinol Metab Clin N Am 27:225–247, 1998.

8. Cooper DS: Hyperthyroidism. Lancet 362: 459–68, 2003.

9. Cooper DS: Antithyroid drugs in the management of patients with Graves' disease: An evidence-based approach to therapeutic controversies. J Clin Endocrinol Metab 88:3474–3481, 2003.

10. Ginsberg J: Diagnosis and management of Graves' disease. Can Med Assoc J 168:575–585, 2003.

11. Kahaly GJ, Nieswandt J, Mohr-Kahaly S: Cardiac risks of hyperthyroidism in the elderly. Thyroid 8:1165–1169, 1998.

12. Ladenson PW: Diagnosis of thyrotoxicosis. In Braverman LE, Utiger RD (eds): Werner & Ingbar's The Thyroid, 8th ed. Philadelphia, Lippincott, Williams & Wilkins, 2000, pp 685–690.

13. McDermott MT, Ridgway EC: Thyroid hormone resistance syndromes. Am J Med 94:424–432, 1993.

14. McDermott MT, Ridgway EC: Central hyperthyroidism. Endocrinol Metab Clin N Am 27:187–203, 1998.

15. Singer PA, Cooper DS, Levy EG, et al: Treatment guidelines for patients with hyperthyroidism and hypothyroidism. Standards of Care Committee, American Thyroid Association. JAMA 273:808–812, 1995.

16. Surks MI, Ortiz E, Daniels GH, et al: Subclinical thyroid disease: Scientific review and guidelines for diagnosis and management. JAMA 291:228–239, 2004.

CHAPTER 35

HYPOTHYROIDISM

Katherine Weber, M.D., and Bryan R. Haugen, M.D.

1. **How common is hypothyroidism?**
   Hypothyroidism is relatively common with a prevalence of 4–8% in the general population. The mean age at diagnosis is the mid-50s. Hypothyroidism is much more common in women, with a female-to-male ratio of 10:1. Postpartum hypothyroidism, a transient hypothyroid phase after pregnancy, is found in 5–10% of women.

2. **What is subclinical hypothyroidism?**
   Subclinical hypothyroidism (now called mild thyroid failure) is a mild and much more common form of hypothyroidism, often with few or no symptoms. Hypercholesterolemia and subtle cardiac abnormalities have been associated. Biochemically, the levels of thyroxine (T_4) or free T_4 are normal, whereas the level of thyroid-stimulating hormone (TSH) is mildly elevated. As many as 10–20% of women older than 50 years have mild thyroid failure.

3. **How is subclinical hypothyroidism treated?**
   When patients are treated with T_4, they have an improved sense of well-being (compared with placebo) and the cardiac and lipid abnormalities improve. Therefore, treatment is generally recommended. Thyroid antibodies, an indicator of autoimmune thyroid disease, may help to predict which patients will progress to clinical hypothyroidism; testing is recommended for patients with a minimally elevated TSH level.

4. **What are the two most common causes of hypothyroidism?**
   Although many disorders can cause hypothyroidism, the two most common causes are chronic lymphocytic thyroiditis (Hashimoto's disease), an autoimmune form of thyroid destruction, and radioiodine-induced hypothyroidism after treatment of Graves' disease (autoimmune hyperthyroidism).

5. **How common is postpartum thyroiditis?**
   Postpartum thyroiditis occurs in approximately 10% of women, two-thirds of whom experience a transient hypothyroid phase (6–12 months) that requires treatment.

6. **List the less common causes of hypothyroidism.**
   - Subacute thyroiditis
   - External irradiation to the neck
   - Medications (antithyroid drugs, amiodarone, lithium, and interferon)
   - Infiltrative diseases
   - Central (pituitary/hypothalamic) hypothyroidism (Fig. 35-1)
   - Congenital defects
   - Endemic (iodine-deficient) goiter, which is fairly common outside the United States

7. **List the symptoms commonly associated with hypothyroidism.**
   Hypothyroidism commonly presents with nonspecific symptoms, such as fatigue, cold intolerance, depression, weight gain, weakness, joint aches, constipation, dry skin, hair loss, and menstrual irregularities.

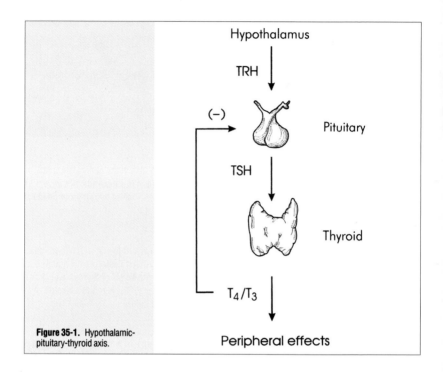

Figure 35-1. Hypothalamic-pituitary-thyroid axis.

8. **What findings on physical examination are consistent with hypothyroidism?**
Physical examination may be normal with mild thyroid failure and should not deter further work-up if clinical suspicions are high. Common signs of moderate-to-severe hypothyroidism include:
- Hypertension (diastolic hypertension is a clue)
- Bradycardia
- Coarse hair
- Periorbital swelling
- Yellow skin (due to elevated levels of beta carotene)
- Carpal tunnel syndrome
- Delayed relaxation of the deep tendon reflexes

9. **What does palpation of the thyroid reveal?**
The thyroid may be enlarged, normal, or small, but thyroid consistency is usually firm.

10. **Summarize unusual presentation of hypothyroidism.**
Unusual presentations of hypothyroidism include megacolon, cardiomegaly, and congestive heart failure (CHF). Severe CHF in one reported patient scheduled for cardiac transplant resolved with thyroid hormone replacement alone.

11. **Describe the laboratory tests that may show abnormal results during hypothyroidism.**
Laboratory clues to hypothyroidism include normochromic, normocytic anemia (menstruating women may also have iron deficiency anemia due to excessive bleeding from irregular menses), hyponatremia, hypercholesterolemia, and elevated levels of creatine phosphokinase.

12. **What tests best confirm the diagnosis of hypothyroidism in the outpatient setting?**
Many thyroid function tests are available to the clinician, including assessments of TSH, T_4, triiodothyronine (T_3), resin uptake, free T_4, free T_3, and reverse T_3. In the outpatient setting only one test is usually necessary: assessment of TSH. TSH, which is synthesized and secreted from the anterior pituitary gland, is the most sensitive indicator of thyroid function in the nonstressed state. Basically, if the TSH is normal (range 0.5–5 mU/L), the patient is euthyroid; if the TSH is elevated (>5 mU/L), the patient has primary gland failure.

13. **How should total T_4 levels be interpreted?**
Care must be taken in interpreting T_4 levels (occasionally done on health-screening panels). Many conditions unrelated to thyroid disease cause low or elevated levels of total T_4 because more than 99% of T_4 is protein-bound, and total T_4 levels depend on the amount of thyroid-binding proteins, which may vary greatly. Total T_4 levels must always be compared with the T_3 resin uptake (T_3RU), which reflects the amount of thyroid hormone-binding protein.

KEY POINTS: HYPOTHYROIDISM ✓

1. TSH level is the best screening test for primary hypothyroidism in the outpatient setting.

2. Levothyroxine (LT_4) is the preferred initial treatment for hypothyroidism and in healthy young patients can be started at a dose of 1.6 μg/k/day.

3. The goal TSH for treatment of primary hypothyroidism is between 0.5 and 2.0 mU/L.

4. Subclinical hypothyroidism (elevated TSH but normal T_4/T_3) is common and treatment can alleviate symptoms, as well as cardiac and lipid abnormalities.

14. **Explain why thyroid function tests are more difficult to interpret in acutely ill inpatients.**
Interpretation of thyroid function tests in acutely ill inpatients is more difficult when hypothyroidism is suspected. Acute nonthyroidal illness may cause suppression of the T_4 and T_3 levels, and TSH may be elevated in the recovery phase (see Chapter 40). Medications, such as dopamine and glucocorticoids, may suppress the TSH. Severe illness may even cause low levels of free T_4.

15. **How do you diagnose hypothyroidism in acutely ill inpatients?**
When hypothyroidism is suspected in the stressed, hospitalized patient, a combination of clinical signs (inappropriate bradycardia, puffy facies, dry skin, and delayed relaxation of deep tendon reflexes) and laboratory tests (TSH and free T_4 levels) is necessary to exclude or confirm the diagnosis of hypothyroidism. If these tests are equivocal, a reverse T_3 level, which is normal or elevated in nonthyroidal illness and low in hypothyroidism, may prove helpful. Inpatient TSH testing also may be confounded by normal diurnal variations in TSH. TSH levels in euthyroid people may exceed the normal range at night, when patients are frequently admitted. A morning test may help to clarify the significance of a mildly elevated TSH.

16. **Which thyroid hormone preparation should you use?**
Since 1891 when sheep thyroid extract was first used to treat myxedema, many preparations have been developed and are still available. Currently the best replacement regimen is LT_4. Brand-name LT_4 (Synthroid, Levothroid, and Levoxyl) is preferred over the generic preparations

because cost is a minor issue (generic LT$_4$ costs $6/month, whereas brand names cost about $10/month) and because generic LT$_4$ may vary 15–20% in bioavailability.

17. **What other thyroid hormone preparations are available?**
Other thyroid hormone preparations include L-triiodothyronine (LT$_3$), which is reserved for special cases because of its potency and short half-life, and desiccated thyroid and thyroglobulin, which give unpredictable concentrations of serum thyroid hormone because of varied content and bioavailability.

18. **What is the recommended dose of LT$_4$ for replacement therapy in a hypothyroid patient?**
Otherwise healthy, young patients may be started on full replacement doses of LT$_4$ (1.6 µg/k/day). Elderly patients and patients with known or suspected cardiac disease should be started on low doses of LT$_4$ (25 µg/day), which are increased by 25 µg/day every 2–3 months until the TSH is normal. In patients with subclinical hypothyroidism, consider starting the patient on 50–75% of the predicted full replacement dose.

19. **What is the appropriate goal for TSH in the treatment of primary hypothyroidism?**
The target TSH in treated hypothyroid patients should be between 0.5 and 2.0 mU/L, which represents the lower end of the normal range reported by most laboratories. When the usual reference ranges for TSH were developed, they included subjects with antithyroid antibodies suggestive of occult autoimmune thyroid disease. The "normal" ranges are therefore thought to be skewed toward higher TSH values. When normal subjects with no antithyroid antibodies are evaluated, most have TSH values below 2.5 mU/L.

20. **Discuss the evidence supporting combination T$_4$/T$_3$ therapy.**
The medical and lay literature has taken a renewed interest in combination therapy. A recent placebo-controlled study suggested that patients taking combination therapy had improved cognitive function and mood scores compared with when they took LT$_4$ alone. Studies in thyroidectomized animals have shown that T$_4$ therapy alone does not restore tissue levels of T$_4$ and T$_3$ to euthyroid levels, even when the TSH is normalized. While these studies are provocative and intriguing, most experts agree that more information is needed before we can recommend combination T$_4$/T$_3$ therapy in most patients. Our current approach is to openly discuss this information with inquiring patients.

21. **When should you consider combination T$_4$/T$_3$ therapy?**
The authors suggest a trial of LT$_4$ alone to normalize TSH within the low normal range (0.5–2.0 mU/L) for a period of 2–4 months. Many patients do extremely well with this approach. Patients who have low-normal TSH while taking LT$_4$ and still feel "hypothyroid" need further evaluation before you consider T$_3$ therapy. We generally exclude anemia and vitamin B$_{12}$ deficiency (associated with Hashimoto's thyroiditis) and inquire about sleep apnea. If this assessment is negative, we decrease the LT$_4$ by 12–25 µg and add 5 µg of Cytomel (T$_3$) in the morning. The goal is to see if the patient's symptoms improve without persistent suppression of the serum TSH (measured in the morning before taking medication). No data clearly support or refute this position; we believe it is a position of "good" medical practice.

22. **How should the clinician approach surgery in the hypothyroid patient?**
There are two broad categories to consider: emergent/cardiac surgery and elective surgery. Hypothyroidism is associated with minor postoperative complications—gastrointestinal (prolonged constipation, ileus), as well as neuropsychiatric (confusion, psychosis); in addition, the incidence of fever with infections is lower. Patients scheduled for elective surgery should wait until TSH is normalized because of the postoperative complications associated with

hypothyroidism. However, rates of mortality and major complications (blood loss, arrhythmias, and impaired wound healing) are similar to the rates in euthyroid patients.

23. **Summarize the current recommendations for emergent surgery.**
Current recommendations are to proceed with emergent surgery in the hypothyroid patient and to monitor for potential postoperative complications while giving replacement therapy with LT_4. Patients with ischemic coronary artery disease requiring surgery should proceed without LT_4 replacement because T_4 increases myocardial oxygen demands and may precipitate worsening cardiac symptoms if given before surgery. Postoperatively the patient should receive replacement therapy with LT_4 at a slow rate and be followed for CHF (increased in hypothyroid patients undergoing cardiac surgery).

24. **How does myxedema differ from hypothyroidism?**
Myxedema is a severe, uncompensated form of prolonged hypothyroidism. Complications include hypoventilation, cardiac failure, fluid and electrolyte abnormalities, and coma (see Chapter 39). Myxedema coma is frequently precipitated by an intercurrent systemic illness, surgery, or narcotic/hypnotic drugs. Patients with myxedema coma should receive replacement therapy with 300–500 mcg of intravenous LT_4 followed by 50–100 mcg each day. Because conversion of T_4 to T_3 (active hormone) is decreased with severe illness, patients with profound cardiac failure that requires pressors or patients unresponsive to 1–2 days of LT_4 therapy should be given LT_3 at 12.5 mcg IV every 6 hours.

WEBSITE

http://www.nacb.org

BIBLIOGRAPHY

1. Arem R, Patsch W: Lipoprotein and apolipoprotein levels in subclinical hypothyroidism. Arch Intern Med 150:2097–2100, 1990.
2. Bunevicius R, Kazanavicius G, Zalinkevicius R, Prange AJ: Effects of thyroxine as compared with thyroxine plus triiodothyronine in patients with hypothyroidism. N Engl J Med 340:424–429, 1998.
3. Canaris GJ, Manowitz NR, Mayor G, Ridgway EC: The Colorado thyroid disease prevalence study. Arch Intern Med 104:526–534, 2000.
4. Cooper DS, Halpern R, Wood LC, et al: L-thyroxine therapy in subclinical hypothyroidism. Ann Intern Med 101:18–24, 1984.
5. Demers LM, Spencer CA: Laboratory medicine practice guidelines: Laboratory support for the diagnosis and monitoring of thyroid disease. Thyroid 13:45–56, 2003.
6. Elder J, McLelland A, O'Reilly SJ, et al: The relationship between serum cholesterol and serum thyrotropin, thyroxine, and tri-iodothyronine concentrations in suspected hypothyroidism. Ann Clin Biochem 27:110–113, 1990.
7. Hay ID, Duick DS, Vliestra RE, et al: Thyroxine therapy in hypothyroid patients undergoing coronary revascularization: A retrospective analysis. Ann Intern Med 95:456–457, 1981.
8. Hollowell JG, Staehling NW, Flanders WD, et al: Serum TSH, T_4, and thyroid antibodies in the United States population (1988 to 1994): National Health and Nutrition Examination Survey (NHANES III). J Clin Endocrinol Metab 87:489–499, 2002.
9. Ladenson PW: Recognition and management of cardiovascular disease related to thyroid dysfunction. Am J Med 88:638–641, 1990.
10. Ladenson PW, Levin AA, Ridgway EC, Daniels GH: Complications of surgery in hypothyroid patients. Am J Med 77:262–266, 1984.

11. Mandel SJ, Brent GA, Larsen PR: Levothyroxine therapy in patients with thyroid disease. Ann Intern Med 119:492–502, 1993.

12. Patel R, Hughes RW: An unusual case of myxedema megacolon with features of ischemic and pseudomembranous colitis. Mayo Clin Proc 67:369–372, 1992.

13. Rosenthal MJ, Hunt WC, Garry PJ, Goodwin JS: Thyroid failure in the elderly: Microsomal antibodies as discriminant for therapy. JAMA 258:209–213, 1987.

14. Roti E, Minelli R, Gardini E, Braverman LE: The use and misuse of thyroid hormone. Endocr Rev 14:401–423, 1993.

CHAPTER 36

THYROIDITIS

Robert C. Smallridge, M.D.

1. Give the differential diagnosis for thyroiditis.
1. Infectious
   (a) Acute (suppurative)
   (b) Subacute (granulomatous; de Quervain's)
2. Autoimmune
   (a) Chronic lymphocytic (Hashimoto's disease)
   (b) Atrophic (primary myxedema)
   (c) Juvenile
   (d) Postpartum
3. Painless (nonpostpartum)
4. Drug-induced
5. Riedel's struma
6. Radiation-induced
7. Traumatic

2. What causes acute thyroiditis?
This rare disease is infectious and usually bacterial; at times, however, fungal, tuberculous, parasitic, or syphilitic infections have been reported. *Pneumocystis carinii* has been observed in patients with AIDS. Treatment involves incision/drainage of the abscess and antibiotics.

3. Describe the four stages of subacute thyroiditis.
- *Stage I:* Patients have a painful (unilateral or bilateral) tender thyroid and may have systemic symptoms (fatigue, malaise, fever). Inflammatory destruction of thyroid follicles allows release of excess thyroxine (T_4) and triiodothyronine (T_3) into the blood, and thyrotoxicosis may ensue.
- *Stage II:* A transitory period (several weeks) of euthyroidism occurs after the T_4 is cleared from the body.
- *Stage III:* With severe disease, patients may become hypothyroid until the thyroid gland repairs itself.
- *Stage IV:* Euthyroid state returns.

4. Summarize the natural history of subacute thyroiditis.
Subacute thyroiditis is probably viral in origin. Histologically, the inflammation is granulomatous. Although patients almost always recover clinically, serum thyroglobulin levels remain elevated and intrathyroidal iodine content is low for many months (Fig. 36-1). Patients requiring steroids are more likely to become hypothyroid at a later time. Such findings suggest persistent subclinical abnormalities after an episode of subacute thyroiditis. About 2% of patients have a second episode many years later.

5. What is the most common cause of thyroiditis?
Autoimmune thyroid disease, which is recognized by the presence of thyroid peroxidase (TPO) antibodies and, less frequently, thyroglobulin antibodies in serum.

6. Give the clinical characteristics of autoimmune thyroid disease.
Chronic lymphocytic thyroiditis (Hashimoto's disease) usually presents as a euthyroid goiter that progresses to hypothyroidism in middle-aged and older persons, especially women.

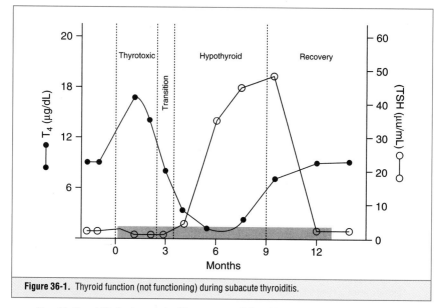

Figure 36-1. Thyroid function (not functioning) during subacute thyroiditis.

Atrophic thyroiditis is characterized by a very small thyroid gland in a hypothyroid patient. Some evidence suggests that thyroid growth inhibitory antibodies may account for the lack of a goiter. Two-thirds of adolescents with goiter have autoimmune (juvenile) thyroiditis.

7. **Does postpartum thyroiditis follow a different clinical course from other types of autoimmune thyroiditis?**
Yes. Postpartum disease develops in women between the third and ninth month after delivery. It typically follows the stages seen in patients with subacute thyroiditis, although histologically patients have lymphocytic infiltration.

8. **How common is postpartum thyroiditis?**
After delivery, 5–10% of women develop biochemical evidence of thyroid dysfunction. About one-third of affected women develop symptoms (either hyperthyroidism, hypothyroidism, or both)

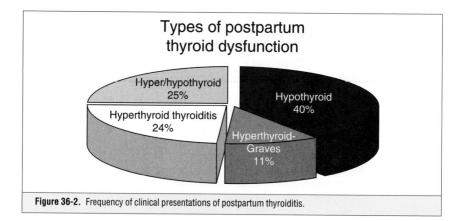

Figure 36-2. Frequency of clinical presentations of postpartum thyroiditis.

and benefit from 6–12 months of therapy with L-thyroxine (LT$_4$). The frequency of each clinical presentation is depicted in Figure 36-2.

9. **Summarize the differences between subacute and postpartum thyroiditis.**
See Table 36-1.

TABLE 36-1. SUBACUTE VERSUS POSTPARTUM THYROIDITIS		
	Subacute Thyroiditis	Postpartum Thyroiditis
Thyroid pain	Yes	No
Sedimentation rate	Increased	Normal
TPO antibody	Transient increase only	Positive
HLA status	B-35	DR3; DR5
Histology	Giant cells; granulomas	Lymphocytes

TPO, thyroid peroxidase; HLA, human leucocyte antigen.

10. **Why do women develop postpartum thyroiditis?**
Women who develop postpartum thyroiditis have underlying asymptomatic autoimmune thyroiditis. During pregnancy, the maternal immune system is partially suppressed, with a dramatic rebound rise in thyroid antibodies after delivery. Although TPO antibodies are not believed to be cytotoxic, they are currently the most reliable marker of susceptibility to postpartum disease.

11. **Does thyroid function in patients with postpartum thyroiditis return to normal, as it does in subacute thyroiditis?**
Not always. Approximately 20% of women become permanently hypothyroid, and a similar number have persistent mild abnormalities.

12. **Do any factors identify women at increased risk of developing postpartum thyroiditis?**
Women with a higher TPO antibody titer are more likely to develop thyroiditis. Approximately 25% of women with type 1 diabetes mellitus develop thyroiditis after delivery. For high-risk patients, screening for thyroid antibodies and careful monitoring of thyroid function are indicated.

13. **What is painless thyroiditis?**
Both men and nonpostpartum women may present with transient thyrotoxic symptoms. As with subacute thyroiditis, they often experience subsequent hypothyroidism. Unlike subacute disease, this disorder is painless. It has been given a variety of names, including hyperthyroiditis, silent thyroiditis, transient painless thyroiditis with hyperthyroidism, and lymphocytic thyroiditis with spontaneously resolving hyperthyroidism. This disease was first described in the 1970s and reached its peak incidence in the early 1980s. It seems to occur less often now.

14. **What causes painless thyroiditis?**
Some investigators believe that it is a variant of subacute thyroiditis because a small percentage of patients with biopsy-proved subacute disease have had no pain (they may have fever and

KEY POINTS: THYROIDITIS ✓

1. In early subacute thyroiditis, the radioactive iodine uptake (RAIU) is suppressed, and sedimentation rate markedly elevated.

2. Approximately 10% of premenopausal women are TPO antibody-positive; many develop postpartum thyroid dysfunction.

3. Amiodarone-induced thyroid disease (AITD) may be due to iodine-induced hyperthyroidism (type 1 AITD) or destruction-induced thyroiditis (type 2 AITD).

4. Subacute thyroiditis may require analgesics (or steroids) and beta blockers early and LT_4 during recovery but usually resolves.

5. Acute infectious thyroiditis requires prompt incision/drainage and antibiotics.

weight loss and may be mistaken for having systemic disease or malignancy). Others believe that painless thyroiditis is a variant of Hashimoto's disease because the histology of the two is similar. Painless thyroiditis can rarely present with thyroid pain.

15. **What is destruction-induced thyroiditis?**
Destruction-induced thyroiditis refers to the three disorders (subacute, postpartum, and painless thyroiditis), in which an inflammatory infiltrate destroys thyroid follicles, and excessive amounts of T_4 and T_3 are released into the circulation.

16. **When a patient presents with hyperthyroid symptoms, an elevated level of T4, and a suppressed level of TSH, what is the next test that should be ordered?**
A 24-hour RAIU should be performed. When the thyroid is overactive (as in Graves' or toxic nodular disease), the RAIU is elevated. In destruction-induced thyroiditis, the RAIU is low, as a result of both suppression of TSH by the acutely increased level of serum T_4 and the diminished ability of damaged thyroid follicles to trap and organify iodine.

17. **What is the appropriate therapy for patients with any type of destructive thyroiditis?**
In the thyrotoxic stage, beta blockers relieve adrenergic symptoms. All forms of antithyroid therapy (drugs, radioactive iodine ablation, and surgery) are absolutely contraindicated. Analgesics (salicylates or prednisone) provide prompt relief of thyroid pain. Thyroid hormone relieves hypothyroid symptoms and should be continued for 6–12 months, depending on the severity of disease. Many patients need no therapy.

18. **Which drugs can induce thyroiditis?**
Amiodarone, an iodine-containing antiarrhythmic drug, may cause thyroid damage and thyrotoxicosis. Interferon alpha (less commonly, interferon beta) and interleukin-2 can cause thyroiditis, and both hyperthyroidism and hypothyroidism have occurred during therapy.

19. **Does amiodarone induce only thyroiditis?**
No. Due to the large amount of iodine in this drug, it can cause either iodine-induced hypothyroidism or hyperthyroidism. Distinguishing hyperthyroidism due to iodine excess (type 1 disease) from amiodarone-induced thyroiditis (type 2 disease) can be difficult. Some differentiating features are listed in Table 36-2.

TABLE 36-2.	TYPE 1 VERSUS TYPE 2 THYROIDITIS	
	Type 1	Type 2
Thyroid size	Goiter; nodules	Normal
RAIU	↓, normal, ↑	↓↓
Thyroid antibodies	↑, negative	Negative
Interleukin-6	Normal, ↑	↑↑
Ultrasound Doppler flow	↑	↓
Therapy	Antithyroid drugs; potassium perchlorate; thyroidectomy	Antithyroid drugs (?); steroids

RAIU, radioactive iodine uptake.

20. **What is Riedel's struma?**
    Riedel's struma is a rare disorder in which the thyroid becomes densely fibrotic and hard. Local fibrosis of adjacent tissues may produce obstructive symptoms that require surgery. In some cases, fibrosis of other tissues (fibrosing retroperitonitis, orbital fibrosis, or sclerosing cholangitis) may occur.

21. **Are there any other causes of thyroiditis?**
    Yes. External beam radiotherapy can cause painless thyrotoxic thyroiditis. Various forms of neck trauma (neck surgery, cyst aspiration, seat belt injury) have also been reported.

WEBSITE

http://www.thyroidmanager.org

BIBLIOGRAPHY

1. Aizawa T, Watanabe T, Suzuki N, et al: Radiation-induced painless thyrotoxic thyroiditis followed by hypothyroidism: A case report and literature review. Thyroid 8:273–275, 1998.

2. Bartalena L, Brogioni S, Grasso L, et al: Treatment of amiodarone-induced thyrotoxicosis, a difficult challenge: Results of a prospective study. J Clin Endocrinol Metab 81:2930–2933, 1996.

3. Berger SA, Zonszein J, Villamena P, et al: Infectious diseases of the thyroid gland. Rev Infect Dis 5:108–122, 1983.

4. de Lange WE, Freling NJ, Molenaar WM, et al: Invasive fibrous thyroiditis (Riedel's struma): A manifestation of multifocal fibrosclerosis? A case report with review of the literature. Q J Med 72:709–717, 1989.

5. Fatourechi V, Aniszewski J, Fatourechi G, et al: Clinical features and outcome of subacute thyroiditis in an incidence cohort: Olmsted county, Minnesota, study. J Clin Endocrinol Metab 88:2100–2105, 2003.

6. Guttler R, Singer PA, Axline SG, et al: *Pneumocystis carinii* thyroiditis. Report of three cases and review of the literature. Arch Intern Med 153:393–396, 1993.

7. Iitake M, Momotani N, Ishii J, et al: Incidence of subacute thyroiditis recurrences after a prolonged latency: 24-year survey. J Clin Endocrinol Metab 81:466–469, 1996.

8. Koh LK, Greenspan FS, Yeo PP: Interferon-alpha induced thyroid dysfunction: Three clinical presentations and a review of the literature. Thyroid 7:891–896, 1997.

9. Meek SE, Smallridge RC: Diagnosis and treatment of thyroiditis and other more unusual forms of hyperthyroidism. In Cooper DS (ed): Medical Management of Thyroid Disease. New York, Marcel Dekker, 2001, pp 93–134.

10. Ross DS: Syndromes of thyrotoxicosis with low radioactive iodine uptake. Endocrinol Metab Clin N Am 27:169–185, 1998.

11. Rotenberg Z, Weinberger I, Fuchs J, et al: Euthyroid atypical subacute thyroiditis simulating systemic or malignant disease. Arch Intern Med 146:105–107, 1986.

12. Roti E, Minelli R, Gardini E, et al: Iodine-induced hypothyroidism in euthyroid subjects with a previous episode of subacute thyroiditis. J Clin Endocrinol Metab 70:1581–1585, 1990.

13. Seminara SB, Daniels GH: Amiodarone and the thyroid. Endocr Pract 4:48–57, 1998.

14. Shigemasa C, Ueta Y, Mitani Y, et al: Chronic thyroiditis with painful tender thyroid enlargement and transient thyrotoxicosis. J Clin Endocrinol Metab 70:385–390, 1990.

15. Smallridge RC: Postpartum thyroid dysfunction: A frequently undiagnosed endocrine disorder. The Endocrinologist 6:44–50, 1996.

16. Smallridge RC: Postpartum thyroid disease: A model of immunologic dysfunction. Clin Appl Immunol Rev 1:89–103, 2000.

17. Smallridge RC: Hypothyroidism and pregnancy. The Endocrinologist 12:454–464, 2002.

18. Smallridge RC, De Keyser FM, Van Herle AJ, et al: Thyroid iodine content and serum thyroglobulin: Cues to the natural history of destruction-induced thyroiditis. J Clin Endocrinol Metab 62:1213–1219, 1986.

19. Volpé R: The management of subacute (de Quervain's) thyroiditis. Thyroid 3:253–255, 1993.

20. Woolf PD: Transient painless thyroiditis with hyperthyroidism: A variant of lymphocytic thyroiditis? Endocr Rev 1:411–420, 1980.

CHAPTER 37

THYROID NODULES AND GOITER

William J. Georgitis, M.D.

1. **What is a goiter?**
   Goiter is a visible swelling in front of the neck due to thyroid gland enlargement. The term is derived from French *goitre*, Middle French *goitron* or throat, a vulgate Latin term *guttrion*, and the Latin terms *guttrio* and *guttur* for throat.

2. **How does a nontoxic goiter develop?**
   The pathogenesis for euthyroid goiter remains an enigma. Proposed mechanisms include:
   - Thyroid-stimulating hormone (TSH)-dependent thyroid enlargement to compensate for diminished thyroid hormone production due to environmental goitrogens.
   - Iodine deficiency.
   - Inherited biosynthetic defects.
   Regression of goiter after iodine supplementation or thyroxine suppression of TSH supports these mechanisms. However, TSH levels are not elevated in endemic goiter. Important genetic variants may involve thyroglobulin, thyroperoxidase, intracellular signaling pathways affecting cell life cycles, and the sodium/iodine (Na^+/I^-) symporter.

3. **Describe the natural history of diffuse nontoxic goiter.**
   Simple goiter tends to become multinodular over time. The nodules are heterogenous in both morphology and function. Autonomous function, defined as TSH-independent production and secretion of thyroid hormone, can evolve. Supplementation programs in iodine-deficient populations, while clearly decreasing the incidence of cretinism and goiter, have also caused some people to develop iodine-associated hyperthyroidism. This jodbasedow hyperthyroidism is more likely to occur in older people with autonomous adenomatous goiters. In the U.S., this form of hyperthyroidism usually results from iodine excess due to radiographic contrast agents or medications rich in iodine. It may be transient and not require ablative therapies, such as thyroidectomy or radioiodine treatment.

4. **How does lithium affect thyroid function?**
   Lithium has diverse effects on thyroid function. It inhibits iodine uptake, dampens iodotyrosine coupling, alters thyroglobulin structure, blocks thyroid hormone secretion, and has mitogenic effects. Both goiter and hypothyroidism can appear during prolonged exposure to lithium (Fig. 37-1).

5. **Describe the mechanism by which lithium produces goiter and hypothyroidism.**
   The inhibitory effect of lithium on thyroid hormone release provokes an increase in TSH even in patients free of thyroid disease. Compensatory thyroid enlargement occurs without hypothyroidism except in patients with an underlying decrease in thyroid functional reserve. In this category of patients, thyroid hormone levels may be normal prior to lithium treatment; but hypothyroidism may appear in patients with chronic lymphocytic thyroiditis, prior to subacute thyroiditis, or partial thyroidectomy. Because hypothyroid signs and symptoms may be difficult to decipher in the presence of depression or bipolar disorder, TSH testing before and during lithium treatment is recommended.

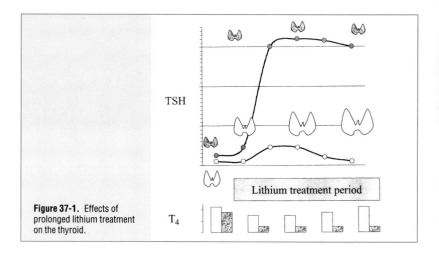

Figure 37-1. Effects of prolonged lithium treatment on the thyroid.

6. **How common are thyroid nodules?**
   Thyroid nodules are common. Prevalence increases as a linear function of age. The cumulative lifetime chance of having a palpable thyroid nodule approaches 6%. The prevalence at autopsy in 90-year-olds is about 60%. The vast majority of thyroid nodules are benign. The yield of thyroid cancer in surgical series before the widespread use of fine-needle aspiration (FNA) averaged about 10%.

7. **List the differential diagnosis for thyroid nodule.**

Adenoma	Thyroiditis	Metastatic cancer
Carcinoma	Thyroid hemiagenesis	Lymphoma/sarcoma
Thyroid cyst	Parathyroid cyst	

8. **Can the nature of a thyroid nodule be determined from the family history?**
   Family history is usually not helpful. An exception is medullary thyroid cancers associated with the multiple endocrine neoplasia syndromes. Inheritance of these tumors is autosomal dominant with almost complete penetrance for the abnormal *ret* oncogene.

9. **Do personal history and physical examination help to determine the nature of a thyroid nodule?**
   In general, no. Most patients with thyroid nodules have no symptoms and normal thyroid function. Hoarseness, dysphagia, dyspnea, or hemoptysis are rare features that suggest malignancy but also occur in benign thyroid disorders. When a patient with a visible goiter reports any of these symptoms, it suggests either rapid growth or involvement of the recurrent laryngeal nerve. An aggressive form of thyroid malignancy, such as lymphoma or anaplastic thyroid cancer, is a consideration, but fortunately it is rare. Thyroid cancer grows without causing pain. Other traits of nodules that suggest malignancy include size greater than 3 cm, fixation to adjacent structures, and palpable cervical lymph nodes.

10. **How are most thyroid cancers discovered?**
    Most thyroid cancers are discovered by chance. Often the patient is the first to notice a lump. A change in the appearance of the neck may be reported by a family member or during a medical visit for some unrelated matter. Ultrasound, magnetic resonance imaging (MRI), and computed tomography (CT) studies for a myriad of indications may first detect a thyroid nodule. Because

they are recognized incidental to the purpose of the procedure, these nodules are often referred to as thyroid incidentalomas.

11. **What diagnosis should be suspected when a thyroid nodule is first discovered due to neck pain?**
Hemorrhagic degeneration of a benign adenoma. Visceral pain fibers are triggered by acute expansion of the nodule, which stretches the thyroid capsule. The resulting deep aching pain may radiate to the jaw or ear. Pain may be mistaken for dental abscess, otitis media, or otitis externa. Aspiration of hemorrhagic fluid can relieve the discomfort and confirms the diagnosis.

12. **If a nodule is cancer, what kind is it likely to be?**
A papillary thyroid cancer or variant of papillary is the most common by far (Table 37-1).

TABLE 37-1. THYROID CANCER CLASSIFIED IN DESCENDING ORDER OF FREQUENCY	
Papillary	50–70%
Follicular	10–15%
Medullary	1–2%
Anaplastic	Rare
Primary thyroid lymphoma	Rare
Metastatic to thyroid	Rarely detected in vivo

13. **How does the appearance of the fluid help in diagnosing thyroid cysts?**
Simple thyroid cysts have yellow-, burgundy-, or chocolate-colored fluid and are generally benign. Complex thyroid nodules with both cystic and solid components contain brown or hemorrhagic fluid. Complex cysts have a higher risk of malignancy than simple cysts. Cytology of cyst fluid is almost always nonspecific and shows histiocytes and crenated erythrocytes. If the fluid removed is crystal-clear like water, the lesion is a parathyroid cyst. Serum calcium should be measured to exclude hyperparathyroidism.

14. **How does the amount of thyroid cyst fluid help guide management?**
One-third of cysts reappear days to weeks after aspiration. If the volume on sequential aspirations does not decrease or the aspirated fluid is grossly bloody, surgical removal of the cyst should be considered.

15. **How important is sampling of the solid component of the complex nodule?**
Fine-needle aspiration (FNA) of any solid component palpable after the fluid has been drained or with ultrasound guidance to ensure sampling of the solid component of the complex nodule can provide diagnostic material.

16. **Is the risk of cancer less in multinodular goiter or Hashimoto's disease than in solitary thyroid nodules?**
Although autopsy series indicate that up to 75% of thyroid nodules are multiple and that malignancy is rare, any thyroid nodule can be cancerous. Contrary to old axioms, a palpable nodule in the presence of multinodular goiter or lymphocytic thyroiditis seems to have the same risk of cancer as a solitary palpable nodule. Size does seem to matter. Palpable nodules are generally at least 1 cm in greatest dimension. Nodules smaller than 1 cm are often not palpable and have a low risk of malignancy.

17. **Summarize the role of FNA in the evaluation of thyroid nodules.**
Fine-needle aspiration (FNA) is a safe, outpatient procedure with an accuracy of 90–95% in adequate specimens interpreted by experienced cytopathologists. FNA should be performed on all readily palpable solitary thyroid nodules and on dominant nodules in a multinodular goiter. After a serum TSH level is shown to be normal, an FNA is really the next evaluation for a thyroid nodule. Most FNAs return benign diagnoses, including adenomatous hyperplasia (benign multinodular goiter), colloid adenoma, and autoimmune thyroiditis. A reading of papillary thyroid cancer helps guide planning for thyroid resection.

18. **Is FNA helpful in diagnosing follicular neoplasms?**
Follicular neoplasms are more vexing. FNA cannot reliably differentiate adenoma from carcinoma since features of capsular or vascular invasion that define follicular carcinoma can be determined only on surgical pathology. Aspirates are inadequate for interpretation in about 15%. This rate can be reduced by using ultrasound guidance, especially for lesions with a cystic component.

19. **Should an FNA be done for a palpable nodule if the TSH is low?**
No. A low TSH indicates hyperthyroidism.

20. **If the TSH is found to be low, what is the next step?**
A thyroid scan, to rule in solitary toxic nodule or toxic multinodular goiter, should be the next test. Although the scan is ordered with the anticipation of finding lesions with autonomous function, a photopenic (cold) nodule may sometimes be encountered.

KEY POINTS: THYROID NODULES AND GOITER ✓

1. The cumulative lifetime chance of having a palpable thyroid nodule is about 6%.

2. Thyroid nodules can be found in about 60% of 90-year-olds.

3. The vast majority of thyroid nodules are benign.

4. Nodules in multinodular goiter are heterogenous in both morphology and function.

5. FNA of the thyroid is a safe outpatient procedure with an accuracy of 90–95% in determining malignancy with adequate specimens interpreted by experienced cytopathologists.

21. **Explain the distinction between cold and hot nodules.**
A cold nodule has diminished uptake of the radioactive agent compared with surrounding normal thyroid tissue. Most cold nodules are benign, but virtually all thyroid cancers are cold on scan. The solitary toxic or hot nodule avidly absorbs tracer, whereas uptake in the remainder of the thyroid is suppressed. Solitary toxic nodules are usually larger than 3 cm in diameter. Most occur in patients older than 40. Toxic adenomas are never cancerous. The majority has gain of function mutations in the thyrotropin receptor.

22. **What is the significance of a warm nodule?**
In contrast, a warm nodule may be malignant. Some hyperfunctional or isofunctional nodules are really cold nodules that appear to concentrate tracer because they are invested by normal thyroid tissue. Other autonomous nodules fail to secrete sufficient thyroid hormone to suppress TSH to dampen tracer uptake by surrounding normal thyroid tissue. Thyroid scanning with the patient taking a TSH-suppressive dose of thyroid hormone can define the autonomous nature of

these nodules. Autonomous nodules may be observed, whereas all others deserve FNA to exclude thyroid cancer.

23. **Who invented the incision used for thyroidectomy?**
Theodor Kocher (1841–1917), a Swedish surgeon, devised the incision. He was an innovator, so be cautious when you ask for a "Kocher" in the operating room. Kocher's name is also associated with a surgical forceps, a wrist operation, and a right subcostal incision for cholecystectomy.

24. **Which treatment was used first for diffuse toxic goiter (Graves' disease): radioactive iodine or antithyroid medications?**
Both were developed in the early 1940s. Thiourea, the first goitrogenic substance to be used, had undesirable toxicities and soon was replaced by methimazole and propylthiouracil. Of the fission products developed during World War II, ^{130}I was used before ^{131}I. Radioiodine became widely available in about 1946.

25. **What goitrous thyroid conditions are treated with radioactive iodine?**
Radioiodine treatment is effective for diffuse toxic goiter, toxic nodular goiter, and solitary toxic nodules. Compressive symptoms from benign multinodular goiters in patients judged to be poor surgical risks can also be relieved by radioactive iodine. Although the goiter shrinks only about 30% or less, relief of symptoms is common.

26. **What does recent evidence reveal about the role of suppression therapy with thyroxine?**
Although thyroxine suppression therapy was widely used in the past in the belief that it reduced the size of thyroid nodules, more recent randomized controlled studies, including some with objective measurements by ultrasound, indicate that suppression therapy is ineffective. For euthyroid patients, thyroid hormone administration to induce regression of thyroid nodules has not proven to be very effective except under special circumstances, such as iodine deficiency or prevention of new nodules after lobectomy in radiation-exposed patients. Used in solitary nodules, the apparent reduction in size judged only by palpation may represent regression of surrounding thyroid tissue rather than the nodule itself. Routine treatment with TSH suppressive doses of thyroid hormone for thyroid nodules or goiter may be associated with more iatrogenic side effects than benefit.

27. **When is suppression therapy with thyroxine useful?**
Suppression therapy may still be of value in selected cases. For example, the patient with an elevated serum TSH and thyroid enlargement may show regression of the goiter with thyroid hormone replacement.

WESITE ⊕

http://www.thyroidmanager.org

BIBLIOGRAPHY

1. Bennedbæk FN, Nielsen LK, Hegedüs L: Effect of percutaneous ethanol injection therapy versus suppressive doses of L-thyroxine on benign solitary solid cold thyroid nodules: A randomized trial. J Clin Endocrinol Metab 83:830–835, 1998.
2. Bennedbæk FN, Perrild H, Hegedüs L: Diagnosis and treatment of the solitary thyroid nodule. Results of a European survey. Clin Endocrinol 50:357–363, 1999.

3. Braverman LE, Utiger RD: Werner and Ingbar's The Thyroid: A Fundamental and Clinical Text Edition, 8th ed. Philadelphia, Lippincott, Williams & Wilkins, 2000.

4. Cheung PSY, Lee JMH, Boey JH: Thyroxine suppressive therapy of benign solitary thyroid nodules: A prospective randomized study. World J Surg 13:818–822, 1989.

5. Dremier S, Coppee F, Delange F, et al: Thyroid autonomy: Mechanism and clinical effects. J Clin Endocrinol Metab 81:4187–4193, 1996.

6. Hegedus L, Nygaard B, Hansen JM: Is routine thyroxine treatment to hinder postoperative recurrence of nontoxic goiter justified? J Clin Endocrinol Metab 84:756–760, 1999.

7. Lazarus JH: The effects of lithium therapy on thyroid and thyrotropin-releasing hormone. Thyroid 8:909–913, 1998.

8. Mazzaferri EL: Management of a solitary thyroid nodule. N Engl J Med 328:553–559, 1993.

9. Mortensen JD: Gross and microscopic findings in clinically normal thyroid glands. J Clin Endocrinol Metab 15:1270–1280, 1955.

10. Ridgway EC: Medical treatment of benign thyroid nodules: Have we defined a benefit? Ann Intern Med 128:403–405, 1998.

11. Rojeski MT: Nodular thyroid disease. N Engl J Med 313:428–436, 1985.

12. Ross DS: Evaluation of the thyroid nodule. J Nucl Med 32:2181–2192, 1991.

CHAPTER 38

THYROID CANCER

Arnold A. Asp, M.D.

1. **Describe the types of thyroid cancer.**
   The thyroid consists predominantly of follicular epithelial cells, which incorporate iodine into thyroid hormone to be stored in follicles, and of smaller numbers of parafollicular cells, which produce calcitonin (CT). Malignant transformation of either type of cell may occur, but the parafollicular malignancy (*medullary* carcinoma of the thyroid [MCT]) is much less common than cancers derived from follicular epithelial cells. Malignancies originating from follicular epithelial cells are designated according to their microscopic appearance and include *papillary*, *follicular*, and *anaplastic* carcinomas (Fig. 38-1).

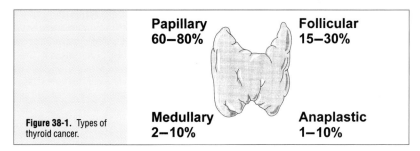

Papillary 60–80%   **Follicular** 15–30%

Medullary 2–10%   **Anaplastic** 1–10%

Figure 38-1. Types of thyroid cancer.

2. **Summarize the frequency of each type of thyroid cancer.**
   Papillary carcinoma and its variants comprise approximately 60–80% of thyroid cancers, whereas follicular carcinoma makes up approximately 15–30% of primary thyroid malignancies. These two forms are frequently referred to as the *differentiated* thyroid carcinomas (DTCs). MCT accounts for 2–10% of thyroid carcinomas, whereas anaplastic forms of thyroid carcinoma account for 1–10%.

3. **Describe the histology of the two differentiated forms of thyroid carcinoma.**
   Papillary and follicular carcinomas are histologically distinct. Papillary carcinoma is generally an unencapsulated tumor marked by enlarged cells with dense cytoplasm and overlapping nuclei that have granular, powdery chromatin, nucleoli, and pseudonuclear inclusion bodies (often called "Orphan Annie eyes"), all arranged in papillary fronds. Follicular carcinoma is generally characterized by atypical-appearing thyroid cells with dense, uniform, overlapping nuclei, and a disorganized microfollicular architecture.

4. **How is follicular carcinoma differentiated from benign follicular adenomas?**
   Follicular carcinoma cannot be differentiated reliably from benign follicular adenomas on cytomorphologic criteria alone; follicular cancer must demonstrate invasion of the tumor capsule or blood vessels.

5. **Summarize the types of papillary carcinoma.**
   Tumors that contain histologic elements of both types of carcinoma are classified as mixed papillary–follicular cancer and are considered to be variants of papillary carcinoma.

Two additional pathologic variants of papillary carcinoma, tall cell and insular cell, may be slightly more aggressive than other papillary forms.

6. **Distinguish the clinical behavior of papillary and follicular carcinomas.**
   Papillary and follicular carcinomas behave as clinically distinct entities. Most endocrinologists consider follicular carcinoma to be the more aggressive of the differentiated cancers, with a higher rate of metastases, more frequent recurrence after therapy, and an exaggerated mortality rate compared with the relatively indolent papillary carcinoma. This view is not universal. Some authors believe that the sharp dichotomy between the clinical courses of papillary and follicular carcinomas is artificial and attribute the apparent aggressiveness of follicular carcinoma to its occurrence in an older population; they argue that when cases are controlled for age, outcomes of patients with either form of DTC are comparable.

7. **Who gets papillary carcinoma?**
   The disease may occur at any age but has a peak incidence during the fourth decade. Women are more commonly affected than men and account for 62–81% of patients in most series.

8. **Describe the clinical course of papillary carcinoma.**
   Papillary carcinoma usually presents as a painless nodule within the thyroid gland or cervical lymphatics. The primary tumor is rarely encapsulated (4–22% in most series) but is less aggressive if a capsule is present. Papillary carcinoma is more commonly multifocal within the thyroid than is follicular carcinoma; 20–80% of glands have multiple lesions at resection. Extrathyroidal invasion through the capsule of the thyroid occurs in 5–16% of cases. Compared with other malignancies, papillary carcinoma is relatively indolent. Cancer-related death occurs in only 4–12% of patients during 20-year follow-up. Prognostic factors at the time of diagnosis that augur a poor outcome include male sex, age > 40 years, extrathyroidal invasion, distant metastases, and large primary tumor (> 1.5 cm diameter).

9. **Discuss the significance of lymph node metastases of papillary carcinoma.**
   Papillary carcinoma frequently metastasizes to regional cervical and high mediastinal lymphatics. At the time of surgery, 35–43% of patients have enlarged regional lymph nodes that harbor cancer. If lymph nodes are systematically "picked" and examined for microscopic foci, the prevalence of cervical metastases increases to 90%. Unlike other neoplasms, the presence of papillary carcinoma in regional lymph nodes does not increase mortality; it does, however, increase the likelihood of recurrence after therapy. Up to 20% of recurrent lesions cannot subsequently be eradicated.

10. **How common is metastasis of papillary carcinoma to sites other than lymph nodes?**
    Although lymphatic metastases are common, only 3–7% of patients with papillary carcinoma manifest distant metastatic lesions during initial therapy. Distant metastases involve the lung (76% of distant foci), bone (23% of distant foci), and brain (15% of distant foci).

11. **Who gets follicular carcinoma?**
    Follicular carcinoma may occur at any age but has a later peak incidence (fifth decade) than papillary carcinoma. Women outnumber men, accounting for approximately 60% of cases. Follicular carcinoma occurs more commonly in areas of iodine deficiency; the incidence of this malignancy has decreased as iodine supplementation has increased.

12. **Describe the clinical course of follicular carcinoma.**
    Follicular carcinoma usually presents as an asymptomatic nodule within the thyroid, but unlike papillary carcinoma, it may present as an isolated metastatic pulmonary or osseous focus without a palpable thyroid lesion. Very rarely metastatic foci of follicular carcinoma retain

hormonal synthetic capability and overproduce thyroid hormones, causing thyrotoxicosis. The tumor is nearly always encapsulated, and the degree of vascular or capsular invasiveness (minimal to extensive) is indicative of malignant potential. Follicular carcinoma is usually unifocal (< 10% multifocal). Death due to follicular carcinoma occurs in 13–59% of patients followed for 20 years. Prognostic factors at the time of initial therapy that portend a poor outcome include age greater than 50 years, male sex (in some settings), marked degree of vascular invasion, and distant metastases.

13. **How common are metastases of follicular carcinomas?**
Hematogenous metastases occur in follicular carcinomas; for this reason, cervical and mediastinal lymphatic involvement is less common than in papillary carcinoma (only 6–13% of patients during initial surgery). In contrast to cases of papillary carcinoma, the presence of cervical metastases indicates advanced disease. Distant metastases to the lung, bone, and central nervous system (in descending order of occurrence) are discovered more commonly in follicular than in papillary carcinoma, occurring in 12–33% of cases.

14. **Discuss the relationship between Graves' disease and DTC.**
DTC is discovered in 5–10% of the surgical resections performed for the treatment of Graves' disease. In some series of patients with Graves' disease, up to 45% of palpable nodules contain papillary carcinoma. Such data have led to the speculation that the thyroid-stimulating immunoglobulins responsible for thyrotoxicosis may potentiate the growth of neoplastic cells and predispose to aggressive forms of DTC.

15. **How is chronic lymphocytic thyroiditis related to DTC?**
Chronic lymphocytic thyroiditis is found concomitantly with papillary carcinoma in 5–10% of cases. Local recurrence and metastatic disease are less common in such cases and may indicate a favorable effect of Hashimoto's disease.

16. **How does metastatic disease affect the prognosis of DTC?**
Distant metastatic disease, as mentioned above, occurs more commonly in follicular carcinoma than in papillary cancer. Regardless of the primary type of cancer, the prognosis associated with distant metastases is dismal. Overall, 50–66% of patients with pulmonary, osseous, or central nervous system lesions die within 5 years. On rare occasions, pulmonary metastases may be compatible with 10 to 20-year survival in younger patients. Metastases to bone are associated with brief survival, despite aggressive therapy.

17. **How are the DTCs treated?**
Simply stated, therapy for DTC is based on surgical removal of the primary tumor and eradication of all metastatic disease with radioactive iodine (^{131}I). Lifelong suppression of thyroid-stimulating hormone (TSH) with exogenous thyroid hormone subsequently reduces the risk of recurrence.

18. **What factors favor limited surgery?**
Opinions about the extent of initial surgical resection have been tempered by the possible complications of thyroid surgery; recurrent laryngeal nerve damage with resultant hoarseness and/or iatrogenic hypoparathyroidism may occur in 1–5% of thyroid resections. Fear of complications, coupled with the relatively low mortality rate associated with DTC, has prompted some surgeons to remove only the thyroid lobe in which cancer is apparent at the time of exploration.

19. **Why do most surgeons favor more extensive surgery?**
Most surgeons are cognizant of the frequency of clinically inapparent multicentric lesions, the increased recurrence rates in patients treated with simple lobectomy, and the low rate of

postsurgical complications; thus they have rejected simple lobectomy and instead prefer near-total thyroidectomy, which entails the removal of the thyroid lobe containing the tumor, the isthmus, and the majority of the contralateral thyroid lobe. The posterior capsule of the contralateral lobe is left undisturbed in an attempt to preserve the underlying parathyroid glands and the recurrent laryngeal nerve. With this procedure, the surgeon is able to remove the primary tumor and the bulk of normal thyroid tissue that may harbor microscopic malignancy.

20. **Are lymph nodes removed surgically?**
Cervical and high mediastinal lymph nodes that appear to harbor metastatic disease are harvested at the time of surgery. Radical neck dissections do not reduce mortality or rate of recurrence and should be avoided, unless there are direct extensions of the tumor throughout the neck. In the event that a single, small (< 1.5 cm) papillary or minimally invasive follicular carcinoma is discovered, lobectomy and isthmusectomy may be curative.

21. **How does ^{131}I therapy benefit the patient?**
Most (but not all) differentiated thyroid malignancies retain the ability to trap inorganic iodine when stimulated by TSH. When ^{131}I is concentrated within normal or malignant thyroid tissue, beta irradiation results in cellular damage or death. If a metastatic lesion is capable of concentrating ^{131}I, it becomes visible with a gamma camera; if it absorbs enough ^{131}I to impart 8000 cGy of irradiation, the tumor focus may be eradicated. This is the basis of postsurgical radioiodine scans (^{131}I or ^{123}I) for whole-body surveillance and the therapeutic use of ^{131}I to treat residual, recurrent, and metastatic disease. Patients with one thyroid lobe intact (after lobectomy and isthmusectomy) concentrate the entire scanning dose of radioiodine within the remaining lobe. Metastatic foci outside the thyroid cannot be detected in these patients, and surveillance scans are therefore uninformative and should be avoided.

22. **How can the efficacy of whole-body scans be optimized?**
To optimize the efficacy of whole-body scans and to maximize the concentration of therapeutic radioiodine in metastatic lesions, serum levels of TSH must be elevated. Withdrawal of exogenous L-thyroxine for 6 weeks before the scan allows the protein-bound fraction of the hormone to be exhausted. To alleviate symptoms of hypothyroidism, liothyronine (Cytomel, 25 mg b.i.d.) is administered for the first 4 weeks of the withdrawal period but discontinued during the 2 weeks before the scan. Liothyronine, with a shorter half-life than thyroxine, is rapidly depleted after withdrawal. During the 2-week period, in which no exogenous thyroid hormone is available, a rapid rise in serum TSH (> 30 mU/L) ensues. Normal remnant thyroid tissue (on the posterior capsule of the thyroid bed) and malignant tissue are maximally stimulated by elevated levels of TSH and usually concentrate any available radioiodine.

23. **How is the whole-body scan performed?**
During the whole-body scan, 2–5 mCi of ^{131}I or 1.5 mCi of ^{123}I is administered orally to the patient, who is subsequently positioned under a gamma camera after the radioiodine is allowed to equilibrate (48–72 hours for ^{131}I; 5 hours for ^{123}I). The resultant image indicates the amount of thyroid tissue remaining in the thyroid bed and the extent of local and distant metastatic diseases. Therapeutic ^{131}I is then administered.

24. **How much ^{131}I is administered to the patient after surgical removal of a single, small papillary tumor without extrathyroidal lesions?**
Generally, in the patient with a single, small papillary tumor (< 1.5 cm) free of extrathyroidal metastases at the time of surgery and on subsequent whole-body scan, many endocrinologists consider the resection curative and do not administer radioiodine. In such cases, the use of adjunctive radioiodine does not alter the course of the disease. The author prefers, however, to administer a small dose of ^{131}I (30 mCi) in an attempt to ablate the thyroid bed and thereby to improve the accuracy of future surveillance scans. This "small" dose ablates up to 80% of

thyroid remnants. Other endocrinologists believe that this dose is insufficient to ablate all residual normal and malignant tissue and prefer a dose of 70–150 mCi of radioiodine.

25. **How much ^{131}I is administered to the patient after surgical removal of a large or aggressive tumor or extrathyroidal lesions?**
Patients with large or aggressive tumors, metastatic disease evident during surgery, or extrathyroidal lesions visible on postsurgical whole-body scans usually receive 100–200 mCi of ^{131}I in an attempt to eradicate the malignancy. These "large" doses of radioiodine have traditionally been administered only in an approved inpatient facility under the auspices of the Nuclear Regulatory Commission (NRC). Patients remain isolated until ambient levels of radioactivity fall to acceptable levels. Radionuclide is excreted renally, but significant amounts are also present in saliva and sweat. Such wastes must be disposed of appropriately. Recently, the NRC has lifted the absolute requirement for inpatient administration of high-dose ^{131}I, and it is now performed in some centers on an outpatient basis.

26. **Discuss the early complications of ^{131}I therapy.**
Radioiodine is absorbed by the salivary glands, gastric mucosa, and thyroid tissue. Within 72 hours of oral administration of ^{131}I, patients may experience radiation sialadenitis and transient nausea. Such symptoms are self-limited. Thyroid tissue may become edematous and tender but rarely requires corticosteroid therapy. Radioiodine, borne in the blood, causes transient, clinically insignificant suppression of the bone marrow. In some centers, dosimetry is used to determine the maximum dose of ^{131}I that can be safely administered at one time to patients with invasive or metastatic disease.

27. **What are the late complications of ^{131}I therapy?**
Late complications of high-dose radioiodine therapy may include gonadal dysfunction and predisposition to nonthyroidal malignancies. Some studies have demonstrated reduced sperm counts in male patients proportional to the administered dose of ^{131}I. Older women may experience temporary amenorrhea and reduced fertility. Two deaths from bladder cancer and three deaths from leukemia have been reported among patients treated with lifetime cumulative doses of radioiodine exceeding 1000 mCi. Most studies suggest that cumulative doses of ^{131}I less than 700–800 mCi, given in increments of 100–200 mCi separated by 6–12 months, are not leukemogenic.

28. **How are bony and pulmonary metastases treated?**
Radioiodine (^{131}I) is often used to treat bony and pulmonary metastases. Multifocal skeletal metastases from differentiated thyroid cancer are generally treated with 200 mCi of ^{131}I. However, isolated bony lesions are often treated instead with surgical resection or curettage or with external beam radiation therapy. Pulmonary metastases present a therapeutic dilemma, because radiation absorbed by the malignant cells often causes fibrosis of the underlying lung parenchyma. For this reason, pulmonary metastases that absorb more than 50% of the scanning dose of radioiodine are usually treated with no more than 75–80 mCi of ^{131}I.

29. **How are patients monitored for recurrent disease?**
Following surgery and radioiodine therapy, all patients are placed on a large enough dose of exogenous thyroid hormone to render serum TSH levels low or undetectable. Most endocrinologists recommend detecting recurrent disease in the asymptomatic patient by annual neck palpation and serum thyroglobulin measurement. This protein, manufactured only by normal or malignant thyroid cells, should be undetectable in the serum of a patient who has undergone complete surgical and radioiodine ablation. Sensitivity of thyroglobulin measurement is enhanced if the patient is withdrawn from exogenous thyroid hormone or stimulated with recombinant TSH (see question 31).

30. **When is a whole-body scan used?**
Evidence of recurrent tumor (rising levels of thyroglobulin or palpable neck mass) warrants the repetition of a whole-body scan. Alternatively, some centers periodically repeat a whole-body scan, after proper preparation, approximately 6–12 months after the initial surgery and ^{131}I therapy. After two serial scans, separated by at least 6–12 months, are free of evident disease, semiannual scans may be discontinued. Some centers subsequently repeat surveillance scans every 5 years, but because the procedure is distinctly uncomfortable for the patient, most centers do not adhere to this schedule.

31. **Discuss the alternative to withdrawal of thyroid hormone prior to a whole-body scan.**
Recombinant human TSH (rhTSH; Thyrogen) has been approved for use in scanning patients with DTC. The rhTSH acts just as native TSH produced by the pituitary, stimulating iodine uptake and thyroglobulin secretion from remnant thyroid tissue and metastatic foci of cancer. The rhTSH (0.9 mg) is administered intramuscularly once daily for 2 consecutive days, followed by a scanning dose of ^{131}I (4 mCi) given orally on the third day. The patient is then imaged under a gamma camera on the fifth day. Serum thyroglobulin levels are drawn before administration of rhTSH and compared with those obtained on the fifth day. The rhTSH stimulated scans, when coupled with concomitant serum thyroglobulin measurements, are generally as accurate as standard whole-body scans, and do not cause the significant hypothyroid symptoms that patients experience with levothyroxine withdrawal scans. Unfortunately, rhTSH has not yet been approved for use in raising serum TSH levels prior to therapeutic ^{131}I administration. Therefore, rhTSH scans should be avoided if recurrent or metastatic thyroid cancer requiring ^{131}I treatment is anticipated.

32. **Which malignancy is associated with prior radiation exposure?**
From 1940 through the early 1970s, external irradiation of the head and neck was used in the treatment of acne, enlarged thymus, enlarged tonsils and adenoids, tinea capitis, and asthma. It was recognized belatedly that such radiation exposure caused neoplastic transformation of thyroid cells; after a 10 to 20-year latency period, 33–40% of exposed individuals developed benign thyroid nodules, and 5–11% developed carcinoma. The carcinomas in irradiated glands mirror those found within the nonirradiated population, with papillary cancer predominating. The tumors are no more aggressive but are more often multicentric (55%) than in nonirradiated individuals (22%).

33. **What is a Hürthle cell?**
Hürthle, or Askanazy, cells are large polygonal cells with abundant cytoplasm and compact nuclei; they are found in benign nodules, Hashimoto's disease, and either form of DTC. Hürthle-cell carcinoma, composed solely of these cells, is believed to be a particularly aggressive variant of follicular cancer that is characterized by frequent pulmonary metastases.

34. **What is anaplastic thyroid carcinoma?**
Anaplastic thyroid carcinoma is one of the most aggressive and resistant forms of human cancer. It accounts for only 1–10% of all thyroid carcinomas in the Western hemisphere but for up to 50% of thyroid carcinomas in some areas of Eastern Europe. Like follicular carcinoma, it is more prevalent in areas of iodine deficiency; the incidence is currently declining throughout North America.

35. **Discuss the histologic variants of anaplastic carcinoma.**
Four histologic variants of anaplastic carcinoma are currently recognized: giant cell, spindle cell, mixed spindle-giant cell, and small cell carcinoma. True small cell carcinoma is extremely rare, and most "small cell" tumors are actually a malignant form of lymphoma that is more amenable to therapy. Microscopic examination of the anaplastic malignancies reveals bizarre fibrous whorls, primitive follicles, and cartilage and osteoid reminiscent of chondrosarcoma.

36. **Who gets anaplastic carcinoma?**

Anaplastic carcinoma occurs more commonly in the elderly (peak age: 65–70 years) and affects equal numbers of males and females. These cancers may arise in preexisting DTCs (dedifferentiation), in benign nodules, or, most commonly, de novo. The minuscule number of anaplastic malignancies within large series of patients followed for decades with DTC may discredit the theory of dedifferentiation of established cancers.

KEY POINTS: THYROID CANCER ✓

1. Papillary and follicular carcinomas comprise the DTCs. Mortality rates are low.

2. DTC is diagnosed by fine needle aspiration (FNA) of a thyroid nodule.

3. Therapy of DTC is based on surgical resection of the primary tumor and removal of all remaining thyroid tissue (bed).

4. Orally administered radioactive iodine is accumulated by thyroid tissue, ablating the thyroid bed and metastatic foci.

5. Thyroglobulin is the most sensitive tumor marker for DTC.

6. Elimination of TSH, a DTC growth factor, by suppressive doses of levothyroxine is the most important therapeutic intervention.

37. **How does anaplastic carcinoma present?**

Anaplastic carcinoma expands rapidly; most patients present with steric symptoms, such as dyspnea, dysphagia, hoarseness, and pain. Nearly one-half of all patients require tracheostomy as a result of explosive tumor growth.

38. **Summarize the prognosis for patients with anaplastic carcinoma.**

The type of histologic variant does not appear to affect outcome; prognosis is dismal in most cases. Surgical extirpation has been combined with external beam irradiation (4500–6000 cGy) or chemotherapy (usually doxorubicin or paclitaxel) in an attempt to eradicate the malignancy. Despite vigorous therapy, average survival is approximately 6–8 months.

39. **What is MCT?**

MCT is a neoplasm that arises from the parafollicular cells (or C cells) of the thyroid. Embryologically, these cells originate in the neural crest and migrate to the thyroid, where, despite close proximity, there is no apparent physical or hormonal interaction with the follicular cells.

40. **Describe the function of parafollicular cells.**

The parafollicular cells elaborate CT, which acts on osteoclasts to modulate release of calcium from skeletal stores. The DNA that contains the genetic code for CT also contains the code for another peptide, CT gene-related peptide (CGRP). Tissue-specific alternative splicing allows parafollicular cells to secrete CT, whereas neural cells produce only CGRP.

41. **How does neoplastic transformation affect the parafollicular cells?**

Neoplastic transformation of parafollicular cells results in unbridled expression of normal cell products (CT) and abnormal products (CGRP, chromogranin A, carcinoembryonic antigen [CEA], adrenocorticotropin [ACTH]). CT serves as an excellent tumor marker for the malignancy, and the abnormal products mediate the clinical syndromes associated with MCT. Accumulation of massive amounts of procalcitonin within the thyroid is detectable histologically as amyloid (AE type).

42. **How common is MCT?**
MCT accounts for approximately 2–10% of all thyroid malignancies and occurs in sporadic and hereditary forms. Sporadic MCT is the more common form.

43. **Describe the presentation of sporadic MCT.**
Most patients present in the fourth or fifth decade, with most series reporting nearly equal numbers of men and women. Sporadic MCT is usually unifocal within the thyroid and may originate in any portion of the gland. One-half of all patients manifest metastatic disease at the time of presentation; metastatic sites include (in descending order) local lymphatics, lung, liver, and bone.

44. **Summarize the forms in which hereditary MCT may occur within kindreds.**
The hereditary form of MCT occurs within kindreds as an isolated condition (familial MCT), as a component of multiple endocrine neoplasia (MEN) 2A (MCT, hyperparathyroidism, pheochromocytoma), as a component of the MEN 2B syndrome (MCT, pheochromocytoma, mucosal neuromas), or in conjunction with pheochromocytoma and cutaneous lichen amyloidosis.

45. **How does hereditary MCT present?**
Hereditary tumors are bilateral and arise in the junction of the upper one-third and lower two-thirds of the thyroid lobes, where the concentration of C cells is highest. Biochemical screening for MCT to detect early disease within affected kindreds enhances the survival of individuals with hereditary MCT compared with those with the sporadic form. An erudite discussion of the MEN syndromes is included in Chapter 53, the belletristic presentation of which will undoubtedly move the reader to tears.

46. **Are extrathyroidal manifestations associated with MCT?**
The wide array of peptides and prostaglandin products secreted by MCT tumors results in multiple extrathyroidal symptoms. The most common is diarrhea, which occurs in up to 30% of patients with MCT. Although CT, CGRP, prostaglandins, 5-hydroxytryptamine, and vasoactive intestinal peptide have been proposed as the causative secretagogue, none has been convincingly implicated.

On rare occasions, Cushing's syndrome may occur in MCT and is attributable to the secretion of either ACTH or corticotropin-releasing hormone (CRH), or both. Successful therapy of the underlying malignancy ameliorates the Cushingoid features. There are no reported cases of hypocalcemia due to the chronic production of CT by MCT.

47. **How can CT be used as a clinically useful tumor marker?**
CT is secreted by normal parafollicular cells and cells undergoing neoplastic transformation. Most certainly in the hereditary form, and probably in the sporadic form of MCT, malignant degeneration of the C cells is preceded by a period of "benign" hyperplasia, during which curative resection is theoretically feasible. The serum level of CT is proportional to the mass of hyperplastic or malignant parafollicular cells. Unfortunately, the Kulchitsky cells of the lung, as well as cells of the thymus, pituitary, adrenal glands, and prostate, also secrete small amounts of CT, as do certain malignancies, such as small cell lung cancer and breast cancer.

48. **How is CT related to MCT distinguished from CT of non-MCT sources?**
The pentagastrin stimulation test is used to distinguish the CT of non-MCT sources from the CT produced by hyperplastic and malignant C cells. The test involves the IV administration of pentagastrin (0.5 mg/kg body weight) with the collection of CT at baseline, 1.5, 2, 5, and 10 minutes after injection. Normal subjects demonstrate little or no response to the infusion, whereas subjects with C-cell hyperplasia or MCT manifest an exaggerated response. Absolute values depend on the assay used for determining CT.

49. **What test may be used if pentagastrin is not available?**
When pentagastrin is unavailable, a calcium infusion (2 mg/kg over 5 minutes) can similarly be used to stimulate CT secretion. As assays for the MEN 2 gene on chromosome 10 become clinically available (see Chapter 53), screening of kindreds for the hereditary form of MCT with stimulation tests may be unnecessary. The test, however, will remain valuable in elucidating residual disease after therapy.

50. **How is MCT treated?**
Therapy for MCT remains frustrating. When MCT is discovered on biopsy or suspected as a result of the screening of kindred members, the entire thyroid should be surgically removed, with care to preserve the parathyroids and laryngeal nerves. A dissection of the lymphatics of the central neck also should be undertaken, because 50–70% of these nodes contain metastases. Because parafollicular cells do not accumulate radioiodine, postsurgical radioablation is not warranted. External beam radiotherapy and chemotherapy do not appear to improve survival, although they are sometimes used in desperation against recurrent disease. Residual disease grows slowly, causing obstructive symptoms and the symptoms listed in question 45.

51. **What are the survival rates of patients with MCT?**
Rates of 10- and 20-year survival in one large series were 63% and 44%, respectively.

52. **Summarize the prevalence and detection of thyroid nodules.**
The prevalence of nodular thyroid disease increases with age and is approximately four times higher in women than in men. By the sixth decade of life, 5–10% of the general population in developed nations has one or more palpable thyroid nodules. Detection by palpation is relatively insensitive, however; ultrasonographic or pathologic (autopsy) examination of the population reveals a much higher prevalence of thyroid nodules (20% by 40 years of age, 50% by 70 years of age). Only 8–17% of surgically resected nodules are cancerous; the remainder is nonmalignant and mandate excision only for obstructive symptoms or cosmesis.

53. **What is the primary responsibility of the internist in regard to thyroid nodules?**
The responsibility of the internist is to steer patients with nodules of malignant potential to resection, but to stay the hand of the surgeon when excision of a benign nodule is proposed.

54. **What is the first test performed on a palpable thyroid nodule?**
FNA is the first test performed by most endocrinologists. Collection of the sample is relatively simple for most sighted individuals; cytologic interpretation of the sample is the limiting factor in this procedure. The diagnostic accuracy of FNA is reported to range between 70% and 97%.

55. **How is the FNA sample interpreted?**
Interpretation of the aspiration sample may indicate that the nodule is malignant, benign, or "suspicious for malignancy." The sample also may be judged to have inadequate material for interpretation, requiring re-aspiration. Papillary carcinoma may be diagnosed with some certainty from FNA samples, but the diagnosis of follicular carcinoma requires the demonstration of vascular invasion. Some large centers boast cytopathologists who can reliably differentiate follicular carcinoma from follicular adenoma; these uncommon, grizzled old demigods have forsaken the company of mortals for the solace of their microscopes. Most cytopathologists designate such samples as "follicular neoplasm" or "suspicious for malignancy."

56. **Discuss the role of radionuclide scans.**
Some endocrinologists advocate the performance of a radionuclide scan to determine the metabolic activity of the nodule and to discern the existence of other unsuspected nodules. Such data are potentially valuable; autonomous or "hot" nodules rarely harbor malignancy but may

yield cytopathologic specimens that mimic malignancy. Detractors of radionuclide scanning, however, criticize the cost and delay in performance of FNA and tout the rare cancer found in autonomous nodules.

57. **How useful is ultrasound?**

Ultrasound of thyroid nodules provides little significant value as a diagnostic tool for an individual nodule but may help detect other nodules that are difficult to palpate because of their posterior or substernal location. Furthermore, ultrasound-guided FNA can be very useful for obtaining tissue from these difficult-to-palpate nodules and from nodules that are discovered incidentally during imaging procedures that were ordered to evaluate other conditions.

58. **How do the results of FNA affect further management?**

Nodules designated as malignant on FNA should be resected. Those designated as "suspicious for malignancy" or "follicular neoplasm" also should be referred for excision, because up to 20% are malignant. Benign nodules should be observed for change in size or obstructive symptoms; the administration of suppressive amounts of exogenous thyroid hormone is controversial because of the attendant risk for osteoporosis and the lack of data demonstrating unequivocal efficacy of this intervention.

59. **Is surgery justified for a nodule judged as benign by FNA?**

The internist occasionally encounters a patient who chooses surgical resection of a nodule despite benign results with FNA. This scenario prompts a final word of advice: "Never stand between a ready surgeon and a willing patient who has been thoroughly apprised of the risks of thyroid surgery." False-negative results of FNA range between 1% and 6%, and up to 35% of thyroids in autopsy series contain clinically insignificant papillary carcinomas, either of which, if discovered at a later date, will engender distrust on the part of the patient.

60. **Has a molecular defect been associated with thyroid carcinoma?**

Mutation of a single protooncogene or tumor suppressor gene has not been associated with thyroid carcinogenesis. Several mutations have been described in thyroid neoplasms; however, none appears to be able to induce malignant changes without concomitant cooperating mutations. Although the practical relevance of these defects is limited at this time, further research may identify these or others as clinical indicators of the malignant potential of individual tumors.

61. **Discuss the potential role of the *ras* protooncogene.**

The *ras* protooncogene code for a family of receptor-associated proteins, named p21, serves as signal transducers between membrane receptors and intracellular effectors. When the receptors are stimulated, p21 becomes complexed with guanosine triphosphate (GTP) and activates MAP kinase. Because excessive kinase activity would be detrimental, native p21 possesses intrinsic GTPase activity, which eventually inactivates the complex and terminates the activity of MAP kinase. Mutation of the *ras* protooncogene results in p21 that lacks GTPase activity, causing uncontrolled accumulation of kinase activity and prompting disordered cellular growth. *Ras* oncogene has been described in 10–50% of follicular carcinomas in iodine-deficient areas.

62. **How may the G-stimulatory (Gs) proteins be related to thyroid cancer?**

Closely related to *ras*-coded p21 are the Gs proteins, which also link transmembrane receptors to intracellular effectors, such as adenyl cyclase. Gs proteins consist of a, b, and g subunits, noncovalently bound together, that become active when GTP complexes to the "a" subunit. Native Gsa possesses intrinsic GTPase activity that functions as a timer, stopping the reaction at an appropriate point. Mutations of the Gsa gene that code for proteins lacking intrinsic GTPase activity have been discerned. These constitutively activated Gs proteins promote both cell growth and function; they have been detected primarily in functioning benign thyroid nodules and rarely in DTCs.

63. **Discuss the potential role of the *ret/ptc* oncogene.**
The *ret/ptc* mutation has been described in DTCs. The *ret* protooncogene is found on chromosome 10 and normally codes a receptor (*ret*) with intrinsic tyrosine kinase activity. The ligand for *ret* is a glial cell derived neurotrophic factor; *ret* is not normally expressed on thyroid follicular cells. The *ret/ptc* mutation results in constitutively activated tyrosine kinase, which causes disordered cellular development and is found in 2–70% of papillary thyroid carcinomas, depending on the ethnic group. Although tumors expressing this mutation are not larger than other papillary cancers, they may be more likely to metastasize.

64. **How is abnormal protein p53 implicated in thyroid cancer?**
A final mutation associated with up to 25% of anaplastic thyroid carcinomas codes for abnormal protein p53. Normal p53 is found in the cytoplasm, where it forms a complex with heat shock protein-70 (hsp70) and crosses the nuclear membrane to interact with nuclear transcription factors. Mutation of the gene coding for p53 results in translation of a protein that cannot interact with these nuclear proteins. Loss of this tumor suppressor causes unrestricted cell growth and, along with other coexisting mutations, malignant degeneration.

WEBSITE ⊕

NCCN thyroid carcinoma practice guidelines. Available at http://www.nccn.org

BIBLIOGRAPHY

1. Baudin E, Cao D, Cailleux AF, et al: Positive predictive value of serum thyroglobulin levels, measured during first year follow-up after thyroid hormone withdrawal, in thyroid cancer patients. J Clin Endocrinol Metab 88:1107–1111, 2003.

2. Brennan MD, Bergstralh EJ, van Heerden JA, McConahey WM: Follicular thyroid cancer treated at the Mayo Clinic, 1946 through 1970: Initial manifestations, pathologic findings, therapy, and outcome. Mayo Clin Proc 66:11–22, 1991.

3. Chua EL, Wu WM, Tran KT, et al: Prevalence and distribution of *ret/ptc* 1, 2, and 3 in papillary thyroid carcinoma in New Caledonia and Australia. J Clin Endocrinol Metab 85:2733–2739, 2000.

4. DeGroot LJ, Kaplan EL, McCormick M, Straus FJ: Natural history, treatment, and course of papillary thyroid carcinoma. J Clin Endocrinol Metab 71:414–424, 1990.

5. Dulgeroff AJ, Herschman JM: Medical therapy for differentiated thyroid carcinoma. Endocr Rev 15:500–515, 1994.

6. Farid NR, Shi Y, Zou M: Molecular basis of thyroid cancer. Endocr Rev 15:202–232, 1994.

7. Fogelfeld L, Wiviott MBT, Shore-Freedman E, et al: Recurrence of thyroid nodules after surgical removal in patients irradiated in childhood for benign conditions. N Engl J Med 320:835–840, 1989.

8. Gagel RF, Robinson MF, Donovan DT, Alford BB: Medullary thyroid carcinoma: Recent progress. J Clin Endocrinol Metab 76:809–814, 1993.

9. Gharib H, McConahey WM, Tiegs RD, et al: Medullary thyroid carcinoma: Clinicopathologic features and long-term follow-up of 65 patients treated during 1946 through 1970. Mayo Clin Proc 67:934–940, 1992.

10. Gharib H: The use of recombinant thyrotropin in patients with thyroid cancer. Endocrinologist 10:255–263, 2000.

11. Kebebew E, Clark OH: Differentiated thyroid cancer: "Complete" rational approach. World J Surg 24:942–951, 2000.

12. Mazzaferi EL, Robbins RJ, Spencer AC, et al: A consensus report of the role of serum thyroglobulin as a monitoring method for low-risk patients with papillary thyroid carcinoma. J Clin Endocrinol Metab 88:1433–1441, 2003.

13. Mazzaferi EL: Management of a solitary thyroid nodule. N Engl J Med 328:553–559, 1993.

14. McConahey WM, Hay ID, Woolner L, et al: Papillary thyroid cancer treated at the Mayo Clinic, 1946 through 1970: Initial manifestations, pathologic findings, therapy, and outcome. Mayo Clin Proc 61:978–996, 1986.

15. Nel CJC, van Heerden JA, Goellner JR, et al: Anaplastic carcinoma of the thyroid: A clinico-pathologic study of 82 cases. Mayo Clin Proc 60:51–58, 1985.

16. Pacini F, Capezzone M, Elisei R, et al. Diagnostic 131-iodine whole-body scan may be avoided in thyroid cancer patients who have undetectable stimulated serum Tg levels after initial treatment. J Clin Endocrinol Metab 87:1499–1501, 2002.

17. Robbins J (moderator): Thyroid cancer: A lethal endocrine neoplasm. Ann Intern Med 115: 133–147, 1991.

18. Wartofsky L. Editorial: Using baseline and recombinant human TSH-stimulated Tg measurements to manage thyroid cancer without diagnostic 131-I scanning. J Clin Endocrinol Metabol 87:1486–1489, 2002.

CHAPTER 39

THYROID EMERGENCIES

Michael T. McDermott, M.D.

1. **What is thyroid storm?**
   Thyroid storm or crisis is a life-threatening condition characterized by an exaggeration of the manifestations of thyrotoxicosis.

2. **How do patients develop thyroid storm?**
   Thyroid storm usually occurs in patients who have unrecognized or inadequately treated thyrotoxicosis and a superimposed precipitating event, such as thyroid surgery, nonthyroid surgery, infection, or trauma.

3. **What are the clinical manifestations of thyroid storm?**
   Fever (> 102 °F) is the cardinal manifestation. Tachycardia is usually present, and tachypnea is common, but the blood pressure is variable. Cardiac arrhythmias, congestive heart failure, and ischemic heart symptoms may develop. Nausea, vomiting, diarrhea, and abdominal pain are frequent features (Fig. 39-1). Central nervous system manifestations include hyperkinesis, psychosis, and coma. A goiter is a helpful finding but not always present.

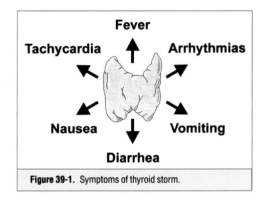

Figure 39-1. Symptoms of thyroid storm.

4. **What laboratory abnormalities are seen in thyroid storm?**
   Serum T_4 (total and free T_4) and T_3 (total and free T_3) are usually significantly elevated, and the serum thyroid-stimulating hormone (TSH) is undetectable. Other common laboratory abnormalities include anemia, leukocytosis, hyperglycemia, azotemia, hypercalcemia, and elevated liver-associated enzymes.

5. **How is the diagnosis of thyroid storm made?**
   The diagnosis must be made on the basis of suspicious but nonspecific clinical findings. Serum thyroid hormone levels are elevated but, if the diagnosis is strongly suspected, waiting for the results of tests may cause a critical delay in the initiation of effective life-saving therapy. Furthermore, thyroid hormone levels do not reliably distinguish patients with thyroid storm from those who have uncomplicated thyrotoxicosis as a coincident disorder. Clinical features are therefore the key.

6. **What other conditions may mimic thyroid storm?**
   Similar presentations may be seen with sepsis, pheochromocytoma, and malignant hyperthermia.

7. **How should patients with thyroid storm be treated?**
The immediate goals are to decrease thyroid hormone synthesis, to inhibit thyroid hormone release, to reduce the heart rate, to support the circulation, and to treat the precipitating condition. Since beta$_1$-adrenergic receptors are significantly increased in patients with this condition, beta$_1$-selective blockers are the preferred agents for heart rate control.

8. **What drugs are used to decrease thyroid hormone synthesis?**
- Propylthiouracil (PTU), 200 mg every 4 hours (orally, rectally, or via nasogastric tube).
- Methimazole (Tapazole), 20 mg every 4 hours (orally, rectally, or via nasogastric tube).

9. **List drugs used to inhibit thyroid hormone release.**
- Sodium iodide (NaI), 1 gm over 24 hours IV.
- Potassium iodide, 5 drops every 8 hours orally.
- Lugol's solution, 10 drops every 8 hours orally.

10. **What drugs are used to reduce the heart rate?**
- Esmolol, 500 μg over 1 minute IV, followed by 50–300 μg/kg/minute infusion.
- Metoprolol, 5–10 mg IV every 2–4 hours.
- Diltiazem, 60–90 mg every 6–8 hours orally, or 0.25 mg/kg over 2 minutes IV, followed by infusion of 10 mg/minute.

11. **List agents used to support the circulation.**
- Dexamethasone, 2 mg every 6 hours IV, or
- Hydrocortisone, 100 mg every 8 hours IV
- Intravenous fluids

12. **What is the prognosis for patients with thyroid storm?**
When thyroid storm was first described, the acute mortality rate was nearly 100%. Today the prognosis is significantly improved when aggressive therapy, as described earlier, is initiated early; however, the mortality rate continues to be approximately 20%.

13. **Define myxedema coma.**
Myxedema coma is a life-threatening condition characterized by an exaggeration of the manifestations of hypothyroidism.

14. **How do patients develop myxedema coma?**
Myxedema coma usually occurs in elderly patients who have inadequately treated or untreated hypothyroidism and a superimposed precipitating event. Important events include prolonged cold exposure, infection, trauma, surgery, myocardial infarction, congestive heart failure, pulmonary embolism, stroke, respiratory failure, gastrointestinal bleeding, and administration of various drugs, particularly those that have a depressive effect on the central nervous system.

15. **What are the clinical manifestations of myxedema coma?**
Hypothermia, bradycardia, and hypoventilation are common; blood pressure, while generally reduced, is more variable. Pericardial, pleural, and peritoneal effusions are often found. An ileus is present in about two-thirds of patients, and acute urinary retention also may be seen. Central nervous system manifestations include seizures, stupor, and coma (Fig. 39-2); deep tendon reflexes are absent or exhibit a delayed relaxation phase. Typical hypothyroid skin and hair changes may be apparent. A goiter, although frequently absent, is a helpful finding; a thyroidectomy scar also may be an important clue.

16. **What laboratory abnormalities are seen in myxedema coma?**

Serum T_4 (total and free T_4) and T_3 (total and free T_3) are usually low, and the TSH is significantly elevated. Other frequent abnormalities include anemia, hyponatremia, hypoglycemia, and elevated serum levels of cholesterol and creatine kinase (CK). Arterial blood gases often reveal carbon dioxide retention and hypoxemia. The electrocardiogram often shows sinus bradycardia, various types and degrees of heart block, low voltage, and T-wave flattening.

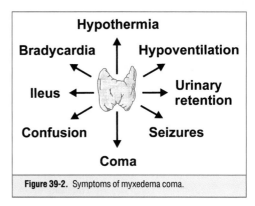

Figure 39-2. Symptoms of myxedema coma.

17. **How is the diagnosis of myxedema coma made?**

The diagnosis must be made on clinical grounds based on the findings described earlier. Serum levels of thyroid hormones are reduced and the TSH level is elevated, but the delay involved in waiting for test results may unnecessarily postpone the initiation of effective therapy.

KEY POINTS: THYROID EMERGENCIES ✔

1. Thyroid storm is a life-threatening form of severe thyrotoxicosis that usually has an identifiable precipitating factor and a high mortality rate if not treated promptly and appropriately.

2. When thyroid storm is diagnosed or suspected, treatment with antithyroid drugs, cold iodine, beta blockers, and stress doses of glucocorticoids, along with management of any precipitating factors, should be promptly initiated.

3. Myxedema coma is a life-threatening form of severe hypothyroidism that often has a precipitating cause and a high mortality rate if not promptly and adequately treated.

4. When myxedema coma is diagnosed or suspected, management should include rapid repletion of the thyroid hormone deficit, stress doses of glucocorticoids, and treatment of any precipitating causes.

18. **How should patients with myxedema coma be treated?**

The goals are to rapidly replace the depleted thyroid hormone pool, to replace glucocorticoids, to support vital functions, and to treat any precipitating conditions. The normal total body pool of T_4 is about 1000 μg (500 μg in the thyroid; 500 μg in the rest of the body).

19. **How are circulating thyroid hormones replaced?**

Whether to use levothyroxine (LT_4), liothyronine (LT_3) or both remains controversial, but the author favors the combination of LT_4 plus LT_3. Regimens for LT_4 alone, LT_3 followed by LT_4, and LT_4 plus LT_3 are listed in the following:

- LT_4 alone: 200–300 μg over 5 minutes IV, followed by 50–100 μg/day orally or IV
- LT_3 followed by LT_4: LT_3, 50–100 μg over 5 minutes IV, followed by LT_4, 50–100 μg/day orally or IV

- LT_4 plus LT_3: LT_4, 200–500 µg over 5 minutes IV, plus LT_3, 20–50 µg over 5 minutes IV, followed by LT_4, 50–100 µg/day, and LT_3, 20–30 µg/day orally or IV

20. **What agent is used for glucocorticoid replacement?**
    Hydrocortisone, 100 mg every 8 hours IV.

21. **What agents and modalities are used to support vital functions?**
    - Oxygen
    - Intravenous fluids
    - Rewarming (blankets or central rewarming)
    - Mechanical ventilation (if needed)

22. **What is the prognosis for patients with myxedema coma?**
    Myxedema coma originally had a mortality rate of 100%. Today the outlook is much improved for appropriately treated patients, although the mortality rate in recent studies has varied from 0–45%.

BIBLIOGRAPHY

1. Brooks MH, Waldstein SS: Free thyroxine concentrations in thyroid storm. Ann Intern Med 93:694–694, 1980.
2. Burch HD, Wartofsky L: Life-threatening thyrotoxicosis: Thyroid storm. Endocrinol Metab Clin N Am 22:263–278, 1993.
3. Dillmann WH: Thyroid storm. Curr Ther Endocrinol Metab 6:81–85, 1997.
4. Jordan RM: Myxedema coma. Pathophysiology, therapy, and factors affecting prognosis. Med Clin N Am 79:185–194, 1995.
5. Nicoloff JT: Myxedema coma: A form of decompensated hypothyroidism. Endocrinol Metab Clin N Am 22:279–290, 1993.
6. Pittman CS, Zayed AA: Myxedema coma. Curr Ther Endocrinol Metab 6:98–101, 1997.
7. Tietgens ST, Leinung MC: Thyroid storm. Med Clin N Am 79 (1):169–184, 1995.
8. Tsitouras PD: Myxedema coma. Clin Geriatr Med 11:251–258, 1995.
9. Yamamoto T, Fukuyama J, Fujiyoshi A: Factors associated with mortality of myxedema coma: Report of eight cases and literature survey. Thyroid 9:1167–1174, 1999.
10. Yeung S-CJ, Go R, Balasubramanyam A: Rectal administration of iodide and propylthiouracil in the treatment of thyroid storm. Thyroid 5:403–405, 1995.

CHAPTER 40

EUTHYROID SICK SYNDROME

Michael T. McDermott, M.D.

1. **What is the euthyroid sick syndrome?**
   The euthyroid sick syndrome refers to changes in serum thyroid hormone and thyroid-stimulating hormone (TSH) levels that occur in patients with a variety of nonthyroidal illnesses, including infections, malignancies, inflammatory conditions, myocardial infarction, surgery, trauma, and starvation. This condition is also called the nonthyroidal illness syndrome. It is not a primary thyroid disorder but instead results from changes in peripheral thyroid hormone metabolism and transport induced by the nonthyroidal illness.

2. **What hormone changes characterize the euthyroid sick syndrome in patients with mild-to-moderate nonthyroidal illness?**
   Serum total T_3 and free T_3 levels decrease as a result of reduced conversion of T_4 to T_3 in peripheral tissues, predominantly the liver. Serum free T_4 and TSH levels usually remain within the reference range.

3. **Describe the hormone changes in patients with moderate-to-severe nonthyroidal illness.**
   Serum total T_3 and free T_3 levels decrease further; total T_4 also decreases, and T_3 resin uptake (T_3RU) increases. The latter changes result from reduced binding of thyroid hormones to their transport proteins due both to impaired protein synthesis and the presence of circulating inhibitors of protein binding. Free T_4 may be normal, decreased or increased. Serum TSH levels remain normal or become slightly decreased at this stage.

4. **Describe the hormone changes associated with recovery from nonthyroidal illnesses.**
   Free T_4 decreases and TSH increases. As hepatic protein synthesis improves and circulating inhibitors of protein binding disappear, serum free T_4 levels drop transiently with a compensatory increase in serum TSH levels before complete normalization occurs.

5. **How can the euthyroid sick syndrome be distinguished from hypothyroidism?**
   In the euthyroid sick syndrome, serum T_3 is decreased proportionately more than T_4, the T_3RU tends to be high, and the TSH is normal or mildly decreased and then mildly increased in the recovery phase. In primary hypothyroidism, serum T_4 is reduced proportionately more than T_3, the T_3RU tends to be low, and the TSH is increased. Other tests also may be helpful. In the euthyroid sick syndrome, free T_4 is usually normal and reverse T_3 (RT_3) is increased; in hypothyroidism, both free T_4 and RT_3 are decreased.

6. **What causes the euthyroid sick syndrome?**
   The euthyroid sick syndrome is believed to be caused by increased circulating levels of cytokines and other inflammation mediators resulting from the underlying nonthyroidal illness. These mediators can inhibit the thyroid axis at multiple levels, including the pituitary (decreased TSH secretion), the thyroid (decreased T_4 and T_3 responses to TSH), peripheral tissues (decreased conversion of T_4 to T_3; decreased responses to T_3), and transport proteins (decreased thyroid hormone binding).

KEY POINTS: EUTHYROID SICK SYNDROME ✓

1. The euthyroid sick syndrome is not a thyroid disorder, but instead a group of changes in serum thyroid hormone and TSH levels that result from cytokines and inflammatory mediators produced in patients with nonthyroidal illnesses.

2. The most common feature of the euthyroid sick syndrome is a decrease in serum T_3 levels due to reduced conversion of T_4 to T_3 in the liver and other tissues.

3. Low serum total T_4, increased T_3RU, and decreased TSH develop in patients with more severe nonthyroidal illnesses because of reduced thyroid hormone binding to transport proteins and suppressed pituitary TSH secretion.

4. A transient elevation of serum TSH levels is sometimes seen in patients as they recover from the nonthyroidal illness.

5. The euthyroid sick syndrome appears to be an adaptive response to reduce tissue metabolism and preserve e nergy during systemic illnesses; therefore, treatment with thyroid hormone is not currently recommended.

7. **Is the euthyroid sick syndrome an adaptive mechanism or is it harmful?**
Many experts consider the euthyroid sick syndrome to be an adaptive mechanism that may reduce peripheral tissue energy expenditure during the nonthyroidal illness. Conversely, others argue that the alterations in circulating thyroid hormone levels may themselves be harmful and may accentuate the effects of the nonthyroidal illness. This issue is likely to remain controversial for years to come.

8. **Should patients with the euthyroid sick syndrome be treated with thyroid hormones?**
Management of the euthyroid sick syndrome is also highly controversial. Currently, there are no consistent or convincing data demonstrating a recovery or survival benefit from treating euthyroid sick syndrome patients with either levothyroxine (LT_4) or liothyronine (LT_3). Experts continue to debate this issue, however, and agree that large, prospective studies are needed to answer this question. In the absence of more definitive data, thyroid hormone therapy cannot be recommended at this time.

9. **Does the euthyroid sick syndrome have any prognostic significance?**
Current evidence indicates that the prognosis for recovery from critical nonthyroidal illnesses may be fairly well predicted from the severity of the reduction in serum levels of T_3 and T_4. Patients with extremely low serum T_3 levels have a very high mortality rate.

10. **Are levels of thyroid hormone ever elevated In patients with nonthyroid diseases?**
The serum T_4 may be transiently elevated in patients with acute psychiatric illnesses and various acute medical illnesses. The mechanisms underlying such elevations of T_4 are not well understood, but may be mediated by alterations in neurotransmitters or cytokines. This condition must be distinguished from true thyrotoxicosis.

BIBLIOGRAPHY

1. Brennan MD, Bahn RS: Thyroid hormones and illness. Endocr Pract 4:396–403, 1998.

2. Brent GA, Hershman JM: Thyroxine therapy in patients with severe nonthyroidal illness and low serum thyroxine concentration. J Clin Endocrinol Metab 63:1–8, 1986.

3. Camacho PM, Dwarkanathan A: Sick euthyroid syndrome. What to do when thyroid function tests are abnormal in critically ill patients. Postgrad Med 105:215–219, 1999.

4. Chopra I: Euthyroid sick syndrome: Is it a misnomer? J Clin Endocrinol Metab 82:329–334, 1997.

5. DeGroot LJ: Dangerous dogmas in medicine: The nonthyroidal illness syndrome. J Clin Endocrinol Metab 84:151–164, 1999.

6. Kimura T, Kanda T, Kotajima N, et al: Involvement of circulating interleukin-6 and its receptor in the development of euthyroid sick syndrome in patients with acute myocardial infarction. Eur J Endocrinol 143:179–184, 2000.

7. McIver B, Gorman CA: Euthyroid sick syndrome: An overview. Thyroid 7:125–132, 1997.

8. Nagaya T, Fujieda M, Otsuka G, et al: A potential role of activated NF-kappa B in the pathogenesis of euthyroid sick syndrome. J Clin Invest 106:393–402, 2000.

9. Peeters RP, Wouters PJ, Kaptein E, et al: Reduced activation and increased inactivation of thyroid hormone in tissues of critically ill patients. J Clin Endocrinol Metab 88:3202–3211, 2003.

CHAPTER 41

THYROID DISEASE IN PREGNANCY

Linda A. Barbour, M.D., M.S.P.H.

1. **How does normal pregnancy affect maternal thyroid function?**
   The hormonal changes of pregnancy and the increased metabolic demands of the fetus cause significant changes in maternal thyroid function (Table 41-1).

TABLE 41-1. THYROID FUNCTION TESTS DURING NORMAL PREGNANCY			
	First Trimester	**Second Trimester**	**Third Trimester**
Total T_4	↑	↑	↑
T_3RU	↓	↓	↓
Free thyroxine index	Normal	Normal	Normal
Total T_3 (RIA)	↑	↑	↑
Free T_4	Normal	Normal	Normal
TSH	Normal or ↓	Normal	Normal

2. **Why must thyroid function tests be interpreted cautiously in pregnancy?**
   The influence of estrogen and human chorionic gonadotropin (hCG) on circulating thyroid hormone levels requires that thyroid function tests in pregnancy be interpreted cautiously. Estrogen increases thyroid-binding globulin (TBG) by 2- to 3-fold beginning a few weeks after conception. The result is a 30–100% increase in serum total T_4 (TT_4) and total T_3 (TT_3) levels since circulating thyroid hormones are highly protein-bound. Measurement of the T_3 resin uptake (T_3RU), which is inversely related to serum thyroid binding capacity, is correspondingly low, so that the free T_4 index (FT_4I; calculated by multiplying the total T_3 by the T_3RU) is usually normal. The free T_4, free T_3, and thyroid-stimulating hormone (TSH) levels, in contrast, are usually normal during all three trimesters, although slight variation in their values can be seen in a number of circumstances at different periods of gestation.

3. **What particular effects may be seen during the first trimester?**
   During the first trimester, high levels of hCG may stimulate thyroid T_4 secretion sufficiently to suppress the serum TSH into the 0.1–0.5 mU/mL range in up to 15% of pregnant women. The beta subunit of hCG has 85% sequence homology in the first 114 amino acids with TSH and can bind to and stimulate the TSH receptor. Levels of hCG above 50,000 IU/L, which may be seen when hCG peaks at the end of the first trimester, can therefore increase the free T_4 level enough to suppress the serum TSH. However, the TSH remains in the low-normal range, and the free T_4 is in the upper-normal range in the majority of cases. A TSH in the high-normal range during the first trimester is therefore suspicious for subclinical hypothyroidism and should be rechecked in 4–6 weeks.

4. **Why must the mother significantly increase thyroid hormone production during pregnancy?**
    - Maternal plasma volume expands 30–40%, requiring a concomitant expansion of the thyroid hormone pool.
    - Placental type III deiodinase activity results in increased maternal T_4 metabolism to reverse T_3.
    - Transfer of T_4 across the placenta to the fetus is limited.
    - High TBG levels decrease the levels of free hormone.
    - GI absorption of thyroid hormone may result from the iron in prenatal vitamins.

5. **What factors may compromise maternal ability to increase thyroid hormone production?**
    Women with limited thyroid reserve due to thyroiditis, partial ablation, or surgical resection may be unable to increase thyroid hormone production and often develop hypothyroidism. Women with inadequate iodide intake may also develop hypothyroidism and a goiter, since iodine requirements increase by ~40% in pregnancy. Women in iodine-replete areas often show a slight increase in TSH and a slight decrease in free T_4 in the third trimester, probably owing to both a 2- to 3-fold increase in TBG and the increasing thyroid hormone requirements during pregnancy. However, TSH and free T_4 in the third trimester are usually maintained in the normal range as long as the functional capacity of the maternal thyroid is normal.

6. **What is the "goiter of pregnancy"?**
    The "goiter of pregnancy" has been well described in iodine-deficient areas of the world but does not generally occur in geographic regions that are iodine-replete. In fact, one of the first pregnancy tests to be developed in these iodine-deficient areas was a loosely braided choker necklace that broke when a woman developed such a goiter. The thyroid gland increased in size with each subsequent pregnancy.

7. **Why do iodine requirements increase in pregnancy?**
    Iodine requirements increase markedly during pregnancy as a result of increased urinary iodine losses due to the 50–100% increase in glomerular filtration rate (GFR) during pregnancy, diversion of iodine to the fetus for thyroid hormone synthesis, and increased maternal thyroid hormone requirements.

8. **What are the recommended iodine intakes during pregnancy?**
    The World Health Organization's (WHO) recommendations for iodine intake are 200 µg/day during pregnancy and 150 µg/day in the nonpregnant state.

9. **What happens if iodine intake is insufficient?**
    If iodine intake is insufficient, thyroid hormone production drops, resulting in increased secretion of TSH, which then stimulates thyroid gland growth. Thyroid volume commonly increases by 30% or more during pregnancy in iodine-deficient regions and often does not completely regress after delivery. Many European and Third World countries with endemic iodine deficiency do not supplement with iodine; therefore, women are at risk of iodine-deficiency goiters during pregnancy. When iodine intake is severely deficient, overt hypothyroidism results both in mother and fetus. Endemic cretinism occurs if severe hypothyroidism due to iodine deficiency goes unrecognized and untreated at birth.

10. **What happens to thyroid gland volume in iodine-replete areas during pregnancy?**
    In iodine-replete areas, such as the U.S., the thyroid gland volume may increase by 10–15%, primarily as a result of pregnancy-induced vascular swelling of the gland. Although this enlargement can be recognized by ultrasound, it cannot usually be appreciated by palpation.

Therefore, any goiter found during pregnancy in an iodine-replete area should be evaluated in the same manner as a goiter occurring outside of pregnancy.

11. **Does thyroid hormone cross the placenta?**
Thyroid hormone crosses the placenta poorly, owing in part to the high placental activity of the type III monodeiodinase that converts T_4 to rT_3 and T_3 to T_2. However, it is now clear that some T_4 does cross the placenta, since fetuses with complete thyroid agenesis have about 30% of the normal amount of thyroid hormone at birth. This amount of thyroid hormone appears to be protective to the brain, and neurologic development usually progresses normally as long as thyroid supplementation is begun immediately after birth. Significant amounts of thyroid hormone also appear to cross in the first trimester before the fetal thyroid begins functioning.

12. **Does iodine cross the placenta?**
Iodine easily crosses the placenta for use by the fetal thyroid, which, after 12 weeks' gestation, takes up iodine even more avidly than the maternal thyroid.

13. **What about thyrotropin-releasing hormone (TRH) and TSH?**
TRH, but not TSH, also crosses the placenta and has been used in experimental protocols to attempt to accelerate fetal lung maturity.

14. **Summarize the ability of thyroid-related antibodies to cross the placenta.**
Immunoglobulin (IgG) TSH receptor-stimulating antibodies (thyroid-stimulating immunoglobulin[TSI]) cross the placenta, especially in the third trimester and can occasionally cause fetal or neonatal hyperthyroidism in infants of women with Graves' disease. Although thyroid peroxidase (TPO) antibodies and antithyroglobulin (TG) antibodies can also cross, they usually have no clinical significance. In rare cases, they may be associated with thyrotropin receptor-blocking antibodies that can cause transient neonatal hypothyroidism.

15. **List common medications that cross the placenta.**
    - Propylthiouracil (PTU)
    - Methimazole
    - Beta blockers

16. **When does the fetus begin making thyroid hormone?**
At about 10–12 weeks, the fetal thyroid gland develops and the hypothalamic-pituitary-thyroid axis begins to function. Because little thyroid hormone synthesis occurs until 18–20 weeks, the fetus is dependent on maternal thyroid hormone in the first trimester.

17. **Is fetal thyroid hormone production independent of the mother's?**
After the first trimester, the fetal hypothalamic-pituitary-thyroid axis is fairly independent of the mother with the exception of its dependence on adequate maternal iodine stores. Antithyroid drugs or high levels of TSI may, however, affect fetal thyroid function or cause goiter development at this stage. Thyroid hormone and TBG levels increase in the fetus and plateau at about 35–37 weeks' gestation. High levels of rT_3 and low levels of T_3 are maintained throughout the pregnancy as a result of the high placental activity of type III monodeiodinase. The axis is relatively immature, however, considering the increased fetal TSH levels relative to the low level of T_4 production at birth. At the time of labor and in the early neonatal period, there is a dramatic increase in the capacity of the liver to convert T_4 to T_3.

18. **What is gestational transient thyrotoxicosis (GTT) or thyrotoxicosis related to hyperemesis gravidarum?**
GTT refers to hyperthyroidism caused by elevated levels of hCG, which binds to the TSH receptor and can stimulate thyroid hormone release. Levels > 75,000 IU/mL, which may be

seen in women with hyperemesis gravidarum, twin gestation, and especially in molar pregnancies, can often cause hyperthyroidism. Posttransitional modification of the sialylation of hCG can change its affinity to the TSH receptor and half-life in the circulation, resulting in elevated thyroid levels in the first half of pregnancy. A woman who presents with hyperthyroidism and a positive pregnancy test should have an ultrasound to exclude a molar pregnancy.

Women with hyperemesis gravidarum (persistent nausea and vomiting accompanied by electrolyte derangements and at least 5% weight loss) commonly have abnormal thyroid function tests. In one of the largest series yet to be published, half of the 57 women with hyperemesis gravidarum had elevated free T_4.

19. **What are the most common causes of hyperthyroidism in pregnancy? During what period of gestation is hyperthyroidism most likely to occur?**
    Hyperthyroidism complicates pregnancy in about 0.2% of women. Graves' disease is the most common cause of hyperthyroidism in pregnancy, accounting for nearly 85% of the cases. Autoimmune thyroid disease is most likely to present in the first trimester or the postpartum period because the immune suppression of pregnancy has been shown to significantly decrease thyroid antibody levels during the second and third trimesters. Other causes include toxic multinodular goiters, solitary toxic adenomas, iodine-induced hyperthyroidism, and subacute thyroiditis. As noted earlier, hCG-induced hyperthyroidism is common in women with hyperemesis gravidarum or hydatidiform moles and also usually presents in the first trimester.

20. **Summarize the diagnostic approach to the pregnant woman with hyperthyroidism.**
    Normal pregnancy can produce clinical features that mimic hyperthyroidism, such as heat intolerance, mild tachycardia, increase in cardiac output, a systolic flow murmur, peripheral vasodilation, and a widened pulse pressure. Weight loss may be obscured by the weight gain of pregnancy. As in the nonpregnant state, hyperthyroidism in pregnancy is usually characterized by low serum TSH levels and increased serum levels of free T_4. However, in interpreting thyroid tests in pregnant women, it is important to realize that serum TSH levels are also frequently low in normal women during the first trimester of pregnancy.

21. **How can the various causes of hyperthyroidism be differentiated with certainty?**
    Radioisotope scans are contraindicated during pregnancy; therefore, the differential diagnosis of hyperthyroidism in pregnant women must be based on the history, physical exam, and laboratory testing. An obstetric ultrasound may be indicated to exclude a hydatidiform mole or to look for twin pregnancies.

22. **What findings help distinguish between Graves' disease and hyperemesis gravidarum?**
    Although a diffusely enlarged thyroid gland with a bruit in a woman with ophthalmopathy and prepregnancy symptoms is strongly suggestive of Graves' disease, the diagnosis is often less clear, since these findings may be absent. If a woman is actively vomiting, the distinction between early Graves' disease and hyperemesis gravidarum may be particularly difficult. It is unusual, however, for women to develop hCG-induced hyperthyroidism at hCG levels less than 50,000 IU/mL. Clues pointing to Graves' disease rather than hCG-induced hyperthyroidism include the presence of a goiter, ophthalmopathy, onycholysis, or preexisting hyperthyroid symptoms antedating the pregnancy. In addition, TSI levels are often positive and T_3 levels are generally higher in Graves' disease because hyperemesis gravidarum results in a compromised nutritional state and decreased conversion of T_4 to T_3 in peripheral tissues.

23. **Why is it important to distinguish GTT from Graves disease?**

It may be difficult to differentiate GTT from other causes of hyperthyroidism, since autoimmune hyperthyroidism also commonly presents during the first trimester of pregnancy and the biochemical profile of the two conditions is similar. However, it is extremely important to determine whether the thyrotoxicosis is due to Graves' disease or hyperemesis gravidarum because the latter usually resolves without antithyroid treatment by ~18 weeks when hCG levels decline. It is rarely necessary to treat with beta-blocker therapy or antithyroid drugs, since the hyperthyroid state is usually self-limited. Hyperthyroidism is probably not the cause of the nausea. Instead, it appears that hCG mediates both the hyperthyroidism and perhaps the nausea by different mechanisms.

24. **Why is the woman's original country of residence significant?**

Women who have goiters from endemic areas of iodine deficiency and who move to the U.S. may develop iodine-induced hyperthyroidism when they suddenly become iodine-replete. Hot nodules can also occur and do not improve in later pregnancy with the immune suppression of pregnancy.

25. **What are the risks of Graves' disease to the mother?**

Inadequately treated hyperthyroidism in the mother can result in preeclampsia, weight loss, tachycarcdia, proximal muscle weakness, anxiety, and atrial fibrillation. Left ventricular dysfunction can occur and is usually reversible but may persist for several weeks after biochemical hyperthyroidism has been corrected. This may place the pregnant woman at risk for the development of congestive heart failure, especially in the presence of superimposed preeclampsia, infection, anemia, or at the time of delivery. Thyroid storm can rarely occur in these women.

26. **What are the risks to the fetus of maternal Graves' disease?**

Inadequately treated maternal hyperthyroidism can result in fetal tachycardia, severe growth restriction, premature births, and a 9-fold increased incidence of low birth weight in the infants. Congenital malformations are probably not increased in babies born to mothers with either treated or untreated hyperthyroidism. Inadequately treated maternal hyperthyroidism can cause suppression of the hypothalamic-pituitary thyroid axis, resulting in temporary hypothyroidsism in the neonate (Kempers, 2003).

27. **Describe the possible effects on the fetus of high levels of TSH-receptor-stimulating antibodies.**

In about 2–5% of cases, fetal or neonatal hyperthyroidism can develop as a result of very high levels of maternal TSH receptor-stimulating antibodies (TSI). Because transplacental passage of IgG is limited, this condition is unusual unless the TSI levels are at least 5-fold elevated in the second and third trimesters.

28. **How are such effects treated?**

Treatment consists of administering higher doses of PTU to the mother so that a sufficient amount of medication is delivered into the fetal circulation. Occasionally, mothers are rendered hypothyroid with these high PTU doses, and maternal T_4 supplementation may be required.

29. **Why is neonatal hyperthyroidism more common than fetal hyperthyroidism?**

Neonatal hyperthyroidism is more common than fetal hyperthyroidism because of the high activity of placental type III monodeiodinase, relatively low serum T_3 levels in utero, and the effects of maternal antithyroid drugs on the fetus. TSH receptor-stimulating antibodies remain at high levels after birth, stimulating the neonata thyroid to produce excess thyroid hormone.

30. **How does fetal hyperthyroidism manifest?**

Neonatal hyperthyroidism may manifest as irritability, failure to thrive, hyperkinesis, diarrhea, poor feeding, jaundice, tachycardia, poor weight gain, thrombocytopenia, goiter, and, less commonly, exophthalmos, cardiac failure, hepatosplenomegaly, hyperviscosity syndrome, or craniosynostosis.

31. **What is the mortality rate of neonatal hyperthyroidism?**
The neonatal mortality rate may be as high as 30% if the condition is unrecognized.

32. **How should hyperthyroid infants be treated?**
They may need to be placed on antithyroid medications until the antibody levels wane, which usually occurs by 12 weeks. If the mother has been receiving antithyroid drugs during pregnancy, it may take 5–10 days for the neonate to manifest symptoms because of the residual effects of these medications. Rarely, women who are euthyroid from previous ablative therapy still have high enough levels of TSI to cause their infants to develop fetal or neonatal hyperthyroidism.

33. **How can pregnant women with Graves' disease be safely treated in pregnancy?**
Treatment of clinical hyperthyroidism is definitely indicated to decrease morbidity in both mother and fetus. Thionamide therapy with the judicious use of beta blockers until thyroid hormone levels are reduced is the preferred treatment because radioiodine readily crosses the placenta and will be concentrated by the fetal thyroid after 10–12 weeks of gestation.

34. **Which is preferable in pregnant and breast-feeding women—PTU or methimazole?**
PTU remains the preferred antithyroid medication in the U.S. because of previous reports that it crosses the placenta less well than methimazole (MMI) and that MMI may be associated with a scalp deformity in the infant (aplasia cutis). Both of these concerns about MMI have been recently challenged, however, and it is currently believed that MMI can be used safely if necessary. Because PTU is more highly protein-bound and crosses less efficiently into breast milk than MMI, it is also considered preferable to use PTU in women who breast-feed their infants.

35. **How are PTU and MMI dosed during pregnancy?**
Because both PTU and MMI cross the placenta, the lowest possible doses should be given with a goal of maintaining the mother's serum free T_4 or T_3 (if the mother is predominantly T_3 thyrotoxic) in the high-normal range. The serum TSH level often remains persistently suppressed in women with free T_4 and T_3 levels in this range and therefore cannot be used to accurately titrate the dose of antithyroid drugs during pregnancy. Approximately 1–3% of newborns exposed to PTU in utero develop transient neonatal hypothyroidism or a small goiter. However, this is rare when PTU doses are titrated appropriately.

36. **When can doses of PTU and MMI be reduced?**
Fortunately, antithyroid drugs can usually be markedly decreased by the third trimester because of the decreasing levels of TSI that accompany the natural immunosuppression of pregnancy. In fact, many women require minimal or no drug at term, especially if they have a small goiter, but it is important to ensure that they are not hyperthyroid at delivery to reduce the risk of hyperthyroid complications to the cardiovascular system. The majority of women have a rebound in their hyperthyroidism, and postpartum thionamide therapy needs to be increased.

37. **Discuss the role of beta blockers during pregnancy.**
Beta blockers are indicated to treat symptomatic hyperadrenergic signs and symptoms until antithyroid drug therapy has rendered the patient euthyroid. However, they should be discontinued when the patient becomes euthyroid because long-term treatment with beta blockers has been associated with intrauterine growth restriction. No compelling data indicate that one beta blocker is safer than another.

38. **Why is radioactive iodine contraindicated in pregnancy?**
    Radioactive iodine is contraindicated in pregnancy because after 12 weeks' gestation the fetal thyroid gland has avidity for iodine that is 20–50 times that of the maternal thyroid. Accordingly, any dose of radioiodine will be more highly concentrated in fetal thyroid tissue and can easily ablate the fetal gland.

39. **Can cold iodine be given during pregnancy?**
    Cold iodine (e.g., Lugol's solution or SSKI) should also be avoided in pregnancy except in women with thyroid storm. If it must be given after 10–12 weeks, the fetus should be monitored for the development of a goiter and the duration should be limited if possible to 3 days.

40. **Does surgery have a role during pregnancy?**
    Surgery is rarely indicated during pregnancy but may be necessary in women who are unable to take antithyroid drugs (i.e., because of agranulocytosis) or who are refractory to high doses of antithyroid medications. If necessary, it is best to perform surgery in the second trimester before fetal viability. The rationale for this timing is that there is a significant increase in the risk of miscarriage in the first trimester and of preterm labor when surgery is done after 24 weeks.

41. **Should a woman be counseled to terminate a pregnancy if she inadvertently receives a ^{123}I scan or an ablative dose of ^{131}I?**
    A woman who receives ^{123}I for a thyroid scan early in pregnancy can be reassured for the most part because the fetus has not developed the ability to concentrate iodine before 10 weeks and the radiation exposure from this test is very low with a half-life of only ~8 hours. An ablative dose of ^{131}I given early in pregnancy, however, is cause for greater concern because the half-life of ^{131}I is 8 days, and the radiation is more destructive to the thyroid gland. Generally, if the dose is given very early, when the fetal thyroid gland is not yet trapping iodine, the relatively low thyroid and total body irradiation dose is probably not sufficient to justify termination of the pregnancy.

42. **How may the risk to the fetus be minimized?**
    It may be useful to give PTU to block the recycling of ^{131}I in the fetal thyroid gland if it can be given within 1 week of ^{131}I treatment. Fetal hypothyroidism can be diagnosed in utero by percutaneous umbilical sampling, and T_4 treatment may be given via amniotic fluid injections, although such treatment is still experimental. Certainly, all women of childbearing age regardless of contraceptive measures should have a pregnancy test before receiving any dose of ^{123}I or ^{131}I.

43. **How should women with Graves' disease be counseled about treatment alternatives before becoming pregnant?**
    Many experts recommend definitive treatment with ^{131}I (after a negative pregnancy test) in a woman of childbearing age who wishes to become pregnant. In a series of nearly 300 women given radioiodine for cancer therapy, no significant difference in stillbirths, preterm births, low-birth-weight infants, or congenital malformations were reported in subsequent pregnancies. Effective birth control needs to be established, and then women should optimally wait for at least 3–6 months after regaining a stable euthyroid status before trying to conceive. Women who are stable on low doses of thionamides should not have a problematic pregnancy, but it is highly likely that thionamide doses will need to be adjusted during pregnancy and the postpartum period. Women requiring high doses or who have large goiters should be counseled about the benefits of definitive therapy before becoming pregnant.

44. **Describe the natural history of Graves' disease in the postpartum period.**
    About 70% of women have a postpartum relapse of Graves' disease, usually within the first 3 months after delivery, as the natural immunosuppression of pregnancy disappears. Antithyroid therapy must almost always be increased during this time.

45. **What treatment options can be recommended for women who wish to breast-feed?**
For the nursing mother, PTU is the preferred antithyroid drug because it is highly protein-bound and crosses less efficiently into breast milk than MMI. Thyroid function in infants appears unaffected by maternal ingestion of therapeutic doses of PTU or MMI, and it is unnecessary to monitor neonatal thyroid function unless dose requirements are unusually high.

46. **Can a nursing mother undergo a diagnostic ^{123}I scan if the cause of the hyperthyroidism is in question?**
A diagnostic ^{123}I scan can be done if the woman is willing to interrupt breast-feeding for 2–3 days. Both ^{123}I and ^{99}Tc pertechnetate are excreted into breast milk with an effective half-life of 5–8 and 2–8 hours, respectively.

47. **Can ablative therapy with ^{131}I be offered to nursing women?**
Ablative therapy with ^{131}I cannot be offered unless the women is willing to give up nursing altogether, because even a 5-mCi dose requires discontinuation of breast-feeding for at least 56 days.

48. **Can beta blockers be used in nursing women?**
Beta blockers can be used if necessary in the breast-feeding mother. However, atenolol may produce higher breast milk concentrations than other beta blockers, and there are rare reports of neonatal bradycardia in mothers who nursed while taking this drug.

49. **When should a nursing woman take antithyroid drugs?**
It is always best if a mother takes antithyroid drugs immediately after nursing to avoid exposing the infant to peak concentrations of the drug.

50. **Does hypothyroidism pose a risk to the pregnant patient?**
Hypothyroidism occurs in ~2.5% of pregnancies and due to maternal and fetal concerns, a case can be made to screen pregnant women in the first trimester. Certainly any pregnant woman with risk factors for hypothyroidism, including a positive family history, should be screened because hypothyroidism can cause maternal anemia, myopathy, congestive heart failure, and an increased risk of preeclampsia, low-birth-weight infants, and postpartum hemorrhage.

51. **How do thyroid hormone requirements change during pregnancy?**
Thyroid hormone requirements often increase during pregnancy with up to 75% of pregnant women, requiring an increase in thyroxine dosage of up to 50 μg over the prepregnancy dose.

KEY POINTS: THYROID DISEASE IN PREGNANCY ✓

1. Approximately 15% of normal pregnant women have a slightly suppressed TSH in the first trimester.

2. Hyperemesis gravidarum can cause overt hyperthyroidism.

3. Graves' disease most often presents in the first trimester with improvement in later pregnancy but commonly exacerbates after delivery.

4. Thyroid hormone requirements usually increase in pregnancy, beginning in the first trimester.

5. Postpartum thyroiditis occurs in ~5% normal women and ~25% of women with type 1 diabetes.

A recent study confirmed that 85% of pregnant woman required an increase in levothyroxine by 47% by 16 weeks gestation (Alexander 2004). Because requirements increased as early as 5 weeks gestation, women who are athyreotic may need to increase their thyroid hormone dose by 25–30% as soon as pregnancy is confirmed.

52. **What causes the rapid increase in thyroid hormone requirements?**
The rapid increase in thyroid hormone requirements that occurs in the first trimester may be due to the sudden increase in the estrogen-stimulated TBG pool associated with pregnancy.

53. **When should serum TSH levels be checked?**
The serum TSH level should be checked as soon as pregnancy is confirmed, and an appropriate increase in thyroid hormone should be given. A recent study suggests that athyreotic women requiring full replacement doses should receive a 25% dose increase as soon as pregnancy is confirmed in spite of a normal TSH (Alexander, 2004). As discussed earlier, the TSH may be mildly suppressed in normal women during the first trimester as a result of the thyrotropic influence of hCG. Therefore, unless a woman is symptomatically hyperthyroid or has frankly elevated serum free T_4 levels, the thyroxine dosage should not be reduced in response to the finding of a low first-trimester TSH level. The TSH should be checked 4–6 weeks after a dose change and at least every trimester to maintain a normal serum TSH concentration. In women who have had a thyroidectomy for thyroid cancer, the goal of maintaining a suppressed serum TSH without rendering the woman thyrotoxic should be adhered to during pregnancy. Thyroid hormone needs to be reduced almost immediately after delivery to prepregnancy doses to avoid hyperthyroidism postpartum.

54. **When should a pregnant woman take her thyroid hormone?**
It is extremely important to advise the pregnant woman to take her thyroid hormone and her prenatal vitamins or iron supplements at different times, since ferrous sulfate can bind to thyroxine and decrease its bioavailability.

55. **What is the risk of abnormal fetal and neonatal intellectual development in infants born to mothers who are hypothyroid during the first trimester of pregnancy?**
All newborns in the U.S. are screened for hypothyroidism, since it is well established that infants who have severe congenital hypothyroidism but receive thyroid hormone replacement at birth appear to have fairly normal intellectual growth and development. However, the fetal effects of maternal hypothyroidism during the first trimester, when the fetal brain is dependent on maternal thyroid hormone, is a subject of ongoing debate. Several recent publications suggest that psychomotor and intellectual development might be impaired in infants born to mothers who were hypothyroid during the first trimester of pregnancy, although the differences from controls in these studies were small and often became insignificant when the infants were tested later in childhood.

56. **What strategies can reduce the risk to the fetus?**
It seems prudent to attempt to identify and appropriately treat hypothyroidism in women of childbearing age who wish to become pregnant (preconception), as well as in pregnant women in the first trimester. It must be remembered, however, that serum TSH levels often decline in the first trimester as a result of the influence of hCG. Thus a TSH level of 4–5 mU/ml in the first trimester may be inappropriately high while a TSH level of 0.1 mU/ml may be appropriately low because of the thyroid-stimulating activity of high levels of hCG.

57. **How should a thyroid nodule be evaluated during pregnancy?**
The evaluation of a solitary or dominant nodule in a pregnant woman is similar to that in nonpregnant women. Fine-needle aspiration (FNA) should be offered when nodules are > 1–2 cm, especially if they are detected before 20 weeks or if there are other risk factors for

malignancy, such as lymphadenopathy or rapid growth. FNA specimens should be evaluated using the same criteria as established for nonpregnant patients.

58. **What is the likelihood that thyroid nodules discovered during pregnancy are malignant?**
Data suggest that thyroid nodules discovered during pregnancy may have a higher risk of being malignant. However, this finding is likely due in part to selection or sampling bias, since many young women do not have systematic health examinations until they become pregnant. Depending on the patient population, the incidence of biopsied nodules being benign is > 80%, whereas differentiated thyroid cancer has been found in 5–40% of cases. The majority of malignant nodules are papillary thyroid carcinoma. FNA cytology is highly accurate in diagnosing papillary carcinoma, whereas cytology showing a follicular or Hürthle-cell neoplasm predicts only a 5–15% risk of malignancy. When the serum TSH is normal, < 20% of FNA specimens are nondiagnostic. In one series of 61 patients with differentiated thyroid cancer (87% papillary), there were no differences in the rates of recurrence, distant spread, or outcomes related to whether neck surgery was performed during or after pregnancy.

59. **How should a thyroid nodule be managed during pregnancy?**
If the cytology is suspicious or confirms papillary thyroid cancer, the best time to offer a thyroidectomy is probably in the second trimester, to avoid the risk of miscarriage in the first trimester and preterm labor in the third trimester. If the nodule is < 2 cm, has not rapidly increased in size, and the patient has no lymphadenopathy, it may be reasonable to postpone thyroidectomy until after pregnancy and place the woman on thyroid suppression therapy in the meantime.

60. **How common is postpartum thyroiditis? Who is at risk?**
Postpartum thyroid dysfunction occurs in approximately 5–10% of women, with a much higher incidence in certain populations. In one series, 25% of women with type 1 diabetes mellitus developed postpartum thyroid dysfunction; it is therefore recommended that this population should be screened in the postpartum period on a routine basis. In another series of 152 women with TPO antibodies detected at 16 weeks' gestation, postpartum thyroiditis occurred in 50%; of these, 19% had hyperthyroidism alone, 49% had hypothyroidism alone, and the remaining 32% had hyperthyroidism followed by hypothyroidism. Women with a family history of thyroid disease are also at increased risk and may be candidates for screening with TPO antibodies during pregnancy or with thyroid function tests in the postpartum period.

61. **Characterize the histopathology of postpartum thyroiditis.**
The disorder is highly associated with circulating TPO antibodies, while the histology is identical to that of Hashimoto's thyroiditis with profuse mononuclear cell infiltration and destruction of thyroid follicles.

62. **Summarize the clinical course of postpartum thyroiditis.**
Classically, the clinical course consists of three phases, but not all women manifest each phase.

63. **Describe phase 1 of postpartum thyroiditis.**
At 1–3 months after delivery, affected women often develop hyperthyroidism as a result of immunologically mediated destruction of thyroid follicles, which results in the release of stored thyroid hormone into the circulation. Such women may experience anxiety, irritability, palpitations, fatigue, and insomnia, but commonly this phase does not come to the attention of the clinician. Symptomatic patients are best treated with beta blockers, which must soon be tapered and discontinued as the thyrotoxic phase spontaneously resolves.

64. **How can phase 1 of postpartum thyroiditis be distinguished from Graves' disease?**

Occasionally, there is a question about the cause of the hyperthyroidism, since Graves' disease commonly appears or exacerbates in the first several months postpartum. Distinguishing between the two conditions is facilitated by measurement of a serum thyroglobulin level and TPO antibodies (both are high in postpartum thyroiditis) and TSH receptor-stimulating antibodies (often elevated with Graves' disease). However, the most definitive test is a ^{123}I-uptake test (low in postpartum thyroiditis and high in Graves' disease), if the mother is willing to interrupt nursing for 2–3 days.

65. **Describe phase 2 of postpartum thyroiditis.**

More commonly, women present with stage 2 of postpartum thyroiditis, which is characterized by hypothyroidism alone at about 4–8 months after delivery. Nonspecific symptoms include fatigue, depression, impaired concentration, poor memory, aches and pains, dry skin, and weight gain, all of which may be overlooked by the clinician. Symptoms may predate the onset of thyroid function abnormalities in women with positive TPO antibodies and may persist for some time after a euthyroid state is achieved.

66. **How is phase 2 of postpartum thyroiditis treated?**

Women with abnormal thyroid function tests and symptoms consistent with hypothyroidism should be treated with thyroxine replacement for approximately 6–12 months or at least until 1 year after delivery. At that time, discontinuation of thyroxine therapy can be attempted to identify the 80% of women who will return to the euthyroid state by 12 months after delivery.

67. **Describe the natural history of postpartum thyroiditis.**

Most women will return to a euthyroid state at 12–18 months postpartum. However, thyroid function testing should then be followed at least annually in women who become euthyroid. In one series of 43 patients with postpartum thyroiditis, 23% of the women were hypothyroid at 2–4 years, and, in a longer series, 48% of women were hypothyroid 7–9 years later. Women with the highest TPO antibody titers and the most severe hypothyroidism appear to be at the highest risk of developing permanent hypothyroidism. If a woman becomes euthyroid within a year postpartum, she has a very high likelihood (70%) of developing postpartum thyroiditis after a subsequent pregnancy.

BIBLIOGRAPHY

1. ACOG Practice Bulletin: Thyroid disease in pregnancy. Int J Gynaecol Obstet 79:171–180, 2002.

2. Alexander EK, Marqusee E, Lawrence E, et al: Timing and magnitude of increases in levothyroxine requirements during pregnancy in women with hypothyroidism. N Engl J Med 351: 241–249, 2004.

3. Azizi F, Khoshniat M, Bahrainian M, Hedayati M: Thyroid function and intellectual development of infants nursed by mothers taking methimazole. J Clin Endocrinol Metab 85:3233–3238, 2000.

4. Caixas A, Albareda M, Garcia Patterson A, et al: Postpartum thyroiditis in women with hypothyroidism antedating pregnancy. J Clin Endocrinol Metab 84:4000–4005,1999.

5. Chopra IJ, Baber K: Treatment of primary hypothyroidism during pregnancy: Is there an increase in thyroxine dose requirement in pregnancy? Metab Clin Exper 52:122–128, 2003.

6. Fisher DA: Fetal thyroid function: Diagnosis and management of fetal thyroid disorders. Clin Obstet Gynecol 40:16–31, 1997.

7. Gerstein HC: Incidence of postpartum thyroid dysfunction in patients with type I diabetes mellitus. Ann Intern Med 118:419–423, 1993.

8. Glinoer D: What happens to the normal thyroid during pregnancy? Thyroid 9:631–635, 1999.

9. Goodwin TM, Hershman JM: Hyperthyroidism due to inappropriate production of human chorionic gonadotropin. Clin Obstet Gynecol 40:32–44, 1997.

10. Hay ID: Nodular thyroid disease diagnosed during pregnancy: How and when to treat. Thyroid 9:667–670, 1999.

11. Kempers MJE, Van Tijn DA, Van Trotensburg ASP, et al: Central congenital hypothyroidism due to gestational hyperthyroidism: Detection where prevention failed. Clin Endocrinol Metab 88: 5851–5857, 2003.

12. Lazarus JH: Clinical manifestations of postpartum thyroid disease. Thyroid 9:685–690, 1999.

13. Lazarus JH. Epidemiology and prevention of thyroid disease in pregnancy. Thyroid 12:861–865, 2002.

14. Mandel SJ, Larsen PR, Seely EW, Brent GA. Increased need for thyroxine during pregnancy in women with primary hypothyroidism. N Engl J Med 323:91–96, 1990.

15. Masiukiewicz US, Burrow GN: Hyperthyroidism in pregnancy: Diagnosis and treatment. Thyroid 9:647–652, 1999.

16. Mestman JH, Goodwin TM, Montoro MM: Thyroid disorders of pregnancy. Endocrin Metab Clin N Am 24(1):41–71, 1995.

17. Momotani N, Yamashita R, Makino F, et al. Thyroid function in wholly breast-feeding infants whose mothers take high doses of propylthiouracil. Clin Endocrinol 53:177–181,2000.

18. Moosa M, Mazzaferri EL: Outcome of differentiated thyroid cancer diagnosed in pregnant women. J Clin Endocrinol Metab 82:2862–2866, 1997.

19. Othman S, Phillips DIW, Parkes AB, et al: A long-term follow-up of postpartum thyroiditis. Clin Endocrinol 32:559–564, 1990.

20. Pop VJ, Kuijpens JL, van Barr AL et al: Low maternal free thyroxine concentrations during early pregnancy are associated with impaired psychomotor development in infancy. Clin Endocrinol 50:149–155, 1999.

21. Terry AJ, Hague WM: Postpartum thyroiditis. Semin Perinatol 22:497–502, 1998.

22. Vulsma T, Gons MH, de Vijlder JJ. Maternal-fetal transfer of thyroxine in congenital hypothyroidism due to a total organification defect or thyroid agenesis. N Engl J Med 321:13–16, 1989.

23. Zimmerman D. Fetal and neonatal hyperthyroidism. Thyroid 9:727–733, 1999.

CHAPTER 42

PSYCHIATRIC DISORDERS AND THYROID DISEASE

James V. Hennessey, M.D.

1. **How well established is the relationship between thyroid disease and psychiatric symptoms?**

   Since the publication of the Clinical Society of London's "Report on Myxoedema" in 1888, it has been recognized that thyroid disease may give rise to psychiatric disorders that can be corrected by re-establishment of normal thyroid function. Later Asher re-emphasized the fact that patients with profound hypothyroidism may present with depressive psychosis. As outlined in Table 42-1, the symptoms of hypothyroidism often mimic those of depression, and the symptoms of hyperthyroidism include anxiety, dysphoria, emotional lability, and intellectual dysfunction, as well as mania or depression, the latter being especially characteristic among the elderly presenting with so-called apathetic thyrotoxicosis.

TABLE 42-1.	CLINICAL FEATURES COMMON TO BOTH THYROID DISEASES AND MOOD DISORDERS		
	Hypothyroidism	Mood Disorders	Hyperthyroidism
Depression	Yes	Yes	Yes
Diminished interest	Yes	Yes	Yes
Diminished pleasure	Yes	Yes	No
Decreased libido	Yes	Yes	Sometimes
Weight loss	No	Yes	Yes
Weight gain	Yes	Sometimes	Occasionally
Appetite loss	Yes	Yes	Sometimes
Increased appetite	No	Yes	Yes
Insomnia	No	Yes	Yes
Hypersomnia	Yes	Yes	No
Agitation/anxiety	Occasionally	Yes	Yes
Fatigue	Yes	Yes	Yes
Poor memory	Yes	Yes	Occasionally
Cognitive dysfunction	Yes	Yes	Yes
Impaired concentration	Yes	Yes	Yes
Constipation	Yes	Sometimes	No

Adapted from Hennessey JV, Jackson IMD: The interface between thyroid hormones and psychiatry. Endocrinologist 6:214–223, 1996.

2. **What abnormalities of thyroid function are found in psychiatric disorders?**
Since patients with thyroid disease may manifest frank psychiatric disorders that are reversible with endocrine therapy, the thyroid axis has been extensively studied in patients presenting with a wide variety of behavioral disturbances. Various abnormalities of thyroid function have been identified, particularly in depression. In most depressed subjects, the basal serum thyroid-stimulating hormone (TSH), thyroxine (T_4), and triiodothyronine (T_3) are within the reference range, although in one report one-third of such patients were observed to have suppressed TSH levels.

3. **What abnormalities of thyrotropin-releasing hormone (TRH) stimulation may be observed in the depressed patient?**
Patients with depression have a "blunted" TSH response to TRH administration (as defined by a TSH rise 5 μU/mL), occurring in approximately 25% of such subjects. A blunted TSH response is more likely in unipolar than bipolar depression, but differentiating these disorders with TRH stimulation has been disappointing. The blunted TSH response is a "state" marker that normalizes upon recovery from the depression.

4. **Describe the mechanism for blunted TSH response in affective disorders.**
The mechanism is not known; however, glucocorticoids, known to inhibit the hypothalamic-pituitary-thyroid axis, are elevated in depression and may be responsible. The suppressed TSH response to TRH is not specific to depression and may be observed in alcohol withdrawal, starvation, normal aging males, renal failure, acromegaly, Cushing's syndrome, and hypopituitarism. The blunting may also be due to medications, such as T_4, glucocorticoids, growth hormone, somatostatin, dopamine, and phenytoin, all of which have been reported to diminish this response.

5. **Can abnormalities in the TSH circadian rhythm be identified in depression?**
In normal subjects, the TSH begins to rise in the evening before the onset of sleep, reaching a peak between 11:00 PM and 4:00 AM. In depression, the nocturnal surge of TSH is frequently absent, resulting in a reduction in thyroid hormone secretion, supporting the view that functional central hypothyroidism might occur in some depressed subjects. Sleep deprivation, which has an antidepressant effect, returns the TSH circadian rhythm to normal. The mechanism responsible for the impaired nocturnal rise of TSH is unknown.

6. **Is autoimmune thyroid disease frequently present in the depressed patient?**
Although the blunted TSH response to TRH is well recognized in depression, it is less clearly appreciated that an enhanced response may occur in up to 15% of depressed subjects with normal baseline thyroid function tests. The majority of such patients have antithyroid antibodies, suggesting that the TSH hyper-response may indicate latent hypothyroidism caused by autoimmune thyroiditis. When autoimmunity is tested utilizing the antithyroid peroxidase antibody (anti-TPO) rather than the less specific antimicrosomal antibody, the prevalence of autoimmune thyroid disease is even higher. Not all studies, however, have found an increased prevalence of antithyroid antibodies in depressed subjects when compared with matched control groups.

7. **What is the frequency of elevated T_4 values in the psychiatric patient?**
Approximately 20% of patients admitted to the hospital with acute psychiatric presentations, including schizophrenia and major affective disorders, but rarely dementia or alcoholism, may demonstrate mild elevations in serum T_4 levels, and less often T_3 levels. The basal TSH is usually normal but may demonstrate blunted TRH responsiveness in up to 90% of such patients. These findings do not appear to represent thyrotoxicosis, and the abnormalities spontaneously resolve within 2 weeks without specific therapy. Such phenomena may be due to

central activation of the hypothalamic-pituitary-thyroid axis resulting in enhanced TSH secretion with consequent elevation in circulating T_4 levels.

8. **What is the most consistent abnormality of the thyroid axis in hospitalized depressed patients?**
   In hospitalized depressed patients, the most consistent abnormality of the thyroid axis may be an increase in serum total or free T_4 levels, although usually within the conventional normal range. This increase generally regresses following successful treatment of the depression.

9. **What is the prevalence of hypothyroid dysfunction in psychiatric populations?**
   Thyroid function test abnormalities are common in older people. In otherwise normal female subjects over 60 years of age, the prevalence of elevated TSH values and/or positive antithyroid antibodies is 10% or more. Subjecting apparently asymptomatic people with slight elevations of serum TSH but normal T_4 and T_3 levels to a battery of psychological tests has revealed significant differences from control subjects on scales measuring memory, anxiety, somatic complaints, and depression. It is becoming increasingly recognized that depression is much more common in elderly people. Whether borderline hypothyroidism plays a role in these behavioral disturbances requires further investigation. Among alcoholics and those suffering from anorexia nervosa, suppressed T_3 levels with elevations in reverse T_3 and normal TSH values are consistent with the "sick thyroid state." These findings likely result from caloric deprivation.

10. **Which medications affect thyroid function and thyroid function tests?**
    Medications commonly used to treat psychiatric illness have been shown to affect thyroid function tests (Table 42-2).

TABLE 42-2.	IMPACT OF PSYCHOTROPIC MEDICATIONS ON THYROID FUNCTION TESTS	
Medication	**Mechanism**	**Test Findings**
Lithium carbonate	$\downarrow$ thyroglobulin hydrolysis $\downarrow$ T_4 and T_3 release	TSH $\uparrow$ (transiently) Hypothyroidism, goiter
Antipsychotics		
Perphenazine	$\uparrow$ T_4-binding globulin (TBG) concentration	$\uparrow$ T_4, nl free T_4
Anticonvulsants		
Phenytoin	$\uparrow$ hepatic clearance of T_4	$\downarrow$ T_4, $\pm$ $\downarrow$ free T_4, nl TSH
Carbamazepine	$\downarrow$ T_4 binding, $\uparrow$ hepatic clearance	$\downarrow$ T_4, $\pm$ $\downarrow$ free T_4, nl TSH
Phenobarbital	$\uparrow$ hepatic clearance	$\downarrow$ T_4, $\pm$ $\downarrow$ free T_4, nl TSH
Valproic acid	$\downarrow$ T_4 binding (?), $\uparrow$ hepatic clearance (?)	$\downarrow$ T_4, $\pm$ $\downarrow$ free T_4, nl TSH
Narcotics		
Heroin	$\uparrow$ TBG concentration	$\uparrow$ T_4, nl free T_4
Methadone	$\uparrow$ TBG concentration	$\uparrow$ T_4, nl free T_4
Miscellaneous		
Amphetamines	$\uparrow$ TSH secretion (?)	$\uparrow$ T_4, $\uparrow$ free T_4

Adapted from Hennessy JV, Jackson IMD: The interface between thyroid hormones and psychiatry. Endocrinologist 6:214–223, 1996.

11. **How does lithium affect the pituitary-thyroidal axis?**
Lithium carbonate, used to treat bipolar disorders, interferes with both the release and organification of thyroid hormone. Therapeutic lithium levels diminish both T_3 and T_4 release from the thyroid gland, while at higher (probably toxic) levels iodine uptake and organification may also be inhibited. Following a 3-week therapeutic course of lithium carbonate, suppression of serum T_4 and T_3 levels and associated elevations of basal serum TSH values and exaggerated TSH responses to TRH administration may be noted; these abnormalities generally return to normal within 3–12 months, even if the medication is continued.

12. **What is the most common thyroid disorder in lithium-treated patients?**
Goiter is the most common thyroid disorder occurring in lithium-treated patients. Hypothyroidism can also occasionally develop, particularly in patients who have thyroid glands that have been compromised by disorders, such as Hashimoto's thyroiditis and Graves' disease previously treated with ^{131}I therapy. However, it is uncommon for hypothyroidism to occur if pretreatment thyroid function is completely normal and patients are thyroid antibody-negative. If considered clinically necessary, lithium may be continued and T_4 added to treat patients who develop goiter or hypothyroidism.

13. **How does phenytoin affect laboratory tests and the function of the thyroid?**
The effects of phenytoin (Dilantin), occasionally used for bipolar disorder, on thyroid function are quite complex. Suppressed values of total and, occasionally, free T_4 are observed in a significant minority of patients who are chronically treated with phenytoin alone and in upward of 75% of those in whom the drug is combined with carbamazepine (Tegretol). The lower total T_4 levels are likely due to displacement of T_4 from TBG, while the reduced free T_4 levels result from enhanced clearance of T_4 through phenytoin-induced hepatic microsomal oxidative enzyme activity. Generally, the suppressed T_4 levels are accompanied by normal T_3 and free T_3 levels and normal TSH concentrations. Normal basal TSH values with diminished TSH responses to TRH have been attributed to potential phenytoin agonism at the T_3 receptor. However, other studies have suggested that this may be an assay artifact because free T_4 values have been found to be normal or mildly elevated in analyses using undiluted serum.

14. **Describe the effects of carbamazepine on thyroid function.**
Carbamazepine (Tegretol) is used increasingly in bipolar disorder. Chronic use with maintenance of therapeutic serum levels suppresses serum T_4 values in more than 50% of patients. This may be due to enhanced hepatic metabolism of T_4. TRH stimulation testing before and after initiation of Tegretol therapy reveals that TSH responsiveness is reduced by the addition of this drug; this has led to speculation that carbamazepine may inhibit thyroid function through effects on the pituitary gland. Displacement of T_4 from TBG, similar to that seen with phenytoin, has additionally been cited as a potential effect.

15. **How do phenobarbital and valproic acid affect thyroid function?**
Both phenobarbital and valproic acid are reported to lower serum levels of T_4 in chronically treated patients, the former via enhanced hepatic T_4 clearance and the latter likely due to protein binding changes. Heroin, methadone, and perphenazine commonly increase serum TBG levels and therefore may elevate serum total T_4 levels, although TSH and free T_4 values remain normal. Amphetamines induce hyperthyroxinemia through enhanced secretion of TSH, an effect that appears to be centrally mediated.

16. **How do antidepressant therapies affect thyroid function?**
Antidepressants do not generally cause abnormal peripheral thyroid hormone levels but may affect thyroid hormone metabolism in the central nervous system (CNS). However, circulating total T_4 and free T_4, but not T_3, levels often show a modest decline, though still within the normal

range, after treatment with various pharmacologic classes of antidepressants, as well as with electroconvulsive therapy (ECT).

17. **What caveats apply to the use of antidepressant usage in patients with thyroid disease?**

The use of tricyclic antidepressants (TCAs) in thyrotoxic patients should be pursued with caution, as cardiac dysrhythmias may be exacerbated or precipitated. Further, the monoamine oxidase (MAO) inhibitors may cause hypertension in thyrotoxic patients, although they generally do not affect thyroid function or serum thyroid hormone levels.

18. **Can T_4 be used as sole treatment for depression?**

Asher's report on "myxoedema madness" demonstrated that thyroid hormone deficiency resulted in depression that reversed with thyroid hormone administration. This finding led to studies of the role of thyroid hormone therapy alone in the treatment of depression and other psychiatric diseases and open studies of high-dose T_4 for refractory bipolar and unipolar depression. Euthyroid patients with typical hypothyroid symptoms, considered depressed on psychological testing, do not improve when treated with T_4. In fact, patients presenting with symptoms of hypothyroidism with normal thyroid function tests respond more positively to placebo. Although initial reports of T_3 as single therapy were promising, these studies were methodologically flawed, and the role of thyroid hormone by itself in the treatment of depression in the absence of abnormalities of thyroid function has not been established.

19. **Are neuropsychiatric abnormalities demonstrable among patients with mild thyroid failure?**

Recent studies have shown that symptomatic patients with subclinical hypothyroidism (slightly elevated serum TSH but normal T_4 and T_3 levels) can have significant impairment of memory-related abilities, and significant differences in anxiety, somatic complaints, and depressive features compared with euthyroid controls. Normalization of the serum TSH with L-thyroxine (LT_4) therapy may completely reverse these neuropsychiatric features. Furthermore, when thyroid hormone is withdrawn from subjects with underlying hypothyroidism, gradually increasing sadness and anxiety symptoms are observed over the ensuing few weeks. These findings indicate that the patient presenting with depression must be assessed for thyroid dysfunction, since the presence of even subclinical hypothyroidism may provide an opportunity for resolution of the depression with thyroid hormone treatment.

20. **How effective is the combination of LT_4 and T_3 in the treatment of neuro-psychiatric symptoms of hypothyroidism?**

Since the 1960s, multiple reports have evaluated the effectiveness of combining T_3 with LT_4 to improve outcomes. The report of Bunevicius et al. seemed to indicate that substituting 12.5 µg of T_3 for 50 µg of the usual LT_4 dose resulted in improvement in mood and neuropsychological function. Several double-blind randomized controlled trials designed to correct design flaws of previous trials have failed to reproduce these positive effects and do not demonstrate improvement in self-rated mood, well-being, or depression scales with the addition of T_3 to LT_4 therapy. In addition, these studies fail to demonstrate differences in cognitive function, quality of life, or subjective satisfaction with treatment, but they do report that anxiety scores were significantly worse in those treated with the LT_4/T_3 combination. At this point it does not appear justified to use combined LT_4 and T_3 treatment in hypothyroid patients who complain of depressive symptoms after biochemical euthyroidism is restored.

21. **Can combination thyroid hormone and antidepressant enhance response to depression treatment?**

Adjuvant therapy has been said to be logical when depression fails to resolve after 6 weeks of adequate antidepressant medication. Such resistance occurs in about 30–45% of cases. The role of adjuvant thyroid hormone with TCAs has been investigated in euthyroid patients with depression over the past 25 years. T_3 doses of 25–50 µg daily will generally increase serum T_3 levels significantly and cause suppression of serum TSH and T_4 values. Two separate therapeutic effects of T_3 therapy have been studied: first, its ability to accelerate the onset of the antidepressant response; second, its ability to augment antidepressant responses among those considered pharmacologically resistant.

22. **How effective is thyroid hormone for the acceleration of the antidepressant response?**
Several reports have detailed the clinical outcomes of starting T_3 (5–40 µg daily) along with varying doses of TCAs at the outset of therapy. The study populations were inhomogeneous, consisting of patients with various types of depression. Furthermore, there were important methodologic limitations, including small sample sizes, inadequate medication doses, lack of serum medication level monitoring, and variable outcomes measures. As a result, it still has not been clearly established that T_3 accelerates the antidepressant effect of TCAs.

23. **Can T_3 augment the clinical antidepressant response?**
The first placebo-controlled, double-blind randomized study reported results in 16 unipolar depressed outpatients who had experienced no improvement in clinical outcomes with TCAs alone. The intervention consisted of adding 25 µg of T_3 or placebo daily for 2 weeks before the patients were crossed over to the opposite treatment for an additional 2 weeks. No beneficial effect of T_3 was apparent. The only other placebo-controlled, randomized double-blind trial investigating this question involved 33 patients with unipolar depression treated with either desipramine or imipramine for 5 weeks prior to random assignment to placebo or 37.5 µg of T_3 daily. After 2 weeks of observation on T_3, during which TCA levels were monitored, significantly more patients treated with T_3 (10 of 17; 59%) had a positive response than did placebo-treated patients (3 of 16; 19%). A subsequent open clinical trial of imipramine-resistant depression, using a prolonged period of TCA treatment preceding the addition of T_3, showed no demonstrable T_3 effect. A recent, large double-blind, placebo-controlled study to determine the role of T_3 as augmentation therapy did not demonstrate an effect of T_3 in augmenting the response of paroxetine (an SSRI) therapy in patients with major depressive disorder.

24. **What evidence indicates that the effect of selective serotonin reuptake inhibitors (SSRIs) and ECT may be enhanced by the addition of T_3?**
The SSRI group of substances (including fluoxetine, sertraline, and paroxetine) is the preferred antidepressant medication in the United States today. Two case reports addressing the role of thyroid hormone as adjuvant therapy for SSRIs suggested that SSRIs behave similarly to TCAs in this regard. A randomized, placebo-controlled trial of paroxetine and two doses of T_3 compared to placebo failed to augment the response or improve the efficacy of the SSRI treatment in patients with major depressive disorder. T_3 has been reported to augment the antidepressant effect of ECT.

25. **Do any psychiatric conditions respond to pharmacologic doses of T_4?**
For the 10–15% of bipolar disorder patients with four or more episodes of manic-depressive psychosis yearly (rapid cyclers), the prevalence of autoimmune thyroid disease may reach 50% or higher. Therapeutic intervention with standard therapy, such as lithium is frequently disappointing. Open-label studies treating such patients with LT_4 in pharmacologic doses sufficient to suppress serum TSH and elevate T_4 levels to approximately 150% of normal may decrease the manic and depressive phases in both amplitude and frequency and has led to remission in some of the patients. Given these encouraging results, controlled studies on the efficacy of LT_4 or T_3 seem warranted.

KEY POINTS: PSYCHIATRIC DISORDERS AND THYROID DISEASE ✔

1. The symptoms of hypothyroidism often mimic those of depression, while the symptoms of hyperthyroidism may be confused with mania or depression.

2. Approximately 20% of patients admitted to the hospital with acute psychiatric presentations, including schizophrenia and major affective disorders, but rarely dementia or alcoholism, may demonstrate mild elevations in serum T_4 levels and, less often, T_3 levels.

3. Normalization of the serum TSH with LT_4 therapy may completely reverse the neuropsychiatric features of hypothyroidism.

4. Based on the results of recent prospective controlled studies, it does not appear justified to use combined T_4 and T_3 treatment in hypothyroid patients who complain of depressive symptoms after biochemical euthyroidism is restored.

5. It is recommended that T_4 therapy be offered to any depressed patient with an elevated serum TSH, especially if accompanied by increased antithyroid antibody titers or low free T_4.

26. **Are mechanisms of thyroid hormone action on the brain known?**
    Thyroid hormones play a critical role in the development and function of the CNS. T_3 receptors are widely distributed throughout the brain, and there is much evidence that thyroid hormone regulates brain function through interaction with the catecholaminergic system. Thyroid hormone action in brain tissue is accomplished through the binding of T_3 to its nuclear receptor. The T_3 is derived from T_4 by the action of (type II) 5′-deiodinase, which is located throughout the CNS.

27. **Should T_4 or T_3 be used in treating the depressed patient?**
    Most studies using thyroid hormone as adjuvant therapy have used T_3 rather than T_4. In reports where the advantages of one over the other were assessed, T_4 was considered superior. In a randomized trial combining T_4 or T_3 with antidepressants, only 4 of 21 patients (19%) treated with 150 μg/day of T_4 for 3 weeks responded, whereas 9 of 17 (53%) responded with 37.5 μg/day of T_3. Further studies of open T_4 treatment in antidepressant-resistant patients have lacked controls, making interpretation difficult. Combination therapy with T_4 rather than T_3 may be indicated when subclinical hypothyroidism or rapid cycling bipolar disease is present. Since T_4 equilibrates in tissues more slowly than T_3, treatment with T_4 for at least 6–8 weeks, and preferably longer, is necessary to determine its efficacy.

28. **Describe the proposed mechanism for linking thyroid function and depression.**
    It has been postulated that type II 5′-deiodinase activity in the CNS is deficient in depression, giving rise to a state of brain hypothyroidism coexisting with systemic euthyroidism.

29. **Do antidepressant medications have a mechanistic connection to the action of thyroid hormone in the brain?**
    It has been shown that desipramine, a TCA, and fluoxetine, a SSRI, both enhance type II 5′-deiodinase activity in the CNS, thus presumably increasing the availability of T_3 in the brain. This could conceivably account for the clinical efficacy of these classes of drugs.

30. **What recommendations can be made for thyroid evaluation in psychiatric patients?**

It seems prudent to check thyroid function tests in psychiatric patients who are at increased risk for developing thyroid disease. Women over 45 years of age, patients with known autoimmune diseases, patients with a family history of thyroid disease, and patients receiving lithium or suffering from dementia should be screened for underlying thyroid abnormalities. Patients receiving medications known to influence the interpretation of thyroid function tests should have these considered when interpreting the results of testing.

31. **Who should receive thyroid hormone with the intent of relieving psychiatric symptoms?**

It is recommended that LT_4 therapy be offered to any depressed patient with an elevated serum TSH, especially if accompanied by increased antithyroid antibody titers or low free T_4. Thyroid hormone replacement may alleviate the depression in these individuals. On the other hand, antidepressant therapy, if required, may be ineffective prior to normalization of thyroid axis parameters. In patients with refractory depression but normal thyroid function, adjuvant T_3 therapy may not be worth considering.

BIBLIOGRAPHY

1. Asher R: Myxoedematous madness. Br Med J 22:555–562, 1949.

2. Bauer, M., Baur H, Berghöfer A, et al: Effects of supraphysiological thyroxine administration in healthy controls and patients with depressive disorders. J Affect Disord 68:285–294, 2002.

3. Bunevicius R, Kažanaviius G, Žalinkeviius R, et al: Effects of thyroxine as compared with thyroxine plus triiodothyronine in patients with hypothyroidism. N Engl J Med 340:424–429, 1999.

4. Chopra IJ, Solomon DH, Huang T-S: Serum thyrotropin in hospitalized psychiatric patients: Evidence for hyperthyrotropinemia as measured by ultrasensitive thyrotropin assay. Metabolism 93:538–543, 1990.

5. Fava M, Labbate LA, Abraham ME, et al: Hypothyroidism and hyperthyroidism in major depression revisited. J Clin Psychiatry 56:186–192, 1955.

6. Fliers E, Appelhof BC, Brouwer JP, et al: Efficacy of triiodothyronine (T_3) addition to paroxetine in major depressive disorder: A randomized clinical trial. In Annual Meeting of the Endocrine Society. Philadelphia, The Endocrine Society, 2003, pp S19–S22.

7. Hein MD, Jackson IMD: Thyroid function in psychiatric illness. Gen Hosp Psychol 12:232–244, 1990.

8. Hennessey JV, Jackson IMD: The interface between thyroid hormones and psychiatry. Endocrinologist 6:214–223, 1996.

9. Jackson IMD, Whybrow PC: The relationship between psychiatric disorders and thyroid function. Thyroid Update 9:1–7, 1995.

10. Monzoni F, Del Guerra P, Caraccio N, et al: Subclinical hypothyroidism: Neuro-behavioral features and beneficial effect of L-thyroxine treatment. Clin Invest 71:367–371, 1993.

11. Nelson JC: Augmentation strategies in depression 2000. J Clin Psychiatry 61(Suppl 1):13–19, 2000.

12. Pollock MA, Shyrock A, Marshall K, et al: Thyroxine treatment in patients with symptoms of hypothyroidism but thyroid function tests within the reference range: Randomized double blind placebo controlled crossover trial. Br. Med J 323:891–895, 2002.

13. Report on myxoedema. Transactions of the Clinical Society of London, 1888.

14. Saravanan P, Chau, W-F, Roberets N, et al: Psychological well-being in patients on "adequate" doses of L-thyroxine: Results of a large, controlled community-based questionnaire study. Clin Endocrinol 57:577–585, 2002.

15. Sarne D, DeGroot LJ: Effects of the environment, chemicals and drugs on thyroid function. Endocrine Education, 2002. Available at www.thyroidmanager.org.

16. Sawka AM, Gerstein HC, Marriott MJ, et al: Does a combination regimen of thyroxine (T_4) and 3,5,3′-triiodothyronine improve depressive symptoms better than T_4 alone in patients with hypothyroidism? Results of a double-blind, randomized, controlled trial. J Clin Endocrinol Metab 88:4551–4555, 2003.

17. Walsh JP, Shiels L, Lim EM, et al: Combined thyroxine/liothyronine treatment does not improve well-being, quality of life, or cognitive function compared to thyroxine alone: A randomized controlled trial in patients with primary hypothyroidism. J Clin Endocrinol Metab 88:4543–4550, 2003.

18. Whybrow PC: The therapeutic use of triiodothyronine and high dose thyroxine in psychiatric disorders. Acta Med Aust 21:47–52, 1994.

DISORDERS OF SEXUAL DIFFERENTIATION

Robert H. Slover, M.D.

CHAPTER 43

1. **Describe the first level of sexual differentiation.**
   Chromosomal sex, or more specifically genetic sex, is the first level of differentiation. The great majority of infants are 46XX females or 46XY males. Genetic sex determines gonadal sex. Gonadal sex is determined by the presence or absence of the testis-determining factor called SRY (sex-determining region of the Y). Coded by a gene on the short arm of the Y chromosome, SRY stimulates the undifferentiated gonad to become a testis. If a 46XY infant has a defective or absent SRY gene on the Y chromosome, testes will fail to develop. If a 46XX infant has had a translocation of the SRY gene onto an X chromosome, testes will develop.

2. **What is the next level of sex determination?**
   The next level of sex determination involves the genital duct structures. In the normal male, testicular Leydig cells produce testosterone, which is necessary to maintain ipsilateral Wolffian duct structures (e.g., vas deferens, epididymis, seminal vesicles). Normal testes also produce Müllerian-inhibiting factor (MIF), which acts ipsilaterally to cause regression of Müllerian duct structures (fallopian tubes, uterus, upper third of the vagina). In the absence of testosterone and MIF—as in normal females and some abnormal males, Müllerian duct structures are preserved and Wolffian duct structures regress.

3. **Discuss the development of the external genitalia.**
   Male and female external genitalia arise from the same embryologic structures. In the absence of androgen stimulation, these structures remain in the female pattern, whereas the presence of androgens causes male differentiation (virilization). For complete virilization, testosterone must be converted to dihydrotestosterone (DHT) by the enzyme 5-α-reductase, and androgen receptors must be functional. Excessive androgens virilize a female, whereas inadequate production of androgen, inability to convert testosterone to DHT, or androgen receptor defects result in undervirilization of a male.

4. **How is the decision about sex assignment made?**
   Exogenous and endogenous hormones are clearly important, as is the appearance of the genitalia. The decision about sex assignment must be carefully made, taking into consideration each "level" of sex determination. That decision frequently requires a multidisciplinary approach, including genetics, endocrinology, urology, neonatology, and psychology. It is vital that parents completely understand and support the decision, since ambivalence about sex of rearing may result in gender confusion and psychological trauma.

5. **What is testis-determining factor?**
   The testis-determining factor (TDF) promotes differentiation of the gonad into a testis. Originally considered the H-Y antigen, then ZFY (zinc finger on Y), SRY was eventually characterized as the TDF. SRY belongs to a family of DNA-binding proteins. Specific manipulations have shown that the introduction of SRY will sex reverse XX mice, and site-directed mutagenesis of the SRY gene in XY mice will yield XY females. Other genes on the sex chromosomes and autosomal chromosomes are involved in the regulation of SRY.

6. **Describe the Lyon hypothesis. In which cells are two X chromosomes needed for normal development?**
Dr. Mary Lyon addressed the question of the extra X chromosomal material in females. Simply put, if two X chromosomes are needed in each cell, how can males be developmentally normal? Lyon suggested that in each cell, one of the two X chromosomes is inactive and that in any given cell line, *which* X is active is determined randomly. In fact, the inactive X may be identified in many cells as a clump of chromatin at the nuclear membrane (Barr body). However, two functional X chromosomes are needed for normal sustained ovarian development. Without two X chromosomes per cell (as in 45XO Turner's syndrome), the ovary involutes and leaves only fibrous tissue.

7. **Discuss normal male sexual differentiation.**
The fetus is sexually bipotential. Figure 43-1 shows schematically how male development is accomplished. The undifferentiated gonad is derived from coelomic epithelium, mesenchyme, and germ cells, which, in the presence of SRY, give rise to Leydig cells, Sertoli cells, seminiferous tubules, and spermatogonia. Testes are formed at 7 weeks. Testicular production of testosterone (Leydig cells) and MIF (Sertoli cells) then leads to Wolffian duct development and Müllerian duct regression, respectively. Conversion of testosterone to DHT by 5-α-reductase and subsequent binding of DHT to androgen receptors cause masculinization of the external genitalia.

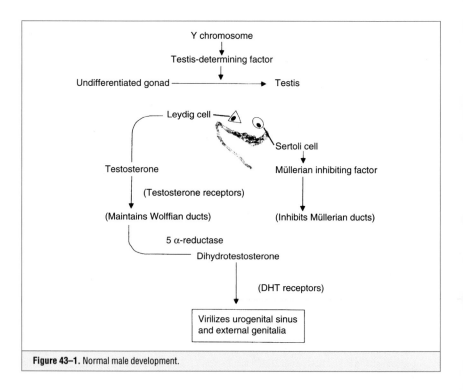

Figure 43–1. Normal male development.

8. **Describe normal female sexual differentiation.**
In the absence of SRY, the undifferentiated gonad gives rise to follicles, granulosa cells, theca cells, and ova. Ovarian development occurs in the 13th–16th weeks of gestation. Lack of

testosterone and MIF allows regression of the Wolffian ducts and maintenance of the Müllerian ducts, respectively. Lack of DHT results in the maintenance of female external genitalia.

9. **How is external genital development determined?**
The external genitalia arise from the urogenital tubercle, urogenital swelling, and urogenital folds. In females these become the clitoris, labia majora, and labia minora, respectively. In males, under the influence of DHT, the genital tubercle becomes the glans of the penis, the urogenital folds elongate and fuse to form the shaft of the penis, and the genital swellings fuse to form the scrotum. Fusion is completed by 70 days of gestation and penile growth continues to term. Female differentiation does not require ovaries or hormonal influence, whereas normal development of male genitalia requires normal testosterone synthesis, conversion to DHT by 5-α-reductase, and normal androgen receptors (see Fig. 43-2).

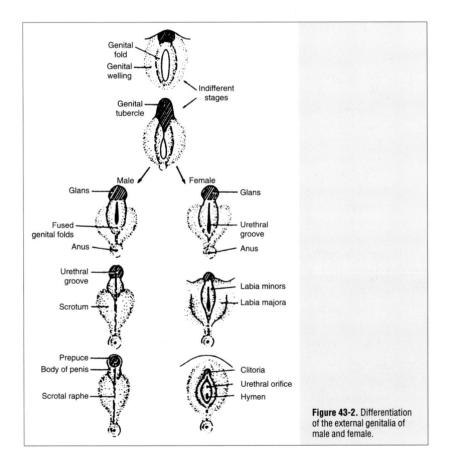

Figure 43-2. Differentiation of the external genitalia of male and female.

10. **The differential diagnosis of sexual differentiation disorders is complex but may be simplified by an approach based on an understanding of the process of sexual differentiation. Can you devise such a classification?**
There are four large categories of ambiguity:
- Virilized 46XX females
- Undervirilized 46XY males

- Disorders of gonadal differentiation
- Unclassified forms, including cryptorchidism, hypospadias, and developmental anomalies

Table 43-1 offers a differential diagnosis based on these categories.

TABLE 43-1. DIFFERENTIAL DIAGNOSIS OF SEXUAL AMBIGUITY

Virilized 46XX females (female pseudohermaphroditism)
    Congenital adrenal hyperplasia (CAH)
        21-hydroxylase deficiency
        11-β-hydroxylase deficiency
        3-β-hydroxysteroid dehydrogenase deficiency
    Maternally derived androgens and synthetic progesterones

Undervirilized 46XY males (male pseudohermaphroditism)
    Testicular unresponsiveness to human chorionic gonadotropin (hCG) and luteinizing
        hormone (LH) (Leydig cell agenesis or hypoplasia)
    Testosterone biosynthesis defects
        Congenital lipoid adrenal hyperplasia (cholesterol side-chain cleavage defect)
        3-β-hydroxysteroid dehydrogenase deficiency
        17-α-hydroxylase deficiency
        17,20-lyase (desmolase) deficiency
        17-β-hydroxysteroid dehydrogenase deficiency
    Peripheral unresponsiveness to androgen
        Androgen insensitivity syndromes (receptor defects)
        5-α-reductase deficiency
    Defects in synthesis, secretion or response to MIF
    Maternal estrogen or progesterone ingestion

Disorders of gonadal differentiation
    46XY partial gonadal dysgenesis
    45X/46XY gonadal dysgenesis
    "Vanishing testes" (embryonic testicular regression; 46XY agonadism; anorchia)
    True hermaphroditism

Unclassified
In males
    Hypospadias
    Cryptorchidism
    Ambiguity secondary to congenital anomalies
In females
    Absence or anomalous development of vagina, uterus, and tubes (Rokitansky syndrome)

---

11. **What is a virilized female?**

A virilized female (previously called female pseudohermaphroditism) is characterized by a 46XX karyotype, ovaries, normal Müllerian duct structures, absent Wolffian duct structures, and virilized genitalia due to exposure to androgens during the first trimester.

12. **What is the most common cause of female pseudohermaphroditism?**
The most common cause of female pseudohermaphroditism is CAH due to 21-hydroxylase deficiency. In fact, this disorder is the single most common cause of sexual ambiguity across the board. The gene responsible for encoding the 21-hydroxylase enzyme is inactive. To produce adequate amounts of cortisol, the fetus makes large amounts of adrenocorticotropic hormone (ACTH), which stimulates increased production of the precursor, 17-hydroxyprogesterone, and of adrenal androgens. Virilization may also be caused by maternal ingestion of androgens or synthetic progesterones during the first trimester of pregnancy.

13. **How do infants with female pseudohermaphroditism present?**
Of importance, affected infants may present with a wide spectrum of ambiguity, ranging from clitoromegaly alone to complete fusion of the labial swellings to form a scrotum and large phallus. Even in the most virilized girls, however, a penile urethra is rare.

14. **What is an undervirilized male?**
An undervirilized male (previously called male pseudohermaphroditism) refers to a 46XY male who has ambiguous or female external genitalia. The abnormality may range from hypospadias to a completely female phenotype. Such disorders result from deficient androgen stimulation of genital development and most often are due to Leydig cell agenesis, testosterone biosynthetic defects, and partial or total androgen resistance (androgen receptor defects).

15. **Which boys with hypospadias should be evaluated for sexual ambiguity?**
First-degree (coronal or glandular) hypospadias as the sole presenting genital abnormality has no apparent endocrine basis and need not be evaluated. The incidence of this anomaly is between 1 and 8 of 1000 births. On the other hand, perineoscrotal hypospadias is a feature of many etiologies of sexual ambiguity, and a child with this finding should be fully evaluated as ambiguous.

16. **What is gonadal dysgenesis?**
Patients with Y-related chromosomal or genetic disorders that cause maldevelopment of one or both testes are said to have gonadal dysgenesis. They present with ambiguous genitalia and may have hypoplasia of Wolffian duct structures and inadequate virilization. MIF may be absent, allowing Müllerian duct structures to persist. Duct asymmetry is therefore common. The Y-containing dysgenetic testes are at risk for developing gonadoblastomas and need to be removed at diagnosis.

17. **An infant is born with ambiguous genitalia, and the sex of the infant is uncertain. How do you approach the parents?**
Honesty and diplomacy are essential. You need to explain that the genitalia are not yet fully developed and that further testing is needed to determine the infant's sex. Reference to more commonly understood birth defects may be useful. Explain that 2–3 days may be necessary to complete the testing, and that a team will participate to make an accurate diagnosis and a considered recommendation. Completion of the birth certificate should be postponed, and the infant should be admitted to the nursery without a sex assignment. You should encourage the family to delay naming the baby and not to give a name applicable to either sex.

18. **What history do you need to evaluate the infant?**
Maternal history is particularly important and should include illnesses, drug ingestion, alcohol intake, and ingestion of hormones during pregnancy. Was progestational therapy used for threatened abortion or androgens for endometriosis? Does the mother have signs of excessive

androgen? Explore family history for occurrence of ambiguity, neonatal deaths, consanguinity, or infertility.

19. **How should you direct the physical examination?**
The diagnosis of the etiology of sexual ambiguity can rarely be made by examination alone, but physical findings can help to direct further evaluation. Look for the following:
   - Are gonads present? Are they normal in size, consistency, and position?
   - What is the phallic length? Measure along the dorsum of the phallus from the pubic ramus to the tip of the glans. At term, a stretched phallic length of 2.5 cm is 2.5 SD below the mean. Assess phallic width and development.
   - Note the position of the urethral meatus, and look for evidence of hypospadias and chordee (ventral curvature secondary to shortened urethra).
   - What is the degree of fusion of the labioscrotal folds? The folds may range from normal labia majora to a fully fused scrotum. In subtle cases, the ratio of the distance from the posterior fourchette to the anus is compared with the total distance from the urethral meatus.
   - Is there an apparent vaginal orifice?

20. **What other areas should be evaluated?**
Certain forms of CAH may cause areolar or genital hyperpigmentation, dehydration, or hypertension. Turner's stigmata may be present, including webbed neck, low hairline, and edema of hands and feet. Other associated congenital anomalies may indicate a complex that includes ambiguity.

21. **Explain which structural studies are needed.**
Structural studies are needed to address the presence of gonads and Müllerian structures. Pelvic ultrasound by qualified personnel should be done as soon as possible to look for a uterus. The presence of gonads, fallopian tubes, and a vaginal vault may also be determined. If necessary, a genitogram may be performed by inserting contrast material into the urogenital orifice (or vaginal orifice) to define vaginal size, presence of a cervix and any fistulas.

22. **Explain the role of karyotyping.**
A karyotype is essential and must be obtained expeditiously. Buccal smears are absolutely contraindicated because they are inaccurate. In many laboratories, a karyotype can be completed within 48–72 hours. Some laboratories can also do FISH analysis for the presence of the *SRY* gene.

23. **What laboratory test is helpful?**
Because 21-hydroxylase deficiency is a relatively common cause of sexual ambiguity, we assess the level of 17-hydroxyprogesterone in all such infants who do not have palpable gonads.

24. **How is further evaluation directed?**
Further evaluation must be directed by information provided through the history, examination, and initial studies. Determining presence or absence of palpable gonads (presumably testes), presence or absence of a uterus, and karyotype allows classification of the infant as virilized female, undervirilized male, a disorder of gonadal differentiation, or one of the unclassified forms.

25. **The infant has no palpable gonads and has fused labioscrotal folds and a prominent phallus. The ultrasound reveals a uterus and tubes with possible ovaries. The karyotype is 46XX. How do you proceed?**
The infant is a virilized female. If there is no history of maternal androgen ingestion or virilization, the infant has one of three forms of CAH. Of these, 21-hydroxylase deficiency is most common and is confirmed by finding an elevated serum level of 17-hydroxyprogesterone.

In 11-β-hydroxylase deficiency, 11-deoxycortisol is elevated, whereas 17-hydroxypregnenolone and dehydroepiandrosterone (DHEA) are elevated in 3-β-hydroxysteroid dehydrogenase deficiency. The baseline levels are usually diagnostic but can be confirmed by an ACTH stimulation test. The electrolyte disturbances seen with such disorders do not usually occur until 8–14 days of life. Many states now screen for CAH.

26. **An undervirilized male represents a more complex diagnostic dilemma. In an infant with palpable gonads, no Müllerian structures and a 46XY karyotype, what is your next step?**
Figure 43-3 outlines the testosterone synthesis pathway. Defects in testosterone synthesis include three enzyme blocks common to the adrenal and testicular pathways (cholesterol side-chain cleavage defect, 3-β-hydroxysteroid dehydrogenase deficiency, and 17-α-hydroxylase deficiency). Enzyme blocks are diagnosed with ACTH stimulation testing and measurement of precursors. Cholesterol side-chain cleavage defects have no measurable precursors but show high levels of ACTH and a low cortisol response. Patients with 17-α-hydroxylase deficiency have elevated levels of progesterone, desoxycorticosterone, and corticosterone, with associated hypertension. Infants with 3-β-hydroxysteroid dehydrogenase deficiency have elevated levels of 17-hydroxypregnenolone and DHEA.

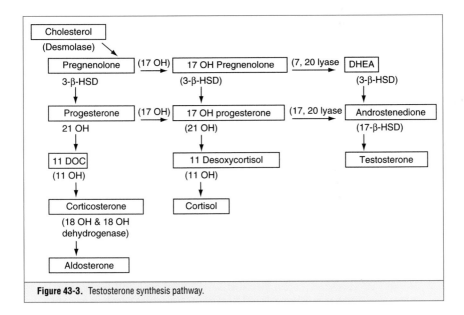

Figure 43-3. Testosterone synthesis pathway.

27. **Discuss the two remaining defects that involve deficiencies of testicular rather than adrenal enzymes.**
The two remaining defects in testosterone synthesis involve deficiencies of testicular rather than adrenal enzymes: 17,20-lyase and 17-β-hydroxysteroid dehydrogenase. Thus, they are not associated with elevations of ACTH or electrolyte disturbances. Both deficiencies are diagnosed by measuring the precursor response to administration of hCG. Infants with 17,20-lyase deficiency have elevated levels of 17-hydroxypregnenolone and 17-hydroxyprogesterone, whereas infants with 17-β-hydroxysteroid dehydrogenase deficiency have elevated levels of DHEA and androstenedione.

28. **What other possibilities should be investigated?**
    - Infants with Leydig cell hypoplasia have low levels of testosterone after hCG stimulation but normal adrenal function. Testicular biopsy reveals normal seminiferous tubules but absent or few Leydig cells.
    - Stimulation with hCG also allows measurement of the testosterone-to-DHT ratio. If the ratio is elevated, 5-α-reductase deficiency should be suspected and may be confirmed by cultures of genital skin fibroblasts.
    - Finally, normal testosterone levels with no abnormalities in ACTH and hCG testing lead to the diagnosis of partial androgen insensitivity (androgen receptor defects). The diagnosis is made by demonstrating abnormal androgen binding in cultures of genital skin fibroblasts in a research laboratory, or molecular analysis.

29. **What is complete androgen insensitivity?**
    The androgen receptor, encoded on the X chromosome, binds testosterone and, more avidly, DHT. Androgen insensitivity results from abnormalities of the androgen receptor. Complete androgen resistance occurs with a frequency of 1 in 20,000 to 1 in 64,000 XY infants.

30. **How do infants with complete androgen insensitivity present?**
    Strictly speaking, complete androgen insensitivity (testicular feminization) rarely presents as ambiguity in the newborn period or early childhood. Unless the testes have descended and are palpable in the labia majora, affected infants appear as phenotypically normal females. Affected children grow as normal females until puberty. They feminize with normal breast development because high levels of testosterone are aromatized to estrogen, but they have no pubic or axillary hair and no menses. Because they produce MIF, they lack Müllerian duct structures. Wolffian duct structures are also rudimentary or absent because they lack normal testosterone receptors. Gender identity is usually female. Patients come to medical attention because of primary amenorrhea. The diagnosis is therefore frequently missed until patients are in their mid- to late teens.

31. **When should the intra-abdominal testes be removed?**
    The intra-abdominal testes are at risk for malignancy, particularly after the onset of puberty. Timing of gonadectomy is debated. Because the risk of malignancy is low until puberty, some prefer to leave the gonads intact until spontaneous pubertal development; on the other hand, because carcinoma in situ has been found in prepubertal patients, others recommend early removal. If the testes are removed before puberty, estrogen therapy is necessary for normal pubertal progression. Because the upper section of the vagina is Müllerian in origin, affected individuals may have shortened vaginas and need plastic surgical repair.

32. **Summarize the physiologic results of 5-α-reductase deficiency.**
    Deficiency of 5-α-reductase impairs the conversion of testosterone to DHT, leading to incomplete virilization and differentiation of the external genitalia. The disorder is particularly well documented in large kindreds in the Dominican Republic and Gaza, in whom it is inherited as an autosomal recessive condition.

33. **Describe the clinical picture of 5-α-reductase deficiency.**
    Male infants with 5-α-reductase deficiency are born with sexual ambiguity. External genitalia range from a penis with simple hypospadias to a blind vaginal pouch and clitoris-like phallus. The most common presentation is a urogenital sinus with a blind vaginal pouch. During puberty, affected boys undergo virilization; affected females are normal. Traditionally, infants with 5-α-reductase deficiency were raised as females until puberty, then continued life as males and, in some cases, achieved fertility. Recently, however, the condition has been recognized early in life, and affected males are now raised from infancy as boys.

KEY POINTS: DISORDERS OF SEXUAL DIFFERENTIATION ✓

1. Sexual ambiguity in a newborn must be seen as a social/psychological emergency requiring a multidisciplinary team approach to assign a sex of rearing.

2. Members of the team include the pediatric endocrinologist, urologist, geneticist, pediatrician, and appropriate counselors.

3. Evaluation of ambiguity must consider the four major categories of children; virilized 46XX females, undervirilized 46XY males, disorders of gonadal differentiation, and unclassified forms (cryptorchidism, hypospadias, developmental anomalies).

4. The most common cause of sexual ambiguity in newborns is CAH, with 21-hydroxylase deficiency as the leading defect.

5. As a general rule, gonadal tissue containing Y chromosomal material is at higher risk for development of malignancy. Consideration must be given to surgical removal of such gonads at some point.

34. **What is a "true hermaphrodite"?**

True hermaphroditism, a disorder of gonadal differentiation, refers to people with both ovarian and testicular elements. Affected children may have bilateral ovotestes, an ovary or testis on one side with an ovotestis on the other, or an ovary on one side and testis on the other. Because the effects of MIF and testosterone on duct structures are ipsilateral and localized, internal duct development is often asymmetrical. Thus, a fallopian tube and unicornuate uterus, with absent or vestigial male duct structures, may develop on the side without testicular elements, whereas epididymis, vas deferens, and seminal vesicles without Müllerian structures may develop on the side with testicular elements. The genitalia may be male, female, or ambiguous, depending on the amount of functioning testicular tissue.

35. **Why is a multidisciplinary team needed in approaching an infant with sexual ambiguity?**

Sexual ambiguity is a complex issue in numerous ways. Accurate diagnosis is essential and may take a fair amount of time. Sex of assignment must be based not only on underlying diagnosis and karyotype but also on potential for adult sexual function, fertility, and psychological health. For these reasons, input from several specialties, including endocrinology, genetics, neonatology, psychology, and urology, is important. All members of the team must communicate adequately with each other. Parents must fully understand the medical recommendation for sex assignment and required therapy. They must whole-heartedly agree and support the assigned sex to avoid ambivalence, which can lead to gender confusion and psychological trauma for the child.

36. **Once the etiology of sexual ambiguity has been determined in an infant, how does karyotype affect gender assignment?**

Arriving at a precise diagnosis provides the treating team an understanding of potential risks and benefits of either sex assignment. Karyotype is not the only important factor. For example, in a poorly virilized male, the difference in outcome among children with defects in testosterone synthesis, complete androgen insensitivity, and 5-α-reductase deficiency is enormous. A child with defective synthesis of testosterone may be raised male or female, depending on other factors; a child with complete androgen insensitivity should be raised female; and a boy with 5-α-reductase deficiency usually is raised male. Yet children affected by any of the three conditions have 46XY karyotypes.

37. **What other factors must be considered?**
What is the potential for unambiguous genital appearance? What is the potential for normal sexual function? Is there a potential for fertility? What was the in utero hormone exposure? What are the factors likely to affect gender identity and psychological health? Phallic size, urethral position, vaginal anatomy, and presence or absence of Müllerian or Wolffian duct structures, as well as gonadal characteristics and karyotype, must be considered.

38. **To which gender are virilized females usually assigned?**
Virilized females are usually assigned a female sex. They have normal ovaries, as well as Müllerian structures and, with surgical correction and steroid replacement, can have normal sexual function and achieve fertility.

39. **How is sex assignment determined in undervirilized males?**
Undervirilized males are often infertile, and sex assignment has usually been based on phallic size. Because a stretched penile length of 2.5 cm is 2.5 SD below the mean, an infant with a phallus smaller than 2.5 cm usually is assigned a female sex of rearing. Deficiency of 5-α-reductase is an obvious exception. If male sex assignment is contemplated, a trial of depot testosterone (50 mg every 3–4 weeks) for 1–3 months indicates whether phallic growth is possible.

40. **Summarize the factors that determine sex assignment in patients with gonadal dysgenesis.**
In patients with gonadal dysgenesis and Y chromosomal material, gonadectomy is necessary and fertility is not possible. Internal duct structure is also frequently deranged. Small phallic size usually leads to a female sex assignment.

41. **How is sex assignment determined in true hermaphrodites?**
True hermaphrodites who have a unilateral ovary and Müllerian structures may have spontaneous puberty and normal fertility and are raised as females. External genital size and structure may allow male assignment, but more commonly, external genitalia are poorly virilized and affected infants are assigned a female sex.

42. **What caveats should be kept in mind when sex assignments are made?**
We need to learn much more about gender identity and consider which decisions might be made later than previously thought. Some surgical interventions are cosmetic, and some affected patients have expressed the wish that they should make the decisions in adolescence or adulthood. This field challenges many of our perceptions of sex and gender and our role as physicians.

BIBLIOGRAPHY

1. Goodall J: Helping a child to understand her own testicular feminization. Lancet 337:33, 1991.
2. Jasso N, Boussin L, Knebelmann B, et al.: Anti-müllerian hormone and intersex states. Trends Endocrinol Metab 2:227, 1991.
3. Kaplan S: Clinical Pediatric Endocrinology. Philadelphia, W.B. Saunders, 1990.
4. Low Y, Hutson JM, for the Murdoch Childrens Research Institute Sex Study Group: Rules for clinical diagnosis in babies with ambiguous genitalia. J Paediatr Child Health 39:406, 2003.
5. McGillivray BC: The newborn with ambiguous genitalia. Semin Perinatol 16:365, 1992.
6. Meyers-Seifer CH, Charest NJ: Diagnosis and management of patients with ambiguous genitalia. Semin Perinatol 16:332, 1992.
7. Mulaikal RM, Migeon CJ, Rock JA, et al.: Fertility rates in female patients with congenital adrenal hyperplasia due to 21-hydroxylase deficiency. N Engl J Med 316:178, 1987.
8. Pagona R: Diagnostic approach to the newborn with ambiguous genitalia. Pediatr Clin North Am 34:1019, 1987.

9. Penny R: Ambiguous genitalia. Am J Dis Child 144:753, 1990.

10. Rangecroft L, for the British Association of Paediatric Surgeons Working Party on the Surgical Management of Children Born with Ambiguous Genitalia: Surgical management of ambiguous genitalia. Arch Dis Child 88:799, 2003.

11. Thigpen AE, Davis DL, Gautier T, et al: Brief report: The molecular basis of steroid 5 alpha-reductase deficiency in a large Dominican kindred. N Engl J Med 327:1216, 1992.

12. Warne GL, Kanumakala S: Molecular endocrinology of sex differentiation. Semin Reprod Med 20(3):169, 2002.

13. Zucker KJ, et al: Psychosexual development of women with congenital adrenal hyperplasia. Hormone Behav 30:300, 1996.

CHAPTER 44

DISORDERS OF PUBERTY

Sharon H. Travers, M.D., and Robert H. Slover, M.D.

1. **What physiologic events initiate puberty?**

   Maturation of the hypothalamic-pituitary axis initiates puberty. The hypothalamus begins to secrete gonadotropin-releasing hormone (GnRH) in pulses during sleep and eventually during waking hours as well. GnRH pulses stimulate the pituitary gland to secrete pulses of gonadotropins, of which there is luteinizing hormone (LH) predominance. In response to the increased secretion of gonadotropins, there is increased secretion of gonadal hormones that lead to the progressive development of secondary sexual characteristics and gametogenesis.

2. **Define adrenarche.**

   Adrenarche refers to the time during puberty when the adrenal glands increase their production and secretion of adrenal androgens. Plasma concentrations of dehydroepiandrosterone (DHEA) and DHEA-sulfate(s), the most important adrenal androgens, begin to increase in children by about 6–8 years. However, the signs of adrenarche, such as pubic and axillary hair development, acne, and body odor, do not typically occur until early to mid-puberty. The control of adrenal androgen secretion is not clearly understood, but it does appear to be separate from GnRH and the gonadotropins.

3. **What is the normal pattern of puberty in males?**

   The mean age of onset of puberty in boys is 11.5 years with a range of 9–14 years. In both sexes, puberty requires maturation of gonadal function and increased secretion of adrenal androgens (adrenarche). The first evidence of puberty in the majority of boys is enlargement of the testes to greater than 4 mL in volume or greater than 2.5 cm in length. It is not until mid-puberty, when testosterone levels are rapidly rising, that boys experience voice change, axillary and facial hair, and the peak growth spurt. Spermatogenesis is mature at a mean age of 13.3 years.

4. **Describe the normal pattern of female pubertal development.**

   Girls normally begin puberty between ages 8 and 13 years (mean age: 10.6 years for white girls and 9.5 years for black girls). The initial pubertal event is typically the appearance of breast buds, although in a small percentage of girls, pubic hair development may appear first. Initial breast development often occurs asymmetrically and should not be of concern. Breast development is primarily under the control of estrogens secreted by the ovaries, whereas pubic and axillary hair growth result mainly from adrenal androgens. Unlike boys, the pubertal growth spurt in girls occurs at the onset of puberty. Menarche usually occurs 18–24 months after the onset of breast development (mean age: 12.8 years). Although most girls have reached about 97.5% of their maximum height potential at menarche, this can vary considerably. Consequently, age of menarche is not necessarily a good predictor of adult height.

5. **What controls the pubertal growth spurt?**

   In both boys and girls, the pubertal growth spurt is primarily controlled by gonadal steroids. Gonadal steroids augment growth hormone secretion and also have direct stimulatory effects on bone and cartilage. At the end of puberty, linear growth is near complete as a result of the effects of gonadal steroids on skeletal maturation and epiphyseal fusion.

6. How is pubertal development measured?

Sexual maturity is determined by examination and is described by a scale devised by John Tanner in 1969 (Table 44-1). Because of the distinct actions of adrenal androgens and gonadal steroids, it is important to distinguish between breast and pubic hair development in girls and between genital and pubic hair development in boys. In all cases, Tanner stage I is prepubertal and Tanner stage V is complete maturation. In addition to the physical examination, the tools to assess pubertal development may include determination of bone age, growth velocity and pattern, and specific endocrine studies.

TABLE 44-1. TANNER STAGES OF PUBERTAL DEVELOPMENT

Stage	Characteristics	Stage	Characteristics
Girls:	*Breast development*		*Pubic hair development*
I	Prepubertal; elevation of papilla only	I	Prepubertal; no pubic hair
II	Breast buds are noted or palpable; enlargement of areola	II	Sparse growth of long, straight, or slightly curly, minimally pigmented hair, mainly of labia
III	Further enlargement of breast and areola, with no separation of their contours	III	Considerably darker and coarser hair spreading over mons pubis
IV	Projection of areola and papilla to form secondary mound above level of breast	IV	Thick, adult-type hair that does not yet spread to medial surface of thighs
V	Adult contour breast with projection of papilla only	V	Hair adult in type and distributed in classic inverse triangle
Boys:	*Genital development*		*Pubic hair development*
I	Prepubertal; testicular length < 2.5 cm	I	Prepubertal; no pubic hair
II	Testes > 2.5 cm in longest diameter scrotum thinning and reddening	II	Sparse growth of slightly pigmented, slightly curly pubic hair, mainly at base of penis
III	Growth of penis in width and length and further growth of testes	III	Thicker, curlier hair, spread to mons pubis
IV	Penis further enlarged; testes larger, with darker scrotal skin color	IV	Adult-type hair that does not yet spread to medial surface of thighs
V	Genitalia adult in size and shape	V	Adult-type hair spread to medial thighs

Data from Marshall WE, Tanner JM: Variations in the pattern of pubertal changes in girls. Arch Dis Child 44:291–303, 1969; and Variations in the pattern of pubertal changes in boys. Arch Dis Child 45:13–23, 1970.

7. **What constitutes sexual precocity in boys and girls?**
   Precocious puberty is defined as pubertal development occurring below the limits of age set for normal onset of puberty. In girls, this is puberty before 8 years of age and for boys, before 9 years of age. Breast development can occur normally as early as 7 years in white girls and 6 years in black girls. Consequently, evaluation and treatment of girls who start puberty between 6 and 8 years should depend on factors such as family history, rapidity of development, presence of central nervous system (CNS) symptoms, and family concern. Girls who are short and start puberty between 6 and 8 years may also benefit from evaluation. In children who present with early pubertal signs, precocious puberty must be distinguished from normal variants of puberty, such as benign premature thelarche and benign premature adrenarche.

8. **What clinical findings are associated with precocious puberty?**
   Precocious puberty, regardless of the cause, is associated with increased linear growth and skeletal maturation secondary to elevated sex steroid levels. Children with precocious puberty are often tall for their age during childhood. However, skeletal maturation may become more advanced than stature, leading to premature fusion of the epiphyseal growth plates and a compromised adult height. In addition to the physical consequences of early puberty, there are social and psychological aspects that the practitioner needs to consider.

9. **In which sex is precocity more prevalent? Why?**
   Precocious puberty predominantly affects girls. The disparity in overall prevalence of precocity is explained by the large numbers of precocious girls with central idiopathic precocity, a condition that is unusual in boys. At least 80% of all precocious puberty in girls is central idiopathic in nature. The prevalence of organic etiologies of precocious puberty (CNS lesions, gonadal tumors, and specific underlying diseases) is similar in both sexes.

10. **Which two common benign conditions in girls are often confused with precocious puberty?**
    - *Premature thelarche* is defined as isolated breast development in girls without accompanying signs of adrenarche, such as pubic/axillary hair, body odor, and acne.
    - *Premature adrenarche*, which occurs in both genders, is defined as the early development of pubic hair with or without axillary hair, body odor, and acne. There are no signs of gonadarche in this condition; thus, girls have no breast development and boys show no testicular enlargement.

11. **How is benign premature thelarche diagnosed?**
    Several characteristics of premature thelarche distinguish it from the breast development that occurs in precocious puberty. First of all, premature thelarche is most common in girls who are either under 2 years or between 6 and 8 years of age. Girls with premature thelarche may have a history of slowly progressing breast development or waxing and waning of breast size. Growth rate and bone age are not accelerated and on physical examination, the breast tissue rarely develops beyond Tanner stages 2–3. GnRH stimulation may provoke a follicle-stimulating hormone (FSH)-predominant response as opposed to the typical LH-predominant response seen in true central precocity.

12. **How is benign premature thelarche treated?**
    The natural course of benign thelarche is for the breast tissue to regress or fail to progress. Because of its benign nature, treatment is not necessary except for reassurance and follow-up. Follow-up is critical because premature thelarche occasionally is the first sign of what later becomes apparent as central precocious puberty.

13. **How is benign premature adrenarche diagnosed? Treated?**
Premature adrenarche is caused by early secretion of the adrenal androgens, primarily DHEA and DHEA-S. A child who has premature adrenarche and Tanner stage 2 pubic hair development will have adrenal androgen values similar to those normally found in a pubertal child at the same stage of development. As in premature thelarche, growth rate and bone age are not accelerated.

14. **How is benign premature adrenarche treated?**
The natural course of premature adrenarche is for the signs to slowly progress without having an effect on the timing of true puberty. Since pubic hair development may be the first sign of puberty, especially in girls, follow-up is necessary to evaluate for evidence of gonadarche (i.e., breast development). If signs of puberty are rapidly progressing or if there is evidence of increased linear growth and advanced bone age, measurement of androgens (DHEA-S, androstenedione, and testosterone) is performed to evaluate for a serious virilizing disorder, such as congenital adrenal hyperplasia (CAH) or an adrenal tumor.

15. **How does GnRH-dependent (central) precocious puberty differ from GnRH-independent (peripheral) precocious puberty?**
Central precocious puberty involves activation of the GnRH pulse generator, an increase in gonadotropin secretion, and a resultant increase in the production of sex steroids. Consequently, the sequence of hormonal and physical events in central precocious puberty is identical to the progression of normal puberty. Peripheral precocious puberty occurs independent of gonadotropin secretion. The causes of precocious puberty are listed in Table 44-2.

TABLE 44-2. CAUSES OF PRECOCIOUS PUBERTY

Central (GnRH-dependent)
Idiopathic true precocious puberty
CNS tumors (hamartomas, hypothalamic tumors)
CNS disorders (meningitis, encephalitis, hydrocephalus, trauma, abscesses, cysts, granulomas, radiation therapy)

Peripheral (GnRH-independent)
Males
Human chorionic gonadotropin (hCG)-secreting tumors (CNS, liver)
CAH (21-hydroxylase, 3-β-hydroxysteroid dehydrogenase, or 11-hydroxylase deficiency)
Adrenal tumors
Leydig cell testicular tumors
Familial gonadotropin-independent Leydig cell maturation (testotoxicosis)
McCune-Albright syndrome (polyostotic fibrous dysplasia)

Females
Follicular cysts
Ovarian tumors
Adrenal tumors
CAH (21-hydroxylase, 3-β-hydroxysteroid dehydrogenase, or 11-hydroxylase deficiency)
Exogenous estrogen
McCune-Albright syndrome (polyostotic fibrous dysplasia)

16. **How is the diagnosis of precocious puberty made?**
The diagnosis of precocious puberty requires the appearance of the physical signs of puberty before the age of 8 years in girls or 9 years in boys. In both boys and girls, a complete history should be taken, with careful consideration of any exposure to exogenous steroids, onset of pubertal signs and rate of progression, presence or history of CNS abnormalities, and pubertal history of other family members. Height measurements should be plotted on a growth chart to determine growth velocity. A physical examination is performed with focus on Tanner staging, presence of café-au-lait spots, and neurologic signs. One of the first steps in evaluating a child with early pubertal development is obtaining a radiograph of the left hand and wrist to determine skeletal maturity (bone age). If the bone age is advanced, further evaluation is typically warranted.

17. **After making the general diagnosis of precocity, how do I proceed to a specific diagnosis?**
It is usually difficult to distinguish GnRH-dependent (central) from GnRH-independent (peripheral) precocity on physical examination. Although the possible causes of peripheral precocious puberty are more numerous (see Table 44-2), central precocity accounts for the overwhelming majority of cases. Sex steroid levels, especially in boys, should be measured; testosterone levels above the prepubertal range (> 10 ng/dL) confirm pubertal status but do not indicate the cause. Estrogen values in girls are not as helpful because slightly elevated levels may indicate either early puberty or benign thelarche.

18. **What is the single most important test in establishing a specific diagnosis?**
The single most important test is a GnRH stimulation test to determine whether gonadotropin responses are consistent with central or peripheral precocious puberty. The diagnosis of central precocious puberty is made by demonstrating an LH response to GnRH greater than 7–10 IU/L. Measurement of random gonadotropins is typically not helpful because of overlap between prepubertal and early pubertal values. If random gonadotropins are measured, a third-generation assay is recommended as it has better discrimination between prepubertal and pubertal levels.

19. **When is an MRI study of the brain indicated?**
In all boys and in girls less than 6 years of age who are diagnosed with central precocious puberty, a magnetic resonance imaging (MRI) study of the brain should be done to evaluate for CNS lesions. It is unlikely that an abnormality will be found in girls between 6 and 8 years, so the need for an MRI in this age group should be individually assessed.

20. **What findings suggest peripheral precocious puberty?**
A suppressed or prepubertal LH response to GnRH suggests that high sex steroid levels (causing negative feedback) are being produced independently of gonadotropin stimulation, a pattern consistent with peripheral precocious puberty. In girls, pelvic ultrasound and serum estradiol levels are obtained in this scenario to evaluate for an ovarian cyst, tumor, or McCune-Albright syndrome. In boys with suspected peripheral precocious puberty, additional laboratory studies should include serum hCG, DHEA-S, and androstenedione levels. Elevated adrenal androgens could indicate an adrenal tumor or CAH. To further evaluate for CAH, measurement of baseline or adrenocorticotropic hormone (ACTH)-stimulated steroid intermediates (e.g., 17-hydroxy progesterone, 17-hydroxy pregnenolone, 11-deoxycortisol) is recommended. Asymmetric or unilateral enlargement of the testes suggests a Leydig cell tumor.

21. **How is central idiopathic precocious puberty treated?**
Children with central precocious puberty can be treated with GnRH analogs, such as leuprolide. GnRH analogs down-regulate pituitary GnRH receptors and thus decrease gonadotropin secretion. With treatment, physical changes of puberty regress or cease to progress, and linear

growth slows to a prepubertal rate. Typically, pubic and axillary hair may persist. Projected final heights often increase as a result of slowing of skeletal maturation. Usually, GnRH analogs are given as a monthly depot intramuscular injection, and side effects are rare. After discontinuation of therapy, pubertal progression resumes, and in girls ovulation and pregnancy have been documented. Therapy is considered for both psychosocial and final height considerations. For example, in a girl who is near the normal age of puberty and who has slowly progressing development, treatment would not necessarily be indicated. However, the same age girl who has already progressed to menarche may benefit psychosocially from treatment. Children on GnRH analogs should be monitored every 4–6 months.

22. **What is the association of hypothyroidism with precocity?**
Rare cases of primary hypothyroidism in children may cause breast development in girls and increased testicular size in boys. The mechanism is most likely related to excessive TSH or alpha-subunit secretion, which can activate gonadotropin receptors. These children generally present with growth deceleration rather than acceleration as typically seen in precocious puberty. Bone ages are typically delayed. Thyroid hormone replacement results in regression of pubertal changes and no other therapy is necessary.

23. **What is McCune-Albright syndrome? How is it treated?**
McCune-Albright syndrome is a triad consisting of irregular (coast-of-Maine) café-au-lait lesions, polyostotic fibrous dysplasia, and GnRH-independent precocious puberty. It affects both sexes but is seen infrequently in boys. In girls, breast development and vaginal bleeding occur with sporadic increases in estradiol. Serum gonadotropin levels are low, and GnRH testing elicits a prepubertal response. With time, however, increased estradiol may mature the hypothalamus, thus leading to true central GnRH-dependent precocity. The syndrome is often associated with other endocrine dysfunction, including hyperthyroidism, hyperparathyroidism, adrenal hyperplasia, Cushing's syndrome, and gigantism. In affected tissues, there is an activating mutation in the gene that encodes the alpha-subunit of Gs, the G-protein that stimulates adenylate cylase. Endocrine cells with this mutation have autonomous hyperfunction and secrete excess amounts of their respective hormones.

24. **How is McCune-Albright treated?**
Girls with McCune-Albright syndrome are generally treated with testolactone, a medication that inhibits the aromatization of testosterone to estrogen. Testolactone, however, is not effective in many girls, and recently there have been trials using tamoxifen, an estrogen receptor antagonist. In boys, treatment consists of either inhibiting androgen production with ketoconazole or a combination of an aromatase inhibitor that blocks the conversion of androgen to estrogen and an antiandrogen that antagonizes androgen at the receptor.

25. **Describe testotoxicosis. How is it treated?**
Familial testotoxicosis is an autosomal dominant, gonadotropin-independent form of male precocity. Boys with this condition begin to develop true precocity with testicular and phallic enlargement and growth acceleration by the age of 4 years. Serum testosterone levels are high, but serum gonadotropins are low and GnRH testing shows a prepubertal response. By mid-adolescence to adulthood, GnRH stimulation demonstrates a more typical LH-predominant pubertal response. The cause, in some families, has been found to be an activating mutation in the gene encoding the LH receptor. The mutant LH receptors in the testes are constitutively overactive and do not require LH binding for their activity but produce testosterone autonomously. Treatment options are the same as for boys with McCune-Albright syndrome.

26. **How does nonsalt-wasting CAH present in boys?**
The most common adrenogenital syndrome is 21-hydroxylase deficiency. Girls usually develop virilization in utero, resulting in a degree of sexual ambiguity. They are discovered at birth

and should be diagnosed within the first few days of life by the finding of greatly elevated serum 17-hydroxyprogesterone levels. In the more common salt-losing form of this disease, boys present with vomiting, shock, and electrolyte disturbances at 7–10 days of age. Fortunately, with neonatal screening for 21-hydroxylase deficiency, boys are being diagnosed prior to developing life-threatening electrolyte abnormalities. A small subset of affected boys and girls do not waste salt and may present in early or late childhood with signs of adrenarche, such as pubic hair, acne, body odor, acceleration of linear growth, and skeletal maturation. A similar presentation occurs in the less common forms of CAH, such as 3-β-hydroxysteroid deficiency and 11-hydroxylase deficiency. 11-Hydroxylase deficiency is also associated with hypertension.

27. **Summarize the treatment of nonsalt-wasting CAH.**
Treatment for all forms of CAH is directed at reducing serum androgen levels by replacing glucocorticoids to reduce pituitary secretion of ACTH. In salt-wasting CAH, the mineralocorticoid, florinef, is required. This is not needed in the nonsalt-wasting forms.

28. **What is adolescent gynecomastia? When and how should it be treated?**
Normal boys often have either unilateral or bilateral breast enlargement during puberty. Breast development generally starts during early puberty and resolves within 2 years. The cause of gynecomastia is not clearly understood but may be related to an elevated ratio of estradiol to testosterone levels. Treatment primarily consists of reassurance and support; however, if resolution does not occur or if the breast enlargement is excessive, surgery may be warranted. Pathologic conditions associated with gynecomastia include Klinefelter's syndrome and various other testosterone-deficient states.

29. **At what age does failure to enter puberty necessitate investigation?**
Delayed puberty should be evaluated if there are no pubertal signs by 13 years of age in girls and by 14 years of age in boys. An abnormality in the pubertal axis may also present as lack of normal pubertal progression, which is defined as more than 4 years between the first signs of puberty and menarche in girls, or more than 5 years for completion of genital growth in boys.

30. **What is constitutional growth delay? How does it affect puberty?**
Constitutional growth delay is the most common cause of delayed puberty. Children with this growth pattern have a fall-off in their linear growth within the first 2 years of life; after this, growth returns to normal, albeit at a lower growth channel than would be expected for parental heights. Skeletal maturation is also delayed, and the onset of puberty is commensurate with bone age rather than chronologic age. For example, a 14-year-old boy with a bone age of 11 years will appropriately start puberty when his bone age is closer to 11.5–12 years. The delay in puberty postpones the pubertal growth spurt and closure of growth plates, so that the child continues to grow after his/her peers have reached their final height. A key feature of this growth pattern is normal linear growth after 2 years of age. There is often a family history of "late bloomers."

31. **How do you distinguish between constitutional delay and hormonal disorders?**
It is often challenging to differentiate between constitutional delay and hormonal disorders of pubertal development, such as gonadotropin deficiency, in the prepubertal period. Time and careful observation are important tools.

32. **When is hypogonadism diagnosed?**
Functional or permanent hypogonadism should be considered when there are no signs of puberty and bone age has advanced to beyond the normal ages for puberty to start. An eunuchoid body habitus is often evident in children with abnormally delayed puberty; a decreased upper to lower body ratio and long arm span characterize this habitus. As a rule, serum gonadotropin levels are measured first to determine whether there is hypogonadotropic hypogonadism (gonadotropin deficiency) or hypergonadotropic hypogonadism (primary

gonadal failure). If a child's bone age is below the normal age for puberty to start, gonadotropin levels are not a reliable means of making an accurate diagnosis.

33. **What hypergonadotropic conditions may cause delayed or lack of pubertal development?**
    - Variants of ovarian and testicular dysgenesis (Turner's syndrome, Klinefelter's syndrome, pure XX or XY gonadal dysgenesis).
    - Gonadal toxins (chemotherapy and/or radiation treatment).
    - Androgen enzymatic defects (17-α-hydroxylase deficiency in the genetic male or female; 17-keto-steroid reductase deficiency in the genetic male).
    - Complete and partial androgen insensitivity syndrome.
    - Other miscellaneous disorders (infections, vanishing testes, traumatic, surgical, torsion).
    - Galactosemia (in girls only)

34. **What hypogonadotropic conditions may cause delayed or lack of pubertal development?**
    - Multiple pituitary hormone deficiencies (empty sella syndrome, pituitary dysgenesis, inflammation, Rathke's pouch cysts, trauma, cranial radiation, tumors [craniopharyngiomas]).
    - Isolated gonadotropin deficiency (Kallmann's syndrome, Laurence-Moon-Bardet-Biedl syndrome, Prader-Willi syndrome).

35. **List the causes of delayed or deferred function that leads to lack of pubertal development.**
    - Constitutional delay of growth and/or puberty
    - Chronic illness
    - Malnutrition/anorexia
    - Drug abuse
    - Excessive energy expenditure/exercise
    - Endocrinopathies (diabetes mellitus, growth hormone deficiency, glucocorticoid excess, hyperprolactinemia, hypothyroidism)

36. **What causes hypogonadotropic hypogonadism?**
    Chronic illnesses, malnutrition, exercise, and anorexia can cause a functional deficiency of gonadotropins that reverses when the underlying condition improves. Hyperprolactinemia can also present as delayed puberty and only 50% of the time will there be a history of galactorrhea. Permanent gonadotropin deficiency is suspected if these conditions are ruled out and gonadotropin levels are low. Gonadotropin deficiency may be associated with other pituitary deficiencies from conditions, such as septo-optic dysplasia, craniopharyngioma, or cranial irradiation. Various syndromes, such as Prader-Willi syndrome, are also associated with gonadotropin deficiency. Isolated gonadotropin deficiency (i.e., occurring without another pituitary deficiency) is often difficult to diagnose, as hormonal tests do not absolutely distinguish whether a child can produce enough gonadotropins or whether he/she simply has very delayed puberty. If gonadotropin deficiency cannot be clearly distinguished from delayed puberty, a short course of sex steroids can be given for 4–6 months. Patients with constitutional delay often enter puberty after such an intervention. If spontaneous puberty does not occur after this treatment or after a second course, the diagnosis of gonadotropin deficiency may be made.

37. **What is Kallmann's syndrome?**
    Kallmann's syndrome is one of a class of disorders referred to as idiopathic hypogonadotropic hypogonadism or idiopathic hypothalamic hypogonadism (IHH). It occurs as frequently as 1:10,000 boys and 1:50,000 girls. The classic form is characterized by hypogonadotropic hypogonadism with hyposmia or anosmia and is associated with hypoplasia or aplasia of other

structures of the rhinencephalon (e.g., cleft lip/cleft palate, congenital deafness, and color blindness). Undescended testes and gynecomastia are common.

38. **What causes hypergonadotropic hypogonadism?**
Elevated gonadotropin levels indicate that there is a failure of the gonads to produce enough sex steroids to suppress the hypothalamic-pituitary axis. These levels are diagnostic for gonadal failure at two periods of time: before 3 years of age, and once the bone age is at or beyond the normal age for puberty to start. Surgery, radiation, and chemotherapy are all potential causes of gonadal failure in both sexes.

39. **Describe the evaluation of gonadal failure with no apparent cause in girls.**
In girls with gonadal failure and no apparent cause, a karyotype evaluation should be performed; Turner's syndrome will be the most likely explanation. 46XX gonadal dysgenesis can also occur and may be inherited as an autosomal recessive trait. A karyotype also identifies 46XY gonadal dysgenesis in a phenotypic female who is actually a genetic male. In this condition, there is complete lack of testicular development and consequently, except for the absence of gonads, normal female genital differentiation occurs.

40. **How is gonadal failure with no apparent cause evaluated in boys?**
Boys may have gonadal failure secondary to testicular torsion, radiation, chemotherapy, or the vanishing testis syndrome. Noonan's and Klinefelter's syndromes (47XXY) are other potential causes of primary testicular insufficiency. Consequently, in a boy with unexplained gonadotropin elevations, a karyotype should be done.

41. **What is Turner's syndrome?**
Any consideration of pubertal delay in girls must include the possibility of Turner's syndrome. An absent or structurally abnormal second X chromosome characterizes Turner's syndrome. The incidence of Turner's syndrome is approximately 1:2000 live female-births. However, the chromosomal abnormality is actually more common than this, as 90% or more of Turner conceptuses do not survive beyond 28 weeks gestation, and the XO karyotype occurs in 1 out of 15 miscarriages. In the absence of a second functional X chromosome, oocyte degeneration is accelerated, leaving fibrotic streaks in place of normal ovaries. Because of primary gonadal failure, serum gonadotropin levels rise and are elevated at birth and again at the normal time of puberty.

42. **What are the clinical findings in patients with Turner's syndrome?**
See Table 44-3.

43. **How is Turner's syndrome treated?**
Approximately 10–20% of Turner girls have some ovarian function at puberty that allows for some breast development. A small percentage of this group also has normal periods, and an even smaller percentage (< 1% of all girls with Turner's syndrome) are actually fertile. Treatment is with unopposed estradiol or conjugated estrogen for a year or more, followed by cycling with estrogen and progestins. The short stature of girls with Turner's syndrome is treated with growth hormone. Final height in girls with Turner's syndrome is related to when growth hormone is initiated, with better outcomes in girls who are started at a young age. Consequently, early diagnosis of Turner's syndrome is essential.

44. **Why do boys with Klinefelter's syndrome have pubertal delay?**
Klinefelter's syndrome, or seminiferous tubular dysgenesis, is the most common cause of testicular failure. It results from at least one extra X chromosome; thus the most common karyotype is 47XXY. The incidence is 1:1000 male births. Eunuchoid proportions are present from early childhood.

TABLE 44-3.   CLINICAL FINDINGS IN PATIENTS WITH TURNER'S SYNDROME

Primary Defects	Secondary Features	Incidence (%)
Physical features		
Skeletal growth disturbances	Short stature	100
	Short neck	40
	Abnormal upper to lower segment ratio	97
	Cubitus valgus	47
	Short metacarpals	37
	Madelung deformity	7.5
	Scoliosis	12.5
	Genu valgum	35
	Characteristic facies with micrognathia	60
	High arched palate	36
Lymphatic obstruction	Webbed neck	25
	Low posterior hairline	42
	Rotated ears	Common
	Edema of hands/feet	22
	Severe nail dysplasia	13
	Characteristic dermatoglyphics	35
Unknown factors	Strabismus	17.5
	Ptosis	11
	Multiple pigmented nevi	26
Physiologic features		
Skeletal growth disturbances	Growth failure	100
	Otitis media	73
Germ cell chromosomal defects	Gonadal failure	96
	Infertility	99.9
	Gonadoblastoma	4.0
Unknown factors— embryogenic	Cardiovascular anomalies	55
	Hypertension	7
	Renal and renovascular anomalies	39
Unknown factors—metabolic	Hashimoto's thyroiditis	34
	Hypothyroidism	10
	Alopecia	2
	Vitiligo	2
	Gastrointestinal disorders	2.5
	Carbohydrate intolerance	40

Data from Hall J, Gilchrist D: Turner syndrome and its variants. Pediatr Clin North Am 37:1421, 1990.

45. **What features help to diagnose Klinefelter's syndrome?**
Associated features include gynecomastia, tall stature, small testes, and elevated serum gonadotropins. Learning disabilities and behavioral problems may also be present. Seminiferous tubular dysgenesis is universal in patients with Klinefelter's syndrome, but Leydig cell function (testosterone production) is variable; thus they may have either delay in pubertal onset or failure to progress normally through puberty. In most patients, testosterone replacement is beneficial.

KEY POINTS: DISORDERS OF PUBERTY ✔

1. Central precocious puberty occurs more frequently in girls than boys. Boys with central precocity, however, have a much higher incidence of underlying CNS pathology.

2. Precocious puberty must be distinguished from normal variants of early development, that is, benign premature thelarche and adrenarche.

3. The most useful diagnostic test to evaluate precocious puberty is a GnRH stimulation test.

4. Children with delayed puberty and normal linear growth will most likely have constitutional growth delay.

5. Bone age assessment is the first step in evaluating a child with delayed puberty.

6. Once it has been determined that a child has abnormally delayed puberty, gonadotropins should be obtained. If gonadotropins are elevated, obtaining chromosomes is generally the next step.

---

46. **Describe the appropriate history for an adolescent with pubertal delay.**
The history should include questions regarding the presence of chronic illnesses, nutritional disorders, exercise history, galactorrhea, family history of infertility, and timing of puberty in parents and siblings. Weight gain or loss should also be noted.

47. **Describe the physical examination of an adolescent with pubertal delay.**
Physical examination should include measurement of arm span and upper-to-lower segment ratio. Eunuchoid proportions occur early in patients with Klinefelter's syndrome and late in those with other forms of hypogonadism. Signs of any chronic illness, malnutrition, anorexia, and features of Turner's syndrome (girls) and Klinefelter's syndrome (boys) should be noted. A careful search should be made for any signs of puberty, such as pubic hair and axillary hair, acne, testicular size and penile length (boys), and breast development (girls). Pubic hair may represent only adrenal androgen production. Testicular length of greater than 2.5 cm indicates gonadotropin stimulation. Estrogen effect is evaluated by breast development and vaginal maturity. In addition, visual field and olfaction should be evaluated (80% of boys with Kallmann's syndrome have reduced, or absent, sense of smell). Signs of hypothyroidism and Cushing's syndrome must also be evaluated. In addition, the growth chart should be analyzed to determine if there is short stature and if linear growth has been normal.

48. **How are gonadotropin levels helpful in the diagnosis of pubertal delay?**
Assessment of bone age is critical in determining biologic age and the time of expected pubertal development. If linear growth is normal and the bone age is less than the normal age for pubertal onset, the diagnosis is likely to be constitutional growth delay. If linear growth is subnormal

with bone age delay, it may be necessary to investigate the poor growth with evaluation of growth hormone or thyroid status. If bone age has advanced to beyond the age for normal puberty, gonadotropin levels are very helpful in distinguishing between gonadotropin deficiency and primary gonadal failure.

49. **What other lab tests may be needed?**
Additional laboratory studies may include chemistry panels, electrolytes, thyroid function tests, estradiol (girls), testosterone (boys), and prolactin levels. If gonadotropins are elevated, chromosome analysis is indicated for both genders to evaluate for Turner's syndrome in girls and Klinefelter's syndrome in boys. In the case of low serum gonadotropins, olfactory testing and cranial MRI are recommended. The GnRH test is difficult to interpret in prepubertal or peripubertal children. Although GnRH testing may suggest the diagnosis of constitutional delay if there is a clear rise in LH levels, the overlap in response among prepubertal, hypogonadotropic, and early pubertal children is significant.

50. **How is delayed puberty managed?**
The treatment of delayed puberty depends on the underlying cause. If the delayed pubertal development is secondary to anorexia, hypothyroidism, or illness, treatment of these underlying conditions results in spontaneous onset of puberty. Puberty also begins spontaneously, albeit late, in constitutional growth delay so that reassurance alone to the patient and family may be sufficient.

51. **When is treatment offered for constitutional growth delay?**
Treatment may be offered for psychological reasons. Both boys and girls may be distressed because of their small size and sexually immature appearance. They are often treated as if they were younger, teased by peers, and denied participation in certain athletic activities.

52. **Describe the treatment for constitutional growth delay in boys.**
A 4- to 6-month course of low-dose depot testosterone (50–100 mg intramuscularly every 4 weeks) can be offered if the bone age is at least 11–12 years. This treatment results in some early virilization without adversely affecting final height. Spontaneous puberty usually begins, as evident by testicular enlargement, 3–6 months after the end of the testosterone course.

53. **How is constitutional growth delay treated in girls?**
Treatment of delayed puberty in girls with constitutional growth delay is more controversial and less frequent. After a thorough initial evaluation, however, some endocrinologists use low doses of conjugated estrogen (Premarin, 0.3 mg) or ethinyl estradiol (5–10 mg) daily for 3–4 months. Therapy is then stopped, and physical changes are evaluated. Withdrawal bleeding is unusual after one course of estrogen therapy but may occur with subsequent courses.

54. **Describe the treatment of boys with hypogonadism.**
In boys with hypogonadotropic hypogonadism for whom fertility is not an immediate issue and in all boys with primary hypogonadism, long-term testosterone therapy is required. While the patient is growing, careful attention must be paid to growth velocity and bone age. Most commonly, depot testosterone esters (enanthate or cypionate) are used in 25–50 mg doses every 3–4 weeks for the first 1–2 years of therapy. By the second or third year, the dose is raised to 50–100 mg intramuscularly every 3–4 weeks. The adult maintenance level is 200–300 mg intramuscularly every 3–4 weeks. Alternatively, the cutaneous testosterone patch or gel may be used.

55. **How is estrogen treatment given for girls with hypogonadism?**
Replacement therapy in hypogonadal girls is begun with estrogen treatment alone, either as ethinyl estradiol (5–10 mg) or as Premarin (0.15–0.3 mg) for 12–18 months. Following this,

progesterone is added for 10–12 days of each month or a birth control pill may be prescribed. Progesterone therapy is needed to counteract the effects of estrogen on the uterus; unopposed estrogen can cause endometrial hyperplasia and carcinoma. Replacement of gonadal steroids in both sexes is also necessary for normal bone mineralization and to prevent osteoporosis.

56. **How do body habitus and lifestyle influence the timing of puberty?**
In the early 1980s, a number of reports suggested that extremely active and thin girls had a high incidence of primary amenorrhea and delay of puberty. Gymnasts, runners, and ballet dancers, among others, were evaluated. A high incidence of primary amenorrhea, secondary amenorrhea, and dysmenorrhea was found among this group of athletes and appears to have been related to their low fat-lean ratios, as well as to the exercise itself. Indeed, when forced by injury to discontinue activity, such athletes gained weight and quickly progressed to menarche.

57. **Does lifestyle influence final height?**
A recent study evaluated the effect of intensive physical training during puberty on final height in girls. Predicted height decreased significantly with time in gymnasts but not in swimmers. The author concluded that heavy training in gymnastics, starting before and lasting through puberty, may reduce final adult height.

58. **Define amenorrhea.**
A girl who has not had menarche by 16 years of age or within 4 years after the onset of puberty is considered to have primary amenorrhea. Secondary amenorrhea is diagnosed if more than 6 months has elapsed since the last menstrual period.

59. **How do you begin to evaluate a girl with amenorrhea?**
To sort out the many causes of amenorrhea, it is helpful to distinguish girls who produce sufficient estrogen from those who do not by performing a progesterone challenge. Girls who are producing estrogen have a withdrawal bleed after 5–10 days of oral progesterone, whereas those who are estrogen-deficient have no or very little bleeding. There are two situations in which girls have sufficient estrogen but do not have a withdrawal bleed. In Rokitansky's syndrome, maldevelopment of the Müllerian structures leads to an absent or hypoplastic uterus and/or cervix. Complete androgen insensitivity syndrome (testicular feminization) in a genetic male results in a phenotypic female who has normal breast development secondary to the aromatization of testosterone to estrogen. However, the production of müllerian-inhibiting factor in these patients leads to regression of the müllerian structures and thus the absence of a uterus. The absence of a cervix is a diagnostic finding in both of these conditions; consequently, a pelvic examination should be considered in all girls who present with amenorrhea, especially primary amenorrhea. The causes of amenorrhea associated with estrogen insufficiency include hypogonadism, which is described in the previous section about delayed puberty.

60. **What causes amenorrhea in girls who are producing estrogen?**
Amenorrhea in girls who are producing normal or even elevated amounts of estrogen is a manifestation of anovulatory cycles. Irregular menses may also be a sign of chronic anovulation; estrogen production, unopposed by progesterone, leads to endometrial hyperplasia and intermittent shedding. Since menarche is normally followed be a period of anovulatory cycles and irregular menses, many adolescents with a pathologic etiology may be missed. Consequently, it is important to evaluate all girls who do not have regular menses by 3 years after menarche. The most common cause of chronic anovulation is polycystic ovarian syndrome (PCOS), a disorder characterized by increased ovarian androgen production. The clinical presentation varies and may include amenorrhea, oligomenorrhea, dysfunctional uterine bleeding, hirsutism, acne, and obesity.

BIBLIOGRAPHY

1. Comite F, Shawker TH, Pescovitz OH, et al: Cyclical ovarian function resistant to treatment with an analogue of luteinizing hormone-releasing hormone in McCune-Albright syndrome. N Engl J Med 311:1032, 1984.

2. Evans SJ: The athletic adolescent with amenorrhea. Pediatr Ann 13:605, 1984.

3. Frisch R, Wyshak G, Vincent L: Delayed menarche and amenorrhea in ballet dancers. N Engl J Med 303:17, 1980.

4. Ghai K, Cara JF, Rosenfeld RL: Gonadotropin releasing hormone agonist (Nafarelin) test to differentiate gonadotropin deficiency from constitutionally delayed puberty in teen-age boys—a clinical research center study. J Clin Endocrinol Metab 80:2980, 1995.

5. Grumbach MM, Styne DM: Puberty: Ontogeny, neuroendocrinology, physiology, and disorders. In Wilson JD, Foster DW, Kronenberg HM, Larsen PR (eds): Williams Textbook of Endocrinology, 9th ed. Philadelphia, W.B. Saunders, 1998, pp 1509–1625.

6. Hall J, Gilchrist D: Turner syndrome and its variants. Pediatr Clin North Am 37:1421, 1990.

7. Herman-Giddens ME, Slora EJ, Wasserman RC, et al.: Secondary sexual characteristics and menses in young girls seen in office practice: A study from the Pediatric Research in Office Setting network. Pediatrics 99(4):505–512, 1997.

8. Ibanez L, Virdis R, Potau N, et al: Natural history of premature pubarche and auxological study. J Clin Endocrinol Metab 74:254, 1992.

9. Kaplan S (ed): Clinical Pediatric Endocrinology. Philadelphia, W.B. Saunders, 1990.

10. Kaplan S, Grumbach M: Pathophysiology and treatment of sexual precocity. J Clin Endocrinol Metab 71:785, 1990.

11. Kappy MS, Ganong CS: Advances in the treatment of precocious puberty. Adv Pediatr 41:223, 1994.

12. Kulin H, Rester E: Managing the patient with a delay in pubertal development. Endocrinologist 2:231, 1992.

13. Levine M: The McCune-Albright syndrome: The whys and wherefores of abnormal signal transduction. N Engl J Med 325:1738, 1991.

14. Pescovitz O: Precocious puberty. Pediatr Res 11:229, 1990.

15. Root AW: Precocious puberty. Pediatr Rev 21(1):10–19, 2000.

16. Rosenfeld R: Diagnosis and management of delayed puberty. J Clin Endocrinol Metab 70:559, 1990.

17. Rosenfield RL: The ovary and female sexual maturation. In Sperling MA (ed): Pediatric Endocrinology. Philadelphia, W.B. Saunders, 1996, pp 75–86.

18. Styne DM: The testes: Disorders of sexual differentiation and puberty. In Sperling MA (ed): Pediatric Endocrinology. Philadelphia, W.B. Saunders, 1996, pp 423–476.

19. Theinz G, et al: Evidence for a reduction of growth potential in adolescent female gymnasts. J Pediatr 122:306, 1993.

20. Wheeler M, Styne DM: Diagnosis and management of precocious puberty. Pediatr Clin North Am 37:1255, 1990.

21. Zachman M: Therapeutic indications for delayed puberty and hypogonadism in adolescent boys. Horm Res 35:141, 1991.

CHAPTER 45

MALE HYPOGONADISM

Derek J. Stocker, M.D., and Robert A. Vigersky, M.D.

1. **Define male hypogonadism.**

   Male hypogonadism refers to the clinical and/or laboratory syndrome that results from a failure of the testis to work properly. The normal testis has two functions: synthesis and secretion of testosterone (from the Leydig cells) and production of sperm (from the seminiferous tubules). Deficiency of one or both functions is termed male hypogonadism. Depending on the stage of development, hypogonadism may have varied manifestations.

2. **What are the manifestations of in utero hypogonadism?**

   In utero androgen deficiency leads to a female phenotype or ambiguous genitalia (male pseudo-hermaphroditism), most commonly caused by a block in the production of testosterone due to congenital testosterone biosynthetic enzyme defects. Rarely, peripheral tissues cannot respond normally to testosterone, resulting in the androgen insensitivity syndromes of testicular feminization (complete) and Reifenstein's syndrome (incomplete). Other manifestations include micropenis, hypospadias, and cryptorchidism.

3. **Describe the manifestations of peripubertal hypogonadism.**

   Childhood androgen deficiency results in delayed or absent pubertal development. Common manifestations include:
   - Eunuchoid proportions (ratio of pubis-to-vertex/pubis-to-floor is < 0.9; arm span is > 5 cm more than height)
   - Small testes (< 20 ml or < 4.5 × 3.0 cm)
   - Decreased body hair
   - Gynecomastia
   - Reduced peak bone mass

4. **Summarize the manifestations of hypogonadism in early adulthood.**

   In early adulthood, a decrease in sperm output (azoospermia/oligospermia) without deficient production of testosterone is common and results in male infertility; thus, infertility is a form of male hypogonadism. A decrease in production of testosterone in adulthood is usually accompanied by a decline in production of sperm. When it is not, the term *fertile eunuch* (eunuchoid proportions, low levels of luteinizing hormone [LH], low levels of testosterone, normal levels of follicle-stimulating hormone [FSH], and spermatogenesis) is appropriately applied. Libido and/or potency may be diminished.

5. **What are the manifestations of hypogonadism in mid-to-late adulthood?**

   The most frequent circumstance in which adult hypogonadism occurs is in the middle-aged or senescent man complaining of decreased libido or potency. Semen analysis is rarely performed in these men since they are usually not concerned with fertility. Other findings may include osteoporosis, diminished androgen production, and small prostate.

6. **How is production of testosterone normally regulated?**

   LH is episodically secreted from the anterior pituitary in response to pulses of gonadotropin-releasing hormone (GnRH), thus stimulating production of testosterone by Leydig cells. Once testosterone is secreted into the bloodstream, it is bound by sex hormone-binding globulin (SHBG). The non-SHBG-bound (or "free") testosterone provides negative feedback to the hypothalamic-pituitary unit and thus inhibits output of LH. This classic endocrine feedback loop serves to maintain serum testosterone at a predetermined level; if serum testosterone falls below the set point, the pituitary is stimulated to secrete LH, which in turn stimulates testicular output of testosterone until serum levels return to the set point. Conversely, if serum testosterone rises above the set point, decreased output of LH results in decreased testicular output of testosterone until serum levels have declined to the set point.

7. **Describe how production of sperm is normally regulated.**
   The regulation of sperm production is complex and less clearly understood than regulation of testosterone production. Both hormonal and nonhormonal factors are important. The Sertoli cells within the seminiferous tubules seem to play an important coordinating role. Sertoli cells respond to FSH by producing inhibin (secreted into the blood) and androgen-binding protein, transferrin, and other proteins (secreted into the seminiferous tubular lumen). Inhibin appears to inhibit the output of FSH from the pituitary gland, thus completing a feedback loop. In theory, if spermatogenesis declines, production of inhibin also should decline; thus the negative feedback effect on the pituitary would be reduced, leading to an increased output of FSH, which then presumably stimulates spermatogenesis. However, not all aspects of this feedback loop (FSH-inhibin-spermatogenesis) have been verified experimentally. Moreover, spermatogenesis depends on intratesticular production of testosterone mediated by androgen receptors within Sertoli cells. Initiation of spermatogenesis during puberty requires both LH and FSH. However, reinitiation of the process if it is disrupted by exogenous factors (see the following), requires only LH (or human chorionic gonadotropin [hCG]), although FSH may be needed to produce a normal number of sperm.

8. **Define primary hypogonadism and secondary hypogonadism.**
   Failure of testicular function may result from a defect either in the testis or at the hypothalamic-pituitary level. Testicular disorders leading to hypogonadism are termed *primary hypogonadism* (Fig. 45-1), whereas disorders of hypothalamic-pituitary function leading to hypogonadism are termed *secondary hypogonadism* (Fig. 45-2).

9. **List the congenital causes of primary hypogonadism.**
   - Klinefelter's syndrome (47XXY and mosaics)
   - Microdeletions of azoospermia factor (AZF) regions of Yp telomere (15% of men with non-obstructive azoospermia; 5–10% of those with oligospermia)
   - Cryptorchidism
   - Myotonic dystrophy
   - Congenital adrenal hyperplasia (3-β-hydroxysteroid dehydrogenase, 17-α-hydroxylase or 17-β-hydroxysteroid dehydrogenase deficiency)
   - Androgen receptor gene mutation (qualitative or quantitative)
   - LH receptor mutations (male phenotype, if mild; female phenotype, if severe)

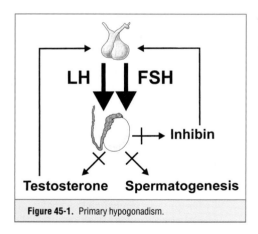

Figure 45-1. Primary hypogonadism.

10. **List the acquired causes of primary hypogonadism.**
    - Cancer therapy: chemotherapy (alkylating agents > cisplatin and carboplatin) and radiation therapy (may be permanent with external radiation; usually transient with radioactive iodine)
    - Drugs (e.g., ketoconazole)
    - Trauma
    - Infiltrative disease (e.g., hemochromatosis)
    - Infections (e.g., HIV [may be multifactorial], mumps orchitis)
    - Systemic illness (e.g., uremia, cirrhosis): may be multifactorial)

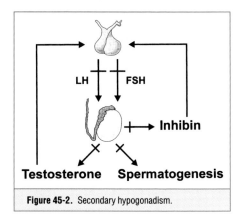

Figure 45-2. Secondary hypogonadism.

11. **Is normal aging associated with primary hypogonadism?**
    A number of cross-sectional studies have noted that older men seem to have mildly reduced levels of total serum testosterone but significantly reduced levels of free testosterone (due to a rise in SHBG with age) compared with younger men. This decline is associated with a rise in LH and FSH and probably reflects an intrinsic part of the aging process on which are superimposed the various chronic diseases that develop as one ages. There is currently considerable controversy over whether or not men with age-associated hypogonadism should be treated with testosterone replacement. While some short-term studies have demonstrated treatment benefits, long-term large studies are lacking and are needed to clarify the criteria for treatment, as well as the risks and benefits associated with testosterone replacement in this population.

12. **Discuss the causes of secondary hypogonadism.**
    Any disease that affects the hypothalamic-pituitary axis can cause secondary hypogonadism. Involvement of the hypothalamus or pituitary stalk interferes with the secretion of GnRH or the ability of GnRH to communicate with the pituitary. Various anatomic lesions of the pituitary cause secondary hypogonadism by interfering with the release of LH and FSH. Such lesions include benign tumors and cysts, malignant tumors (both primary central nervous system tumors and metastatic tumors from distant sources), vascular aneurysms, infiltrative diseases (e.g., hemochromatosis), pituitary hemorrhage, and pituitary trauma. Congenital disorders, in which output of LH and FSH is impaired, such as Kallmann's syndrome, also lead to secondary hypogonadism. Iatrogenic causes, such as the use of narcotic analgesics or the abuse of anabolic steroids by athletes, are other possible causes of hypogonadism.

13. **What is the most common pituitary tumor in adults?**
    The most common pituitary tumor found in adults is a prolactin-secreting adenoma. These tumors primarily cause hypogonadism as a result of local destruction and compression, inhibiting the production and release of LH and FSH. Elevated prolactin levels can also interrupt secretion of GnRH, although this is usually of much less significance in men than the mass effect.

14. **How do other pituitary adenomas cause hypogonadism?**
    Pituitary adenomas that produce growth hormone (acromegaly) or adrenocorticotropic hormone (Cushing's disease) and nonfunctioning pituitary tumors may similarly cause secondary hypogonadism by their mass effects.

15. **What clinical symptoms are seen in male hypogonadism?**
    Loss of the sperm-producing function of the testis leads to infertility, usually defined as failure of a normal female partner to conceive after 12 months of unprotected intercourse. Loss of the

testosterone-producing function of the testis may lead to loss of libido and erectile dysfunction, as well as diminution of secondary sexual characteristics, such as facial and pubic hair. Decreased production of testosterone also may cause more generalized symptoms, such as decreased muscle mass and strength, malaise, and fatigue. In boys who develop hypogonadism before sexual maturation, delay or absence of the onset of puberty is typical. Tender gynecomastia is frequently seen in hypogonadism.

16. **How does hypogonadism affect bone architecture?**
   Osteoporosis is now a well-recognized result of both primary and secondary hypogonadism. Trabecular architecture (and bone strength) is even more severely disturbed than bone density in men with hypogonadism. Thus, it is not surprising that hypogonadism is found in up to 30% of men with vertebral fractures. Estradiol that is aromatized from testosterone may be the most important factor in preserving bone architecture and density in both men and women. However, androgen receptors are also found in bone and may explain the sexual dimorphism of bone density.

17. **What laboratory tests help to confirm a suspected diagnosis of male hypogonadism?**
   The main functions of the testis, production of sperm and production of testosterone, are readily assessed by semen analysis and measurement of serum testosterone, respectively. Normal semen analysis values in men following 2–3 days of abstinence are: 20 million sperm per milliliter and > 60% motility of the sperm. Because sperm density is highly variable from day to day in all men, accurate assessment usually involves several semen analyses done with the same abstinence period each time. The best initial test for testosterone production is measurement of the nonfasting morning serum total testosterone level. Serum testosterone also varies considerably from moment to moment and from morning to night in response to LH secretion; again, several samples may be needed to establish an accurate measurement. In addition, most testosterone in serum is bound to plasma proteins, particularly SHBG; thus, in elderly or obese patients who have increased and decreased SHBG levels, respectively, and in those men in whom plasma protein levels may be disrupted, measurement of the physiologically active "free" testosterone may prove informative. Bone density measurement using a DXA scan may provide helpful baseline information and assist in deciding whether to provide androgen replacement therapy.

KEY POINTS: MALE HYPOGONADISM ✓

1. The manifestations of hypogonadism vary depending on the stage of development of the patient when the hypogonadism occurs.

2. A reduction in testicular volume (below 20 mL) is the most common manifestation of hypogonadism and is seen in nearly all cases of long-standing hypogonadism.

3. The diagnosis of hypogonadism is readily confirmed with a correctly obtained serum testosterone measurement or semen analysis.

4. Hypogonadism should be characterized as primary (a disorder at the level of the testes) or secondary (a disorder at the level of the hypothalamic-pituitary unit).

5. Secondary hypogonadism should be corrected to the mid-normal range with testosterone given in one of the following ways: injection, scrotal or dermal patch, topical gel, or buccal tablet.

6. Patients on testosterone replacement should be monitored for gynecomastia, prostate size and symptoms, polycythemia, sleep apnea, and psychological difficulties.

18. **Can laboratory tests help to distinguish primary from secondary hypogonadism?**

    Primary hypogonadism resulting from a testicular disorder leads to a decline in production of testosterone and sperm, a consequent decrease in the negative feedback effects on the pituitary and a corresponding increase in serum levels of LH and FSH. Conversely, in secondary hypogonadism due to a hypothalamic-pituitary disorder, serum LH and FSH may be subnormal or "inappropriately" normal (explainable, in part, by decreased bioactivity) despite a low testosterone. A subnormal sperm count and normal testosterone level with a normal LH and elevated FSH suggests primary hypogonadism with a dysfunction of the seminiferous tubules and sperm production but intact Leydig cell function.

19. **What other diagnostic tests are useful in defining the cause of male hypogonadism?**

    Additional diagnostic testing should be based on clinical suspicion and the results of preliminary testing. For example, in cases of secondary hypogonadism, measurement of serum prolactin and pituitary radiography, preferably magnetic resonance imaging (MRI) with gadolinium, should be done. Computed tomography (CT) of the sella usually detects macroadenomas (> 1.0 cm) but will miss many clinically significant microadenomas and is therefore less preferable than MRI. Plain skull or sella turcica films are not adequate for diagnosis. Measurement of other pituitary hormones also may be appropriate to assess either possible tumoral hypersecretion (e.g., Cushing's disease, acromegaly) or tumor-related hypopituitarism. Visual field testing is indicated if a macroadenoma is present or there is suprasellar extension. Likewise, the initial findings in primary hypogonadism may suggest additional tests. For example, small firm testes, gynecomastia, azoospermia, modestly reduced serum testosterone, and high levels of serum LH and FSH in a young man may lead to chromosome analysis to confirm a presumptive diagnosis of Klinefelter's syndrome. Measurement of serum estradiol levels may be helpful when feminization is prominent clinically, as with secondary hypogonadism related to production of estrogen by testicular or adrenal tumors. Testis biopsy rarely provides information that is useful in establishing a specific diagnosis, prognosis, or treatment.

20. **Define hermaphrodite.**

    Hermaphrodite refers to someone who has both ovarian and testicular elements in their body. They usually have a 46XX or 46XX/46XY karyotype. Such individuals may have an ovary and a testis or an ovotestis. They most often have ambiguous genitalia.

21. **Define pseudohermaphrodite.**

    Pseudohermaphrodite refers to someone whose external genitalia are not consistent with his or her gonadal sex. A male pseudohermaphrodite, for example, has a 46XY karyotype and testes but has either ambiguous genitalia or a complete female phenotype. Most often this results from genetic disorders of testosterone biosynthetic enzymes, the androgen receptor or the 5-α-reductase enzyme; the severity of the phenotype depends on the severity of the genetic defect. A female pseudohermaphrodite, in contrast, has a 46XX karyotype and ovaries but has ambiguous external genitalia. The most common cause of this is congenital adrenal hyperplasia, which results in virilization of the female fetus in utero.

22. **How is hypogonadism treated?**

    Deficiency of testosterone is easily treated with testosterone replacement therapy (TRT) (see Table 46-2). The treatment goal for all TRT is normalization of the serum LH in primary hypogonadism and a serum total testosterone level in the mid-normal range for secondary hypogonadism. Some older men with testosterone deficiency are unconcerned about sexual function and may not desire testosterone replacement. However, in testosterone-deficient men of any age, low bone density and/or reduced hematopoiesis may be indications for TRT even in the absence of decreased libido or erectile dysfunction. Testosterone preparations are presently designated as schedule III drugs by the Anabolic Steroid Control Act because of their potential for abuse by athletes and others.

23. **What are the potential adverse effects of testosterone treatment?**
Gynecomastia and acne may occur in the first few months after initiating testosterone treatment; these side effects may resolve with continued treatment, although temporary dose reduction may be helpful. Abnormalities in liver function are uncommon with currently used injectable and transdermal preparations. A testosterone-induced increase in hematocrit is common, although clinically significant polycythemia is quite rare unless the drug is being abused. Testosterone treatment may also precipitate sleep apnea; marked increases in hematocrit may be a clue to this side effect. In boys who have not yet gone through puberty, the rapid increase in serum testosterone after initial treatment may lead to considerable psychological difficulties and physically aggressive behavior; initiating treatment with smaller doses may be helpful. TRT has no adverse effect on lipid profiles compared with eugonadal men, but overtreatment can lead to several lipid abnormalities, including decreases in the high-density lipoprotein cholesterol level.

24. **Does testosterone replacement affect the prostate in older men?**
In older men effects of testosterone on the prostate must be considered, including the possibility of precipitating urinary retention due to testosterone-induced enlargement of the prostate. Although no evidence indicates that testosterone treatment causes prostate carcinoma, the potential for testosterone stimulation of occult prostate carcinoma exists. Therefore, it is advisable to perform a digital rectal examination of the prostate and monitor prostate-specific antigen in middle-age and older men before and annually, while they are receiving testosterone replacement.

25. **How does one treat the deficiency of sperm production in primary hypogonadism?**
In men with primary hypogonadism, as manifested by elevated levels of serum FSH, there seems to be no effective pharmacologic treatment for increasing the sperm count. Anatomic lesions, such as varicoceles and ejaculatory duct obstructions, can be corrected surgically, but improvement in spermatogenesis may not result. If one plans to use a medication that is known to cause hypogonadism (e.g., cancer chemotherapeutic agents), it may be desirable to cryopreserve semen specimens before treatment, provided that treatment is not unduly delayed.

26. **How does one treat deficient sperm production in secondary hypogonadism?**
The outlook is much less pessimistic with secondary hypogonadism, particularly if the condition developed after puberty. Treatment with gonadotropins (human chorionic gonadotropin with or without added FSH) may be successful in restoring production of sperm, as well as testosterone. The pretreatment size of the testis is often a clue to prognosis; larger testis size is associated with a better outcome. Production of testosterone and sperm in men with secondary hypogonadism also may be enhanced with pulsatile administration of GnRH via a portable infusion pump, provided that the pituitary retains the capability to make gonadotropins. Treatment with gonadotropins or GnRH tends to be both costly and prolonged.

27. **What reproductive alternative is available to men with hypogonadism who do not respond to therapy?**
In men with primary or secondary hypogonadism who have not responded to specific therapy when appropriate and who have preservation of some germ cells in either ejaculate or testis, intracytoplasmic sperm injection (ICSI) may offer some hope, although at a high financial cost. The prognosis for successful ICSI is dependent on the site and extent of microdeletions on the Y chromosome.

WESTITES

BIBLIOGRAPHY

1. AACE Hypogonadism Guidelines, Endocr Pract 8(6):439–456, 2002.

2. Adamopoulos DA, Lawrence DM, Vassilopoulos P, et al: Pituitary-testicular relationships in mumps orchitis and other viral infections. BMJ 1:1177, 1978.

3. Bagatell CJ, Bremner WJ: Androgens in men—uses and abuses. N Engl J Med 334:707–714, 1996.

4. Baker HWG, Burger HF, DeKretser DM, et al: Changes in the pituitary-testicular system with age. Clin Endocrinol 5:349, 1976.

5. Bannister P, Handley T, Chapman C, Losowsky MS: Hypogonadism in chronic liver disease: Impaired release of luteinising hormone. BMJ 293:1191, 1986.

6. Bhasin S: Androgen treatment of hypogonadal men. J Clin Endocrinol Metab 74:1221, 1992.

7. Byrne M, Nieschlag E. Testosterone replacement therapy in male hypogonadism. J Endocrinol Invest 26(5):481–489, 2003.

8. Castro-Magana M, Bronsther B, Angulo MA: Genetic forms of male hypogonadism. Urology 35:195, 1990.

9. Dada R, Gupta NP, Kucheria K: Molecular screening for Yq microdeletion in men with idiopathic oligospermia and azoospermia. J Biosci 28:163–168, 2003.

10. Gambineri A, Pelusi C, Vicennati V, Pagotto U, Pasquali R. Testosterone in ageing men. Expert Opin Investig Drugs 10(3):477–492, 2001.

11. Griffin JL, Wilson JD: The syndromes of androgen resistance. N Engl J Med 302:198, 1980.

12. Gromoll J, Eiholzer U, Nieschlag E, Simoni M: Male hypogonadism caused by homozygous deletion of exon 10 of the luteinizing hormone (LH) receptor: Differential action of human chorionic gonadotropin. J Clin Endocrinol Metab 85:2281, 2000.

13. Guo CY, Jones TH, Eastell R: Treatment of isolated hypogonadotropic hypogonadism effect on bone mineral density and bone turnover. J Clin Endocrinol Metab 82:658–665, 1997.

14. Harman SM, Metter EJ, Tobin JD, et al: Longitudinal effects of aging on serum total and free testosterone levels in healthy men. Baltimore Longitudinal Study of Aging. J Clin Endocrinol Metab 86:724–731, 2001.

15. Hayes FJ, Seminara SB, Crowley WF: Hypogonadotropic hypogonadism. Endocrinol Metab Clin North Am 27(4):739–763, 1998.

16. Hopps CV, Mielnik A. Goldstein M, et al: Detection of sperm in men with Y chromosome microdeletions on the AZFa, AZFb and AZFc regions. Hum Reprod 18:1660–1665, 2003.

17. Hsueh WA, Hsu TH, Federman DD: Endocrine features of Klinefelter's syndrome. Medicine 57:447, 1978.

18. Lee PA, O'Dea LS: Primary and secondary testicular insufficiency. Pediatr Clin North Am 37:1359, 1990.

19. Lieblich JM, Rogol AD, White BJ, Rosen SW: Syndrome of anosmia with hypogonadotropic hypogonadism (Kallman syndrome): Clinical and laboratory studies in 23 cases. Am J Med 73:506, 1982.

20. Matsumoto AM, Bremner WJ: Endocrinology of the hypothalamic-pituitary-testicular axis with particular reference to the hormonal control of spermatogenesis. Baillieres Clin Endocrinol Metab 1:71, 1987.

21. Schwartz ID, Root AW: The Klinefelter syndrome of testicular dysgenesis. Endocrinol Metab Clin North Am 20:153, 1991.

22. Seminara SB, Hayes FJ, Crowley WF Jr: Gonadotropin-releasing hormone deficiency in the human (idiopathic hypogonadotropic hypogonadism and Kallmann's syndrome): Pathophysiological and genetic considerations. Endocrine Rev 19:521, 1998.

23. Silveira LF, MacColl GS, Bouloux PM. Hypogonadotropic hypogonadism. Semin Reprod Med 20(4):327–338, 2002.

24. Snyder PJ, et al: Effects of testosterone replacement in hypogonadal men. J Clin Endocrinol Metab 85:2670, 2000.

25. Swerdloff RS, Wang C, et al: Long-term pharmacokinetics of transdermal testosterone gel in hypogonadal men. J Clin Endocrinol Metab 85:4500–4510, 2000.

26. Szulc P, Munoz F, Claustrat B, et al: Bioavailable estradiol may be an important determinant of osteoporosis in men: The MINOS study. J Clin Endocrinol Metab 86:192, 2001.

27. Tenover JL: Male hormone replacement therapy including "andropause." Endocrinol Metab Clin North Am 27(4):969–987, 1998.

28. Whitcomb RW, Crowley WF: Male hypogonadotropic hypogonadism. Endocrinol Metab Clin North Am 22:125, 1993.

CHAPTER 46

IMPOTENCE

Robert A. Vigersky, M.D.

1. **What is impotence?**
   Classically, impotence has been defined as the inability to attain and maintain an erection of sufficient rigidity for sexual intercourse in 50% or more attempts. A more descriptive term for impotence is *erectile dysfunction.*

2. **Do men with erectile dysfunction have disturbances in other sexual functions?**
   Most men with erectile dysfunction are able to ejaculate. Premature ejaculation may precede the development of impotence and is sometimes associated with drug therapy. Sexual desire (libido) is also usually preserved; loss of libido is suggestive of hypogonadism or severe systemic or psychiatric illness.

3. **Is impotence common?**
   At least 10 million American men and perhaps as many as 20 million are impotent. Another 10 million may suffer from partial erectile dysfunction. The prevalence of impotence increases with age; about 2% of 40-year-old, 20% of 55-year-old, and 50–75% of 80-year-old men are impotent. Of interest, there is a libido-potency gap in that many elderly men continue to have active libidos, but only 15% of them engage in sexual activity.

4. **How does a normal erection occur?**
   Erection is primarily a vascular event that results from the complex interplay of the hormonal, vascular, peripheral nerve, and central nervous system.

5. **Explain the role of the nervous system in achieving erection.**
   Erection is usually initiated by various psychological and/or physiologic stimuli in the cerebral cortex. The stimuli are modulated in the limbic system and other areas of the brain, integrated in the hypothalamus, transmitted down the spinal cord, and carried to the penis via both autonomic and sacral spinal nerves. (For Latin scholars, these are the nervi erigentes derived from the verb erigo, erigere, erexi, erectus.) Sensory nerves from the glans of the penis enhance the message and help to maintain erection during sexual activity via a reflex arc.

6. **Explain the hormonal aspects of erection.**
   Nervous system stimuli release neurotransmitters that reverse the tonic smooth muscle constriction maintained by norepinephrine, endothelin, and other vasoconstrictive factors. The most important of these are the potent vasodilators, nitric oxide (NO) and prostaglandin E1 (PGE1). In addition to neural sources, NO is derived from endothelial cells, which may explain why endothelial integrity may be necessary for maintenance of an erection. NO works by increasing cyclic guanosine monophosphate (cGMP) and causing a decrease in intracellular calcium. This results in relaxation of vascular smooth muscle cells due to dissociation of actin-myosin.

7. **What vascular changes in the penis result in erection?**
   Within the two spongy corpora cavernosa of the penis are millions of tiny spaces called lacunae, each lined by a wall of trabecular smooth muscle. As neurotransmitters dilate cavernosal and

helicine arteries to the penis and relax the trabecular smooth muscle, the lacunar spaces in the penis become engorged with blood. This results in entrapment of outflow vessels between the expanding trabecular walls and the rigid tunica albuginea that surrounds the corpora cavernosa, thereby greatly reducing venous outflow from the penis. This veno-occlusive mechanism accounts for both rigidity and tumescence. Failure of venous occlusion (venous leak) is one of the intractable causes of impotence.

8. **What types of nerves and neurotransmitters play a role in penile erection?**
   At least three neuroeffector systems play a role in penile erection. Adrenergic nerves generally inhibit erection; cholinergic nerves and nonadrenergic, noncholinergic (NANC) substances enhance erection as follows:
   - Sympathetic nerves (via α-adrenergic receptors): constrict cavernosal and helicine arteries, contract trabecular smooth muscle.
   - Parasympathetic nerves (via cholinergic receptors): inhibit adrenergic fibers, stimulate NANC fibers.
   - NANC messengers (NO, vasoactive intestinal polypeptide, and PGs or other endothelium-derived factors): dilate cavernosal and helicine arteries, relax trabecular smooth muscle.

9. **How does detumescence occur?**
   Phosphodiesterase 5 (PD5), by causing a decrease in cGMP, allows for reversal of the process; that is, detumescence, making PD5 inhibitors, such as sildenafil, vardenafil, and tadalafil, important therapeutic agents for the treatment of impotence (see the following).

10. **What are the common causes of impotence?**
    The frequency of the various causes of impotence is difficult to assess because of the large number of patients who do not report the problem, confusion regarding the diagnosis, and variability in the sophistication of the initial evaluation. Primary causes of impotence in men presenting to a medical outpatient clinic are approximated as follows:
    - Endocrine factors: 30%
    - Diabetes mellitus: 15%
    - Medications: 20%
    - Systemic disease and alcoholism: 10%
    - Primary vascular causes: 5% (Alterations of blood flow are thought to play a role in many causes of impotence, but specific lesions amenable to therapy are relatively rare.)
    - Primary neurologic causes: 5%
    - Psychogenic or unknown causes: 15%

11. **What lifestyles are associated with impotence?**
    - Low levels of physical activity
    - Overeating/obesity
    - Smoking
    - Excessive TV viewing
    - Alcohol consumption

12. **Besides diabetes mellitus, what are the three most common endocrine causes of impotence?**
    - Primary (hypergonadotropic) hypogonadism (increased luteinizing hormone [LH] and decreased testosterone)
    - Secondary (hypogonadotropic) hypogonadism (decreased LH and decreased testosterone)
    - Hyperprolactinemia
      Less common causes include hyperthyroidism, hypothyroidism, adrenal insufficiency, and Cushing's syndrome.

13. **Describe the most common drugs known to induce impotence.**
Nonprescription drugs, such as alcohol (as the porter says to Macduff in Act II, Scene 3 of Macbeth, "It provokes the desire but takes away the performance"), and illicit drugs, such as cocaine, methadone, and heroin, can cause impotence. The prescription drugs most commonly associated with impotence include the following:
   - Antihypertensive agents, especially methyldopa, clonidine, beta blockers, vasodilators (e.g., hydralazine), thiazide diuretics, and spironolactone
   - Antipsychotic medications
   - Antidepressants and tranquilizers
   - Others (especially cimetidine, digoxin, phenytoin, carbamazepine, ketoconazole, and metoclopramide)

14. **Which antihypertensive agents should be used in patients with impotence?**
Virtually every blood pressure medication has been associated with impotence. While there is little overall difference in the rate of erectile problems among the commonly prescribed antihypertensive agents, angiotensin-converting enzyme (ACE) inhibitors, angiotensin-receptor blockers (ARBs), and calcium channel blockers are the agents least likely to affect erectile ability. When beta blockade is required, selective beta antagonists, such as atenolol or acebutolol, are preferred as they have minimal impact on sexual function.

15. **What is "stuttering" impotence? What is its significance?**
Impotence alternating with periods of entirely normal sexual function is termed stuttering impotence. Multiple sclerosis (MS) is the most significant organic cause of stuttering impotence. It may be the initial manifestation of MS and may be present in up to 50% of men with the disease.

16. **What historical information helps to separate organic from psychogenic impotence?**
True psychogenic impotence is uncommon and should be a diagnosis of exclusion. Questions that may help to separate psychogenic from organic impotence are listed in Table 46-1.

TABLE 46-1. ORGANIC VERSUS PSYCHOGENIC IMPOTENCE

	Organic	Psychogenic
Was onset abrupt?	No	Yes
Is impotence stress dependent?	No	Yes
Is libido preserved?	Yes	No
Do you have morning erections?	No	Yes
Do you have orgasms?	Yes	No
Can you masturbate?	No	Yes
Does impotence occur with all partners?	Yes	No

17. **Name the essential components of a physical examination in a man complaining of impotence.**
   - Secondary sexual characteristics, such as muscle development, hair pattern, and presence of breast tissue.
   - Vascular examination, especially of the femoral and lower extremity pulses and the presence of bruits.

- Focused neurologic examination, including assessing the presence of peripheral neuropathy with vibratory and light touch sensation and of autonomic neuropathy using the cremasteric reflex, anal sphincter tone and/or the bulbocavernosus reflex, evaluation of standing and supine blood pressure, and measurement of the heart rate response to deep breathing and Valsalva (diabetics rarely have autonomic neuropathy as a cause of impotence in the absence of peripheral neuropathy).
- Examination of the genitalia to determine penile size, shape, presence of plaque or fibrous tissue (Peyronie's disease); size and consistency of the testes; prostate examination.
- Thyroid examination.

18. **What is the appropriate laboratory assessment for men with impotence?**
Laboratory assessment should be based on history and physical examination findings. It can discover previously unknown disease in 6% of men. Generally, it should include the following:
- Complete blood count
- Urinalysis
- Fasting glucose and (in diabetics) hemoglobin A_{1C} (HbA1C)
- Fasting lipid profile
- Serum creatinine
- Thyroid function tests
- Serum testosterone and LH

19. **Should prolactin levels be measured in all impotent men?**
Whether serum prolactin should be measured in all men with impotence is somewhat controversial. In general, patients with normal levels of testosterone and LH and a normal neurologic examination do not require measurement of prolactin. However, if testosterone is low and associated with low or low-normal LH or if history or examination suggests a pituitary lesion, prolactin should be measured. Because prolactin interferes with the action of testosterone, prolactin status should be assessed in hypogonadal men unresponsive to testosterone replacement therapy. Hypothyroidism and renal failure also may elevate prolactin.

20. **What is a penile brachial index?**
Comparison of the penile and brachial systolic blood pressure allows a general assessment of the vascular integrity of the penis. This technique is not highly sensitive, but it is noninvasive and easy to perform and may help to identify men who require more extensive vascular studies. Penile systolic blood pressure obtained with Doppler ultrasound should be the same as brachial systolic pressure (i.e., ratio approximately = 1.0). An index < 0.7 is highly suggestive of vasculogenic impotence. Diagnostic yield is increased if the penile brachial index is repeated after exercising the lower extremities for several minutes. This maneuver may uncover a pelvic steal syndrome (loss of erection due to pelvic thrusting) that is characterized by a difference of > 0.15 between the resting and exercise ratios.

21. **What is nocturnal penile tumescence monitoring?**
Most men experience 3–6 erections during the night that are entrained to rapid eye movement (REM) sleep. By monitoring such events, one can assess the frequency, duration, and, with some instruments, even the rigidity of erection. This procedure helps to distinguish organic from psychogenic impotence. This can be done at home either semiquantitatively (using a Snap-Gauge) or more quantitatively (using the RigiScan).

22. **What are the therapeutic options in the treatment of impotence?**
Once drugs with a high likelihood of causing impotence are discontinued, lifestyle modifications have been initiated (weight reduction and exercise), and/or other underlying conditions are aggressively treated (e.g., diabetes mellitus, hypercholesterolemia), the broad categories of available therapy are:

- Medical treatment
- Intracavernosal injection
- Transurethral delivery of alprostadil (PG E1)
- External mechanical aids and vacuum/suction devices
- Surgical treatments
- Psychological therapy (especially in the absence of an obvious organic cause)

23. **What options are available for medical treatment?**
    - Testosterone replacement in hypogonadal men
    - Bromocriptine to reduce hyperprolactinemia in men with normal testosterone unresponsive to testosterone treatment
    - PD5 inhibitors, such as sildenafil citrate (Viagra), vardenafil (Levitra), or tadalafil (Cialis)
    - Adrenergic receptor blockers (e.g., yohimbine, 6.5 mg t.d.s.)
    - Herbal remedies (e.g., Korean red ginseng, 90 mg t.d.s.)
    - Selective serotonin reuptake inhibitor for premature ejaculation

24. **Summarize the role of intracavernosal injections.**
    Intracavernosal injection of vasoactive substances (PGE, papaverine, and phentolamine) individually or in combination (Trimix) may be effective for men in whom PD5 inhibitors have failed or are contraindicated.

25. **List the surgical procedures used to treat impotence.**
    - Revascularization procedures
    - Obliteration of venous shunts
    - Surgical penile implants

26. **What are the advantages and disadvantages of the various forms of androgen replacement therapy?**
    Oral forms of testosterone, such as oxandrolone and methyltestosterone, should not be used for long-term therapy because of their propensity to cause hepatotoxicity and hepatic tumors. Fluoxymesterone (Halotestin) cannot be aromatized to estrogens and therefore may not provide protection against osteoporosis. The recommended forms of testosterone with their relative advantages and disadvantages are listed in Table 46-2.

27. **What parameters should be monitored in men on testosterone therapy?**
    The following should be followed at least yearly, once the patient is stabilized:
    - Hematocrit and hemoglobin
    - Prostate size by digital rectal examination
    - Serum prostatic-specific antigen (PSA)
    - Liver function tests
    - Development of gynecomastia, acne, or edema
    - Serum testosterone levels

28. **In what conditions is testosterone therapy contraindicated?**
    - Carcinoma of the prostate
    - Sleep apnea
    - Polycythemia vera
    - Symptomatic and/or severe benign prostatic hypertrophy
    - Breast carcinoma

29. **How effective are PD5 inhibitors?**
    The introduction of the selective PD5 inhibitors [sildenafil citrate (Viagra), vardenafil (Levitra), and tadalafil (Cialis)] has produced a paradigm shift in the approach to the treatment of impo-

TABLE 46-2. RECOMMENDED FORMS OF TESTOSTERONE ADMINISTRATION

	Intramuscular	Scrotal Patch	Dermal Patch	Gel	Buccal
Brand name	Delatestryl/Depo Testosterone	Testoderm	Androderm/ Testoderm TTS	AndroGel/ Testim	Striant
Dose	50–100 mg weekly or 100–200 mg biweekly	4–6 mg q.d.	2.5–5 mg q.d.	50 mg q.d.	30 mg b.i.d.
Reliable delivery/ compliance	4	2	3	3	?
Flexible dosing	4	2	2	2	2
Stable serum levels	1	4	4	4	?
Convenience	1	2	3	3	2
Side effects	2	2	3	1*	?
Cost	1	2	3	3	4

?, data not available; 1, lowest; 4, highest.
*15 minutes of vigorous skin-to-skin contact can transfer significant amounts to testosterone to a female partner.

tence by reducing the relevance of finding a specific cause of the problem. Given 1 hour before anticipated sexual activity (and for Viagra avoiding a fatty meal, which inhibits its absorption by one-third), they are successful in up to 80% of men with organic impotence (although only about 50–70% of diabetic men).

30. **Discuss the side effects of PD5 inhibitors.**
The few side effects associated with PD5 inhibitors (headache, flushing, dyspepsia, and a blue haze in vision) rarely cause discontinuation of their use. Since they cause vasodilatation similar to that of nitrates, they are contraindicated in men taking any form of nitrates. The long half-life of tadalafil (the so-called "week-end pill") may prove to be particularly troublesome if a patient develops angina within 72–96 hours of taking it. In addition, PD5 inhibitors should be given with care in men with a recent myocardial infarction or stroke, resting hypotension, class III or class IV congestive heart failure, and unstable angina.

KEY POINTS: IMPOTENCE ✔

1. Erections are mediated by neural and endothelial NO release, which induce vasodilation.

2. The specific cause of impotence can be diagnosed in 85% of men.

3. The antihypertensives that are least likely to cause impotence are ACE inhibitors, ARBs, and calcium channel blockers.

4. PD inhibitors (sildenafil, vardenafil, and tadalafil) are the most effective drugs in treating nonhormonal impotence.

5. Men treated with testosterone replacement therapy should be monitored yearly by a digital rectal examination and blood tests for hemoglobin, PSA, hepatic function, and testosterone.

31. **What drug interactions are associated with PD5 inhibitors?**
Because PD5 inhibitors are metabolized via *CYP3A4*, any drugs that block that enzyme (e.g., erythromycin and other macrolide antibiotics; ketoconazole and other antifungal drugs; HIV protease inhibitors, such as saquinavir and ritonavir; and cimetidine) increase the plasma concentrations of PD5 inhibitors. In such cases, PD5 inhibitors should be started at one-fourth to one-half of the usual dose. Since PD5 inhibitors may potentiate the hypotensive effect of α-adrenergic blocking agents, they should be given in lower doses (Viagra) or not at all (Levitra) in men on alpha blockers for control of blood pressure or for benign prostatic hypertrophy.

32. **When are intracavernosal or intraurethral injections recommended?**
Injection of vasodilatory substances directly into the corpora cavernosa of the penis should be reserved for men in whom PD5 inhibitors are either ineffective or contraindicated or have produced intolerable adverse effects. Such "PD5 salvage" therapy results in erection satisfactory for intercourse in some men with impotence. PGE1 (Caverject), papaverine, and phentolamine may be used alone or in combination (Trimix).

33. **Discuss the side effects of intracavernosal and intraurethral injections.**
Side effects, which depend on the type and quantity of substances injected, include hypotension, elevation of liver enzymes, and headache. Local complications include hematoma, swelling, inadvertent injection into the urethra, and local fibrosis with long-term use. The most serious local complication is priapism (a sustained erection) for more than 4 hours, which may necessitate injection of α-adrenergic agonists or corpora cavernosal aspiration. PGE1 is also available

as an intraurethral suppository (medicated urethral system for erection [MUSE]) and, since it is less invasive and easier to use, may be a more appropriate second-line agent than intracavernosal injection. No controlled studies have evaluated the success of either approach in PD5 inhibitor failures.

34. **What other modalities are available to treat impotent men?**
Vacuum erection devices provide a noninvasive, mechanical solution for impotence. They are somewhat cumbersome to use and require the placement of an occlusive ring at the base of the penis to prevent venous outflow. They may be particularly effective in those men who have a "venous leak" as the etiology of their impotence. The constrictive ring prevents antegrade ejaculation because of the urethral constriction. Surgical revascularization has a limited place in the treatment of impotent men because of its invasiveness and limited success rate. Similarly, penile prosthesis insertion is rarely done because of the availability of several effective and noninvasive alternatives. In men in whom premature ejaculation is the major problem, intermittent use of selective serotonin reuptake inhibitors (SSRIs) has been efficacious in delaying time to ejaculation.

WEBSITES

1. http://www.endo-society.org/pubrelations/andro_cc_summary.pdf

2. http://www.impotence.org/

3. http://kidney.niddk.nih.gov/kudiseases/pubs/impotence/index.htm

BIBLIOGRAPHY

1. Adams MA, Banting BD, Maurice DH, et al: Vascular control mechanism in penile erection: Phylogeny and the inevitability of multiple overlapping systems. Int J Impotence Res 9:85–95, 1997.

2. Andersson, K-E: Erectile physiological and pathophysiological pathways involved in erectile dysfunction. J Urol. 170:S6–S14, 2003.

3. Bagatell CJ, Bremner WJ: Androgens in men—use and abuses. N Engl J Med 334:707–714, 1997.

4. Cohan P, Korenman SG: Erectile dysfunction. J Clin Endo Metab 86:2391–2394.

5. Cookson MS, Nadig PW: Long-term results with vacuum constriction device. J Urol 149:290–294, 1993.

6. Feldman HA, Goldstein I, Hatzichristou DJ, et al: Impotence and its medical and psychosocial correlates: Results of the Massachusetts male aging study. J Urol 151:54–61, 1994.

7. Goldstein I, Lue TF, Padma-Nathan H, et al: Oral sildenafil in the treatment of erectile dysfunction. N Engl J Med 338:1397–1404, 1998.

8. Goldstein I, Young JM, Fischer J, et al: Vardenafil, a new phosphodiesterase type 5 inhibitor, in the treatment of erectile dysfunction in men with diabetes: A multicenter double-blind placebo-controlled fixed-dose study. Diabetes Care 26:777–783, 2003.

9. Grimm RH Jr, Grandits GA, Prineas RJ, et al (for the TOHMS Research Group): Long-term effects on sexual function of five antihypertensive drugs and nutritional hygienic treatment in hypertensive men and women. Treatment of Mild Hypertension Study (TOHMS). Hypertension 29:8–14, 1997.

10. Hanash KA: Comparative results of goal oriented therapy for erectile dysfunction. J Urol 157: 2135–2139, 1997.

11. Herrmann HC, Chang G, Klugherz BD, Mahoney PD: Hemodynamic effects of sildenafil in men with severe coronary artery disease. N Engl J Med 342:1622–1626, 2000.

12. Hong G, Ji YH, Hong JH, et al: A double-blind crossover study evaluating the efficacy of Korean red ginseng in patients with erectile dysfunction: A preliminary report. J Urol 168:2070-2073, 2002.

13. Krane RJ, Goldstein I, DeTejada JS: Impotence. N Engl J Med 321:1648–1659, 1989.

14. Lerner SF, Melman A, Christ GJ: A review of erectile dysfunction: New insights and more questions. J Urol 149 (5 pt 2):1246–1252, 1993.

15. Linet OI, Ogring FG, and the Alprostadil Study Group:Efficacy and safety of intracavernosal prostaglandin in men with erectile dysfunction. N Engl J Med 334:873–878, 1996.

16. McMahon CG, Touma K: Treatment of premature ejaculation with paroxetine hydrochloride as needed: Two single-blind placebo controlled crossover studies. J Urol 161:1826–1830, 1999.

17. Morley JE, Kaiser FE: Impotence: The internists' approach to diagnosis and treatment. Adv Intern Med 38:151–168, 1993.

18. Neisler AW, Carey NP: A critical reevaluation of nocturnal penile tumescence monitoring in a diagnosis of erectile dysfunction. J Nerv Ment Dis 178:78–79, 1990.

19. NIH Consensus Conference: Impotence. JAMA 270:83–90, 1993.

20. Padma-Nathan H, Hellstrom WSG, Kaiser FE, et al [for the Medicated Urethral System for Erection (MUSE) Study Group]: Treatment of men with erectile dysfunction with transurethral alprostadil. N Engl J Med 336:1–7, 1997.

21. Porst H, Padma-Nathan H, Giuliano F, et al: Efficacy of tadalafil for the treatment of erectile dysfunction at 24 and 36 hours after dosing: A randomized controlled trial. Urology 62:121–125, 2003.

22. Rajfer J, Aronson WJ, Bush PA, et al: Nitric oxide as a mediator of relaxation of the corpus cavernosum in response to nonadrenergic, noncholinergic neurotransmission. N Engl J Med 326:90–94, 1992.

23. Rendell MS, Rajfer J, Wicker PA, et al: Sildenafil for treatment of erectile dysfunction in men with diabetes. A randomized controlled trial. JAMA 281:421–426, 1999.

24. Shabhigh R, Kaufman JM, Steidle JM, Padma-Nathan H: Testosterone replacement therapy with testosterone gel 1% converts sildenafil nonresponders to responders in men with erectile dysfunction and hypogonadism who failed prior sildenafil. J Urol 169:247, 2003 (abstract).

25. Sidi AA: Vasoactive intracavernous pharmacotherapy. Urol Clin N Am 15:95–101, 1988.

26. Witherington R: Mechanical aids for treatment of impotence. Clin Diabetes 7:1–22, 1989.

CHAPTER 47

GYNECOMASTIA

Brenda K. Bell, M.D.

1. **Define gynecomastia.**
   Gynecomastia is defined as the presence of palpable breast tissue in a male.

2. **How does gynecomastia present clinically?**
   Gynecomastia usually presents as a palpable discrete button of tissue radiating from beneath the nipple and areolar region. Gynecomastia will feel "gritty" when the breast is pinched between the thumb and forefinger. Fatty tissue, unlike gynecomastia, will not cause resistance until the nipple is reached. If doubt remains, soap and water on the breast can facilitate the examination by decreasing the skin friction.

3. **What is the significance of painful gynecomastia?**
   Gynecomastia is frequently asymptomatic and incidentally discovered. Pain or tenderness implies recent, rapid growth of breast tissue. This may indicate a pathologic cause for the gynecomastia and should prompt further evaluation.

4. **Is gynecomastia always bilateral?**
   The involvement tends to be bilateral, but asymmetry is common. Unilateral enlargement is present in 5–25% of patients and may be a preliminary stage in the development of bilateral disease. In autopsy studies, unilateral enlargement is often found to be bilateral gynecomastia histologically.

5. **Summarize the pathophysiology of gynecomastia.**
   Gynecomastia results from an imbalance between the stimulatory effect of estrogen on ductal proliferation and the inhibitory effect of androgen on breast development. The imbalance is most commonly caused by increased production of estrogens, decreased production of testosterone, or increased conversion of androgens to estrogens in peripheral tissue. Problems with sex hormone binding globulin and problems with androgen receptor binding and function can also result in gynecomastia.

6. **Where are estrogens produced in the male?**
   Direct testicular production of estrogens accounts for less than 15%. The majority of estrogens come from the conversion of adrenal and testicular androgens to estrogens in peripheral tissues, particularly adipose tissue and the liver.

7. **What is the most common cause of gynecomastia?**
   Asymptomatic palpable breast tissue is common in normal males, particularly in the neonate (60–90%), at puberty (60–70% between the ages of 12 and 15 years), and with increasing age (20–65% over age 50 years). Because of this high prevalence, gynecomastia is considered a relatively normal finding during the above periods of life. Gynecomastia at these ages is often called physiologic or idiopathic.

KEY POINTS: GENERAL APPROACH TO GYNECOMASTIA ✓

1. The most important differentiation is between gynecomastia and breast cancer. If doubt remains after physical examination, obtain a mammogram.

2. Most cases are bilateral, asymptomatic, and incidentally discovered. History, physical examination, and reevaluation in 3–6 months are appropriate for such men.

3. Rapid enlargement, growth greater than 4 cm, pain, and age less than 10 years or between 20 and 50 years correlate with systemic illness/pathologic cause for the gynecomastia. Such men should be evaluated thoroughly if the cause is not apparent after history and physical examination.

4. Malignant tumors, though rare, can cause gynecomastia. Consider testicular, pulmonary and abdominal tumors (pancreatic, adrenal, gastric, renal/bladder).

8. **Why does gynecomastia occur so commonly during these stages of life?**
Neonatal gynecomastia is due to placental transfer of estrogens. During early puberty, production of estrogens begins sooner than production of testosterone, causing an imbalance in the ratio of estrogens to androgens. With aging, production of testosterone decreases, and peripheral conversion of androgens to estrogens often increases because of an age-associated increase in adipose tissue.

9. **What are the other causes of gynecomastia?**
Idiopathic and pubertal gynecomastia makes up the majority of cases. Drugs account for 10–20% of cases and primary hypogonadism for another 10%. Adrenal or testicular tumors account for less than 3% of cases—gynecomastia may precede the development of the testicular tumor. Other causes combined account for less than 10% of cases and include secondary hypogonadism, androgen-resistant disorders, malnutrition, cirrhosis, alcohol abuse, renal disease, congenital adrenal hyperplasia, extragonadal tumors, and hyperthyroidism.

10. **What drugs cause gynecomastia?**
Many drugs have been implicated, some with known steroid effects, others with no clear mechanism:

Anabolic steroids	Methyldopa	Nifedipine	Protease inhibitors
Androgens	Reserpine	Verapamil	Amiodarone
Estrogen creams	Marijuana	Amlodipine	Risperidone
Spironolactone	Heroin	Diltiazem	Amphetamines
Flutamide	Methadone	Captopril	Minocycline
Finasteride	Phenytoin	Enalapril	Ethionamide
Cyproterone acetate	Diazepam	Thalidomide	Isoniazid
Ranitidine	Metronidazole	Fluoxetine	Tricyclic antidepressants
Cimetidine	Ketoconazole	Phenothiazines	Growth hormone
Omeprazole	Chemotherapy	Methotrexate	Theophylline
Digitoxin	Pravastatin	Haloperidol	Auranofin
Domperidone	Atorvastatin	Etretinate	Sulindac
Diethylpropion	Gabapentin	Penicillamine	Dong Quai
Metoclopramide	Alcohol	Melatonin	

11. **How do testicular tumors cause gynecomastia?**
Germ cell tumors can produce human chorionic gonadotropin (hCG). Like luteinizing hormone (LH), hCG increases testicular production of estradiol. Leydig cell tumors may directly secrete estradiol.

12. **What extragonadal tumors cause gynecomastia?**
Pancreatic, gastric, and pulmonary tumors, transitional cell carcinoma of the bladder and renal cell carcinoma have been associated with production of hCG. Hepatomas may have increased aromatase activity that results in excess conversion of androgens to estrogens.

13. **Who should undergo evaluation for gynecomastia?**
History and physical examination are indicated in all cases and will determine the cause in 30–40%. Gynecomastia is so common, however, that many experts are cautious about attaching importance to the detection of a small amount of breast tissue in an otherwise asymptomatic man. In adolescents, there is no reason to consider endocrine testing unless the enlargement is massive or the gynecomastia persists greater than 2 years. Acute development of enlargement and tenderness in males greater than age 20 warrants additional evaluation, as do eccentric, hard masses and lesions greater than 4 cm in size.

14. **What information is significant in the history?**

Age
Duration of enlargement
Breast symptoms (tenderness, discharge)
Other illnesses
Nutritional status and recent changes in weight
Impotence and libido

Thyroid symptoms
Drugs
Alcohol use
Congenital abnormalities
Pubertal progression

15. **What should be noted on the physical examination?**
The most important features include characteristics of the breast tissue (irregular, firm, eccentric; nipple discharge), testes (size, asymmetry), abdomen (liver enlargement, ascites, spider angioma), secondary sexual characteristics, thyroid status (goiter, tremor, reflexes), and any signs of excessive cortisol (buffalo hump, central obesity, hypertension, purple striae, moon facies).

KEY POINTS: TREATMENT OF GYNECOMASTIA ✓

1. Most cases resolve spontaneously or after removal of the offending medication or treatment of the underlying disease.

2. Medical management with tamoxifen can be attempted for 3–6 months if desired.

3. The longer the tissue has been present and the larger the amount of tissue, the less likely the response to tamoxifen. Surgery is indicated for these cases.

16. **Should laboratory tests be ordered?**
Some believe that hormonal testing is not cost-effective and favor checking testicular ultrasound alone to rule out the 3% incidence of feminizing tumors. Most, however, favor measuring liver enzymes, blood urea nitrogen, creatinine, thyrotropin (TSH), and testosterone (total and free). Estradiol, hCG, LH, and follicle-stimulating hormone (FSH) may follow the initial screen. If the hCG or estradiol level is elevated, a testicular ultrasound is indicated. If this is negative, chest radiograph and abdominal computed tomographic (CT) scan should follow. For prepubertal patients, an adrenal CT scan would precede the testicular ultrasound.

17. **What findings raise the suspicion of breast cancer?**
Breast cancer is rare in men (0.2%). The risk is increased in Klinefelter's syndrome (3–6%) and in male relatives of young women with breast cancer. Carcinoma is usually unilateral, painless,

and nontender. Bloody discharge, ulceration, firmness, fixation to the underlying tissue, eccentric location, and adenopathy are suspicious findings. If doubt remains, mammogram or biopsy should be considered. The sensitivity and specificity of mammogram for the diagnosis of male breast cancer approaches 90%. The diagnostic accuracy of fine-needle aspiration cytology is greater than 90%. Excisional biopsy or mastectomy would be recommended for malignant or suspicious cytology or mammogram appearance.

18. **Will gynecomastia spontaneously regress?**
Gynecomastia of recent onset, less than 3 cm in size will regress in 85% of patients. It may take 18–36 months for gynecomastia to resolve during puberty but resolution will occur in greater than 90% of pubertal boys. Persistence is uncommon after age 17. Gynecomastia due to a medication or underlying disease should also resolve after discontinuing the inciting agent or treating the underlying disease. Persistent tissue becomes more fibrous with time, however, and is less likely to remit spontaneously if it has been present for greater than 12 months. More highly developed breast tissue (Tanner stages III, IV, and V) is also less likely to regress.

19. **What is the treatment when gynecomastia does not regress?**
Hormonal therapy can be attempted. Tamoxifen, clomiphene, danazol, dihydrotestosterone, testolactone, and anastrozole have all been used. Tamoxifen has the fewest side effects and the highest response rate for both improvement in tenderness and decrease in size. Medication is more likely to work if gynecomastia has been present less than 4 months and the size of the tissue is less than 3 cm. Tamoxifen is given at a dose of 10 mg twice daily with follow-up in 3 months to assess response. For recurrent or persistent gynecomastia greater than 3 cm, surgery is the recommended therapy. Liposuction/ultrasound guided liposuction, excision or both may be used. Low-dose bilateral breast irradiation can be given prophylactically to prevent the development of gynecomastia caused by estrogens and antiandrogens used to treat prostate cancer.

BIBLIOGRAPHY

1. Bowers S, Pearlman N, McIntyre R, et al: Cost-effective management of gynecomastia. Am J Surg 176:638–641, 1998.
2. Braunstein G: Pathogenesis and diagnosis of gynecomastia. Up to Date in Endocrinology and Diabetes 11(2):1–11, 2003.
3. Braunstein G: Prevention and treatment of gynecomastia. Up to Date in Endocrinology and Diabetes 11(3):1–9, 2003.
4. Ersoz H, Onde M, Terekeci H, et al: Causes of gynecomastia in young adult males and factors associated with idiopathic gynecomastia. Int J Androl 25(5):312–316, 2002.
5. Evans G, Anthony T, Appelbaum A, et al: The diagnostic accuracy of mammography in the evaluation of male breast disease. Am J Surg 181(2):96–100, 2001.
6. Fruhstorfer B, Malata C: A systematic approach to the surgical treatment of gynecomastia. Br J Plast Surg 56(3):237–246, 2003.
7. Gruntmanis U, Braunstein G: Treatment of gynecomastia. Curr Opin Investig Drugs 2(5):643–649, 2001.
8. Ismail A, Barth J: Endocrinology of gynaecomastia. Ann Clin Biochem 38(6):596–607, 2001.
9. Khan H, Blarney R: Endocrine treatment of physiological gynecomastia. BMJ 327:301–302, 2003.
10. Widmark A, Fossa S, Lundmo P, et al: Does prophylactic breast irradiation prevent antiandrogen induced gynecomastia? Urology 61(1):145–151, 2003.
11. Yaturu S, Harrara E, Nopajaroonsri C, et al: Gynecomastia attributable to HCG secreting giant cell carcinoma of the lung. Endocr Pract 9(3):233–235, 2003.

CHAPTER 48

AMENORRHEA

Margaret E. Wierman, M.D.

1. **Define amenorrhea.**

   Amenorrhea is the absence of menstrual periods. Oligomenorrhea refers to lighter, irregular menses. Primary amenorrhea is the failure to ever begin menses, whereas secondary amenorrhea refers to cessation of menstrual periods after cyclic menses have been established.

2. **Describe the normal timing of puberty.**

   In girls, puberty usually begins after age 8 years and is heralded by the initiation of breast development. The average age for girls in the U.S. to begin menses is 12 years. This event generally signals the end of the pubertal process, occurring after the growth spurt and most somatic changes are completed.

3. **Summarize the underlying process of pubertal development.**

   The process is triggered by gonadotropin-releasing hormone (GnRH)-induced episodic secretion of luteinizing hormone (LH) and follicle-stimulating hormone (FSH) from the pituitary gland. The pulsatile release of gonadotropins activates the ovaries, causing maturation of follicles and production of estrogen, and, later, progesterone. These gonadal steroids give feedback at the level of the hypothalamus and pituitary to regulate GnRH and gonadotropin secretion. A final maturation event is the development of positive feedback by estradiol to induce the mid-cycle LH surge that stimulates ovulation. In many adolescents, menstrual cycles are anovulatory and thus irregular for the first 12–18 months. As the hypothalamic-pituitary-gonadal (HPG) axis matures, ovulatory cycles become more frequent. In normal adult women, all but one or two cycles per year are ovulatory.

4. **What types of disorders cause primary amenorrhea?**

   Primary amenorrhea is defined as lack of menses by age 16 or lack of secondary sexual characteristics by age 14. It usually results from abnormal anatomic development of the female reproductive organs or from a hormonal disorder involving the hypothalamus, pituitary gland, or ovaries (Table 48-1). The presence of normal secondary sexual characteristics in such patients suggests an anatomic problem, such as obstruction or failure of development of the uterus or vagina. In contrast, a lack of secondary sexual characteristics indicates a probable hormonal cause.

5. **What are hypothalamic and pituitary causes of primary amenorrhea?**

   GnRH deficiency due to maturational arrest of GnRH-producing neurons in the olfactory placode during embryonic development is a hypothalamic cause of primary amenorrhea. The pituitary gland itself may be compressed by pituitary tumors, craniopharyngiomas, and Rathke's pouch cysts, causing impaired LH and FSH secretion.

6. **Summarize the ovarian causes of primary amenorrhea.**

   The ovaries may be defective because of gonadal dysgenesis due to Turner's syndrome (45XO karyotype) or destruction by chemotherapy or radiation prior to the completion of sexual maturation. The presence of ambiguous genitalia or palpable gonads in the labia or inguinal area may indicate a disorder of sexual differentiation, such as CAH (21-hydroxylase deficiency) or an androgen resistance syndrome (testicular feminization) due to a defect in the androgen receptor.

TABLE 48-1. CAUSES OF PRIMARY AMENORRHEA

Mechanical
- Congenital absence of ovaries, uterus, or vagina
- Cervical stenosis
- Imperforate hymen

Hormonal

Hypothalamic
- GnRH deficiency
- Hypothalamic tumor (craniopharyngioma)

Pituitary
- Prolactinoma
- Rathke's cleft cyst
- Panhypopituitarism from a genetic mutation

Ovarian
- Gonadal dysgenesis (XO)
- Chemotherapy or radiation damage of the ovaries
- Androgen resistance syndromes (XY)

Other: congenital adrenal hyperplasia (CAH)

---

7. **What disorders cause secondary amenorrhea?**

Secondary amenorrhea, which is much more common than primary amenorrhea, occurs post-pubertally. The causes are outlined in Table 48-2. Pregnancy should be excluded in all amenorrheic women. Onset of irregular menses after having regular menses and association with hot flashes should suggest premature menopause. Hypothalamic amenorrhea is a GnRH pulse generator defect that is a diagnosis of exclusion. Hyperprolactinemia is an underlying cause in 10% of women. Pituitary tumors can result in secondary amenorrhea. Hyperandrogenic anovulatory disorders present with oligomenorrhea or amenorrhea and signs and symptoms of excess androgens, such as hirsutism and acne.

TABLE 48-2. CAUSES OF SECONDARY AMENORRHEA

Pregnancy

Hypogonadotropic hypogonadism
- Hyperprolactinemia (from drugs or prolactinoma)
- Pituitary tumor inhibiting gonadotropin production
- Hypothalamic amenorrhea

Hypergonadotropic hypogonadism
- Premature ovarian failure (surgical or autoimmune)
- Gonadotropin producing pituitary tumors

---

8. **How do you evaluate a patient with amenorrhea?**

One must determine whether the disorder is anatomic or hormonal, congenital or acquired, and where the defect is located. A complete history and physical examination provide the first essential clues. Measurement of serum gonadotropin levels (LH and FSH) separates patients into one of two categories. Patients with low or normal levels of LH and FSH (hypogonadotropic hypogonadism) have a disorder at the level of the hypothalamus or pituitary gland. However, patients with high LH and FSH levels (hypergonadotropic hypogonadism) may have a defect at the level of either the ovary or hypothalamic-pituitary unit (e.g., gonadotropin-producing pituitary tumors and polycystic ovary syndrome [PCOS], in which the hypothalamic GnRH pulse generator is abnormally accelerated).

9. **Discuss the major congenital causes of hypogonadotropic hypogonadism.**
   Congenital or idiopathic hypogonadotropic hypogonadism is due to GnRH deficiency. Female patients present with primary amenorrhea. When associated with anosmia, the disorder is termed Kallmann's syndrome. GnRH deficiency occurs in 1/10,000 males and 1/80,000 females and may be X-linked, autosomal dominant, autosomal recessive, or sporadic. The X-linked form is associated with a mutation in the anosmin gene that encodes a neural cell adhesion protein thought to be important in providing the scaffolding for GnRH neurons in their migration from the olfactory placode to the hypothalamus during embryonic development. Thus, GnRH-secreting neurons fail to reach their target in the hypothalamus but instead remain in the olfactory area. All other hypothalamic-pituitary function is normal. Gonadal steroid administration is used to initiate the development of secondary sexual characteristics, and fertility can be attained using pulsatile GnRH or gonadotropin therapy.

10. **What are the acquired forms of amenorrhea due to hypogonadotropic hypogonadism?**
    - Hyperprolactinemia
    - Hypothalamic amenorrhea

11. **How does hyperprolactinemia cause amenorrhea?**
    Elevated prolactin levels may be due to prolactinomas, hypothyroidism, medications (usually psychotropic drugs), and pregnancy. Hyperprolactinemia impairs function of the HPG axis at all levels, but the major site of inhibition is the hypothalamic GnRH pulse generator. As prolactin levels rise, luteal phase defects develop, ovulation ceases, and menstrual cycles become shorter and irregular. Higher elevation in prolactin levels are associated with amenorrhea. Treatment of the underlying cause of the elevated prolactin level usually normalizes menstrual cycles.

12. **What is hypothalamic amenorrhea?**
    Hypothalamic amenorrhea refers to amenorrhea resulting from acquired disorders of the GnRH pulse generator. Excessive stress, exercise, and weight loss have been shown to act centrally to disrupt the GnRH-induced pulsatile gonadotropin secretory pattern. In men, GnRH-induced LH pulses normally occur every 2 hours. In contrast, the LH pulse pattern in women must change across the menstrual cycle, accelerating from every 90 minutes in the early follicular phase to every 30 minutes at ovulation and then slowing from every hour to every 8 hours across the luteal phase. Disruption of this sensitively timed pattern results in anovulation, irregular menses, and, eventually, amenorrhea.

13. **What types of GnRH pulse generator defects cause hypothalamic amenorrhea?**
    Hypothalamic amenorrhea may result from several different types of gonadotropin secretory disorders. Some women with anorexia nervosa have absent LH pulsations (prepubertal pattern), some have pulsations only at night (early pubertal pattern), and still others have LH pulses throughout the 24-hour period but they are significantly reduced in amplitude or frequency.

14. **How do you make a diagnosis of hypothalamic amenorrhea?**
    The diagnosis depends on excluding other causes of amenorrhea and then relies heavily on a history of weight loss and/or high levels of exercise or stress. Supportive findings on

physical examination include evidence of decreased estrogen effects and absence of other major illnesses. Laboratory testing usually reveals low serum estradiol and low or low-normal serum LH and FSH levels; the test for β-hCG is negative, and the prolactin level is normal. Elevated FSH levels with low estradiol levels, in contrast, indicate probable premature ovarian failure.

15. **What are the consequences of estrogen deficiency?**
Short-term consequences of estrogen deficiency may include painful intercourse and hot flashes. Among the more important long-term consequences are osteoporosis and premature coronary artery disease.

16. **What treatment options are available for hypothalamic amenorrhea?**
Interventions to increase body weight and to reduce stress and/or exercise should be attempted initially. If these interventions are unsuccessful, estrogen replacement therapy should be instituted. Fertility, if desired, may be achieved by ovulation induction with clomiphene in mild cases or with human menopausal gonadotropins or pulsatile GnRH administration if the disorder is more severe.

17. **What disorders cause amenorrhea with hypergonadotropic hypogonadism?**
- Premature ovarian failure (high FSH, later high LH)
- PCOS (low FSH, high LH)
- Gonadotropin-secreting pituitary tumors (high FSH and/or LH)

18. **How do you make a diagnosis of premature ovarian failure?**
Premature ovarian failure, which is defined as menopause before the age of 40, may be due to surgical removal or autoimmune destruction of the ovaries. Autoimmune destruction of the ovaries is characterized by a history of normal puberty and regular menses followed by the early onset of hot flashes, irregular menses, and eventual amenorrhea. Elevated serum FSH levels are the laboratory hallmark of gonadal failure. To avoid misdiagnosis, blood for FSH measurement must be drawn in the early follicular phase, if the woman still has menses, because FSH levels rise along with LH at mid-cycle in normally ovulating women. Turner's syndrome mosaics (XO/XX) may have several menses before they undergo menopause; therefore, a karyotype may be helpful if ovarian failure occurs in adolescence or the early 20s.

19. **What other disorders may coexist with premature ovarian failure?**
Both patients and family members are at risk for other autoimmune disorders, including primary adrenal insufficiency (Addison's disease), autoimmune thyroid disorders (Graves' disease, Hashimoto's disease), type 1 diabetes mellitus, pernicious anemia (vitamin B_{12} deficiency), celiac sprue, and rheumatologic disorders.

20. **What are the treatment options for women with premature ovarian failure?**
Estrogen replacement therapy, usually in combination with progesterone, is critical to decrease postmenopausal bone loss and premature coronary artery disease. New options for fertility in women with premature ovarian failure include incubation of donor eggs with the partner's sperm in in vitro fertilization protocols along with hormonal preparation of the patient to enable her to carry the fetus in her uterus.

21. **What is hyperandrogenic anovulation?**
Hyperandrogenic anovulation refers to the cluster of disorders that present with irregular menses or amenorrhea and signs of androgen excess, such as hirsutism and virilization. The disorders in this group include PCOS, androgen-secreting tumors of the ovaries or adrenal glands, CAH (classic or attenuated form), and obesity-induced amenorrhea.

KEY POINTS: AMENORRHEA ✓

1. Amenorrhea with estrogen deficiency can result in osteoporosis and premature cardiovascular disease.

2. Hyperprolactinemia and hypothalamic amenorrhea are the most common causes of amenorrhea with low estrogen and low FSH levels.

3. Premature menopause (high FSH, low E) is an autoimmune disease and patients are at risk for other autoimmune disorders, such as autoimmune thyroid disease, pernicious anemia, celiac sprue, and rheumatologic disorders.

4. Hyperandrogenic anovulation refers to amenorrhea with hirsutism and acne.

5. Polycystic ovarian disease is common, associated with risks of infertility, endometrial cancer, the metabolic syndrome, and type 2 diabetes.

22. **How do tumors cause hyperandrogenic anovulation?**
Tumors are suggested by rapid progression of hirsutism and virilization (temporal hair recession, clitoris enlargement, breast atrophy) and by high serum androgen levels; they may be excluded by a serum testosterone level less than 200 ng/dL or dehydroepiandrosterone sulfate (DHEAS) levels less than 1000 ng/mL.

23. **What clinical and biochemical features suggest a patient with hirsutism has CAH?**
CAH (most commonly due to 21-hydroxylase deficiency) presents in infancy with ambiguous genitalia in girls occasionally with salt wasting syndromes. In adolescence, it is detected with early pubarche and irregular menses. Family history and ethnicity (Ashkenazi Jews, Italians, Hispanics) increase the suspicion of CAH. CAH is diagnosed by high basal (> 2–3 ng/mL) or adrenocorticotropic hormone (ACTH)-stimulated (> 10 ng/ml) levels of 17-hydroxyprogesterone.

24. **When should you suspect obesity-induced amenorrhea?**
Obesity-induced amenorrhea is suggested by a history of normal puberty and menses until progressive weight gain triggers the development of hirsutism, acne, oligomenorrhea, and, later, amenorrhea. Affected women have low serum levels of FSH and LH in the follicular phase in contrast to women with PCOS (see the following).

25. **Describe the pathophysiology of obesity-induced amenorrhea.**
Fat tissue contains aromatase and 5-α-reductase enzymes. Aromatase converts androgens to estrogens; when aromatase is present in increased amounts, as in obesity, constant elevated (rather than normally fluctuating) serum estrogen levels are produced, inhibiting LH and FSH secretion and thereby impairing normal ovulation. Increased activity of 5-α-reductase, which converts testosterone to dihydrotestosterone (DHT), results in excessive DHT production, promoting the development of hirsutism and acne. Primary treatment of obesity results in restoration of normal reproductive function.

26. **How does the patient with PCOS present clinically?**
Most patients with PCOS present in adolescence with a history of early menarche (< 12 years) and persistently irregular menses. Hirsutism and acne beginning in the teenage years are other common features of the disorder. About 60% of patients become overweight in their 20s and 30s. Patients also frequently have signs of insulin resistance, including acanthosis nigricans, a

velvety, hyperpigmented cutaneous lesion on the neck and in the axillae. Irregular, anovulatory menses lead to infertility, and the resultant unopposed estrogen exposure increases the risk of endometrial hyperplasia and carcinoma.

27. **Describe the pathogenesis of PCOS.**

Experts disagree as to whether PCOS is a primary disorder of the central nervous system, the adrenal glands, or the ovaries. Existing data support the presence of an abnormal hypothalamic GnRH pulse generator that, in contrast to hypothalamic amenorrhea, is set too fast. The pituitary gonadotropin response to GnRH is rate dependent; rapid GnRH pulses stimulate LH secretion but inhibit FSH production. The increased LH/FSH secretory ratio results in inadequate ovarian follicle recruitment and/or development, causing anovulation and the appearance of multiple subcapsular cysts. The GnRH pattern triggers constant estrogen and enhanced androgen production by the ovaries. The ovarian androgens—dehydroepiandrosterone (DHEA), androstenedione, and testosterone—may be elevated; for unclear reasons, the adrenal androgens, DHEA and DHEAS, may be increased as well. High levels of circulating androgens decrease hepatic production of sex hormone-binding globulin (SHBG), allowing more free androgen to target the skin and hair follicles, inducing the development of acne and hirsutism. Insulin resistance also plays a role in the ultimate picture because hyperinsulinemia augments ovarian androgen production and further reduces SHBG levels.

28. **What are the treatment options for patients with PCOS?**

The initial goals are to suppress androgen production and action and to ensure regular shedding of the endometrium to decrease the risk of developing endometrial hyperplasia. Birth control pills are the treatment of choice; an antiandrogen, such as spironolactone, may be added if hirsutism is a major problem. Intermittent cycling with medroxyprogesterone (Provera) is an alternative for endometrial protection but does not suppress the elevated androgens and their ultimate impact on ovarian morphology and function. Fertility may be achieved with clomiphene, human menopausal gonadotropins, or pulsatile GnRH administration, but only with difficulty because of the already overactive hormonal environment. Recently designed regimens using progesterone pretreatment to slow the GnRH pulse generator or a GnRH agonist to inhibit endogenous GnRH, coupled with induction of ovulation by human menopausal gonadotropins, have been more successful.

29. **Is there a role for insulin sensitizers in the treatment of women with PCOS?**

Studies have shown that reducing insulin resistance and serum insulin levels with metformin results in modest decreases in serum androgen levels, decreased BP, improved lipids, with some improvement in menstrual regularity, and improved ovulation in response to clomiphene citrate. The thiazolidinedione class of insulin sensitizers has shown promise, but the first-generation agent, troglitazone, was taken off the market. Studies with rosiglitazone and pioglitazone are ongoing. Information on combination therapy with birth control pills, antiandrogens, and insulin sensitizers are not yet available. Predictors of responders to metformin may include patients with a family history of type 2 diabetes, history of rapid weight gain, and lack of severe obesity (body mass index [BMI] < 40).

30. **What are the long-term consequences of PCOS?**

Long-term consequences include infertility, obesity, metabolic syndrome with hypertension, central adiposity, dyslipidemia and increased risk of glucose intolerance, and type 2 diabetes. Epidemiologic studies have not yet defined a clear-cut increase in cardiovascular events, but long-term studies are under way. Oral glucose tolerance testing is recommended in all patients with BMI > 27.

BIBLIOGRAPHY

1. Berga SL: Functional hypothalamic chronic anovulation. In Adashi WY, Rock JA, Rosenwaks Z (eds): Reproductive Endocrinology, Surgery, and Technology. Philadelphia, Lippincott-Raven, 1996, pp 1061–1075.

2. Cumming DC: Exercise-associated amenorrhea, low bone density, and estrogen replacement therapy. Arch Intern Med 156:2193–2195, 1996.

3. Ehrmann DA: Insulin lowering therapeutic modalities for polycystic ovary syndrome. Endocrine Metab Clin North Am 28 (2):423–438, 1999.

4. Kiningham RB, Apgar BS, Schwenk TL: Evaluation of amenorrhea. Am Fam Physician 53:1185–1194, 1996.

5. Pralong FP, Crowley WF Jr: Gonadotropins: Normal physiology. In Wierman ME (ed): Diseases of the Pituitary: Diagnosis and Treatment. Totowa, Humana Press, 1997, pp 203–219.

6. Schlechte JA: Differential diagnosis and management of hyperprolactinemia. In Wierman ME (ed): Diseases of the Pituitary: Diagnosis and Treatment. Totowa, Humana Press, 1997, pp 71–77.

7. Taylor AE, Adams JM, Mulder JE, et al: A randomized, controlled trial of estradiol replacement therapy in women with hypergonadotropic amenorrhea. J Clin Endocrinol Metab 81:3615–3621, 1996.

8. Warren MP: Anorexia, bulimia, and exercise-induced amenorrhea: Medical approach. Curr Ther Endocrinol Metab 6:13–17, 1997.

9. Welt CK, Hall JE: Gonadotropin deficiency: Differential diagnosis and treatment. In Wierman ME (ed): Diseases of the Pituitary: Diagnosis and Treatment. Totowa, Humana Press, 1997, pp 221–246.

10. Wierman ME: Gonadotropin releasing hormone. In Adashi WY, Rock JA, Rosenwaks Z (eds): Reproductive Endocrinology, Surgery, and Technology. Philadelphia, Lippincott-Raven, 1996, pp 665–681.

CHAPTER 49

GALACTORRHEA

William J. Georgitis, M.D.

1. **Define galactorrhea.**
   Galactorrhea is a milk discharge from the breast not associated with breast-feeding. It may also be defined as a milk-like discharge from the breast of a nongravid woman. Milk production persisting for 6 months after nursing has ceased should also be considered galactorrhea and properly investigated for a pathologic cause.

2. **Which hormones affect lactation?**
   Estrogen and prolactin are necessary for milk production. Estrogens promote cellular proliferation and ductular development. Prolactin rises dramatically during pregnancy stimulating further differentiation of acini to prepare the breast for production of milk protein. Paradoxically, high levels of estrogen inhibit milk production during pregnancy. Shortly after delivery, estrogen levels decline and lactation begins. Growth hormone, insulin, and cortisol are necessary permissive factors for breast cell growth in tissue cultures. Androgens inhibit breast growth and differentiation. Galactorrhea rarely occurs in men but can occur in the presence of prolactin excess and an alteration in the normal ratio of androgen and estrogen (see Fig. 49-1).

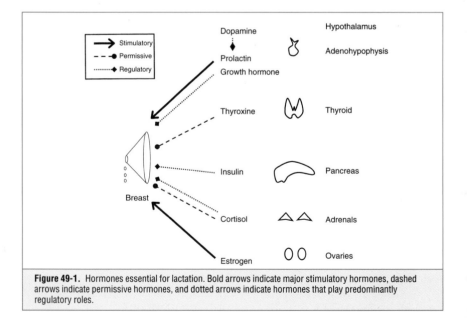

Figure 49-1. Hormones essential for lactation. Bold arrows indicate major stimulatory hormones, dashed arrows indicate permissive hormones, and dotted arrows indicate hormones that play predominantly regulatory roles.

3. **How common is galactorrhea?**
   Quite common. The lifelong cumulative frequency of galactorrhea has been reported to range
   from 2% to 20%. Milk should not be found in nulligravidas, postmenopausal women not receiving hormone replacement, or in men.

4. **Does galactorrhea look like milk?**
   Not always. Breast milk is an emulsion of fat and water. It has over 100 known constituents. The
   fat content of milk varies and the gross appearance may range from milky to opalescent to clear.
   Microscopic examination confirms that a breast secretion is galactorrhea by revealing fat glob-
   ules. Special stains for fat or chemical analysis for lactate or specific milk proteins are rarely
   necessary.

5. **Is galactorrhea always expressed from both breasts?**
   No. Galactorrhea may be unilateral or bilateral. Although many patients report frank leaking or
   staining of garments, some may not notice the discharge. Small amounts of serous fluid can be
   expressed from the breasts of a majority of normal nulliparous women.

6. **List a differential diagnosis for galactorrhea?**
   The differential diagnosis for galactorrhea can be both lengthy and complex. Causes for non-
   puerperal galactorrhea are not easily arranged in a logical sequence. Some lists categorize diagnoses by anatomic location, some by causality, and some by symptoms or signs. Most attempts
   at a structured approach to the differential become less structured as the list progresses. A shift
   in gender often complicates matters. Table 49-1 lists the causes of galactorrhea. Examples are
   given in parentheses.

TABLE 49-1. CAUSES OF NONPUERPERAL GALACTORRHEA	
Idiopathic	Endocrinopathies
Pituitary tumors	Primary hypothyroidism
Prolactinoma	Hyperthyroidism
Somatotropinoma	Primary adrenal insufficiency
Hypothalamic disorders	Endogenous estrogens
Tumor (craniopharyngioma)	Adrenocortical carcinoma
Infiltrative disease (sarcoid)	Reflex arc activation
Infundibular disruption (trauma)	Nipple stimulation
Medications	Thoracic nerve irritation (shingles)
Psychotropic (risperidone)	Miscellaneous associations
Antihypertensive (methyldopa)	Stress
Cannabinoid (morphine)	Empty sella syndrome
Estrogens (oral contraceptives)	Renal or hepatic failure
Antiemetics (metoclopramide)	Polycystic ovary syndrome

7. **Which medications cause galactorrhea?**
   Psychotropic medications are the leading culprits. The most common are phenothiazines, tricyclic antidepressants, haloperidol, benzodiazepines, butyrophenones, amphetamines, and

monoamine oxidase (MAO) inhibitors. Other commonly prescribed drugs implicated as causes include cimetidine, metoclopramide, verapamil, and estrogens in numerous formulations. Prolactin levels can rise 10–20 times above the upper limit of normal with some antipsychotic medications with 17–78% of women experiencing amenorrhea with or without galactorrhea. The pituitary-gonadal axis in men is less affected by psychotropic medications. Risperidone is a particularly noteworthy drug, causing prolactin levels as high as 400 ng/mL.

8. **How often should one obtain a menstrual history from a woman with galactorrhea?**
   Always obtain a comprehensive menstrual history from any woman with galactorrhea. The most common physiologic cause for amenorrhea-galactorrhea is pregnancy. The diagnosis should be considered first. A galactorrheic woman without amenorrhea has only a 20% chance of harboring a pituitary tumor. The prevalence of a pituitary tumor increases to 34% when amenorrhea accompanies galactorrhea.

9. **What percentage of women with hyperprolactinemia have galactorrhea?**
   Women with elevated prolactin levels have a prevalence of galactorrhea ranging from 50% to 80%. The degree of prolactin elevation correlates poorly with the amount of lactation. However, the level of prolactin does provide important clues to etiology.

10. **Discuss the physiologic variations in prolactin levels.**
    Prolactin is a dynamic, not a static, hormone. It rises after meals and in response to hypoglycemia, seizures, intercourse, and vigorous nipple stimulation. Normal levels range as high as 20 ng/mL and show a diurnal variation.

11. **Does degree of elevation in the serum prolactin level help determine the cause for galactorrhea?**
    Drug-induced galactorrhea is usually accompanied by moderately elevated serum prolactin levels. Most medications cause galactorrhea by competitively blocking dopamine receptors. Mild hyperprolactinemia may also result from pituitary, hypothalamic, or parasellar processes. Mass lesions compressing or disrupting normal hypothalamic-pituitary portal connections permit prolactin levels to rise from the loss of the normal restraining influence of dopamine. Both drug-induced and non-prolactin-secreting pituitary region tumors are associated with prolactin levels ranging from 20 to 100 ng/mL. Prolactin levels above 100 ng/mL are most often due to pregnancy or prolactinomas. In a nonpregnant individual, the odds of finding a prolactinoma are proportionate to the degree of hyperprolactinemia. Levels above 300 ng/mL usually indicate the presence of a prolactinoma readily demonstratable with current pituitary imaging methods. Patients with levels ranging from 100 to 300 ng/mL should also have pituitary imaging. If a tumor is not found and treatment not recommended, continued surveillance is necessary because the majority do have microprolactinomas below the resolving power of current imaging modalities.

12. **What other lab tests should be included in the evaluation of galactorrhea?**
    In addition to the mandatory pregnancy test for every potentially fertile woman, a thyroid-stimulating hormone (TSH) should be measured in every patient. Primary hypothyroidism can present as the amenorrhea-galactorrhea syndrome. The accompanying lactotroph hyperplasia in the pituitary may mimic a pituitary adenoma and there are published reports of patients with massive hyperplasia and bitemporal hemianopsia from optic chiasmal compression. Signs of hypothyroidism may be subtle in young women. A TSH level should therefore be measured in every case. It would be a serious disservice to the patient to miss primary hypothyroidism as the cause for amenorrhea-galactorrhea for many reasons. Both the pituitary hyperplasia and the amenorrhea-galactorrhea gradually resolve with thyroxine therapy, which is much less expensive than treatment with dopamine agonists like bromocriptine and cabergoline, associated with

fever, side effects, and correcting hypothyroidism even in the clinically occult case often has benefits recognized by both the physician and the patient in retrospect.

13. **It seems odd that hyperthyroidism is listed as a cause for galactorrhea just below hypothyroidism. How did that come about?**
A single article reported a high prevalence of galactorrhea expressed with breast and nipple compression in hyperthyroid patients. Prolactin levels were normal and the mechanism for the galactorrhea is obscure. Since these patients did not present with symptomatic galactorrhea with subsequent hyperthyroidism defined as the etiology, and it has not been shown that expressible galactorrhea resolves after treatment of the hyperthyroidism, the relevance of this observation to clinical practice is of questionable significance. Perhaps hyperthyroidism should be dropped from the list of disorders included in the differential diagnosis of galactorrhea.

14. **Describe the proposed mechanism for galactorrhea following thoracic surgery or associated with painful chest wall lesions.**
Galactorrhea sometimes appears after major surgery involving both the thorax and the abdomen. In the postoperative period, a woman's prolactin levels may rise while estrogen levels fall—a relationship that favors lactation. There is not a greater frequency of galactorrhea following chest wall surgery compared to other major surgical procedures. Postoperative hyperprolactinemia is not sustained. Galactorrhea also occurs with herpes zoster involving nerves supplying dermatomes in the pectoral region. Prolactin levels are similar to drug-induced hyperprolactinemia ranging up to about 100 ng/mL. The increased prolactin secretion results from stimulation of a neural reflex arc between the breast and the pituitary-hypothalamic unit.

15. **Galactorrhea in renal failure seems odd. What is the connection?**
Hyperprolactinemia in renal failure is modest in degree. It results from decreased metabolic clearance of prolactin but often medications with dopamine inhibitory actions also play a role. Most renal insufficiency patients with elevated prolactin levels do not have galactorrhea.

16. **Can galactorrhea occur in the absence of excessive prolactin?**
Yes. One-third of women with acromegaly have galactorrhea. Galactorrhea results most often from one of two mechanisms but there is a third mechanism. The first is prolactin secretion by the pituitary tumor itself. The second common mechanism is prolactin release due to pituitary stalk disruption and loss of the constant tonic restraint of dopamine inhibition on lactotrophs.

Rarely, an acromegalic patient with galactorrhea will have normal levels of prolactin. The 191-amino-acid human growth hormone molecule has 16% structural homology with the 198-amino-acid human prolactin. Twenty-four percent of the first 50 amino acids are similar. In normoprolactinemic acromegalic patients with galactorrhea, the galactorrhea probably results from cross-activation of breast prolactin receptors by very high levels of growth hormone.

17. **Is galactorrhea associated with an increased risk of breast cancer?**
No. When a breast discharge occurs in breast cancer, a palpable mass is usually present. It is not a common presenting feature of breast cancer. Even bloody breast secretions more often result from benign conditions, including mastitis. Some evidence suggests the risk of breast cancer is reduced in premenopausal women who have lactated.

18. **Are medications often used to treat postpartum galactorrhea?**
Not any more. Dopamine agonists, such as bromocriptine, pergolide, and cabergoline, are still the drugs of choice for patients with prolactinomas. They are also effective for other causes of galactorrhea. In 1994, the manufacturer of bromocriptine withdrew postpartum lactation as a treatment indication following case reports of vascular side effects attributed to bromocriptine, including stroke and myocardial ischemia. Women who choose not to nurse their babies can use

measures, including garments providing firm breast support, analgesics, and ice packs, to relieve the discomfort of postpartum breast engorgement.

19. **What about galactorrhea in men?**

Men rarely present for evaluation of galactorrhea as a primary presenting complaint even though some series have reported that men comprise about 5% of patients evaluated for galactorrhea. Galactorrhea is uncommon even in hyperprolactinemic men due to the lack of estrogen priming necessary for milk production. A man with galactorrhea needs to be examined for feminizing syndromes and a prolactin-producing pituitary tumor.

20. **Does galactorrhea always need treatment?**

Not always. Generally, galactorrhea unaccompanied by amenorrhea, infertility, osteopenia, or a pituitary tumor does not have serious long-term consequences if left untreated. Treatment is indicated to restore fertility and may be indicated when a pituitary tumor is present if the tumor is large or causing symptoms.

KEY POINTS: GALACTORRHEA ✓

1. Prolactin levels rise during pregnancy overlapping with the range of elevation found with prolactinomas.

2. Primary hypothyroidism can cause amenorrhea, galactorrhea, and pituitary enlargement and thus mimic a prolactinoma.

3. The absence of lactation postpartum can signify pituitary necrosis (Sheehan syndrome).

4. Many medications can cause galactorrhea.

5. Painful lesions of the thoracic wall can induce galactorrhea.

6. Estrogen and prolactin are necessary for milk production.

7. High levels of estrogen can inhibit lactation.

21. **Do microadenomas require treatment?**

Microadenomas, which are by definition less than 1 cm in diameter, rarely seem to grow to macroadenomas. Spontaneous improvement with falling prolactin levels and return of menstruation can occur. However, if infertility or estrogen deficiency and osteopenia are present, even microprolactinomas may need treatment. Continued observation is necessary in all cases.

22. **Why should macroadenomas be treated?**

Macroadenomas associated with galactorrhea may need treatment because vision may be threatened or a morbid condition like acromegaly may result from excess cosecretion of another pituitary hormone in addition to prolactin. The most common functional pituitary tumors with galactorrhea are prolactinomas.

23. **How are macroadenomas treated?**

Transsphenoidal surgery for small prolactinomas initially showed postoperative success in about 80% of cases compared with the lower success rate of 50% for macroprolactinomas. Transsphenoidal surgery as the initial treatment of choice for microprolactinomas fell into disfavor when recurrence rates assessed several years postoperatively ranged from 17% to 91%. Now medical therapy with dopamine agonists is first-line therapy for all size categories of prolactinomas.

24. **How do dopamine agonists work in the treatment of macroadenomas?**
Dopamine agonists, including bromocriptine, pergolide, and cabergoline, all lower prolactin levels, shrink tumors, and can restore cyclic menstrual function in premenopausal women with prolactinomas. Serum prolactin levels need to be reduced near or into the normal range to restore menses and control galactorrhea. Galactorrhea can decrease within hours of starting treatment. Some reduction in tumor size occurs in 9 out of 10 patients. A 25% reduction in size occurs in nearly 8 out of 10. Surgery and radiation therapy are effective for tumors failing to respond to medications and occasionally for drug-intolerant patients. Radiation therapy stops tumor growth and results in a gradual decline in prolactin levels over many years. The slow decline in prolactin is accompanied by a progressive increase in the prevalence of radiation-induced hypopituitarism. Surgery and radiation should now be viewed as adjuncts to medical treatment rather than primary treatment modalities for most prolactinoma patients.

25. **What is macroprolactinemia?**
Rarely hyperprolactinemia results from the formation of prolactin multimers in the serum of patients without any sign of reproductive dysfunction or pituitary tumor. This has been called macroprolactinemia. Laboratories can investigate this by several techniques, including the use of polyethylene glycol during assay and serial dilution studies. Proceeding to pituitary imaging in such cases can be misleading because of a significant incidence of unrelated pituitary abnormalities and incidentalomas. This pitfall can be avoided by asking about galactorrhea and taking an adequate menstrual history and then considering the pretest probability of disease before ordering a prolactin level.

26. **What can failure to lactate postpartum indicate?**
It may indicate the presence of Sheehan syndrome. Pituitary necrosis associated with childbirth can lead to the failure to lactate and menstruate postpartum. Loss of pubic and axillary hair can also occur if the deficiencies of prolactin and gonadotropins are accompanied by the loss of corticotropin-dependent adrenal androgen secretion. Pituitary necrosis occurs in deliveries complicated by hypotension from sepsis or hemorrhage. In the United States, pituitary insufficiency from Sheehan syndrome is usually limited to anterior pituitary functions. In some areas of the world, posterior pituitary necrosis can be more extensive resulting in vasopressin deficiency manifesting as neurogenic diabetes insipidus. More prolonged and severe hypotension leads to extension of the pituitary infarction to the neurohypophysis.

27. **Did Hippocrates speak of amenorrhea or galactorrhea?**
His aphorisms show that he did: "If a woman who is neither pregnant nor has given birth produces milk, her menstruation has stopped." (Aphorisms, Section V, No. 39.) Nowadays this woman, having Googled the internet, may come to you requesting pituitary magnetic resonance imaging (MRI) and bearing in hand a negative home pregnancy test and a printout showing the elevated prolactin and normal TSH from a self-serve reference laboratory.
Hippocrates also spoke of early pregnancy and morning sickness: "If the catamenia are suppressed, without being followed by rigor or fever, but by disinclination for food, pregnancy may be suspected." (Aphorisms, Section V, No. 61.) This aphorism reminds us that amenorrhea in women of reproductive age should always make pregnancy a prime consideration.

WEBSITE

Family Practice Notebook. Available at www.fpnotebook.com

BIBLIOGRAPHY

1. Bevan JS, Webster J, Burke CW, Scanlon MF: Dopamine agonists and pituitary tumor shrinkage. Endocr Rev 13:220–240, 1992.

2. Biller BM: Diagnostic evaluation of hyperprolactinemia. J Reprod Med 44(12 Suppl):1095–1099, 1999.

3. Dalkin AC, Marshall JC: Medical therapy of hyperprolactinemia. Endocrinol Metab Clin North Am 18:259–276, 1989.

4. Falkenberry SS. Nipple discharge. Obstet Gynecol Clin North Am. 29:21–29, 2002.

5. Fiorica JV: Nipple discharge. Obstet Gynecol Clin North Am 21:453–460, 1994.

6. Fradkin JE, Eastman RC, Lesniak MA, et al: Specificity spillover at the hormone receptor—exploring its role in human disease. N Engl J Med 320:640–645, 1989.

7. Kapcala LP: Galactorrhea and thyrotoxicosis. Arch Intern Med 144:2349–2350, 1984.

8. Kleinberg DL, Noel GL, Frantz AA: Galactorrhea: A study of 235 cases, including 48 pituitary tumors. N Engl J Med 296:589–600, 1977.

9. Klibanski A, Biller BMK, Rosenthal DI, et al: Effects of prolactin and estrogen deficiency in amenorrheic bone loss. J Clin Endocrinol Metab 67:124–130, 1988.

10. Larsen PR: Physiology and disorders of pituitary hormone axes, Prolactin. Disorders of the female reproductive system. In Williams Textbook of Endocrinology, 10th ed. Philadelphia, Elsevier, 2003, pp 207–208 and 614–620.

11. Luciano AA: Clinical presentation of hyperprolactinemia. J Reprod Med 44(12 Suppl):1085–1090, 1999.

12. Mah PM, Webster J. Hyperprolactinemia: etiology, diagnosis, and management. Semin Reprod Med. 20:365–374, 2002.

13. Mehta AE, Reyes FI, Faiman C: Primary radiotherapy of prolactinomas: Eight- to 15-year follow-up. Am J Med 83:49–58, 1987.

14. Molitch ME, Elton RL, Blackwell RE, et al: Bromocriptine as primary therapy for prolactin-secreting macroadenomas: Results of a prospective multicenter study. J Clin Endocrinol Metab 60:698–705, 1985.

15. Pena KS, Rosenfeld JA. Evaluation and treatment of galactorrhea. Am Fam Physician 63:1763–1770, 2001.

16. Poretsky L, Garber J, Kleefield J: Primary amenorrhea and pseudoprolactinoma in a patient with primary hypothyroidism: Reversal of clinical, biochemical and radiologic abnormalities with levothyroxine. Am J Med 81:180–182, 1986.

17. Rayburn WF: Clinical commentary: The bromocriptine (Parlodel) controversy and recommendations for lactation suppression. Am J Perinatol 13:69–71, 1996.

18. Schlechte JA: Prolactinoma. N Engl J Med 349:2035–2041, 2003.

19. Thomson JA, Davies DL, McLaren EH, et al: Ten-year follow-up of microprolactinoma treated by transsphenoidal surgery. BMJ 309:1409–1410, 1994.

20. Wieck A, Haddad PM. Anti-psychotic-induced hyperprolactinemia in women: Pathophysiology, severity and consequences. Selective literature review. Br J Psychol 182:199–204, 2003.

CHAPTER 50

HIRSUTISM AND VIRILIZATION

Tamis M. Bright, M.D.

1. **Define hirsutism.**
   Hirsutism is the excessive growth of terminal hair in androgen-dependent areas: upper lip, chin, side burns, earlobes, tip of the nose, back, chest, areolae, axillae, lower abdomen, pubic triangle, and anterior thighs. Hirsutism is frequently associated with irregular menses and acne. Hirsutism should be distinguished from hypertrichosis, which is a nonandrogen-dependent increase in vellus hair. Hirsutism affects 5–10% of females.

2. **Define virilization.**
   Virilization consists of hirsutism, acne, and irregular menses along with signs of masculinization: deepening of the voice, increased muscle mass, temporal balding, clitoromegaly, and increased libido. Virilization results from high circulating levels of androgens, close to or in the male range, and is usually due to an androgen-secreting tumor.

3. **Where are androgens produced?**
   Twenty-five percent of testosterone comes from the ovaries, 25% from the adrenal glands, and 50% from peripheral conversion of androstenedione, which is produced by both the ovaries and adrenals. Testosterone is converted into dihydrotestosterone (DHT) by the enzyme 5-α-reductase, which is present in hair follicles, or to estradiol by the aromatase enzyme present in adipose tissue (Fig. 50-1). DHT is responsible for the transformation of vellus into terminal hair. Hair follicles also contain the enzymes that convert dehydroepiandrosterone (DHEA), which is produced by the adrenals, and androstenedione into testosterone.

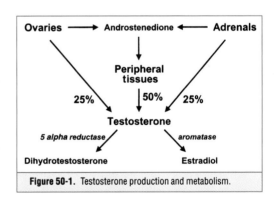

Figure 50-1. Testosterone production and metabolism.

4. **What causes hirsutism?**
   Hirsutism is caused by hyperandrogenism. Androgens transform the fine, downy, minimally pigmented vellus hair in androgen-sensitive areas into coarse, pigmented, terminal hair. An increase in any of the androgenic steroids may cause high levels of DHT in the hair follicle and result in hirsutism.

   Low levels of sex hormone-binding globulin (SHBG), which is produced by the liver, may promote hirsutism. Eighty percent of circulating testosterone is bound to SHBG, 19% is bound to albumin, and 1% is free. Decreases in SHBG increase the free fraction of hormone available to androgen-sensitive hair.

   Increased activity of 5-α-reductase, even with normal circulating androgen levels, also may cause hirsutism by the excessive conversion of testosterone into DHT.

5. **List the conditions that result in hirsutism.**
   - Polycystic ovarian syndrome (PCOS)
   - Congenital adrenal hyperplasia (CAH)
   - Idiopathic/familial hirsutism
   - Cushing's syndrome
   - Prolactinoma
   - Hypothyroidism
   - Ovarian hyperthecosis
   - Medications

6. **Describe the pathophysiology of PCOS.**
   The exact cause of PCOS is unknown, but affected patients have been shown to have an accelerated rate of pulsatile gonadotropin-releasing hormone (GnRH) secretion from the hypothalamus. The gonadotropin secretory profile is highly dependent on the rate of GnRH pulsatility. Rapid GnRH pulses stimulate the secretion of luteinizing hormone (LH), but not follicle-stimulating hormone (FSH), from the pituitary gland. The increased LH/FSH secretory ratio results in arrested ovarian follicle development with cyst formation and hypertrophy of theca cells, leading to constant estrogen and increased androgen production with chronic anovulation.

7. **How does PCOS present?**
   PCOS affects 5–10% of premenopausal women and is a common cause of hirsutism and oligomenorrhea. The hirsutism is gradually progressive, usually beginning at puberty, and most patients have irregular menses from the onset of menarche. However, in a study of hirsute patients with regular menses, 50% had polycystic ovaries. PCOS patients also frequently have insulin resistance and hyperinsulinemia. Because insulin decreases SHBG and increases the ovarian androgen response to LH stimulation, the hyperinsulinemia contributes to the elevated free androgen levels in PCOS. Thus, PCOS presents as a spectrum: some patients have minimal findings, whereas others have the entire constellation of hirsutism, acne, obesity, infertility, amenorrhea or oligomenorrhea, male pattern alopecia, acanthosis nigricans, hyperinsulinemia, and hyperlipidemia.

8. **Describe the pathophysiology of the hyperandrogenism in CAH.**
   CAH results from a deficiency of one of the key enzymes in the cortisol biosynthesis pathway; it often presents with precocious puberty and childhood hirsutism. Partial or late-onset CAH, owing to milder deficiencies of the same enzymes, may cause postpubertal hirsutism. Ninety percent of CAH is due to 21-hydroxylase deficiency, which causes a defect in the conversion of 17-hydroxyprogesterone (17-OHP) to 11-deoxycortisol and of progesterone to desoxycorticosterone (DOC). The resulting low cortisol production rate leads to hypersecretion of pituitary adrenocorticotropic hormone (ACTH), which stimulates overproduction of 17-OHP and progesterone, as well as adrenal androgens, particularly androstenedione (Fig. 50-2). Hirsutism results from the androgen excess.

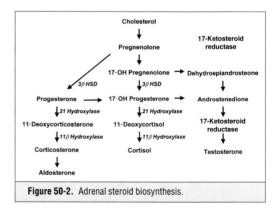

Figure 50-2. Adrenal steroid biosynthesis.

9. **Do any other causes of CAH result in hirsutism?**
   Deficiency of 11-β-hydroxylase decreases the conversion of 11-deoxycortisol to cortisol and of DOC to corticosterone. This stimulates hypersecretion of ACTH, with consequent overpro-

duction of 11-deoxycortisol, DOC, and androstenedione. Patients also frequently develop hypertension from the mineralocorticoid, DOC. *Deficiency of 3-β-hydroxysteroid dehydrogenase* (3β HSD) decreases the conversion of pregnenolone to progesterone and 17-hydroxypregnenolone to 17-OHP. This defect increases pregnenolone, 17-hydroxypregnenolone, and the androgens DHEA, dehydroepiandrosterone sulfate (DHEAS), and androstenediol, which promote the development of hirsutism. *Deficiency of 17-ketosteroid reductase* decreases the conversion of androstenedione to testosterone, DHEA to androstenediol, and estrone to estradiol. Affected patients have elevated basal levels of androstenedione, DHEA, and estrone (see Fig. 50-2).

10. **Describe the pathophysiology of idiopathic and familial hirsutism.**

    Idiopathic hirsutism is believed to be caused by increased cutaneous activity of 5-α-reductase or enhanced skin sensitivity to androgens. Familial hirsutism is an ethnic tendency to have a higher density of hair follicles per unit area of skin. Mediterraneans and Hispanics have increased hair density, whereas Asians have lower density. Patients with idiopathic or familial hirsutism usually have the onset of hirsutism shortly after puberty with a slow subsequent progression. They have normal menses and fertility, as well as a normal hormonal profile.

11. **How do Cushing's syndrome, prolactinomas, and hypothyroidism cause hirsutism?**

    All causes of Cushing's syndrome may result in hypertrichosis because of increased vellus hair on the face, forehead, limbs, and trunk owing to cortisol hypersecretion. Cushing's syndrome due to an adrenal tumor also may produce hirsutism and virilization from increased secretion of androgens with cortisol.

    Hyperprolactinemia suppresses GnRH activity, which diminishes pulsatile LH secretion from the pituitary gland, resulting in decreased ovarian estrogen production and amenorrhea. Prolactin also increases the adrenal androgens, DHEA, and DHEAS. Hypothyroidism decreases SHBG, leading to an increase in free testosterone.

12. **What is the pathophysiology of the hyperandrogenism in ovarian hyperthecosis?**

    Ovarian hyperthecosis is a nonneoplastic condition of the ovaries with proliferating islands of luteinized thecal cells in the ovarian stroma. Hyperthecosis causes overproduction of testosterone, androstenedione, and DHT to an even higher level than is usually seen in PCOS. LH and FSH are either normal or low, and the degree of insulin resistance and hyperinsulinemia is greater than in PCOS.

13. **Which medications can cause hirsutism?**

    Danazol, testosterone, glucocorticoids, metyrapone, phenothiazines, anabolic steroids, and oral contraceptives containing norgestrel and norethindrone can cause hirsutism. Phenytoin, diazoxide, minoxidil, glucocorticoids, streptomycin, penicillamine, and psoralens can cause hypertrichosis.

14. **What conditions cause virilization?**

Ovarian Tumors	Adrenal Disorders
Thecoma	CAH
Fibrothecoma	Adenoma
Granulosa and granulosa-theca cell tumors	Carcinoma
Arrhenoblastoma (Sertoli-Leydig cell tumors)	
Hilus cell tumors	
Adrenal rest tumors of the ovary	
Luteoma of pregnancy	

KEY POINTS: PATHOGENESIS OF HIRSUTISM AND VIRILIZATION ✓

1. Hirsutism is the excessive growth of terminal hair and is frequently associated with irregular menses.

2. Virilization consists of hirsutism and irregular menses associated with signs of masculinization.

3. Hirsutism and virilization usually result from excess androgens.

4. The common causes of hirsutism are PCOS, CAH, idiopathic/familial hirsutism, and medications.

5. The common causes of virilization are ovarian tumors, adrenal tumors, and CAH.

15. **When should a patient be evaluated for hirsutism?**
Any patient with rapid development of hirsutism or coexistence of amenorrhea, irregular menses, or virilization should be evaluated. A patient with regular menses who shows significant concern about hirsutism also may warrant a work-up.

16. **What information is important in the history?**
- Age of onset, progression, and extent of hair growth
- Current measures of hair removal and frequency of use
- Age at menarche, regularity of menses, and fertility
- Family history of hirsutism
- Change in libido or change in voice
- Symptoms of Cushing's disease, prolactinoma, or hypothyroidism
- Medications

17. **What findings are important on physical examination?**
- Distribution and degree of hirsutism
- Increased muscle mass, temporal balding, clitoromegaly, or acne
- Obesity
- Acanthosis nigricans
- Visual field defects
- Moon facies, plethora, buffalo hump, supraclavicular fat pads, striae, or thin skin
- Galactorrhea
- Goiter, loss of lateral eyebrows, periorbital edema, dry skin, or delayed reflexes
- Abdominal or pelvic masses

18. **What laboratory tests should be ordered for a patient with hirsutism?**
Laboratory testing should be guided by the results of the history and physical examination. Many authors advocate against testing in patients with regular menses and only gradual progression of hirsutism. However, serum levels of total testosterone, DHEAS, 17-OHP, LH, and FSH can be useful tests, depending on the individual patient. Patients with signs or symptoms of hypothyroidism, hyperprolactinemia, or Cushing's syndrome also should be evaluated with serum TSH, prolactin, or 24-hour urine cortisol testing, respectively. Otherwise, these tests need not be obtained for every patient.

19. **How are the results of these laboratory tests interpreted?**
For a patient without signs of virilization, it is important to differentiate idiopathic hirsutism, PCOS, and CAH because each is treated differently. Total testosterone, DHEAS, and 17-OHP help

in the differentiation. Idiopathic hirsutism has normal levels on all three tests. PCOS has mildly increased testosterone, normal or slightly increased DHEAS, and normal 17-OHP. CAH has elevated testosterone and DHEAS and mild-to-marked elevation of 17-OHP. An early morning follicular phase level of 17-OHP > 500 ng/dL (normal ≤ 200 ng/dL) is diagnostic. In most patients with PCOS, LH is elevated, FSH is normal or low, and the ratio of LH to FSH should be greater than 2. However, not all patients with PCOS have an elevated LH, particularly those with obesity; thus, LH and FSH are helpful in confirming but not excluding the diagnosis of PCOS.

20. **What do you do if a patient has borderline (200–500 ng/dL) elevations of 17-OHP?**

    A borderline elevated level requires an ACTH stimulation test with assessment of 17-OHP levels at baseline and 60 minutes after stimulation with ACTH. The levels are then plotted on a nomogram to determine normals, heterozygous carriers of the 21-OH gene, and patients with late-onset 21-OH deficiency. Some patients with late-onset 21-OH deficiency have normal baseline 17-OHP levels; however, the ACTH-stimulated levels are usually diagnostic.

21. **What laboratory tests should be ordered in a patient with virilization?**

    A patient with virilization needs to be evaluated to determine if she has an ovarian tumor, an adrenal tumor, or CAH. As in patients without virilization, tests should include serum total testosterone, DHEAS, and 17-OHP. A markedly increased testosterone level (> 200 ng/dL) with normal values on the other tests points to an ovarian tumor. High levels of DHEAS with or without high testosterone levels suggest an adrenal tumor. Increased levels of 17-OHP with modest elevations of DHEAS and testosterone are more consistent with CAH. Laboratory values suggesting tumors need to be followed with a transvaginal ultrasound of the ovaries or computed tomography (CT) of the adrenals or ovaries. If no mass is found, iodocholesterol scanning of the adrenals or venous sampling of the ovaries or adrenals can be performed for localization before surgical removal.

22. **How is PCOS treated in a patient desiring pregnancy?**

    If the patient's primary concern is fertility, clomiphene is the usual drug of choice. If clomiphene fails to induce ovulation, cyclic gonadotropin administration is often useful. Pulsatile GnRH also has been used with some success. In obese patients, weight reduction alone has been shown to increase the spontaneous ovulation rate. If a component of adrenal androgen (DHEAS) hypersecretion appears to be present, low-dose dexamethasone can be added in doses of 0.125–0.375 mg at night. This regimen may improve the ovulation rate, as well as decrease hirsutism.

23. **How is PCOS treated in a patient not desiring pregnancy?**

    If fertility is not the issue, oral contraceptives or cyclic progestins are used to induce regular menses and thereby decrease the risk of endometrial cancer. Preparations containing androgenic progestins, such as norgestrel and norethindrone, should be avoided. Weight reduction should be encouraged. As above, dexamethasone may be added in patients with an elevated DHEAS; however, this may increase glucose in an already glucose-intolerant patient. If hirsutism does not improve with these measures, the agents listed in questions 24 and 27–30 may be needed.

24. **What can be done about the hyperinsulinemia of PCOS?**

    PCOS patients should be evaluated with a fasting blood glucose or an oral glucose tolerance test and a lipid profile because of the high prevalence of glucose intolerance, diabetes, and hyperlipidemia in this disorder. These problems need to be addressed separately because they are not resolved by treating the hyperandrogenism alone. Metformin, rosiglitazone, and pioglitazone have been used in PCOS patients with and without increased glucose levels. The agents improved glucose levels in patients with hyperglycemia and also had benefit in treating other aspects of PCOS, even in euglycemic patients. Metformin resulted in improved regularity of menses, fertility, and hyperandrogenism in some studies. The thiazolidinediones are currently under study but results show an increase in SHBG with rosiglitazone and a decrease in androgens and hirsutism with pioglitazone.

25. **What is the treatment for CAH?**
    Glucocorticoid replacement decreases ACTH secretion and thereby reduces excessive adrenal androgen production. Mineralocorticoid replacement is also required in some causes of CAH. Treatment with the regimens listed in questions 25–29 can hasten improvement of the hirsutism.

26. **Describe how oral contraceptive pills are used for the treatment of hirsutism.**
    Oral contraceptive pills (OCPs) are the most commonly used therapy. They increase serum estrogens and SHBG, which decreases free testosterone levels. Monophasic and triphasic preparations work equally well. Preparations containing the progestins desogestrel, norgestimate, and gestodene are believed to be the best because they are the least androgenic. Potential side effects include weight gain, bloating, nausea, emotional lability, breast pain, and deep venous thrombosis.

27. **Describe how antiandrogens are used for the treatment of hirsutism.**
    Spironolactone is an androgen receptor blocker and a weak inhibitor of testosterone production. Side effects include diuresis, fatigue, and dysfunctional uterine bleeding. Initial doses are 25–100 mg twice daily, tapered to 25–50 mg/day once an effect has been seen. Flutamide, another androgen receptor blocker, is dosed at 125–250 mg once or twice daily. Side effects include increased liver function tests (LFTs) and rare fatal hepatotoxicity. Finasteride, a 5-α-reductase inhibitor, effectively decreases hirsutism. Side effects include headache and depression. Dosage is 2.5–7.5 mg/day. The antiandrogens are usually used in combination with OCPs for additive effects and to give adequate birth control because antiandrogens can feminize a male fetus.

28. **Describe how GnRH agonists are used for the treatment of hirsutism.**
    By providing constant rather than pulsatile GnRH levels to the pituitary, GnRH agonists reduce gonadotropin secretion and thereby decrease ovarian production of both estrogen and androgen. Estrogen replacement must be given to avoid hot flashes, vaginal dryness, and bone density loss. Leuprolide (3.75 mg/month IM), buserelin or nafarelin nasal spray (3 times/day), and goserelin subcutaneous implants effectively reduce hirsutism. Some studies demonstrate an increased effect over OCPs alone, whereas others show similar effects. The preparations are expensive and thus are usually reserved for severe PCOS.

KEY POINTS: DIAGNOSIS AND TREATMENT OF HIRSUTISM AND VIRILIZATION ✔

1. Appropriate laboratory testing includes at least total testosterone, DHEAS, and 17-OHP.

2. Treatment of hirsutism is usually with the combination of OCPs, spironolactone, eflornithine, and cosmetic measures; however GnRH agonists and antiandrogens can be used.

3. PCOS patients may have improvement of symptoms if treated with insulin sensitizers.

4. Treatment of virilization is surgical removal of the tumor or steroid treatment for CAH.

29. **What topical agent is approved for the treatment of hirsutism?**
    Eflornithine HCl 13.9% cream is the newest agent for the treatment of facial hirsutism. Eflornithine HCl irreversibly inhibits ornithine decarboxylase, an enzyme necessary for hair follicle cell division. Inhibition of ornithine decarboxylase results in a decreased rate of hair growth. In clinical trials, 58% of patients had marked improvement or some improvement as compared

with 34% of controls after 24 weeks of treatment. The most common side effects encountered were acne, pseudofolliculitis barbae, burning, tingling, erythema, or rash over the applied area. Generally, side effects resolved without treatment and rarely required discontinuation of the medication. The cream is applied to the face twice daily. The patients' hirsutism returned to baseline by 8 weeks following discontinuation of the medication.

30. **What cosmetic measures can be used for the treatment of hirsutism?**
Bleaching, shaving, plucking, waxing, depilating, and electrolysis are effective measures that can be used alone or in combination with the above treatments. They remove terminal hair that is already present, while the patient waits for medications to decrease new growth and rate of transformation to terminal hair.

Laser-assisted hair removal is an effective treatment for hirsutism. It is an outpatient procedure that uses ruby, alexandrite, diode, or YAG lasers, all of which cause thermal injury to the hair follicle. The techniques result in removal of hair, and a period of 2–6 months before the regrowth of hair, which is thinner and lighter. The side effects include minimal discomfort, local edema and erythema lasting 24–48 hours, rare petechiae, and infrequent hyperpigmentation lasting less than 6 months.

31. **How do you choose the appropriate therapy for the patient's hirsutism?**
Most patients are given a trial of OCPs, with or without spironolactone, and are advised to use cosmetic measures while waiting for the medications to work. The new topical cream, eflornithine HCl, may be used alone or in combination with other measures. Because of their more serious side effects and higher cost, the other medications are reserved for the most severe cases, in which OCPs and spironolactone fail. No matter what therapy is chosen, the patient must be made aware that results will not be seen for at least 3–6 months. Although many different medications and combinations have been used, only topical eflornithine HCl is currently approved by the Food and Drug Administration for treatment of hirsutism. Unfortunately, most patients will have a relapse of hirsutism approximately 12 months after discontinuation of medical therapy.

WEBSITES

1. Atlas of Dermatology. Available at www.dermis.net/bilddb/diagnose/englisch/i704110.htm

2. eMedicine. Available at www.emedicine.com/med/topic1017.htm

BIBLIOGRAPHY

1. Azziz R, Carmina E, Sawaya M: Idiopathic hirsutism. Endocr Rev 21:347–362, 2000.
2. Barman B, Julia A, McClellan K: Topical eflornithine. Am J Clin Dermatol 2:197–201, 2001.
3. Carmina E: A risk-benefit assessment of pharmacological therapies for hirsutism. Drug Saf 24:267–276, 2001.
4. Diamanti E, Zapanti E: Insulin sensitizers and antiandrogens in the treatment of polycystic ovary syndrome. Ann N Y Acad Sci 900:203–212, 2000.
5. Hunter M, Carek P: Evaluation and treatment of women with hirsutism. Am Fam Physician 67:2565–2572, 2003.
6. Moghetti P, Tosi F, Tosti A, et al: Comparison of spironolactone, flutamide, and finasteride efficacy in the treatment of hirsutism: A randomized, double blind, placebo-controlled trial. J Clin Endocrinol Metab 85:89–94, 2000.
7. Speroff L, Glass R, Kase N: Clinical Gynecologic Endocrinology and Infertility, 6th ed. Baltimore, Lippincott Williams & Wilkins, 1999.
8. Vittorio C, Lehrer M: Laser hair removal. Fac Plas Surg 19:131–135, 2003.
9. Yen S, Jaffe R: Reproductive Endocrinology, 4th ed. Philadelphia, W.B. Saunders, 1999.

CHAPTER 51

MENOPAUSE

William J. Georgitis, M.D.

1. **Define menopause.**
The cessation of normal cyclic ovarian function defines menopause. It encompasses approximately one-third of a woman's life and spans the transition from the reproductive years to the final menstruation and then extends for the remainder of life. The final menstruation marks menopause for each woman and, therefore, is established retrospectively.

2. **When do ovulatory cycles decrease in frequency?**
Ovulatory cycles usually decrease in frequency around age 38–42 years.

3. **When does menopause usually occur?**
The median age for the last menses is 51.4 years. The range for menopause is broad, but 90% of women cease menstruating by age 55.

4. **What determines the timing of menopause?**
Menses stop when the ovarian supply of oocytes is exhausted. Oocyte numbers peak in utero. Approximately 80% of the oocytes vanish before birth. It is a curious fact that the destiny of many more eggs is atresia than ovulation (see Fig. 51-1.)

5. **What is premature ovarian failure? What causes it?**
Cessation of cyclic ovarian function before age 35 years is considered premature. It is attributed to either an inadequate complement of follicles from birth or accelerated follicular attrition. Causes for premature ovarian failure include mumps oophoritis, irradiation, chemotherapy, autoimmune destruction, and genetic defects. The incidence of premature ovarian failure in women in the U.S. is about 0.3%. Approximately 146,000 cases occurred in the year 2000.

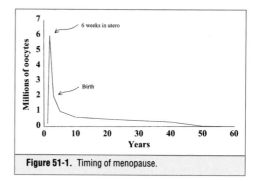

Figure 51-1. Timing of menopause.

6. **Does the age of menopause vary with race, body size, age of menarche, geography, or socioeconomic conditions?**
No. However, the evidence against these factors being significant determinants of menopause onset continues to be sparse. It is known that menopause occurs about 2 years earlier in cigarette smokers, and that nulliparous women tend to experience an earlier menopause than multiparous women. Presumably, the months spent in the gravid state increase the duration of a multiparous woman's reproductive function.

7. **How does the appearance of the ovaries change with menopause?**
The menopausal ovary shrinks and its surface becomes wrinkled. A recent cross-sectional study employing transvaginal ultrasound in 58,673 women found the mean ovarian volume was 4.9 cm^3 in premenopausal women and 2.2 cm^3 in postmenopausal women. Cortical width diminishes, whereas interstitial and hilar cells become more prominent, giving the stroma a hyperplastic appearance.

8. **What is the predominant circulating estrogen in menopause?**
Estradiol is the most abundant serum estrogen during the reproductive years. In menopause, estrone becomes the principal estrogen. Estrone is predominantly derived from adipose tissue conversion of adrenal androstenedione. Estrone is less biologically potent than estradiol. Atrophic changes after menopause affecting breast, vaginal mucosa, and pelvic musculature, especially in leaner women with low adipose tissue mass, can prompt woman to seek assistance for symptoms related to these changes, including dyspareunia, urinary incontinence, and adjustment to changes in body configuration.

9. **What is a hot flash? Or should it be called a flush?**
These terms refer to menopausal spells lasting seconds to minutes or rarely as long as an hour. Symptoms include a sudden reddening of the skin accompanied by a sensation of warmth. In some women, this is followed by profuse sweating. Body surface temperature rises while core temperature falls; this is mediated by hypothalamic-directed, vasomotor dilation of surface blood vessels. The physiology of the flush or flash is complex. Catecholamines, prostaglandins, endorphins, and other neuropeptides all seem to participate.
Both terms, *flash* and *flush,* appear in the medical literature. Each is appropriately descriptive with flush aptly emphasizing vasodilation and flash signifying the abrupt onset and brief duration of the spells. Many menopausal women also describe prodromal auras.

10. **Hot flushes are accompanied by surges in luteinizing hormone. Does excess LH trigger the spells?**
No. The LH surge is an epiphenomenon. Hypophysectomized women lacking LH pulsatility still may experience menopausal hot flushes. Furthermore, women with gonadal dysgenesis have highly elevated levels of gonadotropins, but they fail to manifest hot flushes until after estrogen treatment and subsequent withdrawal. The hypothalamus appears to first require priming with estrogens before later demonstrating episodic vasomotor instability in response to deficient levels of estrogen.

11. **Do all women develop menopausal vasomotor hot flushes? Do they last indefinitely?**
About 85% of women experience vasomotor symptoms. The rate of change in estrogen levels seems to partly explain their severity. Women with abrupt declines in estrogen levels following ovariectomy are often bothered the most. Left untreated, hot flushes tend to diminish after 2–5 years.

12. **Do any menopausal symptoms have an uncertain relation to estrogen?**
Yes. A partial list of symptoms includes fatigue, nervousness, headaches, insomnia, depression, irritability, joint pain, muscle pain, dizziness, palpitations, and formication. Formication is a paresthesia resembling the sensation of ants crawling over the skin.

13. **What important physiologic changes accompany menopause?**
Hot flushes, urogenital atrophy, loss of bone calcium, increased rates of coronary heart disease, and alterations in serum lipids, including rises in low-density lipoprotein (LDL) cholesterol and triglycerides with declines in high-density lipoprotein (HDL) cholesterol, occur during menopause.

14. **What is the principal cause of death in postmenopausal women?**
Cardiovascular disease. One in two women will die of heart disease or stroke, whereas only 1 in 25 will die of breast cancer.

15. **Does male menopause exist?**
Not really. Although hypogonadal men may suffer spells and accelerated loss of bone mineral similar to hypogonadal women, such symptoms do not represent a physiologically programmed event. A man complaining of hot flushes should prompt testing to confirm hypogonadism first, followed by an investigation for the cause.

16. **Historical records indicate the age of menarche has decreased over the centuries, perhaps as a result of improved nutrition and general health. Is this also true for the timing of menopause?**
No. While the average age for first menstruation may have become lower as a result of improved nutrition and general health, a downward shift in the average age of menopause has not been recorded. Perhaps ongoing studies will confirm such changes in the future.

17. **How does one establish a diagnosis of menopause?**
In a woman older than 45 years with secondary amenorrhea of 12 months' duration, historical evidence alone suggests a diagnosis of menopause. Pelvic examination may or may not help confirm the impression by showing signs of vaginal atrophy.
　　Laboratory tests alone are not reliable for diagnosis. Toward the end of a woman's fertile years, serum levels of follicle-stimulating hormone (FSH) gradually rise. Anovulatory periods occur and may be accompanied by menorrhagia. Once amenorrhea is well established, gonadotropins may become tonically elevated. FSH rises 10- to 20-fold, while elevations in LH of 3-fold are more moderate. Levels of FSH above 40 IU/L are generally considered diagnostic of ovarian failure. However, hot flashes and gonadotropin elevations may be prevented by obesity, and, on the other end of the spectrum, elevated gonadotropin levels alone may be misleading because LH and FSH can reach menopausal range values during the mid-cycle surge just prior to ovulation.

18. **What regimens of menopausal hormone replacement are in common use?**
Numerous regimens are currently used for replacement. They vary by route of administration, composition of a variety of estrogens and progestogens, and by timing of administration of the various components. Too many permutations exist to discuss except in generality and by example. ERT refers to estrogen replacement therapy alone and HRT to hormone replacement therapy where some combination or sequence of estrogen is prescribed along with a progestogen. Routes of administration include oral, topical, and vaginal. Schemes for delivering the hormones include sequential dosing of estrogen and progestogen to mimic the normal hormone level variations through the menstrual cycle, continuous combined administration of estrogen and progestogen, and long cycle therapy, in which the progestogen is administered a few times each year rather than on a repeating monthly schedule.

19. **How do you determine which regimen to use for a particular patient?**
It is very difficult to determine which replacement regimen will be acceptable for each patient because individual tolerance varies unpredictably. Breast tenderness and bleeding of endometrial origin are commonly reported by postmenopausal women commencing replacement with any of the regimens. Although bleeding and mastalgia lessen over time, long-term compliance remains poor, perhaps owing to coexisting fear of breast cancer and thrombotic complications. There is at present no ideal treatment for women seeking replacement free from endometrial bleeding.

20. **What regimen is recommended for women who have no endometrium?**
Continuous daily replacement with estrogen alone is appropriate. Conjugated equine estrogens in daily doses ranging from 0.625 to 1.25 mg are commonly prescribed.

21. **What are the choices in women who have not had hysterectomies?**
Combination therapy with estrogen plus progesterone is prescribed for women who have not had hysterectomies to prevent endometrial hyperplasia and neoplasia, both of which increase in incidence with dose and duration of exposure to estrogen unopposed by progestogen. An example of a cyclic combination regimen is conjugated estrogens, 0.625–1.25 mg daily on days 1–25 of each month, and medroxyprogesterone acetate, 5–10 mg daily on days 13–25. During the last 5 days of the month, neither hormone is administered; withdrawal bleeding is common with this type of sequential therapy.

22. **Describe alternative approaches.**
An alternative approach is to use a continuous combination of conjugated estrogens, 0.625–1.25 mg, and medroxyprogesterone acetate, 2.5–5.0 mg, every day of the month. Oral estradiol 1–2 mg/day can be substituted for conjugated estrogens in any of the above regimens. Topical therapy with estradiol patches, applied as a 0.05–0.1-mg/day patch every 3 days or every 7 days, can also be used in either a cyclic or a continuous fashion. Again, spotting may occur with any therapy, including intravaginal estrogen alone. Persistent bleeding, especially early in the cycle of sequential therapy, may necessitate an endometrial biopsy. Intravaginal ultrasound and reliance on the timing of bleeding to assess risk of endometrial disease have proved to be unreliable.

23. **What about testosterone replacement?**
This issue remains controversial. In eugonadal women, circulating testosterone is roughly half ovarian and half adrenal in origin. Serum testosterone declines 50% in premenopausal women following bilateral oophorectomy compared with an 80% decline in serum estradiol. Improvements in sexual function and psychosocial well-being were reported with topical testosterone replacement (patches) in a placebo-controlled dose-response study of middle-aged women with surgical primary hypogonadism. Hot flushes averaged less than two per week at entry and were not affected by testosterone treatment. Adverse effects on lipids, acne, hirsutism, liver function, glucose, insulin, and blood counts were not seen, but serious study-related events, not all attributable to testosterone, occurred in 1 out of 15 subjects in the trial and 1 out of 16 women withdrew from the study. The number needed to treat (NTT) for any specified benefit in this study could not be derived. The placebo response was substantial, and, like prior short-term studies with testosterone implants or injections delivering excessive replacement doses, the long-term risk-benefit ratio of androgen replacement could not be determined and still requires additional investigation.

24. **What are the most common indications for menopausal hormone replacement therapy?**
The most common indications are for relief of vasomotor symptoms or symptoms associated with urogenital atrophy. For relief of these problems, short-term treatment may be sufficient and a commitment to chronic or life-long use may not be necessary.

KEY POINTS: MENOPAUSE

1. Menopause encompasses approximately one-third of a woman's life.

2. The mean ovarian volume determined by transvaginal ultrasound of 2.2 cm^3 for postmenopausal women is less than half the mean ovarian volume found for premenopausal women.

3. The principal cause of death in postmenopausal women is cardiovascular disease.

4. One in two women will die of heart disease or stroke.

5. One in 25 women will die of breast cancer.

25. **What are the benefits of hormone replacement therapy?**

Vasomotor symptoms improve, dyspareunia is reduced, and the frequency of cystitis may be decreased. Deaths attributable to cardiovascular disease in women each year now exceed those for men. Recent surveys show that cardiovascular disease is underdiagnosed and receives less aggressive treatment in women than in men. Women have less favorable outcomes than men following myocardial infarction and even have higher complication rates with coronary revascularization. Whether hormone replacement therapy decreases the risk of vascular disease events, however, remains contentious. Reductions in LDL and increases in HDL cholesterol levels with hormone replacement therapy have been demonstrated in some, but not all, studies. Since lipid intervention trials with cardiovascular endpoints show greater benefit for women than men and since 3-hydroxy-3-methylglutaryl (HMG)-CoA reductase inhibitor therapy is clearly superior to hormone replacement therapy in causing favorable lipids changes, lipid-lowering medications should be used when LDL treatment goals are not met by hormone replacement therapy alone.

26. **How does hormone replacement affect the skeleton?**

There is less controversy about the beneficial effects of hormone replacement on the skeleton, where prevention of bone loss and reductions in the relative risk of osteoporosis-associated fractures are substantial and clinically relevant. The suggestion that estrogen may affect the incidence and natural history of senile dementia deserves further investigation to determine the relevance of those observations in that debilitating disease.

27. **What are the potential detrimental effects?**

Estrogen administration is associated with small increases in the risk of several serious complications, and these risks rise with longer duration of hormone use. Estrogen treatment without the addition of a progestin increases the risk of endometrial hyperplasia or carcinoma 4- to 8-fold. In a reexamination of 51 studies comprised of 150,000 cases and controls, breast cancer risk was found to be increased 1.35-fold for women who had used hormone replacement for 5 years or more. The risk of venous thromboembolic events also increases about 3-fold with estrogen replacement. Progesterone, which markedly decreases the risk of endometrial carcinoma, can cause fluid retention and may also lower HDL and raise LDL cholesterol levels.

28. **How common is long-term compliance with estrogen replacement therapy?**

Long-term compliance is low with estrogen replacement therapy; up to 70% of women refuse it initially or discontinue it on their own accord. Only 30% of women for whom estrogen therapy is prescribed continue it for more than 3 years. Uterine bleeding, breast pain, fear of breast cancer and thromboembolism, and the patient's recognition that treatment alternatives exist for osteoporosis and dyslipidemia, contribute to the poor adherence to treatment.

29. **What about weight gain with hormone replacement therapy?**

Although it is a common perception that hormone replacement causes weight gain, evidence suggests instead that menopause itself is associated with weight gain, in part attributed to reductions in the resting metabolic rate. In hormone treatment trials, untreated controls often gain as much weight as the hormone-treated groups. Furthermore, the distribution of body fat differs in that untreated control subjects tend to develop more androgenous obesity with increases in their waist to hip ratios. This form of obesity carries associations with insulin resistance, dyslipidemia, and hypertension.

30. **Insomnia is a troublesome symptom. Does hormone replacement alter sleep?**

Evidence from objective sleep laboratory studies suggests that estrogen replacement improves sleep quality, decreases the time to onset of sleep, and increases rapid eye movement (REM) sleep.

31. **What levels of estradiol and estrone are achieved with replacement?**
Oral conjugated equine estrogens (0.625 mg), micronized estradiol (1.0 mg), and estrone sulfate (1.25 mg) deliver peak estradiol levels of 30–40 pg/mL and peak estrone levels of 150–250 pg/mL. Intravaginal estrogens yield levels about one-fourth those achieved with oral regimens.

32. **Can gonadotropin levels be used to monitor adequacy of replacement?**
No. Unlike primary hypothyroidism, in which the serum thyroid-stimulating hormone (TSH) can be used to individualize requirements for thyroxine replacement, gonadotropin levels remain elevated despite sex steroid replacement in many postmenopausal women. This elevation may result from a deficiency in inhibin, a polypeptide hormone normally produced by ovarian granulosa cells to inhibit secretion of FSH. Menopausal hormone replacement therapy must be gauged by the response in symptoms and signs, not by gonadotropin levels.

33. **What alternative therapies may be used for the menopausal woman with contraindications for estrogen replacement?**
Clonidine may be tried at bedtime for the relief of hot flushes, but hypotensive side effects may limit its use. Medroxyprogesterone in a daily pill or as a depot injection every 3 months also may relieve hot flushes. Herbal preparations and dietary supplements are not regulated by the FDA and safety and efficacy data are lacking. Widely used alternatives to prescribed hormones for hot flushes include black cohosh and soy, which have benefits attributed to phytoestrogens and side effects that have prompted regulatory agencies of some countries to recommend use for no longer than 6 months.

34. **What web textbook might you recommend for providers seeking information about menopause?**
Endotext.com has a section entitled "Female Reproductive Endocrinology," Robert W. Rebar, Editor, with Chapter 11 devoted to "Menopause and Hormone Replacement" by Michelle P. Warren, M.D., and Jennifer E. Dominguez, BA.

WESBSITES

1. http://www.endotext.com

2. http://www.acog.org

3. http://www.menopause.org

BIBLIOGRAPHY

1. Amundsen, DW, Diers CJ: The age of menopause in medieval Europe. Hum Biol 45:605–612, 1973.
2. Daly E, Gray A, Barlow D, et al: Measuring the impact of menopausal symptoms on the quality of life. BMJ 307:836–840, 1993.
3. Doren M: Hormonal replacement regimens and bleeding. Maturitas 34(Suppl 1):S17–S23, 2000.
4. Pavlik EJ, DePriest PD, Gallion HH, et al: Ovarian volume related to age. Gynecol Oncol 77:410–412, 2000.
5. Schiff I, Regesein Q, Tulchinsky D, Ryan KJ: Effect of estrogens on sleep and psychological state of hypogonadal women. JAMA 242:2405–2407, 1979.
6. Shifren JL, Braunstein GD, Simon JA, et al: Transdermal testosterone treatment in women with impaired sexual function after oophorectomy. N Engl J Med 343:682–688, 2000.
7. Stamm WE, Raz R: Factors contributing to susceptibility of postmenopausal women to recurrent urinary tract infections. Clin Infect Dis 28:723–725, 1999.
8. Walsh BW, Ginsburg ES: Menopause. In Ryan KJ (ed): Kistner's Gynecology & Women's Health, 7th ed., St. Louis, Mosby, 1999, pp 540–569.

9. Walsh BW, Schiff I, Rosner B, et al: Effects of postmenopausal estrogen replacement on the concentrations and metabolism of plasma lipoproteins. N Engl J Med 323:1196–1204, 1990.

10. Wenger NK: Lipid management and control of other coronary risk factors in the postmenopausal woman. J Women's Health Gend Based Med 9:234–243, 2000.

CHAPTER 52

USE AND ABUSE OF ANABOLIC-ANDROGENIC STEROIDS

Jonathan R. Parks, M.D., and Homer J. LeMar, Jr., M.D.

1. **What are anabolic-androgenic steroids (AASs)?**
   AASs are a group of steroid hormones derived from chemical modification of testosterone. Their name is often shortened to anabolic steroids. The term anabolic refers to their ability to promote positive nitrogen balance and accretion of lean body mass. Androgenic refers to masculinization induced by these hormones. Although potency varies among different AASs, all possess both androgenic and anabolic properties.

2. **Summarize the biologic effects of AASs.**
   Endogenous AASs have diverse effects. The most prominent are effects on male sexual differentiation and secondary sexual characteristics, including growth and development of the prostate, seminal vesicles, penis and scrotum, beard, pubic, chest, and axillary hair; thickening of the vocal cords and enlargement of the larynx. AASs promote nitrogen retention, increase lean body mass, and alter fat distribution. They also stimulate release of clotting factors and erythropoietin with a secondary increase in hematocrit.

3. **How do AASs exert their effects?**
   AASs act by binding to a specific receptor known as the androgen receptor. Both androgenic and anabolic effects appear to be mediated through the same receptor. Testosterone may bind directly to the androgen receptor or be converted by 5-α-reductase to dihydrotestosterone, which binds to the receptor more tightly than does testosterone. Some testosterone is converted to estradiol by an enzyme in peripheral tissues called aromatase. Estradiol can then bind to the estrogen receptor.

4. **Where are androgen receptors located?**
   Androgen receptors are present in many tissues, including the reproductive organs, skeletal muscle, bone, kidney, liver, brain, cardiac muscle, skin, fat, hematopoietic tissue, larynx, and thymus.

5. **Why does testosterone need to be modified to make clinically useful AASs?**
   When administered orally, testosterone is rapidly metabolized by the first-pass effect through the gut and liver. The first-pass effect prevents any significant rise in plasma testosterone levels with oral intake of unmodified testosterone. Intramuscular injection of unmodified testosterone is also not very useful because absorption is too rapid and duration of action is too short.

6. **How is testosterone modified to make AASs?**
   Alkylation of testosterone at the 17-α position confers resistance to hepatic metabolism and results in AASs that can be administered orally. Esterification of testosterone at the 17-B hydroxy position results in a hydrophobic molecule, which allows testosterone to be mixed with a fatty vehicle (sesame oil) and given by intramuscular injection. Also, the addition of carbon chains to the ring structure of testosterone increases fat solubility and extends the duration of action.

7. **What routes of administration are available?**
   Testosterone comes in oral, parenteral, patch and gel forms. Sublingual and transbuccal preparations are also now available.

8. **What are the indications for AAS therapy?**

AASs are indicated for use in male hypogonadism, constitutional delay of growth and puberty, hereditary angioneurotic edema, endometriosis, and fibrocystic breast disease; they also can benefit patients with aplastic or hypoplastic anemias. Androgens are useful in the anemia of end-stage renal disease but have been largely replaced by recombinant erythropoietin. Indications of specific agents are listed in Table 52-1.

TABLE 52-1. AASs AVAILABLE IN THE UNITED STATES	
AAS	**Use**
Parenteral agents	
Testosterone cypionate	Male hypogonadism
Testosterone enanthate	Male hypogonadism; delayed puberty; metastatic breast cancer (skeletal) 1–5 years after menopause
Testosterone propionate	Male hypogonadism; delayed puberty
Transdermal testosterone patches	Male hypogonadism; delayed puberty
Transdermal testosterone gel	Male hypogonadism; delayed puberty; concerns for transmission to female partners unlikely but of theoretical risk
Oral agents (17-α-methylated)	
Methyl testosterone	Male hypogonadism; delayed puberty; combined with estrogen for menopausal vasomotor symptoms; metastatic breast cancer (skeletal) 1–5 years after menopause
Oxandrolone	Promotes weight gain after extensive surgery, trauma, chronic infections, prolonged corticosteroid therapy; bone pain in osteoporosis
Stanozolol	Hereditary angioedema
Danazol	Endometriosis; fibrocystic breast disease; hereditary angioedema
Fluoxymesterone	Male hypogonadism; delayed puberty; androgen-responsive breast cancer (recurrent) 1–5 years after menopause
Sublingual agent	
Testosterone cyclodextrin	Male hypogonadism
Buccal agent	
Testosterone buccal system	Male hypogonadism
Under investigation	
Testosterone buciclate	Sustained-released preparation with action up to 12 weeks
Testosterone undecenoate	Sustained-released preparation with action up to 8 weeks

9. **Are there any other potential uses for AASs?**
AASs may help elderly men by increasing body weight and muscle mass, preventing bone loss, and improving the hematocrit. They also may be useful as male contraceptives. Both areas are under investigation. AASs are potentially useful in many other disorders, including severe chronic obstructive pulmonary disease and other wasting syndromes, autoimmune disorders, other hematologic disorders, alcoholic hepatitis, Turner's syndrome (by improving height), and osteoporosis.

10. **Which of the indications in question 8 is the most common use of AASs?**
Most likely none. The illegal use of AASs to enhance sports performance or physical appearance probably represents the single most common use. Abuse is widespread based on the belief that their anabolic properties will enhance the response to physical training, especially weight training.

KEY POINTS: INDICATIONS FOR AASs ✓

1. Male hypogonadism

2. Constitutional delay of growth and puberty

3. Hereditary angioneurotic edema

4. Endometriosis

5. Fibrocystic breast disease

6. Aplastic or hypoplastic anemias

11. **How common is abuse of AASs?**
The true prevalence of AAS abuse is not known. An estimated 2–3 million American athletes have used AASs. Approximately 50–80% of body builders, weight lifters, and power lifters may use AASs.

12. **Who is at risk for using illegal AASs?**
Use is highest among body builders and participants in sports favoring larger and/or stronger athletes. Because AASs increase the hematocrit via enhanced erythropoietin production, they may also be used by athletes participating in endurance-oriented sports. Nonathletes may use AASs solely to improve appearance. Surveys have shown a 5–11% prevalence of use among high school students. Most users are men, although up to 2% may be women. Other risk factors include involvement in school sports, and use of other illicit drugs, alcohol or tobacco.

13. **Do AASs truly help athletes?**
Both athletes and coaches are likely to answer unequivocally, "Yes." AASs used in conjunction with adequate protein and carbohydrate intake, and proper training in experienced athletes seems to induce greater and more rapid gains than training and diet alone. In the past, studies were unable to show consistent gains in size and strength from AAS use in eugonadal men. However, a study comparing supraphysiologic doses of testosterone enanthate with placebo in eugonadal men found clear increases in muscle size and strength, with or without weight-training exercise.

14. **How do AASs help the athletes?**
    Proposed mechanisms for increased size, strength, and performance include the anabolic effects of enhanced nitrogen retention and protein synthesis, anti-catabolic effects of blocking cortisol at its receptor, and the psychological effect of increased motivation.

15. **What doses of AASs are used in attempts to enhance sports performance and appearance?**
    Doses used for illicit purposes are markedly higher (10-fold or more) than therapeutic doses. Furthermore, multiple agents are often used in so-called stacking regimens or arrays. The drugs are often taken in 6–12-week cycles with variable periods off the drugs, but some athletes may use them as long as 1 year or more. Human chorionic gonadotropin may be used at the end of a cycle to stimulate gonadal function. Little is known about precise doses or stacking regimens; however, some anecdotal information is available, and examples of doses are given in Table 52-2 in comparison with the usual therapeutic doses.

TABLE 52-2.	COMPARISON OF DOSES IN THERAPEUTIC USE VERSUS ABUSE OF AASs*	
AAS	**Therapeutic Dose**	**Abuse**
Testosterone cypionate	200 mg every 2 weeks	200–800 mg/week
Testosterone enanthate	200 mg every 2 weeks	200–800 mg/week
Oxandrolone	2.5 mg 2–4 times/day	2.5–8 mg/day or more
Stanozolol	2 mg 3 times/day, then once daily on alternate days	8–12 mg/day

*The doses for abuse are estimates from anecdotal data and may vary considerably in individual users. Two to five or more AASs are often combined at these or higher doses, yielding even higher total doses.

16. **How do athletes get AASs?**
    AASs may be smuggled into the U.S. from countries where they are easily purchased without prescription. Some physicians also may prescribe them, and some AASs may be obtained from veterinarians. A significant black market exists, in which some of the preparations are fraudulent and potentially dangerous.

17. **What are the potential adverse effects of AAS use?**
    A wide range of side effects have occurred with AAS use and abuse. See Table 52-3.

18. **What about side effects in women and children?**
    All of the adverse effects mentioned earlier may occur in women and children. Women may experience oligomenorrhea or amenorrhea with inhibition of gonadotropin secretion. Such effects may reverse with cessation of AAS use. Virilizing effects, including hirsutism, clitoromegaly, and deepening of the voice, may not be reversible. Premature epiphyseal closure with a reduction in final adult height is an additional concern in adolescents using AASs.

19. **Which AASs have the least potential to cause adverse effects?**
    All AASs can cause significant adverse effects. However, hepatic toxicity and lipid derangements are seen predominantly with the oral alkylated AASs. The parenteral esters, patches, and gels are safer in this respect.

TABLE 52-3.   POTENTIAL ADVERSE EFFECTS OF AAS USE AND ABUSE

System Affected	Adverse Effects
Reproductive	Testicular atrophy, oligospermia, azoospermia, and priapism
Hepatotoxicity	Cholestatic hepatitis, pelioses hepatis (hemorrhagic liver cysts), and both benign and malignant hepatic tumors. Predominantly with the 17-alkylated oral agents
Cardiovascular	Stroke and myocardial infarction have been reported in weight lifters
Hematologic	Increases in platelet count and aggregation; ventricular thrombosis and systemic embolism have been reported
Psychological	Aggressive behavior, psychotic symptoms, dependence and withdrawal
Lipid profile	Reduced high-density lipoprotein (HDL) and higher low-density lipoprotein (LDL) cholesterol levels
Skin	Increase sebum production and acne, male pattern baldness
Infectious	Local infections at injection site, septic arthritis, and HIV/hepatitis from needle sharing
Gynecomastia	Caused from aromatization to estradiol; not present with modified androgens that cannot be aromatized (5-α-reduced androgens)
Other effects	Weight gain from fluid retention and increased lean body mass

20. **What has been done on a national and worldwide level to prevent AAS abuse?**
Under Sections 351, 352, 353, and 355 of the Food, Drug, and Cosmetic Act 21 USCA, these substances came under FDA regulation, requiring a prescription from a licensed physician. The Anabolic Steroids Control Act of 1990 made AAS schedule III controlled substances. Possession with an intent-to-sell constitutes a federal felony. Most recently, the World Anti-Doping Agency was established in an effort to coordinate a worldwide strategy for detection of illegal ergogenic aids used by competing athletes.

21. **What has been done on an individual level to prevent AASs abuse?**
With regard to their use by athletes, routine and random drug screening has been implemented. As professional and serious amateur athletes spend vast amounts of energy, time, and

KEY POINTS: EFFECTS AND SIDE EFFECTS OF AASs ✓

1. Biologic effects include growth and development of the prostate, seminal vesicles, penis and scrotum, beard, pubic, chest, and axillary hair and thickening of the vocal cords and enlargement of the larynx.

2. Common side effects of AAS abuse include fluid retention, testicular atrophy, oligospermia, azoospermia, gynecomastia, cholestatic hepatitis, pelioses hepatis, both benign and malignant hepatic tumors, and reduced HDL and higher LDL cholesterol levels.

3. The illegal use of AASs to enhance sports performance or physical appearance probably represents the single most common use.

resources in preparing for and competing in their sport, it is believed that the fear of being pre-cluded from competition will serve as an effective deterrent.

22. **What screening tests are used to detect AASs in athletes?**
Mass spectroscopy and gas chromatography can detect androgens other then testosterone when being used at the time of testing. To detect the use of exogenous testosterone, an increased ratio of urine testosterone to epitestosterone (greater than 6:1) can be confirmatory. Furthermore, urine samples with a high ratio of testosterone to leuteinizing hormone (LH; greater than 30) suggests AAS abuse since LH secretion is suppressed in subjects using testos-terone.

23. **Have androgen precursors, such as androstenedione and dehydroepiandrosterone, been shown to raise serum testosterone levels?**
These compounds are marketed and advertised to be metabolized to testosterone or other active metabolites. The current literature to substantiate these claims is sparse and the results are mixed. However, there is some evidence that these compounds may decrease HDL and raise estradiol levels in young men.

WESTSITES ⊕

1. Anabolic Steroid Abuse. Available at http://www.steroidabuse.org/

2. Anabolic Steroids Information. Available at http://www.steroid-encyclopaedia.com

BIBLIOGRAPHY

1. Bahrke M, Yesalis C, Kopstein A, et al: Risk factors associated with anabolic-androgenic steroid use among ado-lescents. Sports Med 29:397–405, 2000.

2. Basaria S, Wahlstrom J, Dobs A: Clinical review 138: Anabolic-androgenic steroid therapy in the treatment of chronic diseases. J Clin Endocrinol Metab 86:5108–1517, 2001.

3. Bhasin S, Storer TW, Berman N, el al: The effects of supraphysiologic doses of testosterone on muscle size and strength in normal men. N Engl J Med 335:1–7, 1996.

4. Bhasin S, Bremner WJ: Emerging issues in androgen replacement therapy. J Clin Endocrinol Metab 82:3–8, 1997.

5. Brown G, Vukovich M, Martini E, et al: Endocrine responses to chronic androstenedione intake in 30- to 56-year-old men. J Clin Endocrinol Metab 85:4074, 2000.

6. Catlin DH: Anabolic steroids. In DeGroot LJ, et al (eds): Endocrinology, 3rd ed. Philadelphia, W.B. Saunders, 1995, pp 2362–2376.

7. Dickerman RD, McConathy WJ, Zachariah NY: Testosterone, sex-hormone binding globulin, lipoproteins, and vascular disease risk. J Cardiovasc Risk 4(5/6):363–366, 1997.

8. Fudala P, Weinrieb R, Calarco J, et al: An evaluation of anabolic-androgenic steroid abusers over a period of 1 year: seven case studies. Ann Clin Psych 15:121–30, 2003.

9. Griffin J, Wilson J: Disorders of the testes and the male reproductive tract. In Wilson: Williams Textbook of Endocrinology, 10th ed. Philadelphia, W.B. Saunders, 2003, pp 747–751.

10. Hameed A, Brothwood T, Bouloux P: Delivery of testosterone replacement therapy. Curr Opin Invest Drugs. 4:1213–1219, 2003.

11. Hilderbrand R, Wanning R, Bowers L: An update on regulatory issues in antidoping programs in sport. Curr Sports Med Rep 2:226–232, 2003.

12. King DS, Sharp RL Brown GA, et al: Effect of oral androstenedione on serum testosterone and adaptations to resistance training in young men: A randomized controlled trial. JAMA 281:2020–2028, 1999.

13. Kouri EM, Pope HG Jr, Oliva PS: Changes in lipoprotein-lipid levels in normal men following administration of increasing doses of testosterone cypionate. Clin J Sports Med 6:152–157, 1996.

14. Leder BZ, Longcope C, Catlin DH, et al: Oral androstenedione administration and serum testosterone concentrations in young men. JAMA 283:779–782, 2000.

15. Ravaglia G, Forti P, Maioli F, et al: Body composition, sex steroids, IGF-1, and bone mineral status in aging men. J Gerontol A Biol Sci Med Sci 55(9):516–521, 2000.

16. Rhoden EL, Morgentaler A: Risks of testosterone replacement therapy and recommendations for monitoring. N Engl J Med 350:482–492, 2004.

17. Sambrook PN, Eisman JA: Osteoporosis prevention and treatment. Med J Aust 172(5):226–229, 2000.

18. Storer TW, Magliano L, Woodhouse L, et al. Testosterone dose-dependently increases maximal voluntary strength and leg power, but does not affect fatigability or specific tension. J Clin Endocrinol Metab 88:1478–1485, 2003.

19. Wallace MB, Lim J, Cutler A, Bucci L: Effects of dehydroepiandrosterone versus androstenedione supplementation in men. Med Sci Sports Exerc 31(12):1788–1792, 1999.

MULTIPLE ENDOCRINE NEOPLASIA

Arnold A. Asp, M.D.

CHAPTER 53

1. **What are the multiple endocrine neoplasia (MEN) syndromes?**
   There are three well-characterized, inherited pluriglandular disorders in which several endocrine glands simultaneously undergo neoplastic transformation and become hyperfunctional. All of these disorders are genetically transmitted in an autosomal dominant fashion. These disorders include MEN 1, MEN 2A, and MEN 2B.

2. **Define MEN 1.**
   MEN 1 consists of hyperplasia or neoplastic transformation of the parathyroids, pancreatic islets, and pituitary.

3. **Define MEN 2A.**
   MEN 2A consists of hyperplasia or neoplastic transformation of the thyroid parafollicular cells (medullary carcinoma of the thyroid [MCT]), parathyroid glands, and adrenal medulla (pheochromocytoma).

4. **Define MEN 2B.**
   MEN 2B consists of hyperplasia or neoplastic transformation of the thyroid parafollicular cells (MCT) and adrenal medulla (pheochromocytoma) with concomitant development of mucosal neuromas.

5. **How can so many various endocrine organs be affected in these syndromes?**
   This question is a matter of controversy and ongoing research. The cells that comprise many endocrine organs are able to decarboxylate various amino acids and convert the molecules to amines or peptides that act as hormones or neurotransmitters. These cells have been classified as amine precursor uptake and decarboxylation (APUD) cells and are considered to be embryologically of neuroectodermal origin. APUD cells contain markers of their common neuroendocrine origin, including neuron-specific enolase and chromogranin A. Neoplastic transformation of APUD cells long after organogenesis is complete appears to be due to a germline mutation (loss of a tumor suppressor gene in MEN 1 or mutation of a protooncogene to an oncogene in MEN 2A and MEN 2B) in a gene that is expressed only in neuroectodermal cells. When neuroectodermal cells later migrate to specific developing organs, the genetic mutation likewise is distributed to those organs. This may explain the eventual development of tumors in so many diverse tissues.

6. **What is Wermer's syndrome?**
   This is the eponym for the MEN 1 syndrome. Wermer first recognized the association of parathyroid hyperplasia, multicentric pituitary tumors, and pancreatic islet cell tumors in several kindreds and described the syndrome in 1954. Although neoplastic transformation occurs most commonly in the parathyroids, pituitary, and pancreas, hyperplastic adrenal cortical and nodular thyroid disorders have been described. Carcinoid tumors, especially involving the foregut (thymus, lung, stomach, and duodenum), are uncommon but also have been reported in MEN 1 syndrome.

7. **How common is Werner's syndrome?**

   Wermer's syndrome is the most common form of MEN. Its prevalence is estimated to vary between 2 and 20 per 100,000 population. The syndrome is characterized by a high degree of penetrance; expression increases with age.

8. **Is hyperparathyroidism in MEN 1 similar to sporadic primary hyperparathyroidism?**

   No. Hyperparathyroidism associated with MEN 1 results from hyperplasia of all four glands, whereas sporadic primary hyperparathyroidism usually is characterized by adenomatous change in a single gland. Hyperparathyroidism is the most common and earliest manifestation of MEN 1, occurring in 80–95% of cases. It has been described in patients as young as 17 years of age and develops in nearly all patients with MEN 1 by the age of 40.

9. **What causes the hyperplasia of parathyroid glands affected by MEN 1?**

   Hyperplasia of parathyroid glands affected by MEN 1 results from expansion of multiple cell clones, while sporadic parathyroid adenomas result from activation of a single cell clone. Several groups have described a mitogenic factor (probably basic fibroblast growth factor) in the sera of patients with MEN 1. This factor potentiates the hyperplastic growth of parathyroid tissue. Complications of MEN 1 hyperparathyroidism are similar to those of sporadic hyperparathyroidism; they include nephrolithiasis, osteoporosis, mental status changes, and muscular weakness.

10. **Summarize the therapy for hypoplastic parathyroid glands.**

    Therapy of both sporadic adenomas and MEN 1-associated hyperplastic glands depends on surgical resection. In sporadic primary hyperparathyroidism, removal of the solitary adenoma is curative in 95% of cases. In MEN 1-associated hyperplasia, at least 3½ hyperplastic glands must be resected to restore normocalcemia. Only 75% of patients are normocalcemic postoperatively; 10–25% are rendered hypoparathyroid. Unfortunately, the parathyroid remnants in the patient with MEN 1 have a great propensity to regenerate; 50% of cases become hypercalcemic again within 10 years of surgery. This recurrence rate dictates that surgery be delayed until complications of hypercalcemia are imminent or gastrin levels are elevated, as discussed in the following.

11. **How common is neoplastic transformation of pancreatic islet cells in MEN 1?**

    Neoplastic transformation of the pancreatic islet cells is the second most common manifestation of MEN 1, occurring in approximately 66–80% of cases.

12. **What types of pancreatic tumors are found in MEN 1 syndrome?**

    Pancreatic tumors in MEN 1 syndrome are usually multicentric and are often capable of elaborating several peptides and biogenic amines. They are, by convention, classified on the basis of the clinical syndrome produced by the predominant secretory product. This group of tumors characteristically progresses from hyperplasia to malignancy with metastases, making curative resection unlikely. Tumors of the pancreas may arise from normal islet cells (eutopic) or cells that are not normal constituents of the adult pancreas (ectopic).

13. **What is the most common type of pancreatic tumor in MEN 1?**

    Gastrinomas are the most common pancreatic tumors in the MEN 1 syndrome (47–78% of cases). They are ectopic tumors; G cells are normally present in the fetal pancreas only. Gastrinomas also may occur independently of MEN 1 (only 15–48% of all patients with a gastrinoma are later found to have MEN 1). Gastrinomas associated with MEN 1 are multiple and often extrapancreatic, occurring in the duodenal wall and retroperitoneal lymphatics.

14. **Describe the symptoms of gastrinomas associated with MEN 1.**

    Excessive gastrin secretion by these tumors causes prolific production of gastric acid with resultant duodenal and jejunal ulcers and diarrhea. Basal acid output exceeds 15 mmol/h, and basal fasting serum gastrin levels usually exceed 300 pg/mL.

15. **What other conditions may cause hypergastrinemia?**
Hypergastrinemia also may result from any condition that stimulates normal gastrin secretion (hypercalcemia) or that interferes with normal gastric acid production and feedback to the G cells (achlorhydria, gastric outlet obstruction, retained antrum with a Billroth II procedure, vagotomy, and the use of H_2 blockers and proton pump inhibitors). Hyperparathyroidism (see questions 8 and 9) can therefore falsely elevate serum gastrin levels.

16. **How are gastrinomas distinguished from other causes of hypergastrinemia?**
A secretin stimulation test may aid in the differentiation of gastrinomas from other hypergastrinemic states; serum gastrin levels in patients with gastrinomas increase by at least 200 pg/mL. More information about gastrinomas is included in Chapter 55.

17. **What is the second most common type of pancreatic tumor in MEN 1?**
Insulinomas are the second most common pancreatic islet-cell tumor in the MEN 1 syndrome (12–36% of islet-cell tumors) and the most common eutopic type. Persistent or disordered insulin secretion causes severe hypoglycemia; inappropriately elevated concentrations of insulin, proinsulin, and C-peptide are present in the serum. Insulinomas associated with MEN 1 syndrome are more frequently multicentric and malignant than are the sporadic tumors. Approximately 1–5% of all patients with an insulinoma are eventually discovered to have MEN 1. An excellent discussion of the diagnosis and therapy of insulinomas is found in Chapter 55.

18. **What other pancreatic tumors may be seen in MEN 1?**
Pancreatic tumors less frequently associated with MEN 1 include glucagonomas, somatostatin-omas, and vasoactive intestinal polypeptide-secreting tumors (VIPomas). Associated syndromes and therapy are also described in Chapter 55.

19. **How are the most common pancreatic tumors of MEN 1 treated?**
Multicentric gastrinomas are rarely cured surgically (10–15% of cases). Fortunately, symptoms of hypergastrinemia can be pharmacologically controlled with H_2 blocker, proton-pump inhibitor, or octreotide administration. Metastases to the liver become increasingly common when gastrinomas exceed 3 cm in diameter, prompting most surgeons to reserve excision for tumors larger than 3 cm. Gastrinomas express surface receptors for somatostatin, potentiating the use of somatostatin-receptor scintigraphy in combination with annual magnetic resonance imaging (MRI)/computed tomography (CT) surveillance to monitor tumor progression.

20. **Summarize the approach to treatment of hypoglycemia associated with insulinomas.**
Insulinomas, unlike gastrinomas, produce devastating hypoglycemia, which is difficult to counteract medically. Without effective long-term pharmacotherapy, surgical resection of the tumor(s) is required in most patients. Fortunately, when the largest tumor is excised, many of the patient's symptoms are ameliorated. Localization is accomplished preoperatively with endoscopic ultrasonography, MRI/CT, or by comparison of insulin levels in the right hepatic vein following selective infusion of the intrapancreatic arteries with calcium gluconate. Intraoperative ultrasonography may also assist precise localization at the time of surgery.

21. **Which pituitary tumors are associated with MEN 1?**
Pituitary tumors occur in 50–71% of cases of MEN 1. They may result either from neoplastic transformation of anterior pituitary cells with clonal expansion to a tumor or from excessive stimulation of the pituitary by ectopically produced hypothalamic releasing factors elaborated by carcinoids or pancreatic islet cells.

22. **What pituitary tumors are most commonly associated with MEN 1?**
Prolactinomas are the most common pituitary tumors associated with MEN 1, constituting 60% of the total. The symptoms of hyperprolactinemia (galactorrhea and amenorrhea in women;

impotence in men) are the third most common manifestation of MEN 1. The tumors are typically multicentric and large but respond to dopamine agonists, such as bromocriptine. In earlier series, many pituitary tumors described as chromophobe adenomas were, in reality, prolactinomas that contained sparse poorly staining secretory granules. These tumors are also discussed in Chapter 21.

23. What is the second most common pituitary tumor in MEN 1?
The second most commonly encountered pituitary tumor type is the growth hormone-producing tumor, which is reported in 10–25% of patients. Overproduction of growth hormone results in gigantism in children and acromegaly in adults. The tumors are often multicentric and may result from secretion of growth hormone-releasing hormone by pancreatic or carcinoid tumors. Diagnosis and therapy is described in Chapter 22.

24. What other pituitary tumors may be seen in MEN 1?
Corticotropin (adrenocorticotropin [ACTH])-producing tumors that cause Cushing's syndrome may be associated with MEN 1. Such tumors result from neoplastic transformation of the pituitary or elaboration of corticotropin-releasing hormone by pancreatic or carcinoid tumors. Diagnosis and therapy are described in Chapter 24.

25. What causes MEN 1?
The gene predisposing to the development of MEN 1 (MEN 1 susceptibility gene) is located on the long arm of chromosome 11 (11q13) and encodes a protein known as menin, which functions as a tumor suppressor. The proband inherits an allele predisposing to MEN 1 from the affected parent, whereas a normal allele is passed down from the unaffected parent. The gene for this tumor suppressor is unusually susceptible to mutation. When a somatic mutation later inactivates the normal allele, suppressor function is lost, permitting hyperplasia of the gland to occur.

26. How should a kindred be screened after the proband is identified?
Carriers of the genetic defect must first be identified, the extent of their organ involvement determined, and their family screened for additional carriers of the susceptibility gene. As mentioned earlier, mutations in the gene coding for the tumor suppressor, menin, are apparent in patients with MEN 1 and may be used to identify carriers of the disorder in the near future. Because mutational analysis using polymerase chain reaction techniques is currently restricted to research laboratories, periodic measurement of calcium and associated hormones is the next best alternative to detect disease within affected kindreds.

27. At what age should screening begin?
Manifestations of MEN 1 syndrome rarely occur before the age of 15; therefore, people at risk should not undergo endocrine screening before that time. Nearly all people at risk develop the disorder by the age of 40 years; screening may be unnecessary in members older than 50 who are proved to be disease-free.

28. Summarize the tests used for screening of MEN 1 kindreds.
Because hyperparathyroidism is temporally the first manifestation of MEN 1 syndrome, serum calcium concentrations constitute the best screening test to identify asymptomatic carriers. Biochemical evidence of hyperparathyroidism in a member of MEN 1 kindred establishes a presumptive carrier state. Evaluation then should focus on delineation of pancreatic and pituitary involvement. Serum levels of gastrin disclose the presence of a gastrinoma, whereas levels of prolactin most often reveal the presence of pituitary disease (especially in women). The latter two tests are cost-effective only in established disease and should not be used for preliminary screening of the kindred (unless symptoms of hypergastrinemia or prolactinoma are present). The frequency of screening has not been prospectively studied but recommended intervals range from 2–5 years.

KEY POINTS: MEN 1   ✓

1. MEN 1 consists of neoplastic transformation in at least two of these three glands: parathyroids, pancreas, and pituitary.

2. MEN 1 results from a mutation inactivating the menin tumor suppressor on chromosome 11. Routine clinical testing for the mutation is currently impractical.

3. Therapy for MEN 1 includes surgical resection of hyperplastic parathyroid tissue and pituitary adenomas; surgical cure for the associated pancreatic tumors is not usually possible.

29. **What is Sipple's syndrome?**
This is the eponym for MEN 2A. In 1961, Sipple recognized and described a patient who expired with an intracerebral aneurysm and was found at autopsy to have MCT, pheochromocytomas, and hyperparathyroidism. This disorder is inherited in an autosomal dominant fashion and exhibits a high degree of penetrance and variable expressivity. It is less common than MEN-1 syndrome.

30. **Is the form of MCT associated with MEN 2A similar to the sporadic form of MCT?**
No. MCT results from malignant transformation of the parafollicular cells (or C cells) that normally elaborate calcitonin and are scattered throughout the gland. MCT accounts for 2–10% of all thyroid malignancies. The sporadic form of MCT, as described in Chapter 38, is more common (75% of all MCT), occurs in a solitary form (< 20% multicentric), and metastasizes to local lymphatics, lung, bone, and liver early in the course of disease (metastasis may occur with primary tumors less than 1 cm in diameter). Sporadic MCT occurs more commonly in an older population (peak age: 40–60 years) and is usually located in the upper two-thirds of the gland.

31. **Summarize the essential characteristics of MCT associated with MEN 2A.**
MCT associated with MEN 2A is multicentric (90% at the time of diagnosis), occurs at a younger age than sporadic MCT (as young as 2 years of age), and generally has a better prognosis than the sporadic form. MCT occurs in nearly 95% of all cases of MEN 2A and is usually the first tumor to appear.

32. **How common is diarrhea in MCT associated with MEN 2A?**
Calcitonin or other peptides elaborated by the tumor may cause a secretory diarrhea that is present in 4–7% of patients at the time of diagnosis but develops in 25–30% during the course of the disease.

33. **How is MEN 2-associated MCT treated?**
Parafollicular cells in patients with MEN 2A characteristically progress through a state of C-cell hyperplasia to nodular hyperplasia to malignant degeneration over a variable period. It is imperative that patients at risk be diagnosed while still in the C-cell hyperplasia stage; total thyroidectomy precludes malignant degeneration and metastases.

34. **How is C-cell hyperplasia detected?**
Detection of C-cell hyperplasia is facilitated by the pentagastrin stimulation test. MCT also expresses peptides and hormones not commonly elaborated by parafollicular cells, including somatostatin, thyrotropin-releasing hormone, vasoactive intestinal peptide, proopiomelanocortin, carcinoembryonic antigen, and neurotensin.

35. **What is the second most common neoplasm associated with MEN 2A?**
Pheochromocytomas occur in 50–70% of cases of MEN 2A and are bilateral in up to 84% of patients. Compared with the sporadic form, pheochromocytomas associated with MEN 2A secrete greater amounts of epinephrine. Hypertension is therefore less common, and urinary excretion of catecholamines may become supranormal later in the course of the disease.

36. **Summarize the treatment of pheochromocytomas associated with MEN 2A.**
Surgical resection is indicated, but controversy surrounds the need for prophylactic resection of contralateral uninvolved adrenals, 50% of which develop pheochromocytomas within 10 years of the original surgery. The diagnosis and management of pheochromocytomas are discussed in Chapter 29.

37. **Is hyperparathyroidism associated with MEN 2A similar to that found in MEN 1?**
Yes, but it is encountered much less commonly, involving only 40% of cases. No mitogenic factor (as in MEN 1) has been described in the sera of these patients.

38. **What is the genetic basis for the MEN 2A syndrome?**
MEN 2A is caused by an activating mutation of the RET protooncogene located on chromosome 10q11.2. The gene codes for a receptor tyrosine kinase that phosphorylates and activates enzymes critical to cellular development. The ligand that normally activates the tyrosine kinase is glial cell-derived neurotropic factor (GDNF). When GDNF binds, two receptors bind together (homodimerization) and phosphorylation of enzymes occurs downstream. Mutation of the RET protooncogene to an oncogene results in constitutive activation of the enzyme, causing unregulated phosphorylation of other critical enzymes. Inheritance of one RET oncogene from one affected parent is sufficient to cause MEN 2A syndrome in offspring. Five distinct mutations involving exons 10 and 11 have been described in 98% of 203 kindreds with the disorder.

39. **How should a kindred be screened after the proband with MEN 2A is identified?**
As explained in question 26, screening initially entails the differentiation of gene carriers from uninvolved family members and the subsequent delineation of organ involvement in the affected members. But unlike MEN 1, direct DNA sequencing of the RET oncogene causing MEN 2A is clinically available. With appropriate repeat analysis of positive and negative test results, the assay offers near 100% accuracy in identification of affected individuals. Genetic analysis of the kindred should be performed to identify the specific RET oncogene mutation; characterization of the familial oncogene precludes the need for repetitive biochemical screening of noncarriers in subsequent generations.

40. **How is MEN 2A treated?**
Because C-cell hyperplasia has been described in gene carriers as young as 2 years of age, total thyroidectomy is suggested in affected individuals before the age of 5. An alternative to preemptive thyroidectomy is to perform annual pentagastrin stimulation tests and withhold surgery until a positive result is obtained. Because MEN 2A-associated pheochromocytoma may produce large amounts of epinephrine that do not cause hypertension, annual timed urine collections for catecholamines should be obtained in all gene carriers. Serum levels of calcium should be assessed every 2 years. Once the presence of the syndrome is established, screening for adrenal and parathyroid involvement should continue through life.

41. **What comprises the MEN 2B syndrome?**
MEN 2B syndrome is the association of MCT and pheochromocytoma with multiple mucosal neuromas in an affected individual or kindred. Hyperparathyroidism is not associated with MEN 2B. This syndrome is less common than the MEN 2A and is more commonly sporadic than familial, but if inherited, it is transmitted in an autosomal dominant fashion.

42. **What findings raise the suspicion of MEN 2B syndrome?**

The occurrence of multiple mucosal neuromas on the distal tongue, lips, and along the gastrointestinal tract should always raise the possibility of MEN 2B. Other manifestations of MEN 2B include marfanoid habitus (without ectopia lentis or aortic aneurysms), hypertrophic corneal nerves, and slipped femoral epiphysis.

KEY POINTS: MEN 2A AND MEN 2B ✔

1. MEN 2A consists of neoplastic transformation of parathyroids, thyroid parafollicular C cells, and adrenal medulla.

2. MEN 2B consists of neoplastic transformation of thyroid parafollicular C cells, and adrenal medulla, with mucosal neuromas.

3. Genetic testing for the RET mutation causing MEN 2 syndromes is now clinically available.

---

43. **How should MEN 2B be treated?**

The MCT associated with this syndrome is more aggressive than other forms; metastatic lesions have been described in infancy. Because of the propensity toward early metastasis, many advocate that children with the syndrome should undergo total thyroidectomy as soon as surgery can be tolerated. Pheochromocytomas occur in nearly one-half of all patients and follow a clinical course similar to those in the MEN 2A syndrome.

44. **What is the overall mortality rate associated with MEN 2B?**

Overall mortality in MEN 2B is more severe; the average age of death for patients with MEN 2A is 60 years, whereas in patients with MEN 2B the average age of death is 30 years.

45. **Summarize the screening recommendations for MEN 2B.**

Screening of family members with pentagastrin stimulation for MCT should begin at birth and continue through life if thyroidectomy is deferred. Screening for pheochromocytoma should begin at 5 years and continue for life.

46. **What causes MEN 2B?**

Over 95% of the kindreds with MEN 2B have been found to carry a mutation of the RET protooncogene at codon 918 (exon 16). This oncogene codes for a methionine-to-threonine substitution, resulting in activation of the innermost tyrosine kinase moiety of the same receptor associated with MEN 2A.

47. **Have the clinical presentations and prognoses of the MEN syndromes changed since the time of their original descriptions?**

Yes. When the MEN syndromes were initially described, most patients presented with involvement of all of the aforementioned organ systems because diagnostic capabilities were limited. At present, early diagnosis of the proband and aggressive screening of the kindred may permit detection of hyperplasia and prompt prophylactic surgery or medical therapy that limits morbidity and mortality.

BIBLIOGRAPHY

1. Benson L, Ljunghall S, Akerstrom G, et al: Hyperparathyroidism presenting as the first lesion in multiple endocrine neoplasia type 1. Am J Med 82:731–737, 1987.

2. Brandi ML, Auerbach GD, Fitzpatrick LA, et al: Parathyroid mitogenic activity in plasma from patients with familial multiple endocrine neoplasia type 1. N Engl J Med 314:1287–1293, 1986.

3. Brandi ML, Gagel RF, Angeli A, et al: Guidelines for diagnosis and therapy of MEN type 1 and type 2. J Clin Endocrinol Metab 86:5658–5671, 2001.

4. Cadiot G, Laurent-Piug P, Thuille B, et al: Is the multiple endocrine neoplasia type 1 gene a suppressor for fundic argyrophil tumors in Zollinger-Ellison syndrome? Gastroenterology 105:579–582, 1993.

5. Chandrasekharappa SCV, Guru SC, Manickam P, et al: Positional cloning of the gene for multiple endocrine neoplasia type 1. Science 276:404–407, 1997.

6. Eng C: The RET proto-oncogene in multiple endocrine neoplasia type 2 and Hirschsprung's disease. N Engl J Med 335:943–951, 1996.

7. Eng C, Clayton D, Schuffenecker I, et al: The relationship between specific RET proto-oncogene mutations and disease phenotype in multiple endocrine neoplasia type 2. JAMA 276:1575–1579, 1996.

8. Gagel RF: Multiple endocrine neoplasia. In Wilson JD, Foster DW (eds): Williams' Textbook of Endocrinology, 9th ed. Philadelphia, W.B. Saunders, 1998, pp 1637–1649.

9. Gicquel C, Bertherat J, Le Bouc Y, et al: The pathogenesis of adrenocortical incidentalomas and genetic syndromes associated with adrenocortical neoplasms. Endocrinol Metab Clin North Am 29:1–13, 2000.

10. Grauer A, Raue F, Gagel RF: Changing concepts in the management of hereditary and sporadic medullary thyroid carcinoma. Endocrinol Metab Clin North Am 19:613–635, 1990.

11. Herman V, Draznin NZ, Gonsky R, Melmed S: Molecular screening of pituitary adenomas for gene mutations and rearrangements. J Clin Endocrinol Metab 77:50–55, 1993.

12. Marx SJ, Vinik AI, Santen RJ, et al: Multiple endocrine neoplasia type 1: Assessment of laboratory tests to screen for the gene in a large kindred. Medicine 65:2226–2241, 1986.

13. Marx SJ (moderator): Multiple endocrine neoplasia type 1: Clinical and genetic topics. Ann Intern Med 129:484–494, 1998.

14. Phay JE, Moley JF, Lairmore TL: Multiple endocrine neoplasias. Semin Surg Oncol 18:324–332, 2000.

15. Saad MF, Ordenez NG, Rashid RK, et al: Medullary carcinoma of the thyroid. Medicine 63:319–342, 1984.

16. Santoro M, Carlomagno F, Romano A, et al: Activation of RET as a dominant transforming gene by germline mutations of MEN 2A and MEN 2B. Science 267:381–383, 1995.

17. Veldius JD, Norton JA, Wells SA, et al: Surgical versus medical management of multiple endocrine neoplasia (MEN) type 1. J Clin Endocrinol Metab 82:357–364, 1997.

CHAPTER 54

AUTOIMMUNE POLYENDOCRINE SYNDROMES

Arnold A. Asp, M.D.

1. **Define the autoimmune polyendocrine syndromes. How many clinical forms are there?**

   The autoimmune polyendocrine syndromes (APSs) are disorders in which two or more endocrine glands are simultaneously hypofunctional or hyperfunctional as the result of autoimmune dysfunction. It is theorized that a defect in the T-suppressor cell subset inadvertently permits activation of the cellular and humoral arms of the immune system. The nature of this dysfunction is unknown. The two widely recognized clinical forms are appropriately designated APS type 1 and APS type 2. The common clinical link between the syndromes is adrenal insufficiency.

2. **Is evidence of nonendocrine autoimmune dysfunction associated with APSs?**

   Yes. Connective tissue diseases and hematologic and gastrointestinal autoimmune disorders are commonly associated with the APSs.

3. **What constitutes APS type 1?**

   APS type 1 is a pediatric disorder manifested by the presence of a combination of two of the following three disorders: hypoparathyroidism, adrenal insufficiency, and chronic mucocutaneous candidiasis. Usually hypoparathyroidism and candidiasis present by the age of 5 years. Adrenal insufficiency occurs by the age of 12 years, and all manifestations are present by the age of 15 years. Some affected individuals develop only one manifestation. Other endocrine conditions may also occur; the largest series of patients have noted the following endocrine manifestations:

   Hypoparathyroidism: 89%   Thyroid disease: 12%
   Adrenal insufficiency: 60%   Diabetes mellitus type 1: 1–4%
   Gonadal failure: 45%

4. **Are nonendocrine manifestations associated with APS type 1?**

   Yes. Chronic mucocutaneous candidiasis occurs in 75% of patients, celiac disease in 25%, alopecia in 20%, pernicious anemia in 16%, and chronic autoimmune hepatitis in 9%. Dystrophy of the dental enamel, vitiligo, keratopathy, and hypoplasia of the teeth and nails also may occur, prompting the alternative designation for APS type 1: autoimmune polyendocrinopathy-candidiasis-ectodermal dystrophy (APECED).

5. **Explain the etiology of APS type 1.**

   Mutations of the autoimmune regulator (AIRE) gene on chromosome 21 cause APS type 1, which is inherited in an autosomal recessive pattern. There appears to be no human leukocyte antigen (HLA) association. The cause of the candidiasis is not known, although delayed hypersensitivity is defective in affected patients. Antibodies to adrenal enzymes (21-hydroxylase, an enzyme in the biosynthetic pathway for aldosterone and cortisol) and to poorly characterized parathyroid antigens have been described by some groups.

6. **What therapy can be offered?**

   Annual screening of levels of serum calcium, cosyntropin-stimulated cortisol, and liver-associated enzymes is performed in affected sibships until the age of 15 years. Adrenal insufficiency and hypoparathyroidism are treated with glucocorticoids and oral calcium/vitamin D supplementation, respectively. Mucocutaneous candidiasis is treated with fluconazole. Use of prophylactic immunosuppressives, such as cyclosporine, is not recommended.

7. **What disorders are associated with APS type 2?**
APS type 2 occurs in adulthood and consists of autoimmune adrenal insufficiency with autoimmune thyroid disease and/or diabetes mellitus, type 1. The age of onset tends to be between 20 and 30 years; one-half of the cases are sporadic and one-half are familial. Endocrine organ involvement is as follows:

Adrenal insufficiency: 100%   Diabetes mellitus type 1: 50%
Autoimmune thyroid disease: 70%   Gonadal failure: 5–50%

   Very rarely geriatric hypoparathyroidism may be encountered in elderly patients with APS type 2.

8. **What is most common presenting disorder in APS type 2?**
Adrenal insufficiency is the presenting disorder in one-half of cases, whereas adrenal insufficiency with diabetes mellitus or thyroid disease is present at the time of diagnosis in 20% of cases. In the remaining 30%, adrenal insufficiency occurs after other endocrine dysfunction. Between 69% and 90% of patients have circulating antibodies to 21-hydroxylase.

9. **What thyroid disorders are associated with APS type 2?**
Thyroid disorders associated with APS type 2 include Graves' disease (50%) and Hashimoto's disease or atrophic thyroiditis (50%). As expected, thyroid-stimulating immunoglobulins (TSI) are present in cases of hyperthyroidism, whereas antibodies to thyroid peroxidase or thyroglobulin are present in cases of hypothyroidism.

10. **Summarize the significance of cytoplasmic islet-cell antibodies (ICAs) in APS type 2.**
Cytoplasmic ICAs are present in patients with APS type 2 and diabetes mellitus; however, the significance of these antibodies is questionable. APS type 2 patients who have ICAs but not diabetes may have no compromise of beta-cell function and subsequently develop diabetes at a rate of 2% per year, whereas ICA-positive first-degree relatives of non-APS, type 1 diabetic individuals develop diabetes at a rate of 8% per year.

11. **How common is gonadal failure in APS type 2?**
Gonadal failure is more common in women than in men and is associated with antibodies to gonadal tissue.

12. **Are nonendocrine abnormalities described in APS type 2?**
Yes. In about 5% of cases, other autoimmune disorders are found, including vitiligo, pernicious anemia, alopecia, myasthenia gravis, celiac disease, Sjögren's syndrome, and rheumatoid arthritis.

13. **How should kindreds with suspected APS type 2 be screened?**
Because APS type 2 appears in multiple generations and because 20 years may lapse between the development of various endocrine organ failures, affected patients should be screened by assessing levels of serum glucose, thyrotropin (TSH), and vitamin B_{12} every 3–5 years. Symptoms of adrenal insufficiency should be investigated by assessing levels of cosyntropin-stimulated cortisol. First-degree relatives of the proband should be educated about the syndrome and advised to undergo screening every 3–5 years. Antibodies to thyroid peroxidase or thyroglobulin are so common in the general population as to preclude their use as a screening test.

14. **Explain the etiology of APS type 2.**

    The genetic basis of APS type 2 is uncertain, although it appears to be associated with an HLA-DR3 phenotype that may be permissive for the development of autoimmunity. Organ-specific antibodies may cause organ dysfunction, for example, TSI may cause Graves' disease and anti-acetylcholine receptor antibodies may cause myasthenia gravis, or, like antithyroglobulin antibodies, they may be epiphenomena of disease. The only consistent abnormality noted in affected patients is decreased function of T-suppressor cells.

15. **What is POEMS syndrome?**

    POEMS syndrome is a disorder of unknown etiology, unrelated to either APS type 1 or APS type 2, that appears to have an immunologic basis. The acronym highlights the cardinal features of the syndrome: *p*olyneuropathy, *o*rganomegaly, *e*ndocrinopathy, *m*onoclonal component, and *s*kin changes. All of the symptoms are considered to be secondary to a plasma cell dyscrasia (monoclonal gammopathies of undetermined significance; plasmacytoma, osteosclerotic, osteolytic, or mixed myeloma) that produces the monoclonal gammopathy.

KEY POINTS: APSs ✓

1. APS type 1 is a pediatric syndrome marked by hypoparathyroidism, adrenal insufficiency and mucocutaneous candidiasis.

2. APS type 1 is inherited in an autosomal recessive manner and is clinically apparent by 15 years of age.

3. APS type 2 consists of adrenal insufficiency, thyroid dysfunction, and diabetes mellitus type 1.

4. APS type 2 associated organ failure progresses over many years during adulthood and effects multiple generations.

5. Both APS type 1 and APS type 2 manifest nonendocrine organ dysfunction, primarily gastrointestinal and dermatologic diseases.

16. **What eponym is associated with POEMS?**

    Another name for the disorder is Crow-Fukase syndrome.

17. **How does POEMS usually present?**

    The majority of patients are Asian males 45–55 years of age, but any ethnic group of either gender is susceptible. The most common presentation is that of a distal, symmetric peripheral sensorimotor neuropathy. There is usually loss of pin-prick and vibratory sense, and decreased deep tendon reflexes predominantly in the lower extremities. The neuropathy is slowly progressive. Electromyograms and nerve biopsies are most consistent with both demyelination and axonal degeneration. Autonomic neuropathy has not been observed. Papilledema is present in 40–80% of cases. Nerve damage may result from myelin cross-reactivity with monoclonal IgA or IgG M proteins produced by plasmacytomas in sclerotic bone lesions, but evidence of intraneural immunoglobulin deposition has not been found in all series.

18. **How does the organomegaly manifest?**

    Hepatomegaly (uncommon in multiple myeloma) and/or splenomegaly is noted in approximately two-thirds of POEMS cases. The hepatomegaly may be associated with fibrosis and liver dysfunction.

19. **Which endocrine systems are involved?**
Diabetes mellitus type 2 is commonly encountered in either gender (28–48%), as is primary hypothyroidism (45–59%) or, rarely, adrenal insufficiency. Both males and females manifest elevated serum estrogen levels, which may promote hyperprolactinemia with galactorrhea and amenorrhea or impotence. Antibodies to the thyroid or adrenal glands have not been consistently detected.

20. **What skin changes have been encountered?**
Skin changes include sclerosis, hypertrichosis, hyperpigmentation, and hyperhidrosis.

21. **How is POEMS treated?**
Treatment of POEMS is based on elimination of plasmacytomas with radiation or chemotherapy, which, if successful, results in amelioration of the polyneuropathy and reduction in organomegaly. Endocrine deficiencies are treated with replacement hormones.

BIBLIOGRAPHY

1. Ahonen P, Myllarniemi S, Sipila I, et al: Clinical variation of autoimmune polyendocrinopathy–candidiasis–ectodermal dystrophy (APECED) in a series of 68 patients. N Engl J Med 322:1829–1836, 1990.
2. Betterle C, Grehhio NA, Volpato M. Autoimmune polyglandular syndrome type 1. J Clin Endocrinol Metab 83:1049–1055, 1998.
3. Consortium TF-GA: An autoimmune disease, APECED, caused by mutations in a novel gene featuring two PHD-type zinc finger domains. The Finnish-German APECED Consortium. Autoimmune Polyendocrinopathy Candidiasis Ectodermal Dystrophy. Nat Genet 17:399–403, 1997.
4. Eisenbarth GS, Verge CF: The immunoendocrinopathy syndromes. In Wilson JD, Foster DW (eds): Williams' Textbook of Endocrinology, 9th ed. Philadelphia, W.B. Saunders, 1998, pp 1651–1662.
5. Gianani R, Eisenbarth GS: Autoimmunity to gastrointestinal endocrine cells in autoimmune polyendocrine syndrome type 1. J Clin Endocrinol Metab 88:1442–1444, 2003 (editorial).
6. Kutteh WH: Immunology of multiple endocrinopathies associated with premature ovarian failure. Endocrinologist 6:462–466, 1996.
7. Leshin M: Polyglandular autoimmune syndromes. Am J Med Sci 290:77–88, 1985.
8. Mhyre AG, Halonen M, Eskelin P, et al: Autoimmune polyendocrine syndrome. Clin Endocrinol 45:211–217, 2001.
9. Soubrier M, Dubost JJ, Sauvezie B: POEMS syndrome: A study of 25 cases and a review of the literature. Am J Med 97:543–553, 1994.
10. Soubrier M, Sauron C, Souweine B, et al: Growth factors and proinflammatory cytokines in the renal involvement of POEMS syndrome. Am J Kid Dis 34:633–638, 1999.

CHAPTER 55

PANCREATIC ENDOCRINE TUMORS

Michael T. McDermott, M.D.

1. **What are the pancreatic endocrine tumors?**
   These tumors arise from the islet cells of the pancreas and are generally named for the hormones that they secrete. They include tumors that secrete insulin (insulinomas), gastrin (gastrinomas), vasoactive intestinal polypeptide (VIPomas), glucagon (glucagonomas), somatostatin (somatostatinomas), corticotropin releasing factor (CRFomas), adrenocorticotropic hormone (ACTHomas), growth hormone-releasing factor (GRFomas), and pancreatic polypeptide (PPomas) (see Fig. 55-1).

2. **Are pancreatic endocrine tumors usually benign or malignant?**
   Insulinomas are usually benign (80–90%); the other pancreatic endocrine tumors are frequently malignant (50–80%).

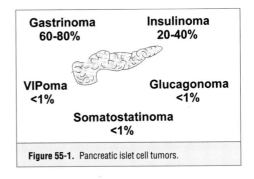

Gastrinoma 60-80%
Insulinoma 20-40%
VIPoma <1%
Glucagonoma <1%
Somatostatinoma <1%

Figure 55-1. Pancreatic islet cell tumors.

3. **Are pancreatic endocrine tumors associated with other endocrine disorders?**
   Up to 10% of pancreatic endocrine tumors occur as part of the multiple endocrine neoplasia type 1 (MEN I) syndrome. This inherited disorder consists of pituitary tumors, pancreatic endocrine tumors, and hyperparathyroidism. Hyperparathyroidism usually precedes the pituitary and pancreatic tumors. The condition is caused by an inherited mutation in the menin gene.

4. **What are insulinomas?**
   Insulinomas are discrete insulin producing tumors within the pancreas. They belong to a larger group of hyperinsulinemic pancreatic beta cell disorders that include insulinomas, islet cell hyperplasia, and nesidioblastosis (neo-proliferation of beta cells along the pancreatic ducts).

5. **What is Whipple's triad?**
   - Hypoglycemia
   - Symptoms during hypoglycemia
   - Relief of symptoms with correction of hypoglycemia

6. **What glucose levels are considered to be hypoglycemia?**
   The exact criteria for hypoglycemia continue to be disputed. However, glucose levels of < 50 mg/dL in men and < 40 mg/dL in women are commonly considered to be hypoglycemia.

7. **What are the symptoms of hypoglycemia?**

   Hypoglycemic symptoms are classified according to the their type and their timing in relation to meals. Symptoms, such as confusion, slurred speech, blurred vision, seizures, and coma, result from inadequate delivery of glucose to the brain (neuroglycopenia). Symptoms, such as tremors, sweating, palpitations, and nausea, result from a counter-regulatory discharge of cate-cholamines (adrenergic). When symptoms occur within 5 hours of the previous meal, they are considered to be "postprandial"; if they occur more than 5 hours after a meal they are considered to be "fasting." Insulinomas most commonly cause fasting neuroglycopenic symptoms, although postprandial and adrenergic symptoms may also occur.

8. **How is the diagnosis of an insulinoma made?**

   The diagnosis requires documentation of symptomatic hypoglycemia and endogenous hyperinsulinemia. Hyperinsulinemic hypoglycemia is defined as hypoglycemia with a insulin:glucose ratio of > 0.33. Some patients present to the provider during a symptomatic episode, but more commonly the physician must attempt to provoke hypoglycemia when the diagnosis is suspected. This often requires a prolonged fast (up to 48 hours) with blood sampling for glucose, insulin and C-peptide levels every 6 hours and during any symptoms that occur. Since proinsulin is normally cleaved into insulin and C-peptide within the pancreas, both C-peptide and proinsulin are markers of endogenous insulin secretion. A drug screen for sulfonylurea and meglitinide use is also recommended.

9. **How can insulinomas be distinguished from other causes of hyperinsulinemic hypoglycemia?**

   Hyperinsulinemic hypoglycemia can be due to insulinomas, surreptitious insulin administration, and medication use. Table 55-1 illustrates how these entities can be distinguished.

TABLE 55-1.	INSULINOMAS VERSUS OTHER CAUSES OF HYPERINSULINEMIC HYPOGLYCEMIA		
Test	Insulinoma	Surreptitious Insulin Use	Sulfonylurea or Meglitinide Use
Insulin	↑	↑	↑
C-peptide	↑	↓	↑
Proinsulin	↑	↓	NI
Drug screen	Neg	Neg	Pos

10. **How can an insulinoma be localized?**

    A computed tomography (CT) scan or magnetic resonance imaging (MRI) is usually the first localization procedure, although the reported sensitivity of these techniques has varied anywhere from 15% to 90% in recent studies. Endoscopic ultrasound of the pancreas has higher sensitivity (56–93%) and can detect tumors as small as 2–3 mm in size. Intra-arterial pancreatic calcium infusions with measurement of insulin changes in the right hepatic vein yields similar or superior results but is clearly a more invasive technique. Intraoperative ultrasound is also highly accurate and is particularly useful for finding small tumors that could not be localized preoperatively. Octreotide scintigraphy (OctreoScan) has proved to be of little value in localizing insulinomas.

11. **What is the treatment for an insulinoma?**

    Surgery is the treatment of choice. When surgery is not desired, or when tumors are unresectable, medical therapy consists of multiple (usually 6 or more) small meals per day and the use of medications that inhibit insulin secretion. The most effective medication for this purpose is oral diazoxide; other drugs that may be useful include propranolol, calcium channel blockers, thiazide diuretics and phenytoin. Octreotide is rarely beneficial. Chemotherapy using streptozotocin with doxorubicin or with 5-fluorouracil reduces symptoms and improves survival in patients with malignant insulinomas.

12. **What are the clinical manifestations of gastrinomas?**
Gastrinomas secrete excessive gastrin, which stimulates prolific gastric acid secretion. Patients develop severe peptic ulcer disease, often associated with secretory diarrhea. This disorder is also known as the Zollinger-Ellison syndrome.

13. **Do gastrinomas always arise from pancreatic islet cells?**
Gastrinomas may arise from the pancreatic islets but also can occur in the duodenum and stomach.

14. **How is the diagnosis of gastrinoma made?**
The diagnosis is made by demonstrating the presence of high gastric acidity (pH < 3.0) in association with a fasting serum gastrin level > 1000 pg/mL or a moderately elevated gastrin that increases by more than 200 pg/mL within 15 minutes after the intravenous administration of secretin.

15. **What is the best way to localize a gastrinoma?**
Localization of the tumor may be pursued with various techniques, including CT scan, MRI, endoscopic ultrasonography, octreotide scanning, transhepatic portal venous sampling, and selective arterial secretin infusions with right hepatic vein gastrin measurements.

16. **How are gastrinomas managed?**
Most benign and some malignant gastrinomas can be cured by surgery. Otherwise, attention should be directed toward reduction of gastric acid overproduction. Proton pump inhibitors are the drugs of choice for this purpose. Octreotide (Sandostatin; 50–500 µg 2 or 3 times/day SQ) or long-acting octreotide (Sandostatin LAR, 10–30 mg every month, intragluteally) are also highly effective agents for this condition. High-dose H_2 blockers may also be useful but are rarely adequate by themselves. Refractory patients may require total gastrectomy and vagotomy for symptom relief.

17. **How do you treat a malignant gastrinoma?**
Since most gastrinomas are malignant, chemotherapy is often necessary. The most effective chemotherapy combinations include the following: streptozotocin, 5-fluorouracil and leucovorin; lomustine and 5-fluorouracil; etoposide, doxorubicin and 5-fluorouracil; cisplatin, dacarbazine and α-interferon. Finally, tumor embolization in conjunction with direct intra-arterial infusions of chemotherapy agents has shown additional promise as a palliative procedure.

18. **What are the characteristics of glucagonomas?**
Glucagon antagonizes the effects of insulin in the liver by stimulating glycogenolysis and gluconeogenesis. Glucagonomas, which secrete excessive glucagon, cause diabetes mellitus, weight loss, anemia, and a characteristic skin rash, necrolytic migratory erythema. Affected patients also have a thromboembolic diathesis. The diagnosis depends on finding an elevated level of serum glucagon (> 500 pg/mL). Techniques similar to those used for gastrinomas are useful for localizing these tumors.

19. **How are glucagonomas treated?**
Treatment options include surgery for localized disease, octreotide to reduce glucagon secretion, and chemotherapy regimens similar to those used for gastrinomas. Chronic anticoagulation to

reduce the risk of thromboembolic events should also be considered. Finally, zinc supplements and intermittent amino acid infusions may help to reduce the skin rash and to improve the patient's overall sense of well-being.

20. **What are the characteristics of somatostatinomas?**
Among its multiple systemic effects, somatostatin inhibits secretion of insulin and pancreatic enzymes, production of gastric acid, and gallbladder contraction. Somatostatinomas secrete excess somatostatin, causing diabetes mellitus, weight loss, steatorrhea, hypochlorhydria, and cholelithiasis. The diagnosis is made by finding a significantly elevated serum somatostatin level.

KEY POINTS: PANCREATIC ENDOCRINE TUMORS ✔

1. Insulinomas most often cause fasting hypoglycemia with neuroglycopenic symptoms.

2. Suspected insulinomas are investigated by measuring serum glucose, insulin, and C-peptide and screening for sulfonylureas and meglitinides during a symptomatic episode or a 48-hour supervised fast.

3. The treatment for an insulinoma is surgery, when possible, or multiple frequent feedings or the use of medications, such as diazoxide.

4. Gastrinomas (Zollinger-Ellison syndrome) cause aggressive peptic ulcer disease, which is sometimes with associated secretory diarrhea.

5. Gastrinomas are diagnosed by finding a markedly elevated serum gastrin or a prominent increase in serum gastrin after intravenous secretin administration in a patient with significant gastric acidity.

6. The treatment for a gastrinoma is surgery, when possible, or reduction of gastric acid production by high-dose proton pump inhibitors or a gastrectomy, if needed.

---

21. **What is the treatment for somatostatinoma?**
Surgery is the treatment of choice. When surgery is not possible, somatostatin secretion and tumor size may be reduced by the same chemotherapy regimens used for other pancreatic endocrine tumors.

22. **What are the characteristics of vasoactive intestinal polypeptide-secreting tumors (VIPomas)?**
VIPomas cause watery diarrhea, hypokalemia, and achlorhydria (WDHA syndrome, pancreatic cholera). This is also known as the Verner-Morrison syndrome. The diagnosis is made by finding an elevated level of serum VIP.

23. **How are VIPomas treated?**
Surgery is the treatment of choice. Octreotide effectively reduces diarrhea in most patients. Radiation therapy and chemotherapy also may effectively reduce diarrhea and tumor size.

24. **Briefly discuss the remaining pancreatic endocrine tumors.**
The remaining pancreatic endocrine tumors are very rare. CRFomas and ACTHomas lead to the development of Cushing's syndrome and GRFomas cause acromegaly. PPomas are initially asymptomatic but may eventually enlarge to produce mass effects without a recognizable hormone hypersecretion syndrome. Localization procedures and treatments are similar to those described earlier for other pancreatic endocrine tumors.

BIBLIOGRAPHY

1. Arnold R, Simon B, Wied M: Treatment of neuroendocrine GEP tumors with somatostatin analogues. Review. Digestion 62(Suppl S1):84–91, 2000.

2. Boukhman MP, Karam JM, Shaver J, et al: Localization of insulinomas. Arch Surg 134:818–822, 1999 (discussion 822–823).

3. Doppman JL, Chang R, Fraker DL, et al: Localization of insulinomas to regions of the pancreas by intra-arterial stimulation with calcium. Ann Intern Med 123:269–273, 1995.

4. Hirshberg B, Livi A, Bartlett DL, et al: Forty-eight hour fast: the diagnostic test for insulinoma. J Clin Endocrinol Metab 85:3222–3226, 2000.

5. Jaffe BM: Current issues in the management of Zollinger-Ellison syndrome. Surgery 111:241–243, 1992.

6. Jensen RT: Pancreatic endocrine tumors: Recent advances. Ann Oncol 10(Suppl 4):170–160, 1999.

7. Krejs GJ, Orci L, Conlon M, et al: Somatostatinoma syndrome: Biochemical, morphologic and clinical features. N Engl J Med 301:283–292, 1979.

8. Leichter SB: Clinical and metabolic aspects of glucagonoma. Medicine 59:100–113, 1980.

9. Moertel CG, Johnson CM, McKusick MA, et al: The management of patients with advanced carcinoid tumors and islet cell carcinomas. Ann Intern Med 120:302–309, 1994.

10. Perry RR, Vinik AI: Diagnosis and management of functioning islet cell tumors. J Clin Endocrinol Metab 80:2273–2278, 1995.

11. Ricke J, Klose K: Imaging procedures in neuroendocrine tumors. Digestion 62(Suppl S1):39–44, 2000.

12. Service FJ: Classification of hypoglycemic disorders. Endocrinol Metab Clin North Am 28:501–517, 1999.

13. Service FJ, McMahon MM, O'Brien PC, et al: Functioning insulinomas—incidence, recurrence, and long-term survival of patients: A 60-year study. Mayo Clin Proc 66:711–719, 1991.

14. Wermers RA, Fatourechi V, Krols LK: Clinical spectrum of hyperglucagonemia associated with malignant neuroendocrine tumors. Mayo Clin Proc 71:1030–1038, 1996.

CHAPTER 56

CARCINOID SYNDROME

Michael T. McDermott, M.D.

1. **What are carcinoid tumors? How are they classified?**
   Carcinoid tumors are neoplasms that arise from enterochromaffin or Kulchitsky cells. They are classified according to their site of origin as foregut (bronchus, stomach, duodenum, bile ducts, pancreas), midgut (jejunum, ileum, appendix, ascending colon), or hindgut (transverse and descending colon, rectum) carcinoids. They also occasionally occur in the ovaries, testes, prostate, kidney, breast, thymus, or skin.

2. **Define carcinoid syndrome.**
   The carcinoid syndrome is a humorally mediated disorder that consists of cutaneous flushing (90%), diarrhea (75%), bronchospasm (20%), endocardial fibrosis (33%), right-heart valvular lesions, and occasionally pleural, peritoneal, or retroperitoneal fibrosis.

3. **What are the biochemical mediators of the carcinoid syndrome?**
   Carcinoid tumors produce a variety of humoral mediators, including serotonin, histamine, prostaglandins, bradykinin, tachykinins, neurotensin, motilin, and substance P. Diarrhea and fibrous tissue formation may be caused by serotonin, whereas flushing and wheezing are likely due to histamine, prostaglandins or kinins (see Fig. 56-1).

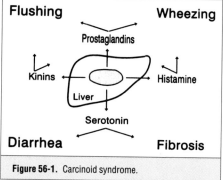

Figure 56-1. Carcinoid syndrome.

4. **Why does pellagra sometimes accompany the carcinoid syndrome?**
   Pellagra is due to niacin deficiency that results when the tumor diverts large amounts of tryptophan from niacin synthesis to produce serotonin.

5. **Why do intestinal carcinoid tumors so infrequently cause carcinoid syndrome?**
   The carcinoid syndrome occurs when humoral mediators enter the systemic circulation in large quantities. Solitary intestinal carcinoids secrete mediators into the portal circulation, where they are almost totally metabolized by the liver and never reach the systemic circulation. Carcinoid syndrome does not usually occur with these tumors unless there are hepatic metastases that impair mediator metabolism or that secrete mediators directly into the hepatic vein. Extra-intestinal carcinoids, however, may cause carcinoid syndrome in the absence of metastases since they secrete mediators into venous systems that do not first pass through the liver.

6. **Do carcinoid tumors cause any other humoral syndromes?**
   Carcinoids may also secrete corticotropin releasing factor (CRF) or corticotropin (adrenocorticotropin [ACTH]), causing Cushing's syndrome, or growth hormone-releasing factor (GRF),

causing acromegaly. These syndromes have been reported mainly with bronchial and pancreatic carcinoid tumors.

KEY POINTS: CARCINOID SYNDROME ✓

1. The carcinoid syndrome results from tumor production of humoral mediators that cause flushing, bronchospasm, diarrhea, and fibrous tissue formation.

2. Most patients with carcinoid syndrome have extensive liver metastases that either impair the metabolic clearance of mediators secreted by the primary tumor or that secrete the mediators directly into the hepatic vein.

3. Carcinoid syndrome is diagnosed by demonstrating increased urinary excretion of 5-hydroxyindoleacetic acid (5-HIAA) or elevated serum levels of serotonin, neurotensin, or substance P.

4. The treatment for carcinoid syndrome is surgery, when possible, or palliation of symptoms by giving medications that reduce secretion of the humoral mediators or antagonize their effects.

5. A carcinoid crisis can be precipitated when a patient with a carcinoid tumor is given an adrenergic medication or a monoamine oxidase (MAO) inhibitor.

6. A carcinoid crisis is best treated with intravenous octreotide and hydrocortisone, while avoiding the use of adrenergic and sympathomimetic agents.

7. **How is the diagnosis of carcinoid syndrome made?**
The diagnosis depends on the finding of increased urinary excretion of 5-HIAA, a breakdown product of serotonin, or increased serum concentrations of serotonin, neurotensin, or substance P. Serum chromogranin A, a nonspecific marker of neuroendocrine tumors, may also be elevated in these patients.

8. **What is the treatment for carcinoid syndrome?**
Surgery can be curative when the carcinoid syndrome results from an extra-intestinal carcinoid tumor that has not metastasized. Most patients with the carcinoid syndrome, however, have extensive metastases at the time of diagnosis. The goal of therapy, therefore, is usually not to cure but to provide palliation and to prolong survival. Medications to control symptoms (flushing, diarrhea, bronchospasm) and chemotherapy to reduce the tumor burden are the most effective general management strategies.

9. **How does one control the symptoms of carcinoid syndrome?**
The most troublesome symptoms patients with carcinoid syndrome experience are intense flushing and frequent diarrhea. Octreotide, a somatostatin analog, is highly effective in controlling most carcinoid symptoms. Table 56-1 lists the various medications or combinations that may be tried for symptom relief.

10. **What chemotherapy regimens are most effective in carcinoid tumors?**
Although not generally curative, chemotherapy may reduce the total tumor burden sufficiently to reduce carcinoid symptoms. The following chemotherapy regimens have thus far shown the greatest efficacy in these patients: streptozotocin, 5-fluorouracil and leucovorin; lomustine and 5-fluorouracil; etoposide, doxorubicin and 5-fluorouracil; cisplatin, dacarbazine and α-interferon. Another promising approach for hepatic tumor debulking has been hepatic artery embolization along with direct intra-arterial chemotherapy infusions.

TABLE 56-1. MEDICATIONS FOR RELIEF OF SYMPTOMS RELATED TO CARCINOID SYNDROME

Medications to control carcinoid flushing

Octreotide (Sandostatin)	50–150 µg 2 or 3 times/day subcutaneously
Octreotide, long acting (Sandostatin LAR)	10–30 mg every month intragluteally
Phentolamine (Regitine)	25–50 mg 1–3 times/day
Phenoxybenzamine (Dibenzyline)	30 mg/day
Cyproheptadine (Periactin)	2–4 mg 3 or 4 times/day
Methysergide (Sansert)	2 mg 3 times/day
Prochlorperazine (Compazine)	5–10 mg every 4–6 hours
Chlorpromazine (Thorazine)	10–25 mg every 4–6 hours
Clonidine (Catapres)	0.1–0.2 mg 2 times/day
Methyldopa (Aldomet)	250 mg 3 times/day
Cimetidine (Tagamet), plus:	300 mg 3 times/day
Diphenhydramine (Benadryl)	50 mg 4 times/day
Glucocorticoids	

Medications to control carcinoid diarrhea

Standard antidiarrheal measures, plus:

Octreotide (Sandostatin)	50–150 µg 2 or 3 times/day subcutaneously
Octreotide, long acting (Sandostatin LAR)	10–30 mg every month intragluteally
Clonidine (Catapres)	0.1–0.2 mg 2 times/day
Cyproheptadine (Periactin)	2–4 mg 3 or 4 times/day
Methysergide (Sansert)	2 mg 3 times/day
Ondansetron (Zofran)	8 mg 3 times/day

11. **What is a carcinoid crisis?**

A carcinoid crisis is an acute episode of severe flushing, bronchospasm, and hypotension. These episodes are most commonly provoked by the administration of adrenergic agents, such as epinephrine and sympathomimetic amines, or MAO inhibitors in patients with underlying carcinoid tumors. Patients need not have previously experienced symptoms of the carcinoid syndrome to have a carcinoid crisis.

12. **How can a carcinoid crisis be prevented?**

Patients with known carcinoid syndrome should not be given epinephrine, sympathomimetic amines or MAO inhibitors. When these patients require a surgical procedure, they should be pretreated with octreotide (Sandostatin) 100 ug subcutaneously 30–60 minutes prior to the operation. Anesthesiologists should be specifically notified that the patient has carcinoid syndrome.

13. **Can a carcinoid crisis be predicted?**

Patients with carcinoid tumors who have not developed carcinoid syndrome can be tested for their potential to have a carcinoid crisis. This is most commonly done with an epinephrine provocation test; patients are given progressive I.V. boluses of epinephrine every 5 minutes, starting with a dose of 1 ug and increasing, if necessary, to 10 ug, while monitoring heart rate and blood pressure every 60 seconds. A positive response consists of flushing or a blood pressure drop of 20 mm systolic or 10 mm diastolic 45–120 minutes after an injection. All patients undergoing this test must have venous catheters and be monitored carefully throughout the test; I.V. phentolamine (Regitine) 5 mg and methoxamine (Vasoxyl) 3 mg preparations must also be available to reverse a crisis should it occur.

14. **Describe the management of a carcinoid crisis.**

An effective treatment for an acute carcinoid crisis is the administration of intravenous octreotide and hydrocortisone. If this does not successfully abort the episode, other options include methotrimeprazine (an anti-serotonin agent), methoxamine (a direct vasoconstrictor), phentolamine (an alpha adrenergic blocker), ondansetron (a serotonin receptor antagonist), and glucagon. It is critical to avoid the use of adrenergic and sympathomimetic agents in patients with suspected carcinoid crisis as these drugs can significantly worsen the condition. Effective medication dose regimens for this condition are listed in Table 56-2.

TABLE 56-2. MANAGEMENT OF CARCINOID CRISIS

Medication	Dose Regimen
Octreotide (Sandostatin)	50 µg IV over 1 minute, then 50 µg IV over 15 minutes
Hydrocortisone (Solu-Cortef)	100 mg IV over 15 minutes
Methotrimeprazine (Levoprome)	2.5–5.0 mg slow IV push
Methoxamine (Vasoxyl)	3–5 mg slow IV push, followed by an infusion
Phentolamine (Regitine)	5 mg slow IV push
Ondansetron (Zofran)	20 mg IV over 15 minutes
Glucagon	0.5–1.5 mg slow IV push

From Warner RRP: Gut neuroendocrine tumors. In Bardin CW (ed): Current Therapy in Endocrinology and Metabolism, 6th ed. St. Louis, Mosby, 1997, pp 606–614.

BIBLIOGRAPHY

1. Fehmann HC, Wulbrand U, Arnold R: Treatment of endocrine gastroenteropancreatic tumors with somatostatin analogues. Recent results. Cancer Res 153:15–22, 2000.
2. Feldman JM: The carcinoid syndrome. Endocrinologist 3:129–135, 1993.
3. Galanis E, Kvols LK, Rubin J: Carcinoid syndrome. J Clin Oncol 16:796–798, 1998.
4. Halford S, Waxman J: The management of carcinoid tumors. Q J Med 91:795–798, 1998.
5. Janmohamed S, Bloom SR: Review: Carcinoid tumours. Postgrad Med J 73:207–214, 1997.
6. Kulke MH, Mayer RJ: Review: Carcinoid tumors. N Engl J Med 340:858–868, 1999.
7. Moertel CG, Johnson CM, McKusick MA, et al: The management of patients with advanced carcinoid tumors and islet cell carcinomas. Ann Intern Med 120:302–309, 1994.
8. Oberg K: Carcinoid tumors: Current concepts in diagnosis and treatment. Oncologist 3:339–345, 1998.
9. O'Toole D, Ducreaux M, Bommelaer G, et al: Treatment of carcinoid syndrome: A prospective crossover evaluation of lanreotide versus octreotide in terms of efficacy, patient acceptability, and tolerance. Cancer 88:770–776, 2000.
10. Soga J, Yakuwa Y, Osaka M: Carcinoid syndrome: A statistical evaluation of 748 reported cases. J Exp Clin Cancer Res 18:133–141, 1999.

CHAPTER 57

CUTANEOUS MANIFESTATIONS OF DIABETES MELLITUS AND THYROID DISEASE

James E. Fitzpatrick, M.D.

1. **How often do patients with diabetes mellitus demonstrate an associated skin disorder?**
   Most published studies report that 30–50% of patients with diabetes mellitus ultimately develop a skin disorder attributable to their primary disease. However, if one includes subtle findings, such as nail changes, vascular changes, and alteration of the cutaneous connective tissue, the incidence approaches 100%. Skin disorders most often present in patients with known diabetes mellitus, but cutaneous manifestations also may be an early sign of undiagnosed diabetes.

2. **Are any skin disorders pathognomonic of diabetes mellitus?**
   Yes. Bullous diabeticorum (bullous eruption of diabetes, diabetic bullae) is specific for diabetes mellitus, but it is uncommon. Bullous diabeticorum most often occurs in patients with severe diabetes, particularly those with associated peripheral neuropathy. In general, all other reported skin findings may be found to some extent in normal individuals. However, some cutaneous conditions (e.g., necrobiosis lipoidica diabeticorum) demonstrate strong associations with diabetes.

3. **What is bullous diabeticorum?**
   Bullous diabeticorum is a blistering disorder that primarily occurs on the distal extremities of patients with diabetes mellitus. They typically develop spontaneous tense blisters that are asymptomatic except for a burning sensation. The exact mechanism is not understood, but a high percentage of patients have peripheral neuropathy, retinopathy, or nephropathy.

4. **What are the skin disorders most likely to be encountered in diabetic patients?**
   The most common skin disorders are finger pebbles, nail bed telangiectasia, red face (rubeosis), skin tags (acrochordons), diabetic dermopathy, yellow skin, yellow nails, and pedal petechial purpura. Less common cutaneous disorders that are closely associated with diabetes mellitus include necrobiosis lipoidica diabeticorum, bullous eruption of diabetes, acanthosis nigricans, and scleredema adultorum (Table 57-1).

5. **What are finger pebbles?**
   Finger pebbles are multiple, grouped minute papules that tend to affect the extensor surfaces of the fingers, particularly near the knuckles. They are asymptomatic and may be extremely subtle in appearance. Histologically finger pebbles are due to increased collagen in the dermal papillae. The pathogenesis is not understood.

6. **What is acanthosis nigricans?**
   Acanthosis nigricans is a skin condition due to papillomatous (wartlike) hyperplasia of the skin. It is associated with various conditions, including diabetes mellitus, obesity, acromegaly, Cushing's syndrome, certain medications, and underlying malignancies. Acanthosis nigricans occurring in patients with insulin-dependent diabetes has been associated with three different mechanisms of insulin resistance: type A (receptor defect), type B (antireceptor antibodies), and

TABLE 57-1. COMMON CUTANEOUS FINDINGS IN DIABETES MELLITUS

Cutaneous Finding	Incidence in Controls (%)	Incidence in Diabetes (%)
Finger pebbles	21	75
Nail bed telangiectasia	12	65
Rubeosis (red face)	18	59
Skin tags	3	55
Diabetic dermopathy	Uncommon	54
Yellow skin	24	51
Yellow nails	Uncommon	50
Erythrasma	Uncommon	47
Diabetic thick skin	Uncommon	30

type C (postreceptor defect). In insulin-resistant states, it is proposed that hyperinsulinemia competes for the IGF receptors on keratinocytes and thereby stimulates epidermal growth. In the case of hypercortisolism as seen in Cushing's disease, there is induced insulin resistance, which is believed to promote epidermal growth.

7. **Describe what acanthosis nigricans looks like.**
   It is most noticeable in axillary, inframammary, and neck creases where it appears as hyperpigmented velvety skin that has the appearance of being "dirty" (Fig. 57-1). The tops of knuckles may also demonstrate small papules that resemble finger pebbles except that they are more pronounced (Fig. 57-2).

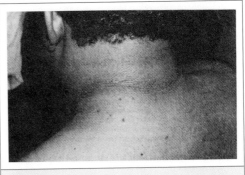

Figure 57-1. Acanthosis nigricans. Characteristic velvety hyperpigmentation of flexural areas.

8. **Define diabetic dermopathy.**
   Diabetic dermopathy (shin spots or pretibial pigmented patches) is a common affliction that initially presents as erythematous to brown to brownish-red macules that typically measure 0.5–1.5 cm in size with variable scale on the pretibial surface (Fig. 57-3). The lesions are typically asymptomatic but are occasionally pruritic or are associ-

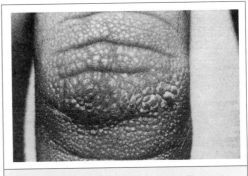

Figure 57-2. Acanthosis nigricans. Typical papillomatous lesions over the knuckles.

ated with a burning sensation. Patients with diabetic dermopathy are more likely to have retinopathy, nephropathy, and neuropathy. They heal with varying degrees of atrophy and hyperpigmentation over 1–2 years. The pathogenesis is unknown but skin biopsies from the lesions demonstrate diabetic microangiopathy characterized by a proliferation of endothelial cells and thickening of the basement membranes of arterioles, capillaries, and venules. Although many physicians attribute these lesions to trauma, this is not supported by an unusual study, in which patients with diabetes mellitus did not develop lesions after being struck on the pretibial surface with a hard rubber hammer! There is no known effective treatment.

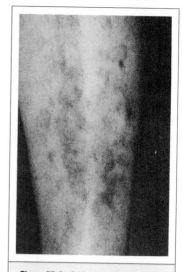

Figure 57-3. Diabetic dermopathy. Characteristic brown macules over pretibial areas.

9. **What is necrobiosis lipoidica diabeticorum?**

Necrobiosis lipoidica diabeticorum is a disease that most commonly occurs on the pretibial areas, although it may occur at other sites. Early lesions present as nondiagnostic erythematous papules or plaques that evolve into annular lesions characterized by a yellowish or yellowish-brown color, dilated blood vessels, and central epidermal atrophy. Developed lesions are characteristic and usually can be diagnosed by clinical appearance. Less commonly, ulcers may develop. Biopsies are usually diagnostic and demonstrate palisaded granulomas that surround large zones of necrotic and sclerotic collagen. Additional findings include dilated vascular spaces, plasma cells, and increased neutral fat. The pathogenesis is not known, but proposed causes include an immune complex vasculitis and a platelet aggregation defect.

10. **Describe the relationship of necrobiosis lipoidica diabeticorum to diabetes mellitus.**

In a major study of patients with necrobiosis lipoidica diabeticorum, 62% had diabetes. Approximately one-half of the nondiabetic patients had abnormal glucose tolerance tests, and almost one-half of the nondiabetics gave a family history of diabetes. However, necrobiosis lipoidica diabeticorum is present in only 0.3% of patients with diabetes. The term "necrobiosis lipoidica" is used for patients who have the disorder without associated diabetes. Because of the strong association between these conditions, patients who present with necrobiosis lipoidica should be screened for diabetes; patients who test negative should be reevaluated periodically.

11. **How should necrobiosis lipoidica diabeticorum be treated?**

Necrobiosis lipoidica occasionally may resolve without treatment. It does not seem to respond to treatment of diabetes in new cases or to tighter control of established diabetes. Early lesions may respond to treatment with potent topical or intralesional corticosteroids. More severe cases may respond to oral treatment with either stanozolol, niacinamide, pentoxifylline, mycophenolate mofetil or cyclosporine. Severe cases with recalcitrant ulcers may require surgical grafting.

12. **Are skin infections more common in diabetic patients than in control populations?**

Yes. But skin infections are probably not as common as most medical personnel believe. Studies show that an increased incidence of skin infections strongly correlates with elevated levels of mean plasma glucose.

13. **What are the most common bacterial skin infections associated with diabetes mellitus?**

   The most common serious skin infections associated with diabetes mellitus are related to diabetic foot and amputation ulcers. One autopsy study revealed that 2.4% of all diabetics had infectious skin ulcerations of the extremities compared with 0.5% of a control population. Even though there are no well-controlled studies, it is felt that staphylococcal skin infections, including furunculosis and staphylococcal wound infections, are more common and serious in diabetics. Erythrasma, a benign superficial bacterial infection caused by *Corynebacterium minutissimum*, was present in 47% of adult diabetics in one study. Clinically it presents as tan to reddish-brown macular lesions with slight scale in intertriginous areas, such as the groin. Because the organisms produce porphyrins, the diagnosis can be made by demonstrating a spectacular coral red fluorescence with a Wood's lamp.

14. **What is the most common fungal mucocutaneous infection associated with diabetes mellitus?**

   The most common mucocutaneous fungal infection associated with diabetes is candidiasis, usually caused by *Candida albicans*. Women are particularly prone to get vulvovaginitis. One study demonstrated that two-thirds of all diabetics have positive cultures for *Candida albicans*. In women with signs and symptoms of vulvitis, the incidence of positive cultures approaches 99%. Similarly, positive cultures are extremely common in diabetic men and women who complain of anal pruritus. Other mucocutaneous forms of candidiasis

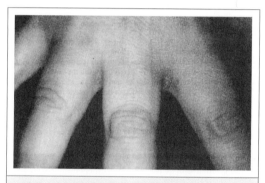

Figure 57-4. Erosio interdigitalis blastomycetica chronica. *Candida* infection in the interdigital spaces in a diabetic patient. A very long name for a very small infection!

include thrush, perlèche (angular cheilitis), intertrigo, erosio interdigitalis blastomycetica chronica (Fig. 57-4), paronychia (infection of the soft tissue around the nail plate), and onychomycosis (infection of the nail). The mechanism appears to be due to increased levels of glucose that serve as a substrate for *Candida* species to proliferate. Patients with recurrent cutaneous candidiasis of any form should be screened for diabetes.

15. **Why are patients with diabetic ketoacidosis especially prone to mucormycosis?**

   Some Zygomycetes, including *Mucor, Mortierella, Rhizopus*, and *Absidia* species, are thermotolerant, prefer an acid pH, grow rapidly in the presence of high glucose levels and are among the few fungi that utilize ketones as a growth substrate. Thus, diabetic ketoacidosis provides an ideal environment for the proliferation of these fungi. Fortunately, these fulminant and often fatal fungal infections are rare.

16. **Are any skin complications associated with the treatment of diabetes mellitus?**

   Yes. Adverse reactions to injected insulin are relatively common. The reported incidence varies from 10% to 56%, depending on the study. In general, these complications may be divided into three categories: reactions due to faulty injections (e.g., intradermal injection), idiosyncratic reactions, and allergic reactions. Several types of allergic reactions have been described, including localized and generalized urticaria, Arthus reactions, and localized delayed hypersensitivity. Oral hypoglycemic agents occasionally may produce adverse cutaneous reactions, including photosensitivity, urticaria, erythema multiforme, and erythema nodosum. Chlorpropamide in particular may produce a flushing reaction when consumed with alcohol.

KEY POINTS: CUTANEOUS MANIFESTATIONS OF DIABETES ✔️ AND THYROID DISEASE

1. Patients with diabetes mellitus demonstrate cutaneous findings attributable to diabetes in almost 100% of cases.

2. The most common cause of acanthosis nigricans is diabetes associated with insulin resistance and obesity.

3. Necrobiosis lipoidica is a granulomatous dermatitis that is typically associated with diabetes mellitus in almost two-thirds of cases.

4. Scleredema adultorum, a disorder characterized by accumulation of collagen and mucin in the skin, is most commonly associated with diabetes mellitus.

5. Generalized myxedema is the most characteristic cutaneous sign of hypothyroidism.

---

17. **What is scleredema adultorum?**
    Scleredema adultorum is a woody induration that most commonly presents on the posterior neck, upper back, and shoulders. Less commonly it may be more extensive and involve the face, abdomen, and extremities. It is most commonly associated with insulin-dependent diabetes and less commonly associated with monoclonal gammopathies and following streptococcal infections. Biopsies demonstrate increased dermal collagen and hyaluronic acid (dermal mucin). The pathogenesis is not understood. When associated with insulin-dependent diabetes, scleredema adultorum is chronic and recalcitrant to therapy.

18. **What are the most important cutaneous manifestations of the hypothyroid state?**
    Generalized myxedema is the most characteristic cutaneous sign of hypothyroidism. Other skin findings include xerosis (dry skin), follicular hyperkeratosis, diffuse hair loss (especially the outer one-third of the eyebrows), dry brittle nails, yellowish discoloration of the skin, and thyroid acropachy (thickening of the distal fingers; see Fig. 57-5). These skin changes are all reversible with appropriate thyroid replacement.

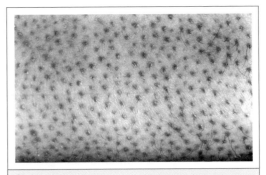

Figure 57-5. Hypothyroidism. Marked follicular hyperkeratosis that quickly disappeared with thyroid replacement.

19. **Why do hypothyroid patients often have yellow skin?**

The yellow color is due to the accumulation of carotene (carotenoderma) in the top layer of the epidermis (stratum corneum). Carotene is excreted by both the sweat glands and sebaceous glands and tends to concentrate on the palms, soles, and face. The increased levels of carotene are probably secondary to impaired hepatic conversion of beta-carotene to vitamin A.

20. **Describe the clinical findings in generalized myxedema.**

Generalized myxedema is characterized by pale, waxy, edematous skin that does not demonstrate pitting. These changes are most noticeable in the periorbital area but may also be observed in the distal extremities, lips, and tongue (Fig. 57-6).

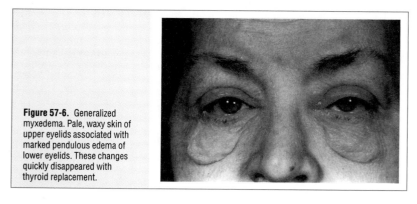

Figure 57-6. Generalized myxedema. Pale, waxy skin of upper eyelids associated with marked pendulous edema of lower eyelids. These changes quickly disappeared with thyroid replacement.

21. **What is the pathogenesis of generalized myxedema?**

The skin demonstrates an increased accumulation of dermal acid mucopolysaccharides, of which hyaluronic acid (ground substance) is the most important. Studies also have demonstrated that an increased transcapillary escape of serum albumin into the dermis adds to the edematous appearance. Neither of these changes is permanent; both are reversible with replacement therapy.

22. **What is the difference between generalized myxedema and pretibial myxedema?**

Generalized myxedema is associated only with the hypothyroid state, whereas pretibial myxedema is characteristically associated with Graves' disease. Patients with pretibial myxedema may be hypothyroid, hyperthyroid, or euthyroid when the skin disorder appears. The pathogenesis has not been proven, but it has been demonstrated that serum from patients with pretibial myxedema will stimulate the production of acid mucopolysaccharides by fibroblasts. Fibroblasts from the pretibial area are more sensitive to stimulation than fibroblasts from other areas, which would account for the tendency for these lesions to occur in pretibial areas. The nature of this circulating factor is unknown but antithyroid immunoglobulins that bind to fibroblasts may be the cause. It has also been postulated that activated T cells can induce fibroblast proliferation and the production of acid mucopolysaccharides.

23. **Describe the clinical manifestations of pretibial myxedema.**

Pretibial myxedema occurs in about 3–5% of patients with Graves' disease. The majority of patients have associated exophthalmos. Thyroid acropachy is also present in 1% of patients with Graves' disease (Fig. 57-7). Clinically pretibial myxedema is characterized by edematous, indurated plaques over the pretibial areas, although other sites of the body also may be involved. The plaques are usually sharply demarcated, but diffuse variants are also reported. The overlying skin surface is usually normal, although it may be studded with smaller papules. The color varies from skin-colored to brownish-red (Fig. 57-8). Overlying hypertrichosis may be present on rare occasions. Histologically, pretibial myxedema demonstrates massive accumulation of dermal hyaluronic acid.

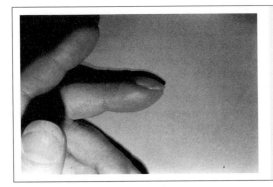

Figure 57-7. Thyroid acropachy. Patient with Graves' disease demonstrating swelling of soft tissue and increased curvature of the nail plate.

24. **How is pretibial myxedema treated?**
Studies comparing different treatment modalities have not been performed. Because the condition is not harmful to patients, and since it may resolve spontaneously, treatment is not always indicated. Many cases respond to potent topical corticosteroids under occlusion or intralesional corticosteroids. More extensive cases may be treated with oral systemic corticosteroids. Treatment of the thyroid disease does not affect the cutaneous findings.

25. **What are the skin manifestations of hyperthyroidism?**
Studies have shown that as many as 97% of all patients with hyperthyroidism develop skin manifestations. Common cutaneous findings include cutaneous erythema, evanescent flushing, excoriations, smooth skin, hyperpigmentation, moist skin (due to increased sweating), pretibial myxedema, pruritus (itching), and warm skin. Nails are often brittle and may separate from the underlying bed (onycholysis). The hair also may be thinner than normal.

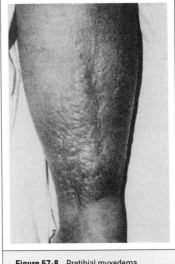

Figure 57-8. Pretibial myxedema. Indurated brownish-red plaque of the pretibial area.

BIBLIOGRAPHY

1. Anderson CK, Miller OF III: Triad of exophthalmos, pretibial myxedema, and acropachy in a patient with Graves' disease. J Am Acad Dermatol 48:970–972, 2003.

2. Bello YM, Phillips TJ: Necrobiosis lipoidica. Indolent plaques may signal diabetes. Postgrad Med 109:93–94, 2001.

3. Ferringer T, Miller F III: Cutaneous manifestations of diabetes mellitus. Dermatol Clin 20:483–492, 2002.

4. Hollister DS, Brodell RT: Finger "pebbles". A dermatologic sign of diabetes mellitus. Postgrad Med 107:209–210, 2000.

5. Jabbour SA: Cutaneous manifestations of endocrine disorders: A guide for dermatologists. Am J Clin Dermatol 4:315–331, 2003.

6. Lipsky BA, Berendt AR: Principles and practice of antibiotic therapy of diabetic foot infections. Diabetes Metab Res Rev 16(Suppl 1):S42–S46, 2000.

7. Niepomniszcze H, Amad RH: Skin disorders and thyroid diseases. J Endocrinol Invest 24:628–638, 2001.

8. Pirotta SS, Johnson JD, Young G, Bezzant J: Bullosis diabeticorum. J Am Podiatr Assoc 85:169–171, 1995.

9. Shemer A, Bergman R, Linn S, Kantor Y, Friedman-Birnhaum R: Diabetic dermopathy and internal complications in diabetes mellitus. Int J Dermatol 37:113–115, 1998.

10. Stoddard ML, Blevins KS, Lee ET, et al: Association of acanthosis nigricans with hyperinsulinemia compared with other selected risk factors for type 2 diabetes in Cherokee Indians: The Cherokee Diabetes Study. Diabetes Care 25:1009–1014, 2002.

CHAPTER 58

AGING AND ENDOCRINOLOGY

Wendy M. Kohrt, Ph.D., and Robert S. Schwartz, M.D.

1. **What effect does aging have on body weight?**

   Aging is associated with important changes in body composition that may be influenced by endocrine status and have important endocrine/metabolic consequences. In cross-sectional studies, body weight increases until about age 55 years and then declines. This may be due to a "die-off" effect in the heaviest patients during middle age. Prospective studies suggest that weight declines after age 65–70 years. This reduction in body weight appears to be associated with an increase in mortality, morbidity, and disability. The untoward effects of weight loss in older people do not appear to be explained simply by unintentional weight loss due to illness or disease, because similar effects have been noted in people who espouse intentional weight loss.

2. **Why is weight loss in elderly people associated with an increase in morbidity and mortality?**

   The explanation is not clear, but it is possible that any sustained weight loss may, in fact, be unintentional, as intentional weight loss is difficult to maintain. Weight loss in the face of illness or disease that raises cytokine levels may predispose to a disproportionate loss of weight as lean mass (muscle mass), thereby exacerbating age-related sarcopenia and leading to a state of cachexia. Small clinical studies (unpublished) of intentional weight loss in *carefully screened* healthy older men have noted a distribution of weight loss that is similar to that seen in younger people on moderate energy restriction.

3. **What changes in lean body mass and muscle mass occur with aging?**

   There is an inevitable loss of lean body mass, mostly skeletal muscle, with aging. This loss has been termed *sarcopenia* and has been blamed for much (but not all) of the age-related decline in muscle strength and power. In cross-sectional studies, a 20–30% loss of lean mass has been detected between ages 30 and 80 years. This finding suggests an even larger loss of muscle mass. The decline in strength is even greater, with longitudinal studies finding up to a 60% loss from age 30 to 80 years. The loss of strength is greatest at the older ages; a 25% decline has been detected between 70 and 75 years. Power (work per unit time) may decline at double the rate of strength. These changes in lean mass, muscle mass, strength, and power have complex but important functional consequences for older people.

4. **Does fat get re-distributed with aging?**

   The changes in adiposity and fat distribution with age have important effects on metabolism. As lean mass declines with age, fat mass increases (at least until ~65 years). Furthermore, the central and intra-abdominal depots of fat increase disproportionately. The increase in central adiposity begins following puberty in men but primarily after menopause in women. This increment in visceral adiposity (along with the decline in physical activity) plays an important role in the age-associated decrement in insulin sensitivity and probably contributes to the high incidence and prevalence of type 2 diabetes mellitus and metabolic syndrome in old age.

5. **Does the menopause trigger an increase in abdominal obesity in women?**

   Cross-sectional comparisons of women across the age spectrum suggest that waist size increases more rapidly in women aged 50 years and older than in younger women. Similarly, comparisons of younger and older women, utilizing soft-tissue scanning techniques (i.e., computed tomography [CT], magnetic resonance imaging [MRI]), suggest that intra-abdominal fat depots do not increase markedly until after the menopause. Premenopausal women treated with gonadotropin-releasing hormone agonists gain fat mass with a disproportionate increase in central body regions. Several randomized, controlled trials have provided evidence that post-menopausal women on hormone replacement therapy gain less weight and have less increase in waist size than the placebo-treated women. The effects seem to be slightly larger with unopposed estrogens. It has not yet been determined whether estrogens specifically prevent or attenuate intra-abdominal fat accumulation.

6. **What changes in bone mass and density occur with aging?**
Prospective data indicate that peak bone mass occurs during the late teen-aged years in women and about a decade later in men. Because of the intimate structural and functional link between muscle and bone, the occurrence of peak bone mass likely corresponds with peak skeletal muscle development. It is generally thought that bone mass is maintained, or decreases slowly (< 0.2% per year), at least through age 40 years in women and age 50 years in men. Intuitively, a decline in physical activity during middle age might be expected to induce an even faster rate of bone loss. However, the increase in body weight that typically also occurs during middle age may counter this to a large extent, by increasing mechanical loading forces acting on the skeleton during weight-bearing activity.

7. **Does menopause have an independent effect on bone mass?**
There is undoubtedly an accelerated decline in bone mineral density around the time of menopause in women. What remains somewhat controversial is whether the menopause-induced increase in resorption diminishes after a few years or persists into old age. In this regard, observational studies of women aged 65 years and older indicate that the rate of bone loss continues to increase with age, particularly in the hip region. This is corroborated by observations that serum markers of bone turnover increase at the menopause and remain elevated into old age. In elderly women and men, the decrease in bone mineral at the hip appears to be accelerated (~1% per year) relative to the changes at the spine. However, vertebral compression fractures and the development of extravertebral osteophytes lead to an increase in bone mineral density, but this does not reflect increased vertebral strength. The utility of spine bone mineral density for the diagnosis of osteoporosis is therefore compromised.

8. **Can weight-bearing exercise prevent the menopause-related loss of bone mineral in women?**
It is unlikely that even vigorous weight-bearing exercise can effectively counteract the deleterious effects of estrogen deficiency on bone mineral density. Older female athletes not on hormone replacement therapy have lower bone mineral density than premenopausal athletes. Moreover, young female athletes with menstrual cycle dysfunction can have bone mineral density levels in the osteopenic (1.0–2.5 SD below the average peak bone mineral density) and even osteoporotic range (> 2.5 SD below the average peak bone mineral density), despite their participation in sports that involve high levels of mechanical loading (e.g., gymnastics, distance running).

9. **Do sex hormones influence the skeletal response to exercise?**
Although the direct effects of estrogens on bone metabolism are well known, growing evidence indicates that the responses of bone cells to mechanical stress involve an activation of estrogen receptor alpha. The effects of age-related sex hormone deficiency on receptor density and/or function in bone remain unknown. In animal models, the effects of mechanical stress in the presence of estrogens (in females) or androgens (in males) on the bone proliferative response have been found to be synergistic (i.e., more than additive). There is also evidence for additive or synergistic effects of exercise and estrogens on bone mineral density in postmenopausal women.

KEY POINTS: AGING AND HORMONE LEVELS ✓

1. Hormone replacement therapy appears to attenuate rather than promote weight gain in postmenopausal women, but the mechanism for this action that is probably estrogen-mediated remains unknown.

2. Exercise, even when weight-bearing and vigorous in nature, may slow age-related bone loss but does not counteract the deleterious skeletal effects of estrogen deficiency.

3. A significant decline in testosterone levels in men begins after about age 30 years. Measurement of dialyzable or "bioavailable" testosterone is recommended.

4. The decline in the entire growth hormone-releasing hormone (GHRH), growth hormone (GH), and insulin-like growth factor 1 (IGF-1) system also begins at about the age of 30 years.

5. As with testosterone, replacement of GH/IGF-1 in deficiency states and supplementation in older patients with low-normal levels appears to be associated with improvements in body composition, but significant positive changes in endurance, strength, power, or function with supplementation have been more difficult to detect.

10. **Describe the changes in the GH/IGF-I axis with aging.**
Aging is associated with a significant decline in the GH area under the curve, as well as number of GH peaks and peak amplitude. These changes in GH secretion are associated with a steady decline in IGF-I after age 30 years. By age 65 years, most individuals have an IGF-I concentration that is near or below the lower limit of normal for young healthy individuals. The decline in the GH/IGF-I axis appears to occur above the level of the pituitary because chronic treatment with GHRH and/or other GH secretagogues (GHS) mitigates much of the decline. The cause of the fall-off in axis activity is not clear but could be explained by age-related changes in GHRH, somatostatin, or ghrelin tone. Ghrelin appears to be the natural ligand for the GHS receptor.

11. **Is the decline in the GH/IGF-I axis related to age-related changes in body composition and function?**
Many of the body compositional changes that occur with aging seem consistent with a GH/IGF-I-deficient state. Indeed, GH-deficient adults have many of the same physiological abnormalities as older individuals, including the following:
- Reduced lean body and muscle mass
- Reduced strength and aerobic capacity
- Excess total, central, and intra-abdominal fat
- High incidence of metabolic syndrome
- Reduced bone mass and density
- Reduced or absent slow-wave sleep
- High incidence of mood disturbance (depression)

12. **Do these abnormalities reverse with GH replacement?**
Most of these abnormalities do in fact reverse with GH replacement. Recently, several clinical trials have examined the role of either GH or GHRH supplementation in older people with low IGF-I concentrations. These studies have consistently demonstrated the ability to increase IGF-I concentrations and lean body/muscle mass and reduce both total and central/intra-abdominal adiposity. However, changes in strength, function, and bone density have been difficult to demonstrate.

13. **Does GH supplementation influence endogenous GH/IGF-I axis activity?**
    It is possible that the potentially most important effects of supplementing the GH/IGF-I axis will be on the brain. The elderly often experience lack of sleep and feeling tired during the day. This may be due to the almost total loss of slow-wave sleep (stages 3 and 4). Of interest, the periods of slow-wave sleep in younger individuals coincide exactly with the nighttime peaks of GH secretion. Indeed, there are animal and some human data that suggest that GHRH supplementation may restart pulsatile GH secretion and stimulate slow-wave sleep. There is also a recent abstract that suggests that chronic GHRH supplementation may improve cognitive function, specifically psychomotor and perceptual processing speed, as well as fluid memory.

14. **What are the adverse effects of GH administration?**
    The adverse effects profile for GH administration (but not GHRH) has been substantial, with development of carpal tunnel syndrome, gynecomastia, edema, and worsening of glucose tolerance, insulin sensitivity, and osteoarthritis. An increase in the risk for certain cancers (breast, prostate) has been postulated but evidence is lacking. While it is possible that the most correct doses of GH, GHRH, or GHS for supplementation have not been defined yet, it would appear reasonable that significant improvements in strength and function may require not only hormone supplementation but also the appropriate stimulus, such as exercise. Nevertheless, considerable interest in supplementation of this axis continues to exist, especially for the treatment or prevention of frailty and recovery from hip fracture.

15. **Describe the changes in testosterone concentration with aging in men.**
    Like IGF-I, testosterone concentration appears to decline steadily after age 30 years in men. However, because of coincident increases in sex hormone binding globulin, the decline in total testosterone concentration is difficult to detect in many studies. When either free or "bioavailable" testosterone is measured, the decline with age is more apparent. Estimates of the prevalence of "hypogonadism" in older men run from 30% to 70%.

16. **Is the decline in the testosterone concentration related to age-related changes in body composition and function?**
    As discussed earlier, there is a close relationship between many of the physiologic findings in young hypogonadal men and older men. Furthermore, reversibility has been noted with testosterone replacement in hypogonadal young men and in patients with acquired hypogonadism associated with human immunodeficiency infection. To date, only a few studies have investigated the effects of testosterone supplementation in older men. The largest published study found improvements in muscle and fat mass but no significant effects on bone mineral density or strength. Unpublished studies suggest that small but detectable changes in strength occur with testosterone supplementation in older men.

17. **Is testosterone or estrogen more important for the maintenance of bone mass in older men?**
    Recently, there has been considerable interest in the effect of testosterone supplementation on bone density in older men. While large clinical trials are still in the planning stages, there is evidence of potential efficacy. However, recent work suggests that much, if not all, of the effect may be due to concomitant elevations of estrogen levels through aromatization. Similarly, it is possible that some of the recently noted cognitive effects of testosterone may be due to estrogen effects on the brain.

18. **What is the appropriate testosterone supplementation dose?**
    The dose of testosterone required for supplementation has not been adequately defined and may vary depending on whether an exercise stimulus is included in the study. The potential side effect profile of testosterone supplementation includes erythrocytosis, prostate enlargement,

stimulation of prostate cancer growth, elevation of liver enzymes, edema, acne, and worsening of obstructive sleep apnea. The appropriate dose is one that minimizes the incidence of these undesirable effects.

KEY POINTS: SIDE EFFECTS OF TESTOSTERONE AND GH/IGF-1   ✓

1. Possible side effects of both: fluid retention, arthritis, carpal tunnel syndrome, hypertension, hyperinsulinemia, and glucose intolerance.

2. Possibly cancer with GRF/GH/IGF-I.

3. Possibly polycythemia, prostate hypertrophy, and development or worsening of sleep apnea with testosterone.

4. The potential risk of increasing the growth of existing prostate cancer is also a real concern with testosterone supplementation.

19. **Does dehydroepiandrosterone concentration change with aging?**
    Dehydroepiandrosterone (DHEA) and its sulfate (DHEAS), collectively referred to as DHEA/S, are the most abundant steroid hormones in humans, with approximately 95% coming from the adrenal glands. DHEAS is one of the best biologic markers of human aging. Peak serum DHEAS levels are reached early in the third decade and then decline steadily. By age 60–70 years, circulating levels are only about 20% of peak levels. The decrease in DHEAS with aging does not represent a general decline in adrenal function, as similar changes in other adrenal hormones do not occur.

20. **Are the biologic effects of DHEA/S known?**
    Despite the abundance of DHEA/S and their distinctive age-related changes, little is known about the biologic effects of DHEA/S in humans. Because it can be converted to testosterone and aromatized to estrogens, the decline in DHEA/S with aging may contribute to physiologic changes that occur as a result of sex hormone deficiency (e.g., the loss of bone and muscle mass). DHEA administration has potent antiobesity, antidiabetogenic, and antiatherogenic effects in rodents. However, it is not clear that these findings are relevant to humans because physiologic DHEA/S levels in rodents are negligible.

21. **Summarize the controlled studies of DHEA administration to humans.**
    Studies of DHEA *supplementation* in young adults have typically involved pharmacologic doses (1600 mg/day). An early study indicated that DHEA use at this dose by young, healthy men for 1 month resulted in a large increase in lean mass and a large decrease in fat mass. However, a subsequent similar study of obese young men by the same investigators found no such effects. Several other studies of short-term DHEA supplementation in young and middle-age individuals had negative outcomes. More recently, studies of DHEA *replacement* in older adults with low DHEA/S levels suggest that DHEA can increase lean mass and bone mineral density and decrease fat mass. Other reports suggest that DHEA replacement in the elderly has beneficial effects on immune and cognitive function. The replacement dose for women and men 60 years and older is ~50 mg/day. Most of the studies in older adults have involved small numbers of subjects, and not all have been randomized, placebo-controlled trials. Larger clinical trials of DHEA replacement in humans are currently in progress.

22. **Are the effects of DHEA mediated by the conversion to testosterone or estrogens?**

The mechanisms for the observed changes in body composition and other outcomes in response to DHEA replacement are not clear. The reported increases in serum IGF-1 and testosterone that occur in both women and men in response to DHEA could have anabolic effects on lean mass and bone mineral density. Serum levels of estrogens do not appear to increase markedly in response to DHEA, but a shift toward more estradiol and less estrone and a decrease in sex hormone binding globulin could result in increased biologic activity of estrogens.

BIBLIOGRAPHY

1. Bassey EJ, Fiatarone MA, O'Neill, et al: Leg extensor power and functional performance in very old men and women. Clin Sci 82:321–327, 1992.
2. Bhasin S: Testosterone supplementation for aging-associated sarcopenia. J Gerontol 58A:1002–1008, 2003.
3. Carr MC: The emergence of the metabolic syndrome with menopause. J Clin Endocrinol Metab 88:2404–2411, 2003.
4. Cheng M, Zaman G, Rawlinson SC, et al: Enhancement by sex hormones of the osteoregulatory effects of mechanical loading and prostaglandins in explants of rat ulnae. J Bone Miner Res 12:1424–1430, 1997.
5. Ensrud KE, Palermo L, Black DM, et al: Hip and calcaneal bone loss increase with advancing age: Longitudinal results from the study of osteoporotic fractures. J Bone Miner Res 10:1778–1787, 1995.
6. Espeland MA, Stefanick ML, Kritz-Silverstein D, et al: Effect of postmenopausal hormone therapy on body weight and waist and hip girths. J Clin Endocrinol Metab 82:1549–1556, 1997.
7. Gruenewald DA, Matsumoto AM: Testosterone supplementation therapy for older men: Potential benefits and risks. J Am Geriatr Soc 51:101–115, 2003.
8. Kohrt WM: Abdominal obesity and associated cardiovascular comorbidities in the elderly. Coronary Artery Dis 9:489–494, 1998.
9. Kohrt WM, Ehsani AA, Birge SJ: HRT preserves increases in bone mineral density and reductions in body fat after a supervised exercise program. J Appl Physiol 84:1506–1512, 1998.
10. Labrie FA, Belanger A, Luu-The V, et al: DHEA and the intracrine formation of androgens and estrogens in peripheral target tissues: Its role during aging. Steroids 63:322–328, 1998.
11. Lamberts SWJ, van den Beld AW, van der Lely A-J: The endocrinology of aging. Science 278:419–424, 1997.
12. Merriam GR, Buchner DM, Prinz PN, et al: Potential applications of GH secretagogues in the evaluation and treatment of the age-related decline in growth hormone secretion. Endocrine 7:49–52, 1997.
13. Newman AB, Haggerty CL, Goodpaster B, et al: Strength and muscle quality in a well-functioning cohort of older adults: The Health, Aging and Body Composition Study. J Am Geriatr Soc 51:323–330, 2003.
14. Rosen CJ, Strom BL: Effect of testosterone treatment on body composition and muscle strength in men over 65 years of age. J Clin Endocrinol Metab 84:2653, 1999.
15. Schwartz RS: Trophic factor supplementation: Effect on the age-associated changes in body composition. J Gerontol Biol Sci Med Sci 50:151–156, 1995.
16. Snyder PJ, Peachey H, Hannoush P, et al: Effect of testosterone treatment on body composition and muscle strength in men over 65 years of age. J Clin Endocrinol Metab 84:2647–2653, 1999.
17. Tobias JH: At the crossroads of skeletal responses to estrogen and exercise. Trends Endocrinol Metab 14:441–443, 2003.
18. Villareal DT, Holloszy JO, Kohrt WM: Effects of DHEA replacement on bone mineral density and body composition in elderly women and men. Clin Endocrinol 53:561–568, 2000.
19. Wallace JI, Schwartz RS: Involuntary weight loss in elderly outpatients: Recognition, etiologies, and treatment. Clin Geriatr Med 13:717–735, 1997.

CHAPTER 59

ENDOCRINE SURGERY

Christopher D. Raeburn, M.D., Thomas N. Robinson, M.D., and Robert C. McIntyre, Jr., M.D.

THYROID

1. **Can operative management of thyroid nodules be based solely on fine-needle aspiration (FNA)?**

   Sometimes. FNA of thyroid nodules is a powerful means of assisting in preoperative surgical decision-making. Possible results of FNA include the following:

   - *Nondiagnostic*: Repeat once.
   - *Benign*: A lesion found to be benign by FNA can be safely followed. The false-negative rate for FNA is < 5%.
   - *Malignant*: Patients with FNA findings of cancer can undergo a definitive cancer operation. The false-positive rate for FNA is < 5%.
   - *Suspicious*: Patients with an FNA result of "suspicious" for papillary cancer should undergo surgery with an intraoperative frozen section; if frozen section confirms papillary cancer, a definitive procedure is done.
   - *Follicular*: An FNA result of follicular neoplasm requires at least a lobectomy. A frozen section rarely can distinguish between benign and malignant follicular tumors. The diagnosis of follicular cancer requires the finding of capsular, vascular, or lymphatic invasion on permanent section. If the final pathology is consistent with follicular carcinoma, then completion thyroidectomy may be done if indicated.

2. **Should ultrasound guidance be used to improve diagnostic accuracy for FNA of thyroid nodules?**

   Ultrasonography is useful for FNA of nonpalpable thyroid nodules and for biopsy of the solid component of complex cystic lesions. However, the sensitivity, specificity, and nondiagnostic rate for ultrasound-guided FNA of palpable nodules is equivalent to FNA performed without ultrasound guidance. Thus, ultrasound guidance for FNA of palpable thyroid nodules increases cost without improving diagnostic accuracy and should not be used routinely.

3. **What is the appropriate extent of thyroidectomy for differentiated thyroid carcinoma?**

   Well-differentiated thyroid cancer (WDTC) (papillary and follicular) can be stratified into low-, intermediate-, and high-risk groups by patient and tumor factors. Patient factors are age and gender, and tumor factors include size, local invasion, and distant metastases.

4. **Characterize the high-risk group. What treatment is required?**

   Factors related to high risk include male gender (age > 45, tumor size > 4 cm, and local invasion or distant metastases). Near-total (leaving less than 1 gm of visible thyroid tissue) or total thyroidectomy should be performed.

5. **Characterize the low-risk group. What treatment is recommended?**

   Factors related to low risk include minimal or occult papillary thyroid cancers (size < 1 cm, no local invasion, and no distant metastases) and minimally invasive follicular carcinoma (fewer than three areas of capsular microinvasion). Patients have good outcomes with lobectomy alone.

6. **What treatment is recommended for the intermediate-risk group?**

Total or near-total thyroidectomy lowers local recurrence rates with minimal additional morbidity. This approach allows postoperative ^{131}I ablation and improved postoperative cancer surveillance.

7. **Describe the appropriate surgical management for medullary thyroid carcinoma.**

Total thyroidectomy is the only treatment for medullary thyroid carcinoma because the tumor is not sensitive to radioiodine or thyroid-stimulating hormone (TSH) suppression. Due to the propensity for spreading to regional lymph nodes early in the course of disease, surgical management includes routine central neck dissection, with the addition of modified radical (lateral) neck dissection for clinically positive nodes. Some surgeons advocate routine bilateral modified neck dissection because of the high incidence of lateral nodal metastases (approximately 75% ipsilateral and 50% contralateral to the thyroid tumor). This therapeutic approach, when implemented early in the course of medullary thyroid carcinoma, results in normalization of calcitonin levels in up to 25% of patients.

8. **Discuss the role of surgery in anaplastic carcinoma of the thyroid.**

Anaplastic carcinoma of the thyroid is one of the most aggressive solid tumors known, with 50% of patients having distant metastases and 95% having local invasion at the time of diagnosis resulting in a dismal outcome regardless of therapeutic strategy. Surgery is rarely curative and in most cases should be restricted to a diagnostic or palliative role. Attempts at curative total thyroidectomy with postoperative chemotherapy may be indicated for the rare patient with localized disease. Palliative surgical debulking and tracheostomy should be reserved for symptoms of dysphagia or airway compromise, respectively, as they do not prolong survival.

9. **What is the role of surgery for primary lymphoma of the thyroid?**

Primary lymphoma of the thyroid is uncommon (< 1% of all thyroid malignancies). Lymphoma of the thyroid most often develops in patients with a history of Hashimoto's thyroiditis. A rapidly enlarging thyroid mass accompanied by compressive symptoms is a common presentation of this tumor. Most tumors are of the large B-cell type and typically are sensitive to both chemotherapy (cyclophosphamide, doxorubicin, vincristine, and prednisone) and radiation. Thus, combined modality therapy is the standard treatment, with surgery being relegated to a purely diagnostic role. FNA or core biopsy is often adequate for diagnosis, but incisional biopsy is sometimes necessary; when it is performed, a fresh specimen should be sent directly to the pathologist so that immunohistochemical analysis can be performed as needed.

10. **What is a central and modified neck dissection?**

A central neck dissection removes all the perithyroidal and tracheoesophageal groove nodes (level IV) from the thyroid notch superiorly down to the thoracic inlet. Laterally, the dissection extends from carotid to carotid artery. The lateral spread of disease usually involves high, middle, and low jugular lymph nodes (levels II–IV) and occasionally lateral (level V) nodes. A modified neck dissection, sometimes referred to as a functional dissection, spares the internal jugular vein, sternocleidomastoid muscle, and spinal accessory nerve, because sacrificing these structures does not improve outcome.

11. **What are the indications for neck dissection in well-differentiated (papillary and follicular) thyroid cancer (WDTC)?**

- All patients with clinically palpable nodes require a compartment (central and/or lateral) dissection.
- A central neck dissection in patients undergoing thyroidectomy with malignant cytology avoids a repeat operation for recurrence with its attendant increased operative risks.

- Preoperative ultrasound in patients with malignant nodule FNA cytology can find suspicious, nonpalpable lateral nodes prompting FNA biopsy, then dissection if positive.

12. **When should formal node dissection be performed versus "berry-picking"?**
Berry-picking (removing only the obviously abnormal nodes) is associated with increased local recurrence compared with formal node dissection and disrupts surgical planes, making subsequent dissection more difficult.

13. **When is surgery indicated for recurrent thyroid cancer?**
Suspected recurrent disease in the neck consisting of either palpable nodes or sonographically suspicious nodes should have FNA biopsy. Confirmed nodal recurrence should be treated with neck dissection followed by radioiodine therapy. Percutaneous ethanol injection of cervical nodal metastases is an alternative for patients who are poor surgical candidates. Radioiodine is the standard therapy for distant metastatic disease but isolated metastases can be surgically resected or treated with external beam radiation.

14. **What is the role of serum thyroglobulin (Tg) in detecting recurrence in patients with low-risk papillary thyroid cancer?**
Serum Tg levels are frequently used to monitor patients who have undergone total thyroidectomy or near-total thyroidectomy with ^{131}I ablation for papillary thyroid cancer. However, an undetectable serum Tg level obtained while patients are on thyroid hormone suppression therapy can be misleading. Approximately 20% of these patients will demonstrate a rise in Tg to above 2 ng/mL when stimulated with recombinant human TSH (rhTSH) and 36% of these patients are found to have recurrent disease. Multiple studies have shown that rhTSH-stimulated serum Tg levels are sufficiently sensitive (90–100% sensitive) to be used as the principal test in the follow-up of low-risk patients with papillary cancer. Routine use of whole body ^{131}I scanning is unnecessary when rhTSH-stimulated Tg levels are negative.

15. **How many times should a thyroid cyst be aspirated if it reaccumulates fluid? Should the cyst fluid be sent for cytology?**
Thyroid cysts are most often benign. The initial diagnostic and therapeutic procedure is aspiration. The complete disappearance of a palpable lesion is adequate therapy for thyroid cysts; however, about 50% will reaccumulate fluid. If the cyst recurs after repeat aspiration, it should be considered for surgical excision. Fluid cytology results are typically nonspecific; however, it may be prudent to perform cytology on cysts that reaccumulate fluid. If the nodule does not completely disappear after aspiration, it may be a complex cyst, which is associated with higher malignant potential. Therefore, FNA of the solid component should be performed.

16. **List the indications for thyroidectomy in hyperthyroidism.**
In the United States, thyroidectomy is not commonly performed for hyperthyroidism unless secondary to a single hyperfunctioning adenoma or because of a goiter containing a suspicious nodule. Despite the excellent success, low recurrence rate, safety, and more rapid return to a euthyroid state, fewer than 10% of patients with hyperthyroidism undergo thyroidectomy.

17. **List possible indications for thyroidectomy in patients with hyperthyroidism.**
- Failure of antithyroid medications
- Large goiter and low iodine uptake
- Compression symptoms, such as dysphagia, stridor, or hoarseness
- Nodules suspicious for cancer
- Children
- Pregnant patient who is difficult to treat medically
- Young female who wants to become pregnant in the near future
- Noncompliance

- Cosmetic concerns
- Severe Graves' ophthalmopathy

18. **How should patients with hyperthyroidism be prepared for surgery?**
It is important to render patients euthyroid prior to surgery for hyperthyroidism to avoid peri-operative thyroid storm. Antithyroid medications administered for 4 weeks prior to surgery are usually adequate. Some surgeons use saturated solution of potassium iodide (SSKI or Lugol's solution 3–5 drops 3 times a day) for 3–5 days prior to surgery to decrease the vascularity of the goiter and reduce the risk of bleeding. Patients who are very symptomatic may benefit from preoperative beta-blockade. For more rapid induction of a euthyroid state, patients may also be given dexamethasone, which can return T_4 and T_3 to within the normal range in < 7 days.

19. **What is the extent of thyroidectomy for hyperthyroidism?**
The controversy over the appropriate extent of thyroidectomy for hyperthyroidism resides in the desire to render the patient euthyroid without inducing hypothyroidism while balancing the risk of recurrence. Many surgeons prefer to perform near-total thyroidectomy, which successfully cures hyperthyroidism in nearly 100% of patients; however, it does so with the drawback of uniform hypothyroidism. Patients willing to accept the risk of recurrent hyperthyroidism may undergo subtotal thyroidectomy, which leaves approximately 4–8 gm of visible thyroid tissue with an adequate blood supply. A recent meta-analysis revealed subtotal thyroidectomy to result in a euthyroid state (no need for postoperative thyroid replacement therapy) in approximately 60% of patients, but it has a 5–10% incidence of persistent or recurrent hyperthyroidism.

20. **What are the complications of thyroidectomy?**
Thyroidectomy is a safe procedure with a mean length of hospitalization in large series of < 1.5 days. The incidence rates of specific complications after thyroidectomy are listed in the following:
- Cervical hematoma: 1%
- Recurrent laryngeal nerve injury: 1%
- Superior laryngeal nerve injury: 1%
- Temporary hypocalcemia: 10–15%
- Permanent hypoparathyroidism: 1%
- Mortality: 0.3%

21. **What is the significance of an incidentally noted thyroid hot spot on positron emission tomography (PET) scan?**
Fluorodeoxyglucose (FDG) whole body PET scan is increasingly being used in the diagnostic work-up or follow-up of patients with various types of cancer. An unexpected hot spot within the thyroid region is incidentally noted in up to 2% of PET scans. A recent study found that ultrasound-guided FNA of these lesions identified an indication for surgery in eight consecutive patients. Five of seven patients who agreed to surgery had a thyroid malignancy. This study suggests that thyroid incidentalomas noted on PET scans have a high rate of malignancy and warrant appropriate diagnostic evaluation.

22. **What is the appropriate therapy for an intrathoracic goiter?**
Intrathoracic goiters are typically cervical goiters with mediastinal extension, although primary intrathoracic goiters do occur secondary to abnormal descent of the thyroid during development. The incidence of carcinoma residing in intrathoracic goiters is reported as high as 17%; moreover, approximately 40% of patients present with compressive symptoms resulting from impingement on the airway, esophagus, vascular structures, or nerves. Radioiodine ablation is not typically recommended because of the risk of transient enlargement of the goiter during initiation of therapy, potentially resulting in life-threatening airway compromise. Thus, the presence of an intrathoracic goiter is generally accepted as an indication for thyroidectomy. Since the

arterial supply of intrathoracic goiters originates in the neck, the vast majority of these tumors can be resected through a cervical approach. Extension into the posterior mediastinum, malignancy, or compression of the vena cava may necessitate a combined cervical and sternotomy approach, although this is required in < 5% of cases.

23. **When should thyroglossal duct cysts be removed? Describe the operation.**
During the embryologic development of the thyroid, a diverticulum forms from the foramen cecum at the base of the tongue and descends as the thyroglossal duct to the future anatomical position of the thyroid overlying the anterolateral surface of the upper tracheal rings. The thyroglossal duct normally disappears during further development but in rare cases will persist as a patent duct or as a thyroglossal duct cyst. Patients may complain of infection, pain or compressive symptoms, or may have cosmetic concerns. Because of the risk of infection, thyroglossal duct cysts should be removed; this requires excision of the entire cyst and cyst tract from the origin at the foramen cecum down to the cyst itself. Since the tract nearly always passes through the hyoid bone, the center of the hyoid should be resected to lower the risk of recurrence; this causes no disability and requires no repair.

24. **What are the indications for minimally invasive video-assisted thyroidectomy?**
Minimally invasive video-assisted thyroidectomy (MIVAT) is an alternative method for thyroidectomy that is performed through a short incision that does not require neck extension or subcutaneous flap formation. Selection criteria for this new approach include a small thyroid volume (less than 15 mL by ultrasound), thyroid nodule less than 3.5 cm, no previous neck surgery or irradiation, and the absence of thyroiditis. While a few centers have found MIVAT to be as safe as conventional thyroidectomy and to have improved cosmetic results, the number of eligible patients is low, operative times are longer, and the procedure is more costly. Furthermore, long-term results for nerve injury, hypoparathyroidism, and recurrence are not yet known. At present, it is unclear what role this technically challenging approach will play.

KEY POINTS: THYROID SURGERY ✓

1. FNA is the single most important diagnostic test in the evaluation of a thyroid nodule.

2. Near-total or total thyroidectomy (as opposed to thyroid lobectomy) is the preferred treatment for most differentiated thyroid cancers.

3. Lymph node involvement in thyroid cancer should be treated with a systematic compartment node dissection.

4. A TSH stimulated Tg level is the preferred test to detect clinically inapparent recurrence of papillary thyroid cancer.

5. Incidental thyroid hot spots discovered on PET scans have a high rate of malignancy and should be evaluated by ultrasound-guided FNA.

PARATHYROID

25. **Discuss the indications for parathyroidectomy.**
Patients with classic symptoms of hyperparathyroidism (nephrolithiasis, severe bone disease or fractures, or overt neuromuscular syndrome) should undergo parathyroidectomy. A 2002 workshop at the National Institutes of Health (NIH) revised the 1990 recommendations for operation in asymptomatic patients with HPT as follows:

- Calcium > 1.0 mg/dL above normal
- 24-hour urine calcium > 400 mg
- Creatinine clearance reduced by > 30%
- Bone mineral density reduced > 2.5 standard deviations below age-matched control
- Age < 50 years
- Patients who do not desire or cannot undergo surveillance

Nonspecific symptoms, such as fatigue, mental slowing, and depression, were not included in the indications for surgery but several studies indicate improvement in patient-reported outcomes after curative operation.

26. **When should preoperative parathyroid localization studies be performed?**
    The 2002 NIH workshop confirmed the 1990 consensus that an experienced parathyroid surgeon does not require preoperative localization prior to an initial bilateral neck exploration. However, preoperative localization enables minimally invasive parathyroidectomy (directed, unilateral, radio-guided, or endoscopic). Patients with a prior history of neck surgery and certainly all patients with persistent or recurrent hyperparathyroidism should undergo preoperative localization studies prior to planned re-exploration. The best localization study available is the 99m technetium sestamibi scan, although ultrasound, computed tomography (CT) scan, magnetic resonance imaging (MRI), and arteriography with or without venous sampling may all be useful in certain situations, especially persistent or recurrent hyperparathyroidism.

27. **Define minimally invasive parathyroidectomy.**
    The combination of accurate preoperative localization studies and intraoperative intact parathyroid hormone (ioPTH) assay has fostered the development of minimally invasive approaches to parathyroidectomy as an alternative to conventional parathyroidectomy (identifying all four glands). Minimally invasive parathyroidectomy is a viable option for patients found to have a single adenoma on preoperative imaging (up to 95% of patients). A directed unilateral approach utilizes preoperative imaging to limit the dissection to one side. If one normal gland and one adenomatous gland are identified, the adenoma is removed and the surgery is terminated.

28. **What other function may ioPTH serve?**
    Many surgeons also utilize an ioPTH assay to exclude the possibility of multiglandular disease. Minimally invasive radio-guided parathyroidectomy is a second alternative to conventional parathyroidectomy and involves a 99m technetium sestamibi scan the morning of the surgery and an intraoperative gamma probe to localize the abnormal gland. A directed incision is performed and the gland removed. A third option is endoscopic parathyroidectomy, but this technique is only performed in a few centers.

29. **Summarize the advantages of minimally invasive approaches.**
    All minimally invasive approaches appear to be as safe and effective as conventional parathyroidectomy but may be more time- and cost-efficient because they limit the amount of dissection required and can be done without hospitalization.

30. **Describe when an ioPTH assay should be utilized.**
    A rapid assay for ioPTH allows intraoperative assessment of the functional success of the operation. This test is performed by drawing a sample of blood before the operation and 10 minutes after the suspected abnormal gland(s) has/have been removed. The test typically takes 10–15 minutes to run. A reduction of the ioPTH to 50% of the preoperative level and into the normal range predicts successful removal of all abnormal glands, and the surgery is terminated. ioPTH is most useful in patients with hyperplasia, those undergoing reoperation, and during minimally invasive parathyroidectomy.

31. **What is the expected success of surgery for primary hyperparathyroidism?**
Parathyroidectomy is highly successful for primary hyperparathyroidism, correcting hypercalcemia in more than 95% of patients when performed by an experienced surgeon. Bone density increases in the vast majority of patients. Successful parathyroidectomy significantly decreases the risk of kidney stone recurrence. Nearly all patients experience improvement in the vague nonspecific symptoms of hyperparathyroidism.

32. **Describe the appropriate management of a "missing" parathyroid.**
Despite meticulous operative technique during conventional parathyroidectomy (identification of all four glands), the surgeon occasionally encounters a "missing gland." Up to 20% of parathyroid glands are ectopic. A systematic search of the most common ectopic locations is required for successful outcome in these patients. When three normal glands have been identified and the fourth gland is not in a normal position, the most likely ectopic location depends on whether it is a missing upper or lower gland.

33. **List the likely locations for an ectopic inferior parathyroid gland.**
   - Thyrothymic ligament
   - Thymus
   - Mediastinum outside thymus
   - Undescended gland

34. **List the likely locations for an ectopic superior parathyroid gland.**
   - Posterior to thyroid
   - Tracheoesophageal groove
   - Posterosuperior mediastinum
   - Intrathyroid

35. **When should autotransplantation of parathyroid tissue be performed?**
A single adenoma is by far the most common cause of primary hyperparathyroidism; however, 10–15% of patients have hyperplasia. Patients with sporadic hyperplasia, a multiple endocrine neoplasia (MEN) syndrome, or secondary and tertiary hyperparathyroidism must undergo either subtotal (removal of 3½ glands [SPTx]) or total parathyroidectomy with autotransplantation of parathyroid tissue (TPTx + AT). The success of either approach depends on finding all four glands.

36. **How is autotransplantation performed?**
Autotransplantation is performed by placing 10–15 grafts of 1-mm pieces of parathyroid into two or three separate pockets formed in either the sternocleidomastoid muscle or a forearm muscle and marked with a nonabsorbable suture for easy identification.

37. **Discuss the advantages and disadvantages of SPTx versus TPTx + AT.**
It is generally thought that SPTx has a lower incidence of postoperative hypocalcemia. The advantage of TPTx + AT is that persistent or recurrent hypercalcemia can be treated by partially or completely removing the grafts under local anesthesia, while the same complication occurring after SPTx requires repeat neck operation with higher morbidity. One very small prospective, randomized trial demonstrated a clear benefit of TPTx + AT for secondary hyperparathyroidism in renal failure patients; in those it resulted in a more rapid return of normal calcium homeostasis and relief of symptoms.

38. **List the complications of parathyroidectomy and their prevalence.**
   - Persistent or recurrent hyperparathyroidism: 1–12%
   - Transient hypocalcemia: 10–25%
   - Permanent hypoparathyroidism: 2–5%

- Permanent recurrent laryngeal nerve injury: < 1%
- Temporary recurrent laryngeal nerve injury: 3%
- Mortality: < 0.5%

39. **Define persistent or recurrent hyperparathyroidism.**
Persistent hyperparathyroidism is defined as failure of calcium and PTH levels to normalize or remain normal in the initial 6 months after operation, whereas recurrent hyperparathyroidism is defined by recurrence of hypercalcemia after 6 months.

40. **Discuss the approach to patients with persistent or recurrent hyperparathyroidism.**
The approach to patients with persistent or recurrent hyperparathyroidism requires confirmation of the diagnosis, estimation of disease severity, careful review of the operative and pathology reports, and preoperative localization. Causes of failure include missed adenoma in a normal location, ectopic glands, inadequate resection in multiglandular disease, and supernumerary glands.

41. **Discuss the options for treatment of persistent or recurrent hyperparathyroidism.**
Preoperative localization is usually achieved by 99m technetium sestamibi scan. Repeat cervical exploration is successful in normalizing PTH levels in about 85% of patients and may be aided by intraoperative ultrasound and ioPTH assay. Mediastinal parathyroid tissue is most often removed via the transcervical approach, but thoracoscopy or median sternotomy may be required 1–2% of the time. Angiographic ablation of mediastinal parathyroid tissue using high doses of ionic contrast may be successful in selected patients with high surgical risk.

42. **How does one recognize parathyroid cancer?**
Parathyroid cancer is the rarest of all endocrine tumors, with a reported incidence of < 1% in patients with primary hyperparathyroidism. Patients may present with a palpable mass and typically have symptomatic hypercalcemia that is often severe (> 14 mg/dL) and of rapid onset. Successful outcome requires early recognition and appropriate treatment.

43. **Describe the management of parathyroid cancer.**
The diagnosis is rarely confirmed preoperatively and is often not obvious at the initial operation. Local invasion and pathologic nodes should be assumed to represent cancer. Any suspicious parathyroid lesions should be carefully removed without disrupting the parathyroid capsule, since this may result in tumor spillage and local recurrence. If a parathyroid gland is obviously abnormal and infiltrating other tissues, those tissues should be resected en bloc with the tumor whenever possible, including the ipsilateral thyroid lobe when necessary. Removal of the central nodes on the side of the tumor is indicated at the initial operation. Any obviously enlarged lateral nodes should be resected in an appropriate neck dissection. Prophylactic neck dissections have shown no benefit. The histopathologic diagnosis of this cancer is also difficult; thus, intraoperative frozen section is rarely useful other than to confirm parathyroid tissue.

44. **Give the recurrence and survival rates for parathyroid cancer.**
Recurrence rates are high, but prolonged survival is still possible. The National Cancer Database reports 5- and 10-year survival rates of 85.5% and 49.1%, respectively.

ADRENAL GLANDS

45. **What imaging studies are available for evaluating adrenal pathology?**
The appropriate imaging study for adrenal lesions depends on the diagnosis. Aldosteronomas are typically < 2 cm in diameter, and therefore the sensitivity of CT scans is only 85%. When CT

KEY POINTS: PARATHYROID SURGERY ✓

1. Indications for parathyroidectomy in primary hyperparathyroidism include the classic symptoms of nephrolithiasis and overt bone or neuromuscular syndrome.

2. Indications in asymptomatic patients include high serum calcium (> 1.0 mg/dL above normal), age under 50 years, osteoporosis, high urinary calcium (> 400 mg/day), and reduced creatinine clearance.

3. Surgery for primary hyperparathyroidism results in normocalcemia in greater than 95% of patients when performed by an experienced parathyroid surgeon.

4. Parathyroid cancer is rare but should be suspected in patients with a palpable mass and symptomatic hypercalcemia that is severe and of rapid onset.

scanning fails to demonstrate an adenoma, adrenal venous sampling is useful to differentiate small adenomas from bilateral hyperplasia. For cortisol-producing adenomas, CT scans are very accurate. Most pheochromocytomas are of considerable size by the time they are diagnosed, so CT scans are very accurate. MRI is essentially equivalent to CT for adrenal tumors; however, it may be superior in recurrent or metastatic disease and for pheochromocytomas. Meta-iodobenzylguanidine scans are best utilized for recurrent or nonadrenal pheochromocytomas.

46. **Should all incidentally discovered adrenal masses be resected?**
A recent NIH consensus conference set forth guidelines for the evaluation and treatment of incidentally discovered adrenal tumors. The prevalence of clinically inapparent adrenal masses discovered at autopsy is 1–7% and increases with age. The decision to surgically remove an adrenal incidentaloma is based on tumor size, imaging characteristics, and biochemical activity. Adrenal cortical carcinoma accounts for 2% of tumors less than 4 cm but 25% of tumors greater than 6 cm. Up to 20% of adrenal incidentalomas are found to have subclinical hormonal dysfunction.

47. **Summarize the appropriate laboratory evaluation of an adrenal mass.**
   - 1 mg overnight dexamethasone suppression test
   - Fractionated urinary or plasma free metanephrines
   - In hypertensive patients: serum potassium and plasma aldosterone-plasma renin activity ratio

48. **What findings on CT or MRI help to distinguish between benign and malignant tumors?**
   - Benign tumors are typically < 4 cm, homogeneous with smooth borders, and have low attenuation (less than 10 Hounsfield units [HU]).
   - Malignant tumors are typically > 6 cm, heterogeneous with irregular borders, and have increased attenuation (> 10 HU).

49. **Discuss the role of FNA in the evaluation of an adrenal mass.**
FNA is rarely indicated. It is reserved for patients with a history of cancer to evaluate for metastasis and is performed only if the result will influence therapy. It is always necessary to exclude pheochromocytoma first.

50. **List the indications for surgery.**
   - Unilateral tumor with signs or symptoms of hormonal dysfunction
   - Subclinical hormone dysfunction

- Size > 6 cm
- Size < 6 cm with worrisome radiographic signs (rapid growth, heterogeneous appearance, irregular borders, and high attenuation (> 20 HU)

51. **Describe the open technique for adrenalectomy.**
There are many different surgical approaches to the adrenal glands. Conventional open adrenalectomy can be performed through an anterior (transperitoneal), an anterolateral (extraperitoneal), or a posterior (retroperitoneal) approach. Rarely, a combined thoracoabdominal approach is required for extremely large or malignant lesions.

52. **Discuss the role of laparoscopic surgery.**
Advances in laparoscopic surgical techniques have been applied to adrenalectomy; currently, most endocrine surgeons agree that laparoscopic adrenalectomy is the procedure of choice for benign adrenal tumors, with open adrenalectomy reserved for malignant tumors. Laparoscopic adrenalectomy has been associated with decreased hospital stay, less postoperative pain, less blood loss, shorter recovery, and overall increased patient satisfaction compared with the open techniques.

53. **What approaches are used for laparoscopic surgery?**
Just as with open adrenalectomy, several different laparoscopic approaches are available. The most common technique is via an anterolateral approach, which provides excellent exposure but does not allow removal of both glands without repositioning the patient. An anterior approach provides access to both adrenal glands but exposure is more difficult. A posterior endoscopic approach avoids entering the peritoneal cavity altogether; however, this approach provides a limited working space and may hinder removal of larger lesions.

54. **Summarize the long-term success of adrenalectomy for functional tumors.**
Adrenalectomy for aldosteronomas is at least 95% successful in normalizing the aldosterone level and correcting hypokalemia, but the long-term resolution of hypertension is variable. For younger patients with relatively recent onset hypertension, adrenalectomy usually results in normotension. In older patients with severe, long-standing hypertension associated with renal dysfunction, adrenalectomy may not normalize the blood pressure but often results in easier control of hypertension with fewer or lower-dose medications. Unilateral adrenalectomy is 95% effective in treating cortisol-producing adenomas; bilateral adrenalectomy in patients failing hypophysectomy for adrenocorticotropic hormone-dependent Cushing's syndrome is slightly less effective, with approximately 25% of patients having persistent symptoms, hypertension or diabetes. These patients must also deal with hormone replacement. Adrenalectomy for nonfamilial benign pheochromocytomas is curative in most cases; however, a 5–10% late recurrence rate has been reported, and therefore these patients should undergo lifelong observation.

55. **Describe the appropriate management of adrenal malignancy.**
Adrenocortical carcinoma is a rare and aggressive cancer that is frequently metastatic by the time of diagnosis. Approximately 60% of adrenocortical carcinomas are functioning tumors. The overall 5-year survival rate is around 25%. The only chance for cure is surgery, which should be offered to all patients without metastases with a reasonable surgical risk. Surgery should also be considered for young patients with an isolated, easily resectable metastasis.

56. **Describe the appropriate management of pheochromocytoma.**
Approximately 10% of pheochromocytomas are malignant, and the 5-year survival is approximately 40% with surgical resection offering the only chance for cure. The adrenal glands are a relatively common site for metastases from other malignancies, but surgical resection is restricted to patients with isolated lesions.

KEY POINTS: ADRENAL SURGERY ✓

1. Adrenal tumors smaller than 4 cm are rarely malignant; however, 25% of tumors larger than 6 cm are malignant.

2. Cortisol-producing adenoma is the most common functional adrenal tumor.

3. Laparoscopic adrenalectomy is now the preferred approach for most adrenal tumors; however, recurrence rates may be higher than the open approach if the tumor is malignant.

PANCREATIC ENDOCRINE AND CARCINOID SURGERY

57. **How should pancreatic islet cell tumors be imaged?**
Due to the small size of most islet cell tumors, preoperative localization is often difficult, and the extent of preoperative imaging needed is controversial. Ultrasound, CT, MRI, and angiography have reported sensitivities around 60%. Octreotide scans are highly sensitive (85%), especially for metastases, in locating most islet cell tumors, with the exception of insulinomas (50% sensitivity), which are the most common type. Provocative arterial stimulation (secretin for gastrinomas and calcium for insulinomas) and hepatic venous sampling have a higher sensitivity and have replaced portal vein sampling, but their invasiveness and ability to only regionalize a tumor make them less desirable. Recent reports have shown endoscopic ultrasound to be the most sensitive preoperative test for localizing pancreatic islet cell tumors, although it is invasive and highly operator dependent.

58. **How important is it to localize islet cell tumors before surgery?**
Due to the above difficulties, many surgeons believe that exhaustive efforts to localize islet cell tumors preoperatively are unwarranted. They prefer to obtain a preoperative ultrasound or CT scan to identify obviously invasive or metastatic tumors and then rely on intraoperative palpation (90% sensitivity) with intraoperative ultrasound (sensitivity approaches 100%) to localize the tumor. All patients undergoing re-exploration for islet cell tumors should undergo preoperative localization studies.

59. **What is the appropriate surgical approach for insulinomas?**
Insulinomas account for approximately 90% of nonfamilial islet cell tumors. The small size of these tumors and the rarity of malignancy allow simple enucleation (60% of cases) or distal pancreatectomy (35% of cases) in the vast majority of cases. Rarely, formal pancreaticoduodenectomy is required (< 5% of cases), most typically for malignant tumors. Laparoscopy for enucleation or distal pancreatectomy is used selectively in some centers.

60. **Describe the surgical approach to gastrinomas.**
The surgical approach to gastrinomas is more complex because these tumors are more frequently malignant and occur outside the pancreas in up to 50% of cases. Tumors occurring distal to the pancreatic neck should be removed by formal pancreatic resection because of the high incidence of malignancy. Tumors in the pancreatic head can often be enucleated, reserving formal pancreaticoduodenectomy for more invasive tumors or those in close proximity to the pancreatic duct. Careful evaluation of the duodenum by palpation, endoscopic transillumination, or duodenotomy is necessary to identify the tumor within the duodenal wall. Small submucosal lesions can be enucleated, but a full-thickness resection of the duodenal wall may be necessary. The propensity for these tumors to metastasize to lymph nodes necessitates a regional lymph node dissection in all patients.

61. **How should other sporadically occurring islet cell tumors be managed?**
Other sporadically occurring islet cell tumors are typically large, and 50% are malignant, requiring an individualized surgical approach in these rare cases.

62. **Should islet cell tumors occurring in patients with MEN type I be approached differently than those occurring sporadically?**
Yes. Approximately 70% of patients with MEN type I develop pancreatic islet cell tumors, with gastrinoma being the most common tumor. Due to the multifocal nature and diffuse islet cell dysplasia seen in these patients, aggressive surgery rarely results in biochemical cure. The morbidity and mortality rates of aggressive surgical resection combined with low cure rate and the availability of effective palliative treatment options for symptomatic patients sway many clinicians to treat patients medically unless there is suspicion of malignancy. Other surgeons take a more aggressive approach, citing the incidence of malignancy. Further, the larger tumors seen on preoperative imaging (> 3 cm) often account for symptoms, and therefore surgical extirpation of these tumors may be beneficial. Formal resection of the distal pancreas accompanied by enucleation of tumors in the pancreatic head is necessary. Search for duodenal tumors and resection of the lymph nodes must accompany resection of pancreatic tumors.

63. **Discuss the role of surgery for liver metastases from neuroendocrine tumors.**
Patients who undergo resection of isolated liver metastases from neuroendocrine tumors experience symptomatic improvement in 95% of cases and have prolonged survival (60–75% versus 25–30% 5-year survival rates) compared with patients with similar tumor burdens not undergoing hepatic resection. Patients with unresectable liver metastases or those with prohibitive surgical risks may benefit from either cryosurgical or radiofrequency thermal ablation.

64. **How are carcinoid tumors localized?**
Carcinoid tumors develop from enterochromaffin tissue and can be divided into those arising in the foregut, midgut, or hindgut. The most common locations of carcinoid tumors are:
- Small intestine (35%)
- Appendix (35%)
- Rectum (15%)
- Bronchial system (10%)

65. **Describe the presentation of carcinoid tumors.**
Bronchial carcinoids may present with hemoptysis or carcinoid syndrome, while tumors developing in the small intestine are typically diagnosed incidentally or after carcinoid syndrome develops secondary to metastases. Hindgut carcinoids do not usually produce active hormones and are typically found incidentally during endoscopy performed for other reasons.

66. **Once a patient is diagnosed with carcinoid syndrome, what is the next step?**
The tumor must then be localized. This goal may be difficult because of the small size of most carcinoid tumors. Tumors arise in the small bowel and appendix in nearly 70% of patients, and therefore a small bowel contrast study or abdominal CT scan is often the initial study performed. If these tests fail to localize the tumor, a chest x-ray and/or chest CT scan should be obtained to exclude a bronchial carcinoid. Metaiodobenzylguanidine or octreotide scintigraphy is sometimes able to localize tumors not found by conventional methods.

67. **Describe the appropriate surgical management for carcinoid tumors.**
Bronchial carcinoids tend to spread locoregionally and therefore should be resected by formal lobectomy when possible. Gastric and small intestinal carcinoids without metastases should be excised by segmental resection and lymph node dissection. Appendiceal carcinoids are typically incidentally discovered and occur most commonly at the appendiceal tip. Distal lesions < 2 cm are adequately treated by appendectomy. The presence of a carcinoid near the appendiceal base,

size > 2 cm, or grossly involved lymph nodes require formal right hemicolectomy. Rectal carcinoids often present with bleeding or are incidentally found on endoscopy. Extensive surgery for rectal carcinoids offers no survival advantage over local excision.

68. **Discuss the role of surgery in carcinoid syndrome.**
Patients with surgically resectable hepatic tumors experience improvement in symptoms and survival comparable to that for islet cell tumors metastatic to the liver. The development of somatostatin analogs has allowed successful control of symptoms in most patients with carcinoid syndrome and diffuse hepatic metastases. Systemic chemotherapy and hepatic artery embolization have not been very effective in palliating these patients; however, selective hepatic artery chemoembolization has been successful in decreasing tumor burden and alleviating symptoms in up to 80% of patients. Patients who do not respond to medical palliation may benefit from aggressive tumor debulking by resecting the primary tumor and as many of the liver metastases as feasible. As with liver metastases from islet cell tumors, cryosurgical or radiofrequency thermal ablation may be useful for unresectable lesions in patients not responding to medical palliation.

KEY POINTS: PANCREATIC ENDOCRINE AND CARCINOID SURGERY ✔

1. Insulinoma is the most common islet cell tumor, is usually benign, and can be treated by enucleation.

2. Gastrinoma is usually malignant and can occur in the pancreas, duodenum, and lymph nodes.

3. Octreotide scintigraphy and endoscopic ultrasound are the most useful preoperative imaging studies for gastrinoma.

4. Arterial stimulation with hepatic venous sampling has replaced portal venous sampling for localization of islet cell tumors.

5. Islet cell tumors in patients with MEN are frequently multifocal and are treated medically due to the low cure rate following surgery.

6. Resection of isolated liver metastasis from neuroendocrine tumors improves symptoms and prolongs survival.

BARIATRIC SURGERY

69. **Define obesity. How common is it?**
The incidence of obesity in the United States exceeds 30% and is steadily increasing. Morbid obesity is defined as a body mass index (BMI; weight in kilograms divided by height in meters squared) in excess of 40 and is known to cause or worsen many diseases, including diabetes mellitus, hypertension, obstructive sleep apnea, hyperlipidemia, and osteoarthritis.

70. **How successful is nonsurgical treatment of obesity?**
Evidence suggests that nonsurgical treatment (diet/behavior modification, exercise programs, and psychological support) for morbid obesity has a more than 90% failure rate. Similarly, pharmacologic therapy for morbid obesity has been hampered by serious side effects and, overall, has met with disappointing results.

71. **What are the indications for surgery for obesity?**
An NIH Consensus Conference held in 1991 recommended that the following patients be considered for bariatric surgery:
- BMI > 40
- BMI of 35–40 if associated with other severe medical problems that are likely to improve with weight reduction.

72. **List the contraindications to bariatric operations.**
- Endocrine disorders that cause morbid obesity
- Psychological instability
- Alcohol or drug abuse

73. **Categorize the various surgical options for weight reduction.**
Surgical options for weight reduction can be divided into either restrictive or malabsorptive; however, some procedures utilize a component of both.

74. **List the options for restrictive surgery.**
- *Vertical-banded gastroplasty:* A stapling device is used to divide the stomach vertically along the lesser curve starting at the angle of His to create a small (20 mL) pouch. A prosthetic device is then wrapped around the outlet of the pouch to prevent it from dilating over time.
- *Gastric banding:* This procedure is now commonly performed laparoscopically and involves placement of an adjustable band around the top of the stomach to create a small (20-mL) pouch. The band is connected to a reservoir placed in the subcutaneous tissue that enables band adjustment.

75. **What is the option for malabsorptive surgery?**
Biliopancreatic bypass. A subtotal gastrectomy is performed leaving a gastric remnant of 500 mL. The small bowel is divided at the junction of the jejunum and ileum. The ileum is anastomosed to the stomach and the jejunum is connected to the side of the ileum approximately 50–100 cm from the ileocecal valve. This procedure results in malabsorption by creating a short common channel for digestion and absorption of food.

76. **Explain the combined option.**
Known as the *Roux-en-Y gastric bypass,* the top of the stomach is stapled (and commonly divided) horizontally to create a small 15–30 mL proximal stomach pouch. This small reservoir restricts the amount of food that can be ingested at one time. The jejunum is then divided just distal to the ligament of Treitz and the distal end anastomosed to the proximal stomach pouch. The proximal end of the jejunum is then anastomosed to the side of the jejunum 50–110 cm distal to the gastrojejunostomy. The length of this Roux limb determines the degree of malabsorption and is typically made longer for patients with very high BMIs. This procedure is now commonly performed using laparoscopic technique.

77. **How much weight do patients lose following bariatric surgery?**
Success following bariatric surgery is determined by both weight lost and improvement in obesity-related comorbidities. However, many surgical studies report outcome as percentage excess weight loss and consider loss of at least 50% of excess weight as a minimum criterion for success. Although the 1991 NIH Consensus Conference endorsed gastric restriction as an acceptable option for surgical weight reduction, recent studies suggest that it is less effective in maintaining long-term weight loss. An 80% failure rate at 10 years has been reported following vertical-banded gastroplasty. Both gastric bypass and biliopancreatic bypass result in the loss of 65–85% of excess weight, which is maintained at 3–5 years after surgery.

KEY POINTS: BARIATRIC SURGERY

1. Surgery is the only therapy that consistently results in significant, long-term weight loss in morbidly obese patients.

2. Laparoscopic Roux-en-Y gastric bypass is currently the most common bariatric operation performed in the U.S. and results in loss of 65–75% of excess weight.

3. Surgical weight loss significantly reduces obesity-related comorbidities and is a surgical cure for diabetes mellitus.

78. **What are the effects of bariatric surgery on obesity-related comorbidities?**
Long-term weight loss following bariatric surgery has been shown to significantly reduce obesity-related comorbidities. Approximately 85% of patients with diabetes, hyperlipidemia, and obesity hypoventilation syndrome will be improved or cured at 2 years after surgery. Hypertension also improves or resolves in over two-thirds of patients after successful weight loss. Salutary effects on other comorbidities, such as sleep apnea, depression, arthritic pain, and unemployment are frequently observed following surgery.

79. **What are the complications of bariatric surgery?**
Perioperative mortality in most series of bariatric surgery is less than 0.5%. A laparoscopic technique has changed the pattern of perioperative complications. While wound complications are less frequent, anastomotic stenosis, gastrointestinal (GI) bleeding, and bowel obstruction occur more frequently with laparoscopic compared to open techniques. Mean hospital stay following laparoscopic bariatric surgery is 2–3 days, which is significantly shorter than after open surgery (5–7 days). Each procedure has its own unique risk of complications.

80. **Give the incidence of complications following laparoscopic bariatric procedures in general.**
   - Anastomotic leak (1–2%)
   - Anastomotic stenosis (5–10%)
   - Postoperative bowel obstruction (3%)
   - GI bleed (2%)
   - Gallstones (>50%)
   - Protein-calorie malnutrition (3–5%)
   - Anemia (30%)
   - Vitamin deficiency (30%)
   - Wound complication (infection, dehiscence, and hernia) (4–5%)
   - Band slippage or erosion into stomach (5%)

WEBSITE

http://endocrinesurgeons.org/home.html

BIBLIOGRAPHY

THYROID SURGERY

1. Chen H, Zeiger MA, Clark DP, et al: Papillary carcinoma of the thyroid: Can operative management be based solely on fine-needle aspiration? J Am Coll Surg 184:605–610, 1997.
2. Cohen MS, Arslan N, Dehdashti F, et al: Risk of malignancy in thyroid incidentalomas identified by fluo-rodeoxyglucose-positron emission tomography. Surgery 130:941–946, 2001.
3. Fleming J, Lee J, Bouvet M, et al: Surgical strategy for the treatment of medullary thyroid carcinoma. Ann Surg 230:697–707, 1999.
4. Mazzaferri EL, Kloos R: Current approaches to primary therapy for papillary and follicular thyroid cancer. J Clin Endocrinol Metab 86:1447–1463, 2001.
5. Mazzaferri EL, Robbins RJ, Spencer CA, et al: A consensus report of the role of serum thyroglobulin as a moni-toring method for low-risk patients with papillary thyroid carcinoma. J Clin Endocrinol Metab 88:1433–1441, 2003.
6. Moley JF, DeBenedetti MK: Patterns of nodal metastases in palpable medullary thyroid carcinoma: Recommendations for extent of node dissection. Ann Surg 229:880–887, 1999 (discussion 887–888).
7. Palit TK, Miller CC III, Miltenburg DM: The efficacy of thyroidectomy for Graves' disease: A meta-analysis. J Surg Res 90:161–165, 2000.

PARATHYROID SURGERY

8. Allendorf J, Kim L, Chabot J, et al: The impact of sestamibi scanning on the outcome of parathyroid surgery. J Clin Endocrinol Metab 88:3015–3018, 2003.
9. Bilezikian JP, Potts JT Jr, Fuleihan Gel H, et al: Summary statement from a workshop on asymptomatic primary hyperparathyroidism: A perspective for the 21st century. J Clin Endocrinol Metab 87:5353–5361, 2002.
10. Burney RE, Jones KR, Coon JW, et al: Assessment of patient outcomes after operation for primary hyper-parathyroidism. Surgery 120:1013–1018, 1996 (discussion 1018–1019).
11. Denham DW, Norman J: Cost-effectiveness of preoperative sestamibi scan for primary hyperparathyroidism is dependent solely upon the surgeon's choice of operative procedure. J Am Coll Surg 186:293–305, 1998.
12. Gasparri G, Camandona M, Abbona GC, et al: Secondary and tertiary hyperparathyroidism: Causes of recurrent disease after 446 parathyroidectomies. Ann Surg 233:65–69, 2001.
13. Hundahl SA, Fleming ID, Fremgen AM, Menck HR: Two hundred eighty-six cases of parathyroid carcinoma treated in the U.S. between 1985-1995: A National Cancer Data Base Report. The American College of Surgeons Commission on Cancer and the American Cancer Society. Cancer 86:538–544, 1999.
14. Molinari AS, Irvin GL III, Deriso GT, Bott L: Incidence of multiglandular disease in primary hyperparathyroidism determined by parathyroid hormone secretion. Surgery 120:934–936, 1996 (discussion 936–937).
15. Silverberg SJ, Shane E, Jacobs TP, et al: A 10-year prospective study of primary hyperparathyroidism with or without parathyroid surgery. N Engl J Med 341:1249–1255, 1999.
16. Sywak MS, Knowlton ST, Pasieka JL, et al: Do the National Institutes of Health consensus guidelines for parathy-roidectomy predict symptom severity and surgical outcome in patients with primary hyperparathyroidism? Surgery 132:1013–1019, 2002 (discussion 1019–1020).

ADRENAL SURGERY

17. Dackiw AP, Lee JE, Gagel RF, et al: Adrenal cortical carcinoma. World J Surg 25:914–926, 2001.
18. Gagner M, Pomp A, Heniford BT, et al: Laparoscopic adrenalectomy: Lessons learned from 100 consecutive pro-cedures. Ann Surg 226:238–246, 1997 (discussion 246–247).
19. Goldstein RE, O'Neill JA Jr, Holcomb GW III, et al: Clinical experience over 48 years with pheochromocytoma. Ann Surg 229:755–764, 1999 (discussion 764–766).
20. Grumbach MM, Biller BM, Braunstein GD, et al: Management of the clinically inapparent adrenal mass ("inciden-taloma"). Ann Intern Med 138:424–429, 2003.

21. Icard P, Goudet P, Charpenay C, et al: Adrenocortical carcinomas: Surgical trends and results of a 253-patient series from the French Association of Endocrine Surgeons study group. World J Surg 25:891–897, 2001.

22. Lo CY, Tam PC, Kung AW, et al: Primary aldosteronism. Results of surgical treatment. Ann Surg 224:125–130, 1996.

23. Sawka AM, Young WF, Thompson GB, et al: Primary aldosteronism: Factors associated with normalization of blood pressure after surgery. Ann Intern Med 135:258–261, 2001.

PANCREATIC ENDOCRINE AND CARCINOID SURGERY

24. Chung MH, Pisegna J, Spirt M, et al: Hepatic cytoreduction followed by a novel long-acting somatostatin analog: A paradigm for intractable neuroendocrine tumors metastatic to the liver. Surgery 130:954–962, 2001.

25. Hiramoto JS, Feldstein VA, LaBerge JM, et al: Intraoperative ultrasound and preoperative localization detects all occult insulinomas. Arch Surg 136:1020–1025, 2001 (discussion 1025–1026).

26. Jensen RT: Carcinoid and pancreatic endocrine tumors: Recent advances in molecular pathogenesis, localization, and treatment. Curr Opin Oncol 12:368–377, 2000.

27. Norton JA, Fraker DL, Alexander HR, et al: Surgery to cure the Zollinger-Ellison syndrome. N Engl J Med 341:635–644, 1999.

28. Sarmiento JM, Heywood G, Rubin J, et al: Surgical treatment of neuroendocrine metastases to the liver: A plea for resection to increase survival. J Am Coll Surg 197:29–37, 2003.

29. Wiedenmann B, Jensen RT, Mignon M, et al: Preoperative diagnosis and surgical management of neuroendocrine gastroenteropancreatic tumors: General recommendations by a consensus workshop. World J Surg 22:309–338, 1998.

BARIATRIC SURGERY

30. Anthone GJ, Lord RV, DeMeester TR, Crookes PF: The duodenal switch operation for the treatment of morbid obesity. Ann Surg 238:618–627, 2003 (discussion 627–628).

31. Biertho L, Steffen R, Ricklin T, et al: Laparoscopic gastric bypass versus laparoscopic adjustable gastric banding: A comparative study of 1,200 cases. J Am Coll Surg197(4):536–544, 2003 (discussion 544–545).

32. Brolin RE: Bariatric surgery and long-term control of morbid obesity. JAMA 288:2793–2796, 2002.

33. Schauer PR, Burguera B, Ikramuddin S, et al: Effect of laparoscopic Roux-en Y gastric bypass on type 2 diabetes mellitus. Ann Surg 238:467–484, 2003 (discussion 84–85).

ENDOCRINOLOGY IN THE MANAGED CARE ENVIRONMENT

Elliot G. Levy, M.D.

CHAPTER 60

1. **Define managed care.**
   The American College of Physicians/American Society of Internal Medicine has defined managed care as "a system of health-care delivery provided by contracted providers in which the entities responsible for financing the cost of health care exert influence on the clinical decision-making of those who provide the health care in an attempt to provide health care that is cost effective, accessible, and of acceptable quality."

2. **Is there only one type of managed care?**
   Managed care is actually a spectrum of health care delivery systems ranging from managed indemnity insurance through preferred provider organizations (PPOs) and point-of-service (POS) plans to various types of health maintenance organizations (HMOs). Collectively, these organizations are called managed care organizations (MCOs). To a greater or lesser extent, all managed care systems attempt to shift financial risk in one way or another to the providers of care.

3. **Who is the patient's initial contact in a managed care environment?**
   In most cases, the patient's initial contact is with a health care provider, conveniently called a "primary care provider" (PCP). This person is usually a physician, such as a family medicine, family practice, or general practice physician, but often may be a physician who has specialized in internal medicine or an internist with a subspecialty (such as endocrinology) who enjoys practicing primary care in addition to his or her subspecialty or does not have enough subspecialty work to fill his or her schedule. The PCP can also be a physician extender, such as a nurse practitioner or a physician assistant. Some MCOs utilize physicians in large clinic type settings in an effort to control costs. In other situations, PCPs function out of their usual private practice offices—in a sense, mixing their private (or non-MCO) patients with their HMO or PPO patients.

4. **Do pediatricians and gynecologists function as PCPs?**
   There has been a movement over the past few years to allow pediatricians to become PCPs for children and for obstetrics and gynecology specialists to become PCPs for women of childbearing years, who often have no need to see other types of physicians.

5. **How does the patient make contact with a subspecialist?**
   A patient is allowed to see a subspecialist, such as an endocrinologist, only with the recommendation of a PCP. Usually, an endocrinologist is not allowed to function as both a PCP and a subspecialist within a given HMO. In these situations, when a fully trained endocrinologist is serving as a PCP, he or she cannot even perform specialty-type procedures and must refer them to another endocrinologist.

6. **What is a meant by the MCO's "panel" of providers?**
   Once an MCO has established itself in a community, it begins to develop a "panel" of all the providers it needs, including PCPs, medical subspecialists, surgeons and surgical subspecial-

ists, pediatricians, obstetricians-gynecologists, and dermatologists. Simultaneously, the MCO contracts with hospitals (strategically located around the community that it wants to "penetrate"), nursing homes, home health agencies, physical therapy centers, dialysis centers, outpatient diagnostic centers, clinical (commercial) laboratories, and, sometimes, even outpatient diabetes education centers, or dietitians.

7. Explain the MCO directory.

The panel of providers is published yearly in a directory that goes by a variety of names (e.g., preferred provider list) and is distributed to all participants of the MCO. This directory is sometimes called the "list." It is used by patients to determine which PCP is available for them to use (although in some HMOs the new patients are immediately assigned to a PCP of the HMO's choice). It is used by a PCP to know which subspecialists, diagnostic center, and laboratory to use. It is also used by the MCO itself as a marketing tool to solicit business for itself by proudly showing which subspecialists belong to its panel of providers. It is, therefore, necessary to be on "the list" to receive referrals from this HMO. However, your presence on the list as a subspecialist does not mean that you will ever receive referrals. The health care for the MCO is then provided by this entire group of health care providers, all of whom are under contracts with the HMO to provide the care in the manner and for the price that is negotiated. Thus, the MCO has managed to do what the health care system was never able to do by itself—organize all the health care into one unit.

8. Explain the "POS" option.

In some cases, the POS option allows the patient to see any specialist, although the reimbursement schedule is different. In addition, the patient's out-of-pocket expenses (co-payment) are often much larger. The POS option differs greatly among insurance companies that offer it.

9. How do MCOs compare with other business units?

When one looks at the managed care system from afar, it is not so different from any other business unit that has to negotiate with vendors to provide services that it cannot provide on its own. Think of a business unit as the cruise ship industry, which negotiates with its own employees, as well as entertainers, doctors, food suppliers, fuel suppliers, ports, and travel agents, to provide for its customers (passengers) a total package for their enjoyment. So have the MCOs attempted to organize the United States health care system. It is clearly a private, nongovernment-regulated, for-profit (in most cases) system whose primary goal is to earn a profit for its shareholders, while attempting to contain costs for the entire health care system. Not-for-profit MCOs are not necessarily any more efficient in providing the care to its members and often have the same fiscal problems as for-profit MCOs.

10. What is the difference between a PPO and an HMO?

Preferred provider organization (PPO) is a plan, as originally conceived 10–20 years ago, which contracts with independent providers at a discounted fee for service. When the PPO systems first started, their representatives would approach a PCP or a specialist and offer a discounted fee schedule to a physician in exchange for the potential of being specifically referred a group of patients who otherwise would not be able to see that physician. There developed the concept of "panels" (i.e., the "lists" discussed earlier), in which a list of accepted providers would be given to patients covered by the plan, who must agree to use only the physicians on such a panel in order for their care to be covered by the plan. This concept has been modified many times (see question 12).

HMO was originally defined as a prepaid organization that provided comprehensive health care services to voluntarily enrolled members in return for a prepaid fixed amount of money. Nowadays, an HMO can be a health plan that places some providers at risk for medical expenses or a health plan that uses PCPs as gatekeepers.

11. **Are there other types of MCO plans?**
    As pressure was placed on businesses with large numbers of employees who were not happy with the original types of plans and the costs involved with the yearly premiums of certain plans, many other different insurance options were created.

12. **What are blended policies?**
    Blended policies include PPO with an assigned PCP and full coverage for specialty referral within the network of contracted providers but partial payment for use of specialists outside the network. Plans can have different deductibles for office visits, hospitalizations, and brand name versus generic medications. In some HMOs an entire clinic provides all of the health care, and referrals must be made internally. Other HMOs may contract with certain physicians within a community to be PCPs and with other physicians to be the specialists. Referrals may be scrutinized very carefully, and PCPs may be indirectly penalized by withholding bonuses or even reprimanded when they refer too many patients to specialists. There are many more plans as insurance companies try to provide options to employers that meet the needs of the employees but keep the cost down to the employer. In many MCOs, a physician must provide care for both HMO and PPO patients, although some times with different fee schedules. Some MCOs allow physicians to participate in one or the other.

13. **How does an endocrinologist join an HMO?**
    As many options are there for a physician to practice, such are the options for joining MCOs. In some cases, an endocrinologist is employed by a faculty group practice of a large medical center or a large group practice, in which all members are participants in the specific plan. He or she is most likely to become a provider as soon as his or her credentials are approved by the MCO. In areas of the country with a shortage of endocrinologists, you will be approached by many MCOs to participate immediately. For the most part, if an endocrinologist decides to practice solo or joins a group practice in an area where the MCO is satisfied with the doctors already on the panel, joining the HMO can be very difficult; in some cases, it may be impossible. Trying to open a solo office for general endocrinology in an area of great HMO penetration may be extremely difficult and frustrating. Sometimes, however, the MCO is under pressure to increase the number of endocrinologists, especially in certain geographic areas, and welcomes the applications of new doctors. At other times MCOs receive specific requests from patients or employers to include in their panels certain groups of doctors who were not previously participants. In general, the process of application, review of application, and final approval for participation can be quite long, maybe even more than 6 months. During this time, a physician cannot see patients for the MCO.

14. **How does an HMO patient get to your office?**
    Once a PCP determines that he or she does not have the experience or expertise to treat a certain endocrine problem, the patient is referred to your office. Sometimes the referral is made by the patient's HMO or "center," as it is often called. The patient must have in hand some kind of a referral form, either an authorization form or a special slip of paper giving you the specific authority to evaluate and treat the patient. Without the referral form or some kind of definite referral from the center, you will not be compensated for the consultation visit. Each subsequent visit must also be authorized in the same manner, or payment will be withheld. It can be frustrating when a patient arrives for follow-up at the physician's office without the authorization form. Naturally the doctor wants to see the patient and has blocked out the time in his or her schedule for the visit. Nonetheless, HMO will definitely refuse to back-issue a referral form, and, most likely, the doctor will receive no compensation for the visit.

15. **What can you expect to be able to do for the patient at the initial consultation or at subsequent follow-up visits?**
    In general, you will be allowed to perform a history and physical examination and order simple diagnostic tests without hassle. Blood tests should be allowed, although the samples usually

have to be sent to the laboratory with which the MCO has contracted (see question 17). Other tests have to be approved in writing by the HMO center or by the main HMO office, depending on the individual company's policy. Approval for simple procedures, such as thyroid scans, ultrasound studies, radioactive iodine treatment, and even fine-needle aspiration (FNA) biopsies can take from hours to days. Some HMOs require that PCPs schedule all tests, which can be a problem since you may not know when or where the study is scheduled or when to have the patient return to discuss the results. The more expensive a test is (such as an MRI), the more difficult it is to arrange.

16. **Can you use your own physician office laboratory (POL) for HMO patients?**
Although many endocrinologists have their own laboratories, accredited to perform certain endocrine tests, you usually cannot utilize them for HMO patients. Often the HMO has arranged special fees with commercial labs. This situation can create logistical problems in your office if you work for several different HMOs, all of which use different commercial labs. Your laboratory technicians must keep straight which specimens go where. In addition, some HMOs require that the patients have all blood tests drawn at the office of the PCP. This requirement is especially a problem because sometimes you will never know if your patient went to the PCP's office to have the blood drawn, and the test results may not be returned to you until the patient returns for a follow-up visit. You may have to call the PCP's office to have the results given to you over the phone or by fax.

17. **What potentially serious problem may arise in regard to pathology?**
Endocrinologists often perform FNA biopsy of a thyroid nodule. Most endocrinologists trust the interpretations by one particular laboratory, often at a university setting. The MCO may not have a contract with that laboratory and may require you to use a totally different laboratory for FNA cytology interpretation. Sometimes the pathologists at that laboratory may not be used to interpreting thyroid FNAs, and the results you receive may not be as accurate. This particular problem is being addressed at present by the American Thyroid Association and the College of American Pathologists.

18. **What happens if your patient changes jobs and receives health insurance from a company for which you are not providing services, or if the patient's employer switches insurance because the price of the original plan was too high?**
Obviously, this problem is highly frustrating for both patient and physician. The concept of long-term loyalty has been changed. Occasionally a POS option may be available in the new plan, but often the patient gets tired of paying the extra copayment. Sometimes a physician will give the patient a discount to continue their professional relationship. At other times patients feel so strongly about the opinion of their doctor that they pay the fee out of pocket to the doctor, especially if the patient only has to be seen once or twice a year. There are movements in Congress to allow the continuation of the patient–physician relationship. Until such time, the physician has to understand that losing patients in this way may be unavoidable. He or she should always welcome the patient back to his or her practice when the insurance situation changes.

19. **Describe the process by which the endocrinologist submits the bill for patient services.**
Once endocrinologists finish seeing the patient, they usually complete a "superbill" by entering the type of office visit performed, any diagnostic tests ordered that are performed in house, and the proper diagnosis code covering the patient's medical condition. The doctor then turns the chart and superbill over to a clerical person, thus ending the patient–physician interaction of the day. What happens thereafter is usually a total mystery to most doctors. A secretary or administrative assistant usually enters the charges and the diagnosis into some type of Physician Management System, where an insurance claim is generated and sent electronically or by paper to the insurance carrier. The carrier examines the claim, and eventually a check is cut covering

what the carrier feels is appropriate. The check returns to the physician's office after some period of time and a clerical person posts the payment received in the patient's account. There was somewhat of an "honor system" in the past, whereby the insurance company trusted the physician explicitly. This is no longer the case.

20. **Why are payments often delayed?**
MCOs are notorious for holding back payments. There are all kinds of excuses:
   - Deliberate down-coding (i.e., stating that the service provided was really a level 3 service, even though the claim was submitted at level 4).
   - Bundling (e.g., including the charges for the physician component of treatment for a hyperthyroid patient with the cost of the radiopharmaceutical).
   - Delayed payments (holding on to the claim for 6–8 rather than 2–3 weeks).
   - Wrongful denial of claims (such as stating, inappropriately, that there is no coverage, no authorization, a nonexistent preexisting condition, or improper completion of the insurance form).

21. **What problems may result from such practices?**
These problems result in inappropriate payments (always less than expected), prolonged time before the claims are finally resolved, and endless amounts of paper work, secretary time, and loss of income. In fact, there is an ongoing lawsuit against five MCOs, filed on behalf of the Florida Medical Association, California Medical Association, Texas Medical Association, and Medical Association of Georgia, for using such practices. For this reason physicians must understand all of the potential problems before they enter into contract to see patients for a specific HMO or continue seeing their patients without checking with their billing offices to find out what kinds of problems may exist.

22. **Is it advisable to continue seeing patients for MCOs if such problems exist?**
This becomes a personal and financial decision that each physician or group practice has to make. Some doctors work for a company strictly on a salary basis. Seeing all patients is just part of what they have to do. Physicians who are in solo practice or small groups need to be aware of all the problems so that the decision to begin or continue seeing patients is made for the right economic reasons. Many doctors react out of fear and anger, the worst emotions to invoke when an economic decision has to be made.

23. **Explain why doctors need to be involved in all aspects of the MCO relationship.**
Doctors need to be involved in all aspects of the MCO relationship, from contract negotiation to ongoing monitoring of day-to-day problems in seeing patients for the particular MCO and awareness of reimbursement problems. The practice needs to monitor collections, to be on top of claims, and to resubmit claims that were rejected, down-coded, or held for a long time without payment. The doctor needs to make sure that the collection of claims is not forgotten and that all claims are actively pursued, especially when third-party payment (i.e., from an insurance company) is involved. Doctors or their staff must have a policy in force to ensure that referrals are obtained, claims submitted on time, and proper payments received.

24. **What special concerns apply to doctors in small groups?**
Doctors in small groups must make sure that the MCO in question is contributing a significant amount to the gross revenue of the practice to be worth the "hassle" involved in seeing its patients. As a particular doctor gets busier and busier, it might be more worthwhile to replace patients from an HMO with a low reimbursement schedule with patients from HMOs with higher schedules. Perhaps the doctor can see only patients covered by higher-paying PPOs or choose not to be involved in MCOs at all, if there are enough patients to fill his or her schedule. For those new in practice, it may be worthwhile to see more and more patients, despite the associated problems.

25. **What pitfalls should doctors avoid in making decisions about participation in MCOs?**

The decision to join MCO panels or to resign from a particular panel should not be an emotional one, such as fear that if you do not accept a contract with what you consider an inadequate reimbursement schedule, another endocrinologist will do so. In addition, do not make a decision in anger, when a company denies payment or down-codes a series of claims without good reason. Work out the economics associated with leaving rather than resign out of anger. In fact, first try to work it out with the MCO, then look at all the above issues and decide whether resignation is appropriate for economic reasons, not emotional ones.

26. **What factors should be taken into account in deciding whether to renew a specific MCO contract?**

Contracts for most HMOs come up for renewal each year. Doctors have a chance to decide whether the contract should be continued. The decision to continue should be based on facts rather than feelings: revenue tracking, handling of claims, and fee schedule.

27. **Explain revenue tracking.**

Doctors should track their revenue during each year from all payers to make sure that no one MCO becomes such a large percentage of their practice that dropping the company or, even worse, being dropped by the company may result in a gigantic loss of revenue. No one can say for sure what the ideal percentage should be, but some physicians use 10%.

28. **What factors are relevant to handling of claims?**

Practice management software should be able to provide information, such as how many claims for each MCO were down-coded, bundled, or denied. How many claims were delayed in payment for more than 3 weeks? How many times did a billing clerk have to call the company before payment was finally received? Each time a claim is not paid properly or promptly, administrative costs are associated with collecting these fees. These extra costs effectively reduce the expected amount of reimbursement. In addition, talk to the secretaries to find out what kinds of hassles are encountered in receiving referrals, scheduling procedures, and getting laboratory tests done promptly. They can guide you in your decision.

29. **How do you evaluate the fee schedule?**

Once the decision is made to continue seeing the patients for an MCO, the physician must look at the fee schedule. Try not to sign a document that expresses reimbursement in terms of a percentage of Medicare or some other baseline. Try to be specific in providing a list of office visit codes that will be used and agree on a criteria for judging what documentation is required for each level. Also provide the company with a list of procedures and tests that you perform in your office and agree on a fee schedule. Make sure that the company signs off on the reimbursement expected for each item. This strategy will save a major hassle later when down-coding or denials appear.

30. **Should doctors consult a lawyer before signing an MCO contract?**

Yes. Do not expect to understand the contract that is provided to you. Have an attorney review it and point out the potential problems. Many physicians are reluctant to spend the money to do so, but this reluctance is very shortsighted.

31. **Can doctors negotiate the terms of MCO contracts?**

Contracts are always up for discussion. Do not feel that you cannot negotiate for terms other than those initially provided.

32. **Does the physician have to be a good business person to survive in the managed care environment?**

Unfortunately, yes. Most physicians go to medical school to learn how to become a good doctor. They work hard during their residency and fellowship to learn as much internal medicine and then endocrinology as they can. Most likely, nothing is taught about practice management, contract negotiation skills, and cost-effective medical care. In addition, the traditional role of a physician as a healer of the sick without concern for compensation because doctors "always made a good living" is no longer applicable. It is becoming too expensive to run an office without being aware of the costs of every aspect of the practice, the revenue stream, and the "bottom line." Some doctors sell their practices in order to not have to deal with these problems, only to find out that working for a physician management company or a hospital that acquires practices, or very large groups creates an entirely different set of problems that they never expected.

To have a financially successful practice, the doctor must have a totally different attitude from that of physicians of a generation ago. The doctor has to view practice as a business, with the provision of health care as only one part of the practice. It takes time, effort, experiential learning, and even mistakes to be successful. Doctors have high intellectual abilities. They need to apply these abilities to learning the business aspects of their practices. Combining a career in clinical endocrinology with a successful income stream is certainly possible and should be the goal of all practicing endocrinologists.

BIBLIOGRAPHY

Levy EG: On entering private practice: A personal perspective. A guide for the young endocrinologist about to embark on a career in private practice. Endocrinologist 9:119, 1999.

CHAPTER 61

ENDOCRINE CASE STUDIES

Michael T. McDermott, M.D.

1. A 34-year-old woman has new-onset hypertension. Her serum potassium level is 2.7 mEq/L. Initial hormone screening shows a plasma aldosterone (PA) of 55 ng/dL (nL, 1–16) and a plasma renin (PR) of 0.1 ng/mL/h (nL, 0.15–2.33). Subsequent testing reveals the following: PA after a saline infusion = 54 ng/dL (nL, 1–8), 4-hour upright PA = 32 ng/dL (nL, 4–31), 4-hour upright PR = 0.1 ng/mL/h (nL, 1.31–3.95), and serum 18-hydroxycorticosterone = 108 ng/dL (normal < 30). What is the probable diagnosis?

   The presence of hypertension and hypokalemia suggests primary aldosteronism (Conn's syndrome). The PA level is elevated, the PR is suppressed, and the PA/PR ratio is greater than 20, supporting this diagnosis. It is confirmed by the failure of PA to suppress after volume expansion with saline. The next step is to determine if the cause is an aldosterone-producing adenoma or bilateral adrenal hyperplasia. The very low basal serum potassium, the drop in PA during the 4-hour posture test, and the elevated 18-hydroxycorticosterone level are consistent with an adrenal adenoma. An abdominal computed tomography (CT) scan should be done next. The treatment for an aldosterone-producing adrenal adenoma is surgical removal. Spironolactone should be given to control blood pressure and to normalize the serum potassium preoperatively (see Chapter 28).

2. A 32-year-old business executive develops amenorrhea. She has not recently lost weight but states that her job is very stressful. Evaluation reveals the following laboratory results: serum estradiol = 14 pg/mL (nL, 23–145), luteinizing hormone (LH) = 1.2 mIU/mL (nL, 2–15), follicle-stimulating hormone (FSH) = 1.5 mIU/mL (nL, 2–20), prolactin = 6.2 ng/mL (nL, 2–25), thyroid-stimulating hormone (TSH) = 1.2 mU/L (nL, 0.5–5.0), and a serum pregnancy test is negative. A magnetic resonance imaging (MRI) scan of her pituitary gland is normal. What is the probable diagnosis?

   The patient has secondary amenorrhea with low levels of estradiol and gonadotropins. This clinical picture is most consistent with hypothalamic amenorrhea, which sometimes occurs in women who exercise excessively or who have stressful jobs. The disorder results from reduced frequency of gonadotropin-releasing hormone (GnRH) pulses in the hypothalamus. Treatment consists of stress management and, if menses do not resume, estrogen replacement therapy (see Chapter 48).

3. A nulliparous 48-year-old woman presents with symptoms of thyrotoxicosis. She has a modest, nontender goiter and no exophthalmos. She takes no medications and has had no recent radiology procedures. The following results are found on thyroid evaluation: free T_4 = 3.5 ng/dL (nL, 0.7–2.7), TSH < 0.1 mU/L, 24-hour radioactive iodine uptake (RAIU) = 1% (nL, 20–35%), thyroglobulin = 35 ng/mL (nL, 2–20), and sedimentation rate = 10 mm/h. What is the likely diagnosis?

   The patient has clinical and biochemical thyrotoxicosis but the RAIU is low. The differential diagnosis includes postpartum thyroiditis, silent thyroiditis, subacute thyroiditis, factitious thyrotoxicosis, and iodine-induced thyrotoxicosis. She has never been pregnant and denies medication use and recent iodine exposure. The nontender gland, elevated thyroglobulin, and normal sedimentation rate are most consistent with silent thyroiditis. A transient (1–3 months) thyrotoxic phase followed by a transient (1–3 months) hypothyroid phase is expected before the condition resolves; 20% of patients, however, remain hypothyroid. If symptomatic, the thyrotoxic phase is best treated with beta blockers and the hypothyroid phase can be managed, if necessary, with levothyroxine (see Chapter 36).

4. **A 38-year-old man has coronary artery disease, xanthomas of the Achilles tendons, and the following serum lipid profile: cholesterol = 482 mg/dL, triglycerides (TG) = 152 mg/dL, high-density lipoprotein (HDL) cholesterol = 42 mg/dL, and low-density lipoprotein (LDL) cholesterol = 410 mg/dL. What is the probable diagnosis?**
    Significant elevations of total cholesterol and LDL cholesterol, normal TG, tendon xanthomas, and premature coronary artery disease are most consistent with a diagnosis of heterozygous familial hypercholesterolemia. This disorder is due to deficient or abnormal LDL receptors or an abnormal apoprotein B-100 molecule. Aggressive lipid lowering with combinations of statins, ezetimibe, bile acid resins and/or niacin, and occasionally plasmapheresis is indicated (see Chapter 7).

5. **A 28-year-old man presents because of infertility. He is found to have small, firm testes and gynecomastia. Laboratory testing shows the following abnormalities: testosterone = 2.6 ng/mL (nL, 3.0–10.0), LH = 88 mIU/mL (nL, 2–12), and FSH = 95 mIU/mL (nL, 2–12). What is the likely diagnosis?**
    The patient has hypergonadotropic hypogonadism with small firm testes and gynecomastia, which is most consistent with a diagnosis of Klinefelter's syndrome. Such patients usually have a 47XXY karyotype. Androgen replacement therapy is the treatment of choice (see Chapter 45).

6. **A 38-year-old nurse presents in a stuporous state; the blood glucose level is 14 mg/dL. Additional blood is drawn and the patient is quickly resuscitated with intravenous glucose. Further testing on the saved serum reveals the following: serum insulin = 45 mU/mL (normal < 22), C-peptide = 4.2 ng/mL (nL, 0.5–2.0), and proinsulin = 0.6 ng/mL (nL, 0–0.2). A sulfonylurea screen is negative. What is the probable diagnosis?**
    The patient has hyperinsulinemic hypoglycemia. The differential diagnosis includes insulinoma, surreptitious insulin injection, and oral sulfonylurea ingestion. The elevated serum C-peptide and proinsulin levels are most consistent with an insulinoma. After an appropriate localizing procedure, surgical removal is the treatment of choice (see Chapters 6 and 55).

7. **A 28-year-old woman with type 1 diabetes mellitus develops amenorrhea. Further testing reveals the following serum hormone values: estradiol = 15 pg/mL (nL, 23–145), LH = 78 mIU/mL (nL, 2–15), FSH = 92 mIU/mL (nL, 2–20), prolactin = 12 ng/mL (nL, 2–25), TSH = 1.1 mU/L, and a pregnancy test is negative. What is the most likely diagnosis?**
    The patient has secondary amenorrhea with low levels of estradiol and elevated gonadotropins. The differential diagnosis includes premature ovarian failure and the resistant ovary syndrome. In a patient with another autoimmune disease (type 1 diabetes mellitus), the most likely diagnosis is premature ovarian failure. Hormone replacement therapy is the treatment of choice (see Chapter 48).

8. **A 34-year-old woman presents with galactorrhea, amenorrhea, headaches, fatigue, and weight gain. Laboratory evaluation reveals the following: prolactin = 58 ng/mL (nL, 2–25), free T_4 = 0.2 ng/dL (nL, 4.5–12), and TSH > 60 mU/L**

(nL, 0.5–5.0). She has an enlarged pituitary gland on MRI scan. What is the probable diagnosis?

The patient has moderately increased serum prolactin levels, pituitary enlargement, and severe primary hypothyroidism. Her entire clinical picture is most likely explained solely by the hypothyroidism, which is well known to cause secondary hypersecretion of prolactin and pituitary enlargement due to thyrotroph hyperplasia. All abnormalities should resolve after adequate thyroid hormone replacement is established (see Chapters 21 and 49).

9. A 6-year-old girl has recently developed breast enlargement and some pubic hair. She has not complained of headaches and has had good health otherwise. Her older sister entered puberty at about 8 years of age. Her height is at the 90th percentile for her age, and her physical examination reveals Tanner stage 3 breast development and stage 2 pubic hair growth. Abdominal and pelvic examinations are normal. Laboratory tests show the following results: LH = 7 mIU/mL (nL, 2–15), FSH = 8 mIU/mL (nL, 2–20), prolactin = 6 ng/mL (nL, 2–25), TSH = 1.9 mU/L (nL, 0.5–5.0), and a normal pituitary MRI scan. Her bone age is 1.8 years ahead of the chronologic age. What is the probable diagnosis?

The patient has gonadotropin-dependent true precocious puberty. The etiology includes pituitary and hypothalamic tumors, but most cases in girls are idiopathic. The normal pituitary MRI points to a diagnosis of idiopathic precocious puberty. A long-acting GnRH analog should successfully arrest her premature development and allow her to enter puberty at a later, more appropriate time (see Chapter 44).

10. A 19-year-old man presents with excessive thirst and urination. Laboratory evaluation shows the following: serum glucose = 88 mg/dL, serum sodium = 146 mEq/L, serum osmolality = 298 mOsm/kg, and urine volume = 8800 mL/24 h. A water deprivation test is performed, and it shows a urine osmolality of 90 mOsm/kg with no response to water deprivation and an increase in urine osmolality to 180 mOsm/kg after the administration of vasopressin. What is the likely diagnosis?

The patient has polyuria and polydipsia with maximally dilute urine. The differential diagnosis includes central diabetes insipidus, nephrogenic diabetes insipidus, and primary polydipsia. The lack of response to water deprivation and the more than 50% increase in urine osmolality after administration of vasopressin are most consistent with central diabetes insipidus. This may be caused by inflammatory or mass lesions in the hypothalamus but is often idiopathic. An MRI of the pituitary-hypothalamic region should be performed. The treatment of choice is desmopressin (DDAVP) nasal spray (see Chapter 28).

11. A 25-year-old woman presents with a cushingoid appearance. The results of hormone testing are as follows: 24-hour urine cortisol = 318 mg (nL, 20–90), morning serum cortisol = 28 µg/dL (nL, 5–25), and morning plasma adrenocorticotropic hormone (ACTH) = 65 pg/mL (nL, 10–80). After an 8-mg oral bedtime dose of dexamethasone, the morning serum cortisol = 3 µg/dL. What is the probable diagnosis?

Cushingoid features and elevated urinary excretion of cortisol confirm the diagnosis of Cushing's syndrome. The cause is usually an ACTH-secreting pituitary adenoma (65–80%), ectopic production of ACTH (10–15%), or a cortisol-producing adrenal adenoma (10–15%). The normal plasma level of ACTH, which is inappropriate for the elevated serum cortisol level, and suppression of serum cortisol with high-dose dexamethasone are most consistent with a pituitary adenoma (Cushing's disease). This should be confirmed with an MRI of the pituitary gland and/or inferior petrosal sinus sampling. Transsphenoidal surgical removal is the treatment of choice (see Chapter 24).

12. An 8-year-old boy with known adrenal insufficiency complains of paresthesias of the lips, hands and feet, and intermittent muscle cramps. He has a positive Chvostek's and Trousseau's sign on examination. Results of blood testing are as follows: calcium = 6.2 mg/dL (nL, 8.5–10.2), phosphorous = 5.8 mg/dL (nL, 2.5–4.5), intact parathyroid hormone (PTH) = 6 pg/mL (nL, 10–65), and 25-hydroxyvitamin D = 42 ng/mL (nL, 16–74). What is the most likely diagnosis?

Hypocalcemia, hyperphosphatemia, and a low serum PTH level are diagnostic of primary hypoparathyroidism. This disorder, which is often autoimmune in nature, may occur in association with adrenal insufficiency as part of the polyendocrine failure type I syndrome. The treatment of this condition is calcium supplementation along with calcitriol administration. Calcitriol is necessary because the lack of PTH makes these patients unable to convert 25 hydroxyvitamin D into 1,25 dihydroxyvitamin D in the kidneys and the latter vitamin D metabolite is necessary for normal intestinal calcium absorption (see Chapters 17 and 54).

13. A 52-year-old man has a personal and family history of early coronary artery disease, minimal alcohol consumption and no xanthomas on examination. He has the following results on serum testing: cholesterol = 328 mg/dL, TG = 322 mg/dL, HDL = 35 mg/dL, LDL = 229 mg/dL, apoprotein B = 178 mg/dL (nL, 60–130), apoprotein E phenotype = E3/E3, TSH = 2.1 mU/L (nL, 0.1–4.5), and glucose = 85 mg/dL. What is the probable diagnosis?

The patient has elevations of both serum cholesterol and TG and no detected disorders that cause secondary dyslipidemia. The differential diagnosis includes familial combined hyperlipidemia and familial dysbetalipoproteinemia. The elevated level of apoprotein B and the normal apoprotein E phenotype are most consistent with familial combined hyperlipidemia. The top treatment priority is LDL reduction with a statin. Once LDL cholesterol is under the NCEP goal, persistent TG elevations should be addressed with the possible addition of a fibrate or niacin (see Chapter 7).

14. A 58-year-old man has recently developed diabetes mellitus, weight loss, and a skin rash that is most prominent on the buttocks; a dermatologist diagnoses this as necrolytic migratory erythema. What is the probable underlying diagnosis?

Diabetes mellitus, weight loss, and necrolytic migratory erythema are virtually diagnostic of a glucagon-secreting pancreatic endocrine tumor (glucagonoma). The diagnosis can be confirmed by finding an elevated serum level of glucagon. After appropriate localizing procedures, surgery is the treatment of choice, if possible. Chemotherapy should be considered for unresectable malignant tumors or tumor remnants (see Chapter 55).

15. A 29-year-old woman has asymptomatic hypercalcemia. Her mother and a sister also have hypercalcemia and have had failed neck explorations for presumed parathyroid tumors. Further testing results: serum calcium = 11.0 mg/dL (nL, 8.5–10.2), phosphorous = 3.0 mg/dL (nL, 2.4–4.5), creatinine = 0.9 mg/dL, intact PTH = 66 pg/mL (nL, 10–65), 25-hydroxyvitamin D = 42 ng/mL (nL, 16–74), 24-hour urine calcium = 13 mg (nL, 100–300), and creatinine =1100 mg. What is the probable diagnosis?

The vast majority of patients with hypercalcemia and a mildly elevated serum PTH level have hyperparathyroidism. But here, the very low urinary calcium excretion and family history of unsuccessful parathyroidectomies point to a likely diagnosis of familial hypocalciuric hypercalcemia. The diagnosis is confirmed by finding a calcium/creatinine clearance ratio (urine calcium × serum creatinine/serum calcium × urine creatinine) of < 0.01. This autosomal dominant disorder results from a heterozygous inactivating mutation in the gene that encodes the calcium receptor. The mutant receptors, present in parathyroid and renal tubular cells, have a raised threshold for calcium recognition. The result is a physiologic equilibrium, in which hypercalcemia coexists with mild elevations of PTH and low urinary calcium excretion. The disorder causes no morbidity and does not require treatment (see Chapters 14 and 15).

16. **A 39-year-old HIV-positive man with *Pneumocystis carinii* pneumonia has the following serum thyroid hormone values: T_4 = 4.0 µg/dL (nL, 4.5–12.0), T_3 = 22 ng/dL (nL, 90–200), T_3 resin uptake = 48% (nL, 35–45%), and TSH = 1.3 mU/L (nL, 0.5–5.0). What is the most likely endocrine diagnosis?**
The very low T_3, mildly low T_4, elevated T_3 resin uptake, and normal TSH are most consistent with the euthyroid sick syndrome. This is not a primary thyroid disorder but is instead a set of circulating thyroid hormone abnormalities that occur in the presence of nonthyroidal illnesses; it corrects when the underlying illness resolves. Treatment of the condition with thyroid hormone administration, though controversial, is not currently recommended (see Chapter 40).

17. **An 18-year-old girl has not yet begun menstruating. She has a height of 56 inches, a small uterus, and no breast development. The results of hormone tests are as follows: estradiol = 8 pg/mL (nL, 23–145), LH = 105 mIU/mL (nL, 2–15), FSH = 120 mIU/mL (nL, 2–20), prolactin = 14 ng/mL (nL, 2–15), and TSH = 1.8 mU/L (nL, 0.5–5.0). What is the probable diagnosis?**
Primary amenorrhea, short stature, a low serum estradiol level, and elevated gonadotropins are most consistent with a diagnosis of Turner's syndrome. This disorder, which is characterized by ovarian dysgenesis, is associated with a 45XO karyotype. These patients should be given hormone replacement therapy with estrogen and progesterone. GH therapy should also be considered as it has been shown to improve longitudinal growth and final height (see Chapter 48).

18. **A 62-year-old woman presents for evaluation of recent nephrolithiasis and low back pain. Her estimated calcium intake is 800 mg/day and she takes no vitamins. Her physical examination is unremarkable. Spinal x-rays reveal osteopenia and a compression fracture at L2. Laboratory evaluation shows the following: serum calcium = 13.0 mg/dL (nL, 8.5–10.5), phosphorus = 2.3 mg/dL (nL, 2.5–4.5), albumin = 4.4 g/dL (nL, 3.2–5.5), intact PTH = 72 pg/mL (nL, 11–54), and 24-hour urine calcium = 312 mg (nL, 100–300). What is the most likely diagnosis?**
Hypercalcemia, hypophosphatemia, and elevated serum PTH levels are characteristic of primary hyperparathyroidism. The only other cause of hypercalcemia with increased serum PTH levels is familial hypocalciuric hypercalcemia. Hyperparathyroidism is usually due to a solitary parathyroid adenoma, but familial cases and those associated with multiple endocrine neoplasia (MEN) syndromes more often have 4-gland hyperplasia. Surgical indications include serum calcium levels > 1 mg/dL above the normal range, urine calcium > 400 mg/24 h., kidney stones, renal impairment, osteoporosis, or symptoms related to hyperparathyroidism. Observation alone or bisphosphonate therapy may be appropriate for patients with mild, asymptomatic disease, or only mild bone loss (see Chapter 16).

19. **A 32-year-old woman presents with the recent onset of fatigue, palpitations, profuse sweating, and emotional lability. She gave birth to her second child 8 weeks ago. Her pulse is 100/minute, and she has mild lid retraction, a fine hand tremor, and a slightly enlarged, nontender thyroid gland. Laboratory tests are as follows: TSH < 0.03 mU/L (nL, 0.5–5.0), free T_4 = 3.8 ng/dL (nL, 0.7–2.7), and RAIU is < 1% at 4 and 24 hours. What is the probable diagnosis?**
Postpartum thyrotoxicosis is most often due to Graves' disease or postpartum thyroiditis. The RAIU will distinguish the two, being high in Graves' disease and very low in postpartum thyroiditis. This patient has postpartum thyroiditis, a condition caused by lymphocytic inflammation with leakage of thyroid hormone from the inflamed gland. There is often a thyrotoxic phase (lasting 1–3 months) followed by a hypothyroid phase (lasting 1–3 months) and eventual return

to euthyroidism, although nearly 20% remain permanently hypothyroid. Treatment consists of beta blockers, if needed, for symptom control in the thyrotoxic phase, and levothyroxine, if needed, for symptom control in the hypothyroid phase and for those who remain permanently hypothyroid (see Chapter 36).

20. **A 70-year-old man complains of a 1-year history of weakness, weight loss, and hand tremors. He has been treated with amiodarone for nearly 3 years for a diagnosis of paroxysmal atrial flutter. Laboratory tests show the following: TSH < 0.01 mU/L (nL, 0.5–5.0), free T_4 = 3.35 ng/dL (nL, 0.7–2.7), and the RAIU was 2.7% at 6 hours and 4.1% at 24 hours. Thyroid scan showed scant patchy tracer uptake. What is the likely diagnosis?**

    This man most likely has amiodarone-induced thyrotoxicosis (AIT). This condition occurs in up to 10% of patients using amiodarone, which has very high iodine content. There are two subtypes: type 1 AIT results from iodine overload and occurs mainly in patients with underlying goiters; type 2 AIT results from drug-induced thyroid follicular damage. Both are associated with a low RAIU. There are no tests to reliably distinguish the two subtypes, although an underlying goiter and a detectable RAIU are more common in type 1 AIT. Treatment of type 1 AIT consists of administering thionamides with or without potassium perchlorate, whereas type 2 AIT may respond to steroid therapy. Difficult cases may require plasmapheresis, dialysis, or thyroidectomy (see Chapter 34).

21. **A 20-year-old man presents for failure to enter puberty. He has small, soft testes, no gynecomastia, normal visual fields, and decreased sense of smell. Laboratory evaluation is as follows: serum testosterone = 0.7 ng/mL (nL, 3.0–10.0), LH = 2.0 mIU/mL (nL, 2–12), FSH = 1.6 mIU/mL (nL, 2–12), prolactin = 7 ng/mL (nL, 2–20), and TSH = 0.9 mU/L (nL, 0.5–5.0). An MRI of the pituitary gland is normal. What is the probable diagnosis?**

    This picture is most consistent with idiopathic hypogonadotropic hypogonadism, also known as Kallmann's syndrome. This disorder is due to a deficiency of GnRH, resulting from failure of fetal migration of the GnRH secreting neurons from the olfactory placode to the hypothalamus. Mutations of the *Kal* gene have been detected in some patients. Maldevelopment of the olfactory lobe causes the associated anosmia. Androgen therapy is indicated to promote appropriate masculinization. When desired, these patients can also become fertile by receiving treatment with GnRH or gonadotropin preparations (see Chapters 44 and 45).

22. **A 32-year-old man complains of impotence and retro-orbital headaches intermittently for the past year. He is adopted and does not know his natural family history. He has bitemporal visual field loss but his examination is otherwise normal. Laboratory tests reveal the following: serum calcium = 11.8 mg/dL (nL, 8.5–10.5), phosphorous = 2.5 mg/dL (nL, 2.5–4.5), albumin = 4.8 g/dL (nL, 3.2–5.5), intact PTH = 58 pg/mL (nL, 11–54), and prolactin = 2650 ng/mL (nL, 0–20). What is the likely diagnosis?**

    This patient has a prolactinoma, manifested by impotence, headaches, bitemporal hemianopsia, and a significantly elevated serum prolactin level. Hypercalcemia with an elevated serum PTH level indicates that he also has hyperparathyroidism. The MEN type 1 syndrome (MEN 1), which consists of hyperparathyroidism, pituitary tumors, and pancreatic endocrine tumors, results from an inherited mutation in the menin gene. This patient should be screened for a gastrinoma and insulinoma by measuring serum gastrin, insulin, proinsulin, and glucose following an overnight fast. After pituitary imaging studies, he should be treated with a dopamine agonist and/or transsphenoidal surgery, and subsequently parathyroid surgery (see Chapters 21 and 53).

23. **A 52-year-old woman complains of a 1-year history of progressive fatigue, puffy eyes, dry skin, and mild weight gain. She had acromegaly treated with**

transsphenoidal surgery and radiation therapy 10 years ago. Physical examination shows normal visual fields, mild periorbital edema, and dry skin. Laboratory testing reveals the following: GH = 1.2 ng/mL (nL, < 2.0), insulin-like growth factor 1 (IGF-1) = 258 µg/mL (nL, 182–780), TSH = 0.2 mU/L (nL, 0.5–5.0), and free T_4 = 0.6 ng/dL (nL, 0.7–2.7). What is the most likely cause of this patient's symptoms?

This patient has central hypothyroidism due to pituitary damage from the combined effects of surgery and radiation treatment of her pituitary tumor 10 years earlier. Such a lengthy delay in the development of this condition is not uncommon. The diagnosis of central hypothyroidism is based on the presence of symptoms of thyroid hormone deficiency, a low serum free T_4 and a low or low-normal serum TSH. Treatment consists of levothyroxine replacement in doses sufficient to relieve symptoms and to maintain the serum free T_4 level in the mid-normal or upper-normal range. Because TSH secretion is impaired, the serum TSH level cannot be used to monitor this patient's response to therapy. Assessment of her pituitary-adrenal axis is also indicated (see Chapters 19 and 35).

24. A 32-year-old woman complains of deep pain in both thighs. She was diagnosed as having type 1 diabetes mellitus at age 20. She currently has 2–3 bowel movements each day. Her menses are regular. Her diet is well balanced with adequate calcium intake and she takes a multivitamin. Physical examination is normal. Laboratory studies show the following: serum calcium = 8.2 mg/dL (nL, 8.5–10.5), phosphorous = 2.3 ng/dL (nL, 2.5–4.5), alkaline phosphatase = 312 U/L (nL, 25–125), PTH = 155 pg/mL (nL, 11–54), and 25 hydroxyvitamin D = 7 ng/mL (nL, 16–74). Explain the findings in this patient and suggest a probable underlying diagnosis.

Her biochemical profile of hypocalcemia, hypophosphatemia, elevated alkaline phosphatase, and significant secondary hyperparathyroidism suggests vitamin D deficiency, which is confirmed by the low serum 25-hydroxyvitamin D level. Lactose intolerance can cause chronic diarrhea but seldom results in vitamin D and calcium malabsorption. Celiac disease (gluten sensitive enteropathy), which occurs with increased frequency in patients with type 1 diabetes mellitus, should be suspected. The diagnosis can be confirmed by the measurement of tissue transglutaminase, antiendomysial or antigliadin antibodies, or by a small bowel biopsy. The treatment is elimination of gluten (wheat, rye, barley, and oats) from the diet and supplementation with calcium and vitamin D (see Chapter 12).

25. A 42-year-old man presents for evaluation of a skin rash that has recently developed. He has known type 2 diabetes mellitus. He drinks 2–3 alcoholic beverages several nights each week. Physical examination shows eruptive xanthomas (red papules with golden crowns) all over his body, most prominently on the buttocks, thighs, and forearms. Laboratory studies reveal the following: glucose = 310 mg/dL, hemoglobin A_{1C} (HbA1C) = 12.9%, cholesterol = 1082 mg/dL, and TG = 8900 mg/dL. Discuss the cause and treatment of this lipid disorder.

The patient has severely elevated serum TG. This condition usually results from combining a secondary cause of TG elevation (uncontrolled diabetes mellitus, excess alcohol use) with an inherited TG disorder (familial hypertriglyceridemia or familial combined hyperlipidemia). His LDL cholesterol cannot be assessed until the serum TG levels are < 400 mg/dL. Because he is at high risk of developing acute pancreatitis, the priority is to quickly lower his serum TG level to less than 1000 mg/dL. This goal can be achieved most effectively with a temporary very low fat (< 5% fat) diet, blood glucose control, and discontinuation of alcohol. TG levels will fall by about 20% a day on this regimen. Fenofibrate or gemfibrozil should then be added and he should be switched to an American Heart Association diet. Diabetes control must be continued and further alcohol intake should be discouraged (see Chapter 7).

26. A 26-year-old woman requests to be tested for a type of thyroid cancer that has recently been found in her mother and two of five siblings. She notes that she has had intermittent headaches and palpitations for the past year. Her blood pressure is 164/102. She has a 1-cm, left-sided thyroid nodule without associated lymphadenopathy. Laboratory testing shows the following results: serum calcium = 11.2 mg/dL (nL, 8.5–10.5), phosphorus = 2.4 mg/dL (nL, 2.5–4.5), albumin = 4.5 g/dL (nL, 3.2–5.5), intact PTH = 55 pg/mL (nL, 11–54), calcitonin = 480 pg/mL (nL, 0–20), and 24-hour urine catecholamines = 1225 μg (nL, 0–200). Discuss her diagnosis and management.

    The thyroid nodule, elevated serum calcitonin, and family history make medullary thyroid cancer likely. Her hypertension, headaches, palpitations, and elevated urinary catecholamines indicate a probable pheochromocytoma. She also has hyperparathyroidism. MEN type 2A (MEN 2A) consists of medullary thyroid carcinoma, pheochromocytoma, and hyperparathyroidism. It is an autosomal dominant syndrome that results from a germline mutation in the *Ret* gene. After alpha blocker administration and blood pressure control, treatment of this patient would consist of removal of the pheochromocytoma(s) followed by later removal of the abnormal thyroid and parathyroid glands. Screening at-risk family members for the Ret/MCT oncogene should also be done (see Chapters 38 and 53).

27. A 68-year-old man complains of a 10-year history of progressive pain in the shins, knees, and left arm. He also notes progressive hearing loss. Physical examination reveals tenderness above the left elbow and enlarged, bowed shins. Bone scan shows intense uptake in both tibias and the left humerus. Skeletal x-rays show enlargement with multiple focal lytic and sclerotic areas in the tibias and the distal left humerus. Laboratory evaluation reveals: serum calcium = 9.8 mg/dL (nL, 8.5–10.5) and alkaline phosphatase = 966 U/L (nL, 25–125). What is the probable diagnosis?

    Bone pain and deformity, reduced hearing, and markedly elevated serum alkaline phosphatase levels suggest a diagnosis of Paget's disease. Intense radioisotope uptake on bone scanning supports this diagnosis and the characteristic findings on skeletal radiographs confirm it. Treatment options include analgesics, intermittent oral or intravenous bisphosphonates, and calcitonin, all of which may control but will not cure the disease (see Chapter 13).

28. A 19-year-old man has experienced fatigue, muscle weakness, and dizziness for the past 3 weeks. This morning he fainted when he went outdoors to exercise. His blood pressure is 95/60, and his pulse is 110. His skin is cool, dry, and tanned. His thyroid feels normal. Laboratory testing shows the following: hematocrit = 36%, glucose = 62 mg/dL, sodium = 120 mEq/L, potassium = 6.7 mEq/L, creatinine = 1.4 mg/dL, and blood urea nitrogen (BUN) = 36 mg/dL. What endocrine disorder should be considered and evaluated?

    Hyponatremia with hyperkalemia always suggests adrenal insufficiency (Addison's disease). Fatigue, weakness, hypotension, tanned skin, anemia, azotemia, and hypoglycemia are also consistent with this diagnosis. The most common cause is autoimmune destruction of the adrenal glands. The diagnosis is made by a Cosyntropin stimulation test that shows a low basal serum cortisol level that fails to increase after ACTH administration. During an adrenal crisis, however, one does not have time to wait for the test results. When this diagnosis is suspected, one should draw blood for a serum cortisol measurement and then start treatment with intravenous fluids and glucocorticoids (hydrocortisone, 100 mg every 6 hours). Precipitating conditions should be actively sought and treated. Once the patient is stable, he can be switched to oral hydrocortisone and Florinef for chronic maintenance. The diagnosis is likely if the serum cortisol measured during the crisis was low but this should be confirmed by repeat Cosyntropin stimulation testing upon recovery from the acute event (see Chapter 31).

CHAPTER 62

FAMOUS PEOPLE WITH ENDOCRINE DISORDERS

Kenneth J. Simcic, M.D.

1. **Despite his type 1 diabetes, this former National Hockey League star led the Philadelphia Flyers to back-to-back Stanley Cup championships in 1973–1974 and 1974–1975.**
Bobby Clarke. Clarke's diabetes was diagnosed at age 13.

2. **This female track star recovered from Graves' disease and went on to win the title of "Fastest Woman in the World" at the 1992 Summer Olympics in Barcelona. Who is she?**
Gail Devers. Devers repeated as champion in the women's 100 meters at the 1996 Olympics in Atlanta.

3. **Name the dwarf actor who gained fame for his role as Tattoo on the television series *Fantasy Island (1977–1984)*.**
Herve Villechaize (1943–1993). Villechaize's short stature was due to achondroplasia. His adult height was only 3 ft 2 in.

4. **Television and film actress Mary Tyler Moore has what endocrine disorder?**
Type 1 diabetes. Moore was diagnosed at age 33. Her diabetes has been complicated by retinopathy and recurrent foot infections.

5. **George Bush and his wife Barbara were both diagnosed with Graves' disease during his presidency (1989–1993). How did the President's Graves' disease present clinically?**
Atrial fibrillation. (Mrs. Bush's Graves' disease was also complicated by ophthalmopathy. In addition to radioactive iodine for her hyperthyroidism, she required treatment with glucocorticoids and orbital radiation therapy for her eye disease.)

6. **Pulitzer Prize winning film critic Roger Ebert was diagnosed with what endocrine disorder at age 59?**
Papillary thyroid cancer (treated with thyroidectomy and radioactive iodine). Ebert has a major risk factor for papillary thyroid cancer. As a child, he was given radiation treatment for an ear infection.

7. **Name the acromegalic giant who played the character Jaws In the James Bond films *The Spy Who Loved Me* and *Moonraker*.**
Richard Kiel (Kiel is 7 ft 2 in. tall).

8. **Name the 2 ft 8 in. dwarf actor best known for his role as Mini-Me in the film *Austin Powers: The Spy Who Shagged Me (1999)*.**
Vern Troyer. Troyer's dwarfism is secondary to achondroplasia. He has had acting roles in more than 15 feature films.

9. **Which late actor, who appeared in the film *Young Frankenstein (1974)*, had obvious Graves' ophthalmopathy?**
Marty Feldman (1933–1982).

10. **Ancient Egyptian sculptures and paintings suggest that Tutankhamun (1357–1339 B.C.) and other pharaohs of the Eighteenth Egyptian Dynasty had what endocrine disorder?**
Gynecomastia. Familial aromatase excess syndrome is a possible explanation for this historical finding.

11. **Which male ice-skater overcame growth failure related to a childhood illness to win the gold medal at the 1984 Winter Olympics in Sarajevo?**
Scott Hamilton. As a child, Hamilton suffered from Shwachman syndrome, a rare disorder of the pancreas. His adult height is 5 ft 3 in. (Hamilton was also diagnosed with testicular cancer at age 38.)

12. **In 1999, Tipper Gore, the wife of former Vice President Al Gore, had surgery for what endocrine disorder?**
Thyroid nodule (benign).

13. **Name the late professional wrestler (and actor) who was well known for his acromegalic features.**
Andre "The Giant" Rousimoff (1947–1993).

14. **Charles Sherwood Stratton (1838–1883) reached an adult height of only 3 ft 4 in. What was his circus name?**
General Tom Thumb. In 1863, Stratton married fellow diminutive circus performer Lavinia Warren whose height was only 2 ft 8 in.

15. **Actress Catherine Bell, who stars as Lt. Col. Sarah "Mac" MacKenzie on the television series *JAG (1995–)*, has been treated for what thyroid disorder?**
Thyroid cancer (probably papillary).

16. **Oscar award winning actress Halle Berry was diagnosed with what endocrine disorder at age 21?**
Type 1 diabetes.

17. **After successful treatment for Graves' disease, this professional golfer captained the United States team to the 1999 Ryder Cup in what has been called the greatest comeback in Ryder Cup history. Who is he?**
Ben Crenshaw.

18. **Vocalist Rod Stewart has had surgery for what endocrine disorder?**
Thyroid cancer (most likely papillary). It took 9 months for Stewart's voice to recover from the surgery.

19. **Ron Santo won six Golden Glove Awards and played in nine All Star games while playing third base for the Chicago Cubs. He was diagnosed with type 1 diabetes at what age?**
Eighteen years, just after signing his first contract to play major league baseball. Since his retirement from baseball, Santo has suffered the following macrovascular complications of his diabetes: coronary artery disease requiring a quadruple coronary artery bypass operation and implantation of an automatic cardiac defibrillator device; bilateral below the knee amputations for peripheral vascular disease.

20. Name the 3-ft, 7-in., 65-lb midget who batted one time for the St. Louis Browns on August 19, 1951.
Eddie Gaedel (1925–1961). Gaedel was walked on four pitches by Detroit Tigers' pitcher Bob Cain.

21. Gheorghe Muresan of the Washington Bullets is the tallest player in the history of the National Basketball Association, NBA (7 ft, 7 in.). What treatments has he received for his acromegaly and gigantism?
Transphenoidal pituitary surgery, pituitary radiation, and somatostatin injections. (*Note:* Shaquille O'Neal is 7 ft, 1 in. tall.)

22. In his 6-year NBA career (Washington Bullets 1993–1997; New Jersey Nets 1998–2000), Muresan twice led the league in what category?
Field goal percentage (1995–1996 season: .584; 1996–1997 season: .604).

23. Regardless of their acting ability, it seems like every famous giant gets an acting role in a movie. Gheorghe Muresan starred in what movie with Billy Crystal?
My Giant (1998).

24. The late actor Rondo "The Creeper" Hatton had severe acromegalic facial features. He played the villain in numerous horror films such as *The Pearl of Death* (1944), *House of Horrors* (1946), and *The Brute Man* (1946). How old was Hatton at the time of his death?
Hatton died of a myocardial infarction at age 51. At the time of his death, he also reportedly suffered from diabetes and loss of vision. All of these conditions were probably sequelae of his untreated acromegaly.

25. Nicole Johnson was 24 years old when she was crowned Miss America 1999. At age 19, she was diagnosed with what endocrine disorder?
Type 1 diabetes.

26. Comedian/actor Joe Piscopo has been treated for what type of thyroid cancer?
Medullary thyroid cancer.

27. Grammy award winning vocalists Johnny Cash (1932–2003), Ella Fitzgerald (1917–1996), Waylon Jennings, and Luther Vandross had/have what endocrine disorder?
Type 2 diabetes.

28. Track star Carl Lewis competed in five consecutive Olympics. He is one of only two athletes who have won nine gold medals in an Olympic career. With what endocrine disorder was he diagnosed at age 35?
Primary hypothyroidism (secondary to Hashimoto's thyroiditis).

29. Name the American swimmer who was diagnosed with type 1 diabetes 18 months before he won two gold medals at the 2000 Olympics in Sydney, Australia.
Gary Hall, Jr. At the age of 29, Hall repeated as gold medalist in the 50-meter freestyle swim at the 2004 Olympics in Athens.

30. **Carla Overbeck, women's soccer star and captain of the United States 1996 gold medal Olympic team, was diagnosed with what endocrine disorder at age 32?**
Graves' disease.

BIBLIOGRAPHY

1. Dawson LY: Skating at the cutting edge: Bobby Clarke. Diab Forecast 16–19, March 1994.
2. Drimmer F: Very Special People. New York, Carol Publishing Group, 1991.
3. Falcon M, Shoop SA: Roger Ebert reviews his thyroid cancer. April 5 2002. Accessed at www.usatoday.com/news/health/spotlight/2002/03/20-ebert.htm on 23 November 2003.
4. Famousheights.com. Accessed at www.famousheights.com on 23 November 2003.
5. Ford-Martin P. Famous People Who Have Diabetes. Accessed at http://diabetes.about.com//cs/diabetesfame/ on 23 November 2003.
6. Mandernach M: Short hitter, long memory. Sports Illustrated (September) 2:5, 1996.
7. Mazur ML: Here she is—Miss America. Diab Forecast (July):49–51, 1999.
8. Montville L: Giant. Sports Illustrated (October) 2:50–56, 1995.
9. Paulshock BZ: Tutankhamun and his brothers: Familial gynecomastia in the eighteenth dynasty. JAMA 244:160–164, 1980.
10. Shomon M: Famous People with Thyroid Conditions. Accessed at www.thyroid.about.com/cs/amouspeople/ on 23 November 2003.

CHAPTER 63

INTERESTING ENDOCRINE FACTS AND FIGURES

Michael T. McDermott, M.D.

1. **Who is the tallest man on record?**
   The man with the greatest medically documented height was Robert Wadlow of Alton, Illinois. He was 7 ft, 1.75 in. at age 13 years and 8 ft, 11.1 in. when he died in 1940 at the age of 22 years. He weighed 439 lb. His condition was the result of a growth hormone-secreting pituitary tumor that developed before closure of the skeletal epiphyseal plates (gigantism).

2. **Name the tallest woman on record.**
   Zeng Jinlian of Hunan Province, China, is the tallest woman on record. She was 7 ft, 1.5 in. tall at age 13 years and reached 8 ft, 1.75 in. just before her death at age 17 in 1982. She also had a growth hormone-secreting tumor that developed during childhood.

3. **How tall was the shortest man on record?**
   Calvin Phillips of Bridgewater, MA, was 26.5 in. tall and weighed 12 lb at the age of 19 years. He died at age 22 in 1812. He had progeria, which is characterized by dwarfism and premature senility.

4. **Who is the shortest woman on record?**
   The shortest adult woman on record was Pauline Musters of The Netherlands. She was 23.2 in. tall and weighed 9 lb shortly before her death at age 19 years in 1895. Because of her relatively normal proportions, she is believed to have had pituitary growth hormone deficiency, although growth hormone measurements were clearly not available in 1895.

5. **Who had the most variable adult stature?**
   Adam Rainer of Austria was a 3-ft, 10.45-in. dwarf at the age of 21 years but rapidly grew into a 7-ft, 1.75-in. giant at age 32 years in 1931. He was 7 ft, 8 in. tall when he died in 1950 at age 51 years.

6. **Which is the tallest tribe in Africa?**
   The Watusi (or Tutsi) tribe of Sudan, Rwanda, Burundi, and Central African Republic are the tallest in the world. The men average 6 ft, 5 in., and the women average 5 ft, 10 in. Their tall stature is believed to be a genetic adaptation.

7. **Which is the shortest tribe?**
   The Mbutl pygmies of central Africa have the lowest mean height. The men average 4 ft, 6 in., and the women 4 ft, 5 in. Their short stature is thought to result from genetic resistance to growth hormone, possibly due to deficient growth hormone receptors.

8. **Who was the heaviest man on record?**
   Jon Brower Minnoch of Bainbridge Island, WA, was 6 ft, 1 in. tall and weighed approximately 1400 lb when he was admitted to the hospital at age 37 years of congestive heart failure. He remained in the hospital for 2 years on a 1200-calorie diet and was discharged at 476 lb.; his weight loss of 924 lb is also a record. He weighed 798 lb when he died at age 42 years in 1983. His wife weighed 110 lb.

9. **How much did the heaviest woman on record weigh?**
The heaviest woman on record was Rosalie Bradford, who weighed 1199 lb in 1987. She also holds the record for weight loss, having shed 917 lb over the subsequent 7 years.

10. **What is the greatest rate of weight gain ever recorded?**
Arthur Knorr of the U.S. gained 294 lb during the last 6 months of his life; this is an average weight gain of 1.6 lb a day. Since a pound of fat has about 3500 kcal, this represents an excess intake (above caloric expenditures) of 5600 kcal a day. Doris James holds the record for women, having gained 328 lb in the last year of her life (3150 kcal/day excess) before she died at age 38, weighing 675 lb.

11. **What is the largest recorded waist size?**
Walter Hudson of New York, who stood 5 ft, 10 in., had a peak weight of 1197 lb and a waist size of 119 in.

12. **Who are the heaviest twins on record?**
Billy McCrary and Benny McCrary of Hendersonville, NC, weighed 743 and 723 lb, respectively. Both had 84-in. waists. One brother died in a motorcycle accident, but the other is alive at the time of this printing.

13. **What is the longest anyone has ever survived without food or water?**
Andreas Mihavecz of Austria was put in jail in 1979. The guards forgot about him and gave him no food or water for 18 days, after which he was found still alive, but barely.

14. **What is the greatest known number of children born to one woman in a lifetime?**
A peasant woman from Shuya, east of Moscow, Russia, gave birth to 69 children from 1725 to 1765. She had 27 pregnancies, producing 16 pairs of twins, 7 sets of triplets, and 4 sets of quadruplets. Sixty-seven of the children survived infancy. Her husband had 18 more children with a second wife.

15. **Who is the oldest known woman to give birth?**
In 1956, Ruth Alice Kistlen of California gave birth to a daughter at the age of 57 years, 129 days. She is the oldest medically verified mother to have become pregnant and delivered a child without a medically assisted reproductive method. Newer technologies have allowed this record to be eclipsed. In 1996, a 63-year-old woman gave birth to a healthy baby following implantation of an ovum from a younger woman.

16. **What is the highest reported number of multiple births for a single gestation?**
Ten births (decaplets) were reported in Brazil (1946), China (1936), and Spain (1924). Nine births (nonuplets) were recorded in Australia (1971), Philadelphia (1972), and Bangladesh (1977). The largest number to survive a multiple gestation is seven (septuplets), born at 31 weeks gestation to Bobbie McCaughey of Nebraska, in 1997.

17. **What is the highest single birth weight ever recorded?**
Anna Bates of Canada, gave birth to a 23 lb, 12 oz baby boy who died 11 hours later in 1879. Anna was 7 ft, 5.5 in. tall.

18. **What is the highest blood glucose level ever reported?**
A 12-year-old boy with new-onset diabetes mellitus was still conscious when he was discovered to have a blood glucose level of 2350 mg/dL in 1995.

19.   **What is the record for most kidney stones produced by one individual?**
Don Winfield of Canada passed 3711 kidney stones over a 15-year period (1986–2001).

20.   **What is the largest tumor ever reported?**
A 328-lb ovarian cyst was removed from a woman in Texas in 1905.

21.   **What is the longest hair ever recorded?**
Hoo Sateow of Thailand had his hair measured at 16 ft, 11 in. in 1997. He had not cut his hair for 70 years.

22.   **What is the record distance walked by an individual in 24 hours?**
The record for men is 142.25 miles, by Jesse Castenda of the United States in 1976. The record for women is 131.27 miles by Annie Van der Meer-Timmerman of the Netherlands in 1986. The 24-hour record for an individual in a wheelchair is 77.58 miles by Nik Nikzaban of Canada in 2000.

23.   **Did King David of Israel have an endocrine disorder?**
"When King David was old and advanced in years, though they spread covers over him, he could not keep warm. His servants therefore said to him, 'Let a young virgin be sought to attend you, lord king, and to nurse you. If she sleeps with your royal majesty, you will be kept warm.'...The maiden, who was very beautiful, nursed the king and cared for him, but the king did not have relations with her" (I Kings 1:1–4). Some speculate King David was afflicted with hypothyroidism.

24.   **What endocrine disorder might Goliath of Gath have had?**
Goliath of Gath, who was killed by a stone from David's sling (I Samuel 17:1–51), probably stood about 6 ft, 10 in. His tall stature may have resulted from a growth hormone-secreting pituitary tumor. Others add that the ease with which David's stone became embedded in Goliath's skull may have been due to hyperparathyroidism and his bizarre behavior may have resulted from hypoglycemia due to an insulinoma. He may thus be the earliest known case of MEN 1 syndrome.

25.   **What endocrine disorder did President John F. Kennedy have?**
Kennedy had primary adrenal insufficiency—Addison's disease. He was sustained throughout the later years of his life and his presidency by therapy with oral glucocorticoids.

WEBSITE

http://www.guinessworldrecords.com

BIBLIOGRAPHY

1.   Baumann G, Shaw MN, Merimee TJ: Low levels of high affinity growth hormone-binding protein in African Pygmies. N Engl J Med 320:1705–1709, 1989.
2.   Farlan D (ed): The Guiness Book of World Records. New York, Bantam Books, 1991.
3.   Folkard C (ed.): The Guiness Book of World Records. New York, Bantam Books, 2003.
4.   The New American Bible. Catholic Publishers, Inc., 1971.

INDEX

Page numbers in **boldface type** indicate complete chapters.